BIOPSY INTERPRETATION SERIES

BIOPSY INTERPRETATION OF THE HEAD AND NECK

Third Edition

BIOPSY INTERPRETATION SERIES

BIOPSY INTERPRETATION OF THE HEAD AND NECK

Third Edition

Edward B. Stelow, MD
Professor of Pathology
University of Virginia School of Medicine
Charlottesville, Virginia

Stacey E. Mills, MD
Professor and Director
Surgical Pathology and Cytopathology
University of Virginia School of Medicine
Charlottesville, Virginia

Wolters Kluwer

Philadelphia • Baltimore • New York • London
Buenos Aires • Hong Kong • Sydney • Tokyo

Acquisitions Editor: Nicole Dernoski
Development Editor: Ariel S. Winter
Editorial Coordinator: Anthony Gonzalez
Editorial Assistant: Maribeth Wood
Marketing Manager: Phyllis Hitner
Production Project Manager: Catherine Ott
Design Coordinator: Joseph Clark
Manufacturing Coordinator: Beth Welsh
Prepress Vendor: TNQ Technologies

Third edition

9 8 7 6 5 4 3 2 1

Printed in China

Library of Congress Cataloging-in-Publication Data

ISBN-13: 978-1-975139-36-0

Cataloging in Publication data available on request from publisher.

---

shop.lww.com

RRS2004

PREFACE

There continue to be great advances in our understanding of lesions of the tract. We have certainly come to better understand the role of human papillomavirus in upper aerodigestive tract disease. We also now know many of the genetic abnormalities that can be seen with some previously described diseases, and our understanding of these abnormalities has allowed us to better classify previous entities. We have endeavored here to improve our descriptions of these lesions so that they can be readily diagnosed using the most modern techniques.

PREFACE TO THE FIRST EDITION

Biopsy Interpretation of the Upper Aerodigestive Tract and Ear uses the most recent World Health Organization classification schema for tumors of the head and neck, soft tissues, and hematolymphoid tissues. Included are more than 300 color images in the text itself and an additional 350 color images in the accompanying online image bank. Tables are included to assist the reader in working through differential diagnoses for biopsies taken at different sites and for biopsies showing nonspecific features.

As most of the neoplasms that we discuss are found throughout the head and neck region, we have structured the chapters dealing with neoplasia based on histologic types, for example, salivary gland–type neoplasms and soft tissue tumors, rather than anatomic location. Nonneoplastic disease is discussed in chapters related specifically to site, for example, nonneoplastic diseases of the nasal cavity, paranasal sinuses, and nasopharynx. The separation of the numerous lesions that can be found throughout the area is not always perfect, however, and we have endeavored to best retain continuity based on diagnostic differential. Thus, nonneoplastic lymphoid proliferations are discussed in the chapter devoted to hematolymphoid tumors, rather than in the chapters devoted to nonneoplastic diseases.

Because of the complexity of the region, we are forced to exclude some lesions, namely, primary tumors of the bones of the head and neck and odontogenic lesions. Complete discussions of these would have exceeded the goals of this book and, likely, our page limit! This is especially true if one considers the amount of discussion that would be necessary regarding radiology, since a detailed understanding of this is required for the interpretation of both bone and odontogenic lesions. We invite the readers to use other more exhaustive texts when faced with these lesions.

Finally, a text devoted to the pathology of the upper aerodigestive tract could include most of the pathologic entities found throughout the body. Some very uncommon lesions are not discussed, and we ask for the readers' patience if they find themselves faced with an upper aerodigestive tract biopsy of an entity that we have not included.

CONTENTS

BIOPSY INTERPRETATION SERIES

BIOPSY INTERPRETATION OF THE HEAD AND NECK

Third Edition

1

NORMAL ANATOMY AND HISTOLOGY

The upper aerodigestive tract and ear are unified by location and function. Because this region does not represent a single organ, per se, a discussion of the anatomy and histology will be somewhat complicated. That said, understandings of the two are essential for surgical pathologists as they struggle to interpret biopsies from these sites. The correct interpretation of lesional histology presupposes an understanding of normal histology. Furthermore, such an understanding also enhances one's awareness of how certain lesions tend to occur throughout the system (e.g., squamous cell carcinoma and salivary gland–type neoplasms), while others only develop at specific sites (e.g., olfactory neuroblastoma and schneiderian papilloma).

THE NASAL CAVITY

The nasal cavity is bounded anteriorly by the external nares and posteriorly by the nasal choana. It is composed of the left and right nares which are separated by the nasal septum. The septum is both osseous and cartilaginous and is composed of the vomer (inferior and posterior), the ethmoid bone (superior), and septal cartilage (anterior). Laterally the "scroll-shaped" superior, middle, and inferior turbinates or conchae are present. Openings to the paranasal sinuses are present laterally and include the openings to the sphenoid sinuses (located behind the superior turbinate), the frontal sinus ostia (located in the anterior region of middle turbinate), the primary (and accessory) maxillary ostia (located in the hiatus semilunaris), and openings to the anterior, middle, and posterior ethmoid air cells (located in the middle turbinate and behind the superior turbinate). The superior portion of the nasal cavity is bounded by the cribriform plate.

The vast majority of the nasal cavity is lined by ectodermally derived tissue.[1] The most anterior mucosa, that of the vestibule, is lined by a keratinized, stratified squamous epithelium. This epithelium is continuous with that of the external nose and the mucosa includes adnexal structures such as hair follicles and sebaceous and sweat glands (Fig. 1.1, eFig. 1.1). As one progresses posteriorly, this epithelium is replaced by nonkeratinizing squamous cells and ciliated columnar cells with occasional mucous or

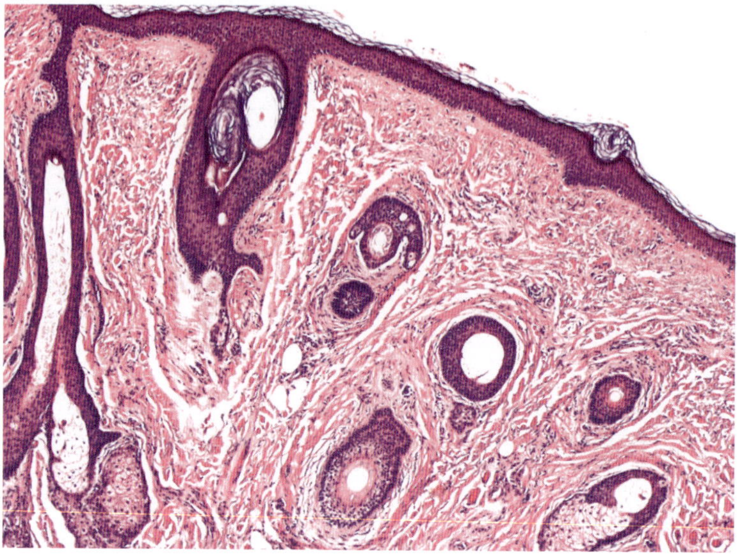

FIGURE 1.1 Squamous mucosa of the nasal vestibule.

goblet cells and intermediate cells (schneiderian mucosa) (Figs. 1.2–1.4, eFigs. 1.2–1.4). Seromucinous glands are present beneath the epithelium within a loose stroma. Occasional melanocytes may be present within the surface epithelium or underlying glands, and may even be seen in the lamina propria overlying the septum and turbinates. At the lower, anterior septum, a small tubular sac lined by nonciliated columnar cells (the vestigial

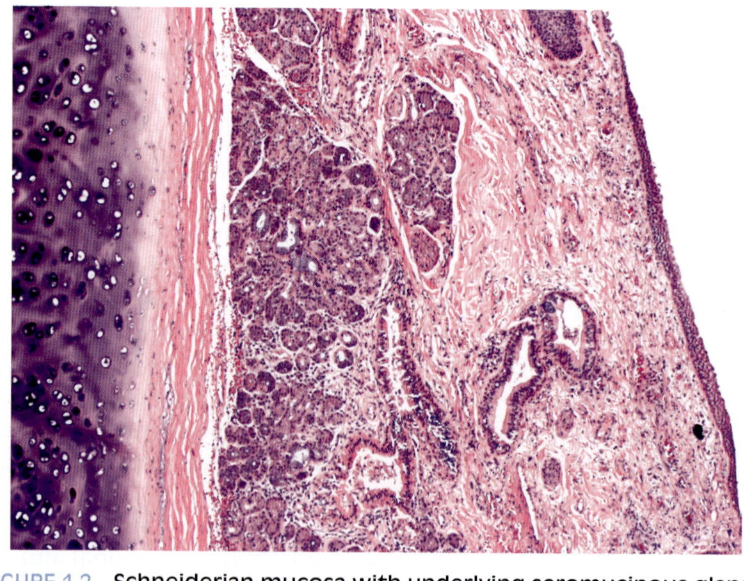

FIGURE 1.2 Schneiderian mucosa with underlying seromucinous glands.

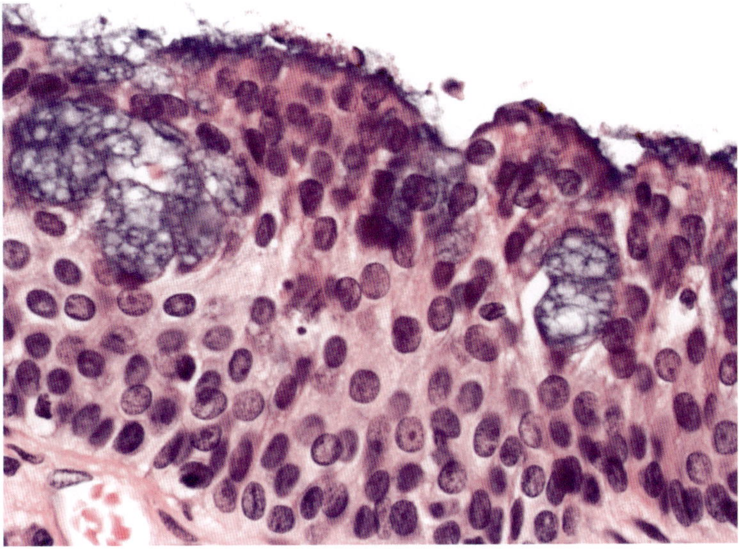

FIGURE 1.3 Schneiderian epithelium with mucous cells.

vomeronasal organ of Jacobson) may be seen.[1] This organ is better developed in the more olfactory-inclined animals. Dense, muscular vascular tissue is present beneath the seromucinous glands and is sometimes noted to appear "erectile" (Fig. 1.5, eFig. 1.5). Lymphatic channels, small nerves, and occasional, scattered inflammatory cells can also be present.

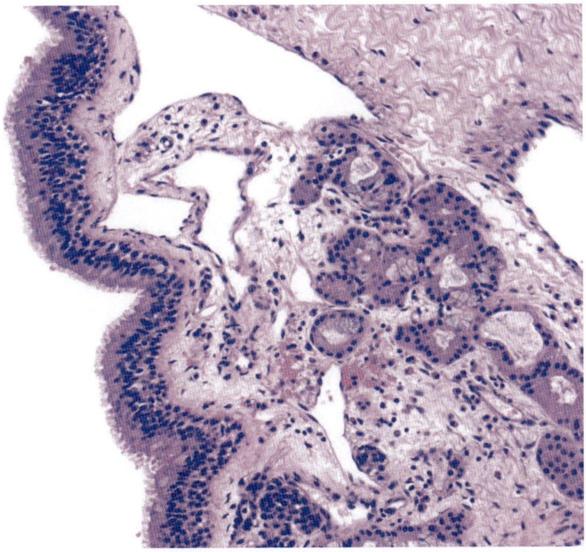

FIGURE 1.4 Proximal schneiderian mucosa. The epithelium is composed mostly of ciliated, columnar cells.

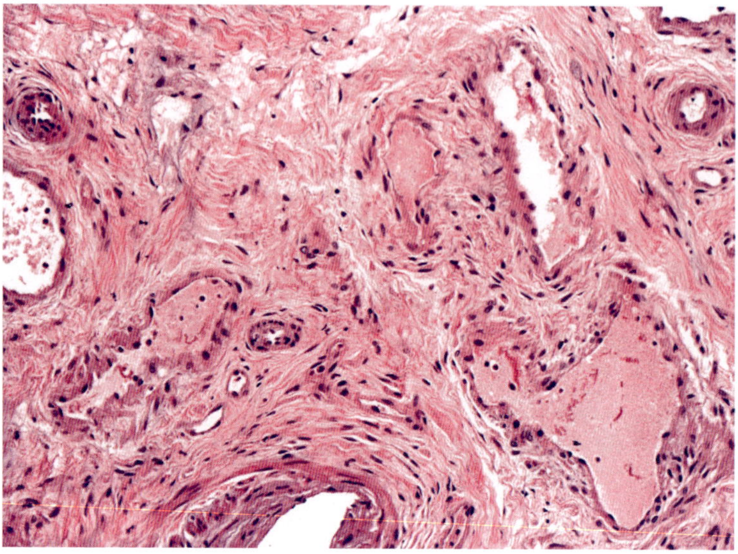

FIGURE 1.5 Fibromuscular vascular tissue.

The cribriform plate, the medial superior turbinate, and the superior one-third of the nasal septum all may be lined by olfactory mucosa (Fig. 1.6, eFig. 1.6). This specialized mucosa is composed of tall, eosinophilic sustentacular or supporting cells, elongated, ciliated olfactory neurons,

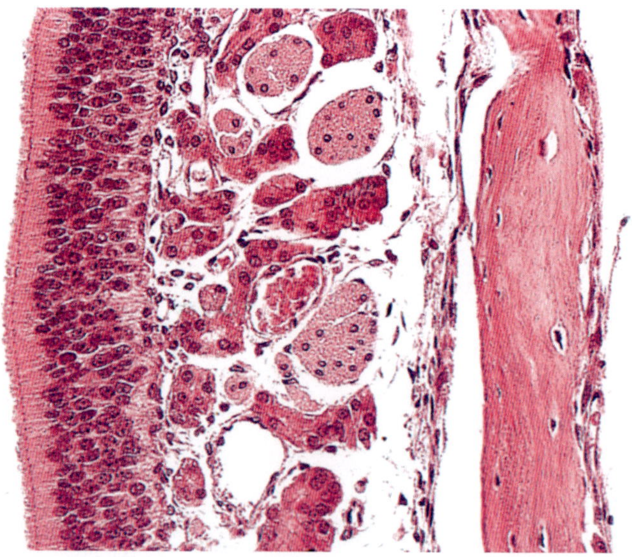

FIGURE 1.6 Olfactory epithelium. (Reproduced from Balogh K, Pantanowitz L. Mouth, nose, and paranasal sinuses. In: Mills SE, ed. *Histology for Pathologists*. 3rd ed. Philadelphia, PA: Lippincott-Williams & Wilkins; 2007:403-430.)

and small basally located cells. The sustentacular cells can sometimes contain lipofuscin which may give the area a yellow appearance, clinically.[2] Beneath the mucosa are serous glands (the glands of Bowman). Focally, olfactory mucosa may be intermixed and replaced by schneiderian mucosa.

THE PARANASAL SINUSES

The paranasal sinuses include the frontal, maxillary, sphenoid, and ethmoid sinuses. The ethmoid sinuses are composed of numerous (usually 3–18) ethmoid air sacs. The sinuses are each in communication with the nasal cavity and may be considered "diverticula" of the nasal cavity. They grow until adulthood and are usually somewhat asymmetrical in shape and size.

The paranasal sinuses are lined by ciliated columnar cells with occasional mucinous cells (Fig. 1.7, eFig. 1.7). These cells tend to be less tall than those of the nasal cavity and the mucosa is only half as thick as the nasal mucosa. Between the epithelium and bone is only a thin layer of fibrous tissue. Seromucinous glands are rare and are present primarily near the ostia to the nasal cavity.

ORAL CAVITY

The mouth begins at the vermillion border of the lips. It is encircled by the hard and soft palates (superior), cheeks (lateral), and anterior two-thirds of the tongue and floor of mouth (inferiorly). The posterior

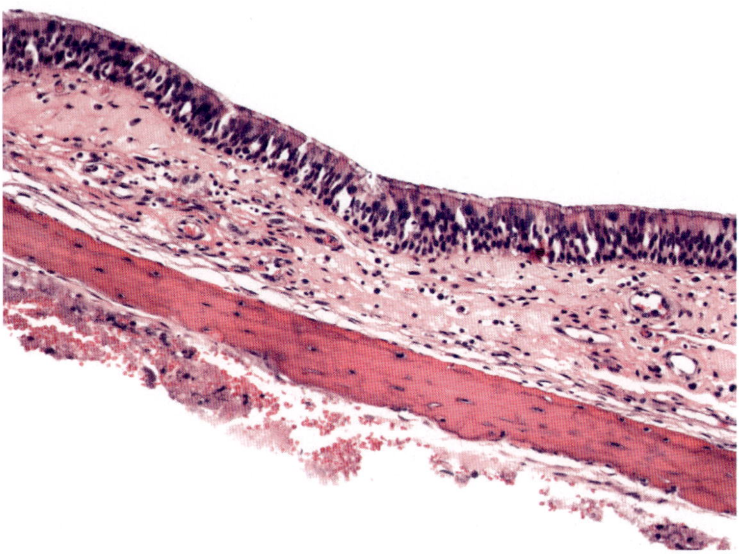

FIGURE 1.7 Mucosa of the paranasal sinus.

junction with the oropharynx (the fauces) is located superiorly at the posterior edge of the soft palate and uvula, laterally at the tonsillar pillars, and inferiorly at the circumvallate papillae of the tongue (the sulcus terminalis).

Although there are some regional differences, the majority of the oral cavity is lined by a nonkeratinizing squamous epithelium (Fig. 1.8, eFig. 1.8). Varying degrees of keratinization may be present overlying the gingiva and hard palate as they are exposed to mastication. Melanocytes and Merkel cells may be present and, although they are difficult to identify, they are generally scattered throughout the oral mucosa. The tongue is lined by filiform, fungiform, foliate, and circumvallate papillae which may have taste buds along the sides of their invaginations (Fig. 1.9, eFig. 1.9). These are composed of gustatory, sustentacular, and basal cells akin to olfactory mucosa of the nasal cavity. Immediately beneath the epithelium throughout the mouth is a basal lamina which is composed of type IV collagen, heparan sulfate, laminin, and enactin.[2] Beneath the epithelium of the tongue, a small amount of loose connective tissue overlies skeletal muscle (Fig. 1.10, eFig. 1.10). The remainder of the oral cavity has prominent seromucinous glands which may be especially prominent overlying the hard palate (Fig. 1.11, eFig. 1.11). The proportion of mucous to serous glands varies throughout the mouth. Surrounding these glands is the dense and loose connective tissue lamina propria and

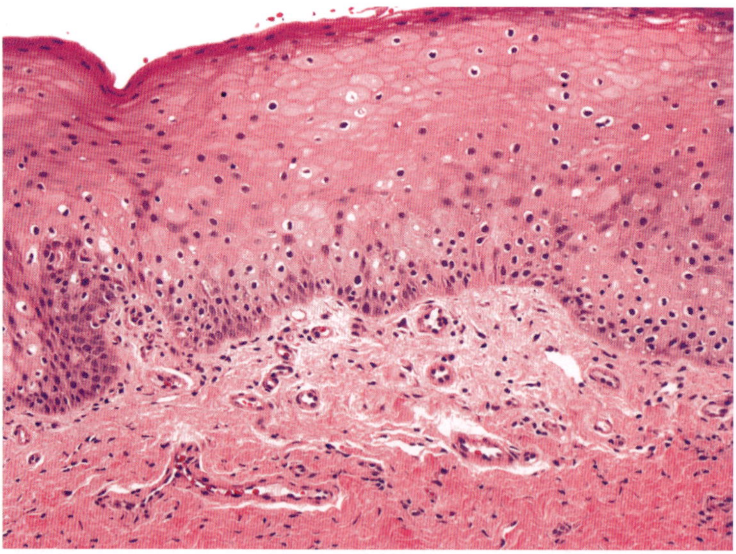

FIGURE 1.8 Squamous epithelium of the mouth.

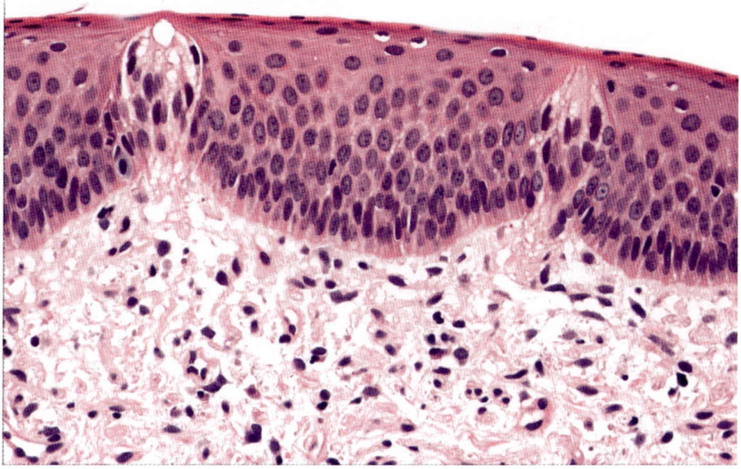

FIGURE 1.9 Circumvallate papillae are sometimes sampled with so-called blind biopsies of the base of the tongue. Taste buds can be seen extending through the squamous epithelium.

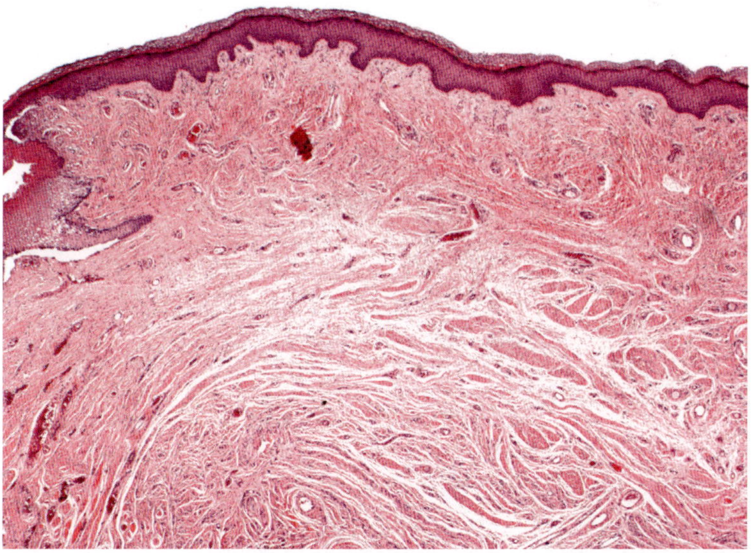

FIGURE 1.10 Squamous mucosa of the tongue with underlying skeletal muscle.

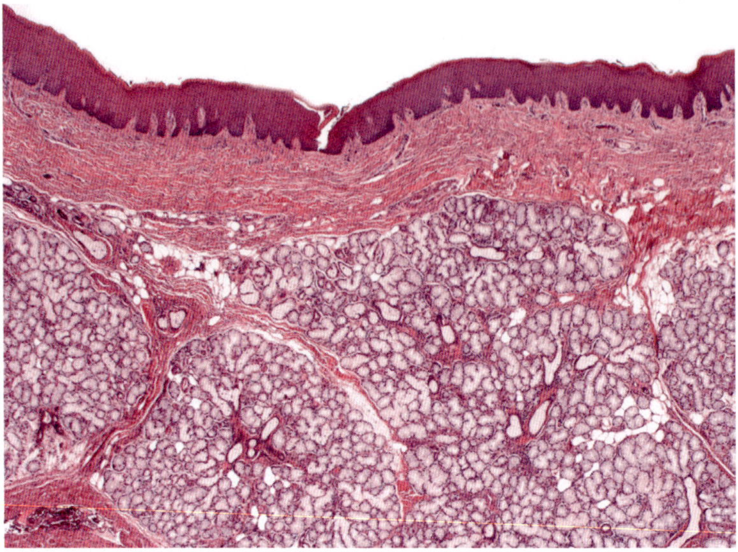

FIGURE 1.11 Palate mucosa with abundant seromucinous glands.

submucosa. Adipose tissue is sometimes seen within the submucosa. In the region of the retromolar trigone, nests of nonkeratinizing squamous cells (the organ of Chievitz) may be found within the stroma (Fig. 1.12, eFig. 1.12).[2] It is important that these not be confused with invasive malignancy.

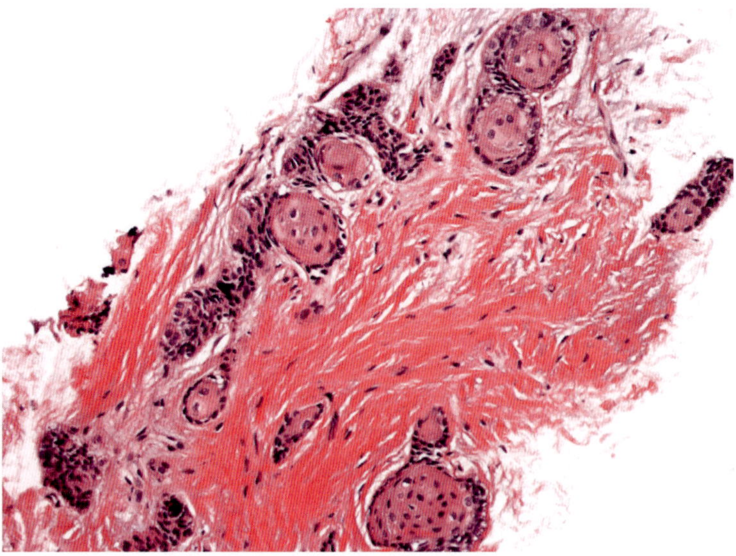

FIGURE 1.12 Organ of Chievitz.

THE PHARYNX

The pharynx as a whole includes the nasopharynx, oropharynx, and hypopharynx. The nasopharynx extends from its border with the nasal cavity at the nasal choana to its border with the oropharynx at the soft palate. The roof and posterior wall are arch-shaped and lie just beneath the base of the skull. The oropharynx is bordered by the nasopharynx at the soft palate, the oral cavity at the fauces, and the hypopharynx at upper edge of the epiglottis. The hypopharynx then includes the pyriform sinuses and borders with the larynx at the aryepiglottic folds. Inferiorly, it joins with the uppermost portion of the esophagus.

The eustachian tubes open into the posterior-lateral nasopharynx anterior to a small depression called the pharyngeal recess or fossa of Rosenmüller. Waldeyer ring of pharyngeal lymphoid tissue includes the pharyngeal tonsils or adenoids located in the superior nasopharynx, the palatine tonsils located laterally at the border of the oropharynx and oral cavity, and the lingual tonsils located in the base of the tongue.

The nasopharynx is lined by ciliated respiratory epithelium and stratified squamous epithelium which covers the lower portions of the nasopharynx. The junction between these often appears metaplastic. Within tonsillar tissue, the epithelium becomes extremely convoluted as it extends into the tonsillar crypts. It is surrounded throughout by dense lymphoid tissue with numerous germinal centers (Figs. 1.13 and 1.14, eFigs. 1.13 and 1.14). Numerous lymphocytes can be seen extending into the epithelium. Because of the convolutions, occasional groups of epithelia will appear

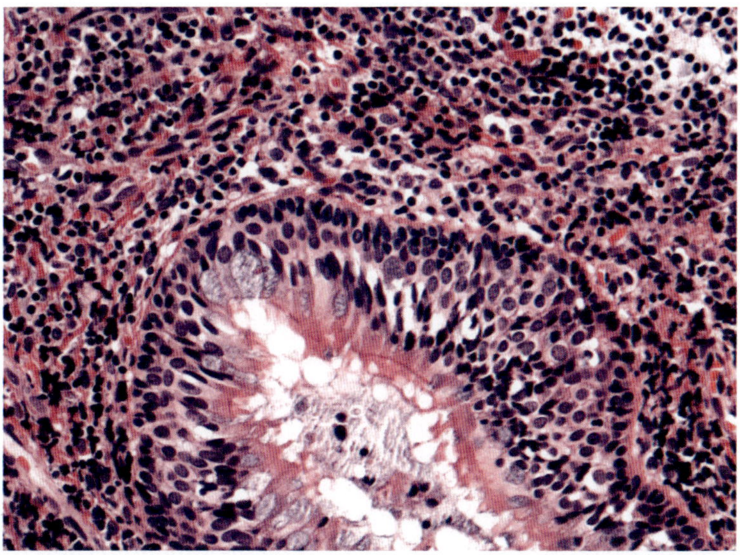

FIGURE 1.13 Nasopharyngeal tonsil with respiratory-type epithelium.

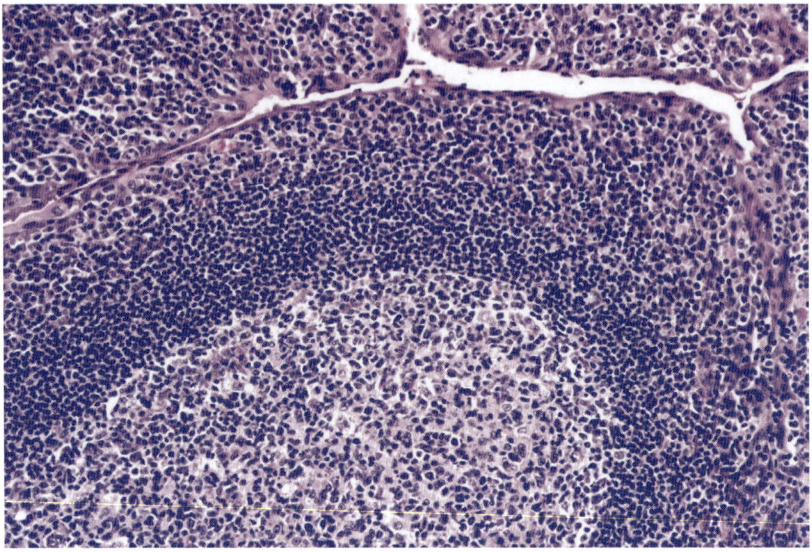

FIGURE 1.14 Oropharyngeal tonsil with squamous epithelium.

as "islands" surrounded by lymphocytes. Often, keratinization and squamous pearl formation may be present with abundant debris (eFig. 1.15). Although most lymphoid tissue is present within the tonsils, other areas throughout the pharynx will normally contain at least some lymphoid tissue. This is especially true in the areas surrounding the openings to the eustachian tubes. It is important to be aware that the irregular and thin nonkeratinized squamous epithelium of the oropharynx is often immunoreactive with antibodies to p16 so as to not confuse this normal finding with human papillomavirus–related neoplasia (Fig. 1.15, eFig. 1.16).

Seromucinous glands are present within the lamina propria throughout the nasopharynx. Some epithelial cells may appear large and eosinophilic, especially in older individuals (oncocytic metaplasia).[3] At the roof of the nasopharynx, epithelial remnants of Rathke pouch may be observed within the deep mucosa or within underlying periosteum.[3] Remnants of pharyngeal bursa may also be identified in the superior nasopharynx.

Nonkeratinizing, stratified squamous epithelium lines the nontonsillar tissue of the oropharynx and hypopharynx. Seromucinous glands are abundant throughout its lamina propria. Occasional lymphoid aggregates may be seen.

THE LARYNX

The larynx is a complex structure that is bordered superiorly by the hypopharynx at the tip of the epiglottis and the aryepiglottic folds and inferiorly by the trachea which begins at the inferior margin of the cricoid cartilage.

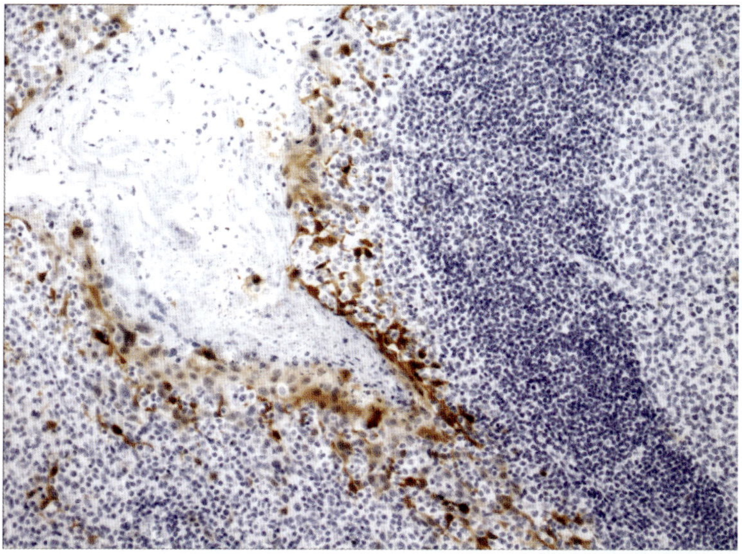

FIGURE 1.15 Normal crypt epithelium of the oropharyngeal tonsil is often immunoreactive with antibodies to p16.

Anteriorly, the larynx merges with soft tissues of the subcutaneous neck and is considered to contain the thyroid and cricoid cartilages and the thyrohyoid and cricothyroid membranes. Posteriorly, the larynx merges with the submucosal tissues of the hypopharynx and esophagus and is considered to contain the posterior portion of the cricoid cartilage and the

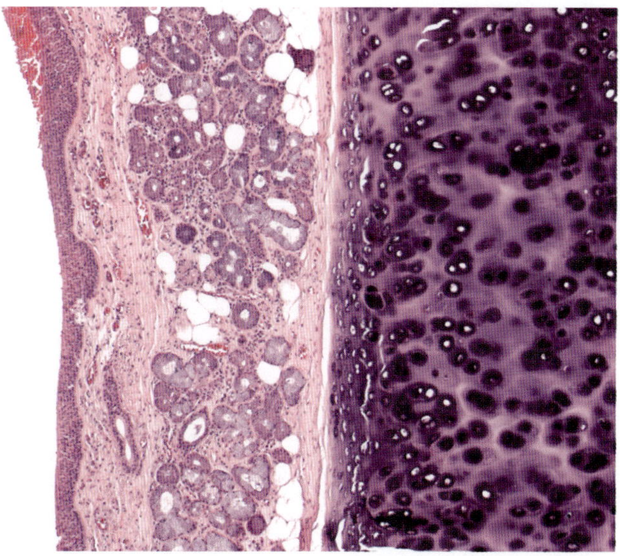

FIGURE 1.16 Squamous epithelium overlying the epiglottis.

arytenoids. The cricoid, thyroid, and arytenoid cartilages are hyaline cartilage and ossify in adulthood. Other cartilages of the larynx do not ossify.

Traditionally, the larynx is divided into the supraglottis, glottis, and subglottis. The supraglottis is considered the larynx above the superior edge of the true vocal cord. The false cords and laryngeal ventricles are thus considered part of the supraglottis. The glottis consists of the true vocal cords and the anterior and so-called posterior commissure. The subglottis extends from the inferior portion of the true vocal cords to the trachea.

The newborn's larynx is lined by a ciliated respiratory epithelium in all areas except at the true vocal cords where it is lined by nonkeratinizing stratified squamous epithelium.[3] In adults, the posterior epiglottis and portions of the supraglottis and subglottis will have patchy areas of squamous epithelium (Fig. 1.16, eFig. 1.17). In smokers, the entire larynx may be lined by squamous epithelium.[3] The ciliated cells may appear tall, with loss of nuclear polarity, and thus pseudostratified or may appear more cuboidal. Intervening mucinous cells or goblet cells can vary in their numbers. The transition between ciliated and squamous cells may be abrupt or may show a transitional metaplastic appearance (Fig. 1.17, eFig. 1.18).

The squamous epithelium of the larynx may vary in thickness but should mature normally. Mitotic figures should be located only in the basal cell layer. Keratosis is not normally present. Occasional, scattered melanocytes may be present.

Aside from at the true vocal cords, seromucinous glands are present throughout the lamina propria of the larynx (Fig. 1.18, eFig. 1.19). They empty onto the surface via ducts lined by ciliated, columnar cells.

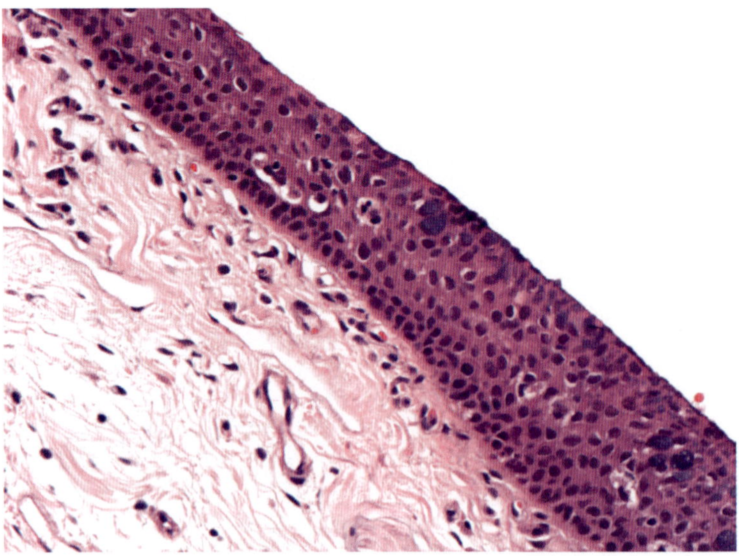

FIGURE 1.17 "Transitional" epithelium of the larynx.

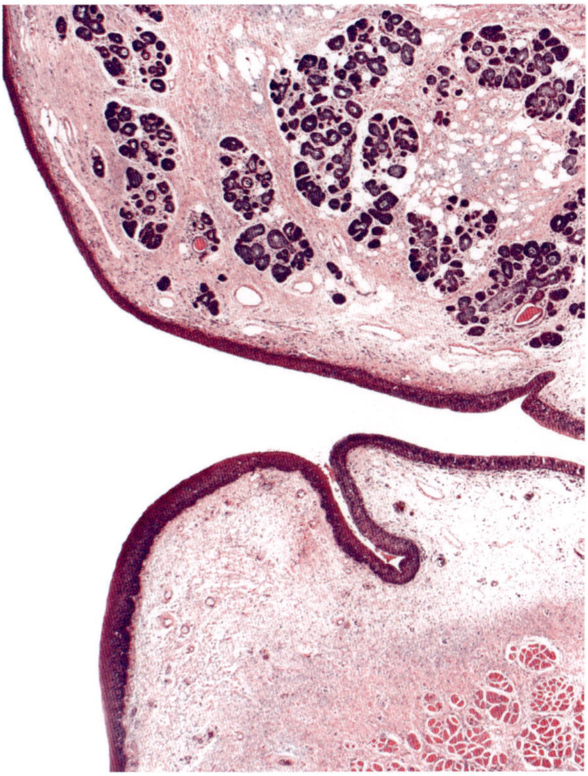

FIGURE 1.18 The vocal cords (note the absence of seromucinous glands within the true cord).

Squamous metaplasia may be present throughout the glands and should not be confused with neoplasia. The lamina propria of the true vocal cords is composed of loose, fibromyxoid connective tissue which overlies the vocal cord ligaments. Vascular and lymphatic channels tend to be more sparse in this area than they are in the remaining larynx. It should be noted that at the posterior portion of the true vocal cord, there is a well-circumscribed, elastochondroid nodule, the vocal process of the arytenoid cartilage (Fig. 1.19, eFig. 1.20).[3] This should not be confused with a chondroid neoplasm. Also, the larynx contains two pairs of paraganglia which may be sampled at biopsy and should not be confused with neoplasms (eFig. 1.21).

THE EAR

The ear is anatomically divided into the external, middle, and inner ear (Fig. 1.20, eFig. 1.22). The external ear includes the auricle or pinna and the external auditory meatus and canal. It ends at the tympanic membrane which separates it from the middle ear. The auricle is structurally

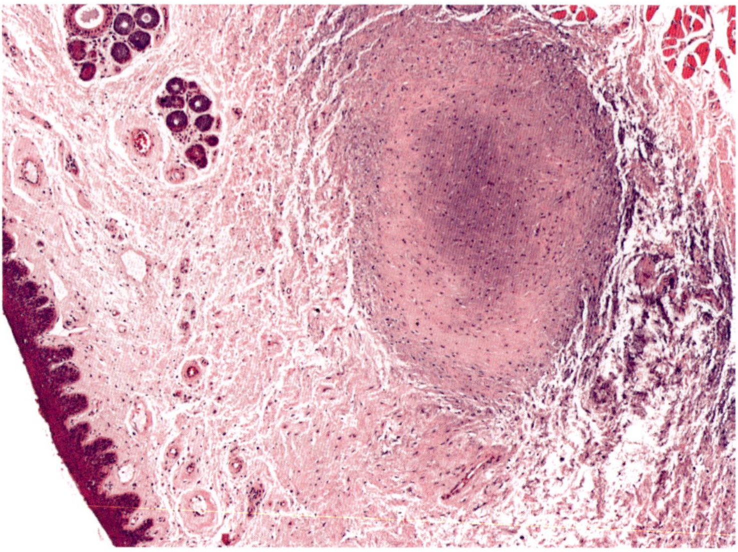

FIGURE 1.19 Elastochondroid nodule of the true vocal cord.

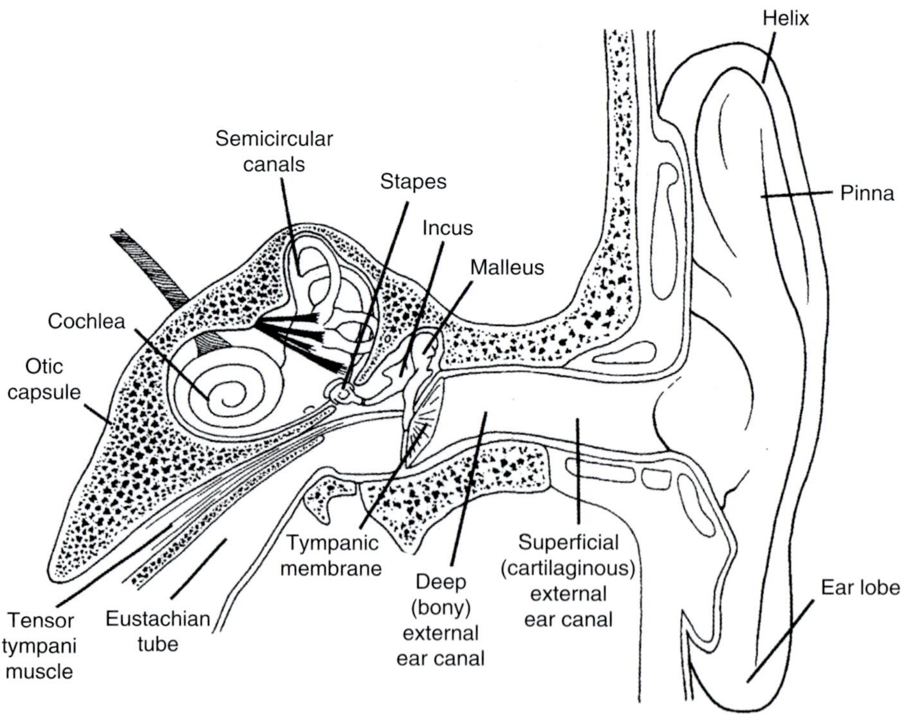

FIGURE 1.20 Anatomy of the ear. (From Michaels L. The ear. In: Sternberg SS, ed. *Histology for Pathologists*. 2nd ed. Philadelphia, PA: Lippincott–Raven; 1997:337-366, with permission.)

formed by underlying cartilage which extends into and partially encircles the outer one-third of the external auditory canal. Only a small portion of the superior and posterior canal is devoid of cartilage and underlain with dense fibrous tissue instead.[4,5] The remaining external canal is encircled by bone.

The middle ear lies between the tympanic membrane, the inner ear, and the nasopharynx. It includes the malleus, incus, and stapes (the three ossicles) and tympanic cavity; the eustachian tube; the epitympanic recess; and the mastoid cavity. The malleus attaches to the tympanic membrane and is then connected via the incus and stapes to the fenestra vestibuli. The epitympanic recess then extends superiorly and posteriorly and is in continuity posteriorly with the mastoid antrum and air cells located in the petrous portion of the temporal bone. The eustachian tube extends from the tympanic cavity to the posterior-lateral nasopharynx.

The external ear is covered with skin, a keratinized, stratified squamous epithelium, and underlying dermis replete with hair follicles, sebaceous glands, sweat glands, and apocrine glands. Adipose tissue is present only within the lobe. The remaining auricle has cartilaginous tissue juxtaposed with the overlying dermis. Skin extends into the external auditory canal with adnexal structures located primarily in the outer one-third of the canal. Lobules of ceruminous glands are present within the external canal and closely resemble apocrine glands (Fig. 1.21, eFigs. 1.23 and 1.24). They have an inner layer of eosinophilic, secretory cells which have abundant cytoplasm and yellow pigment granules. These cells often have apocrine snouts at their luminal surface and small, bland nuclei. An outer

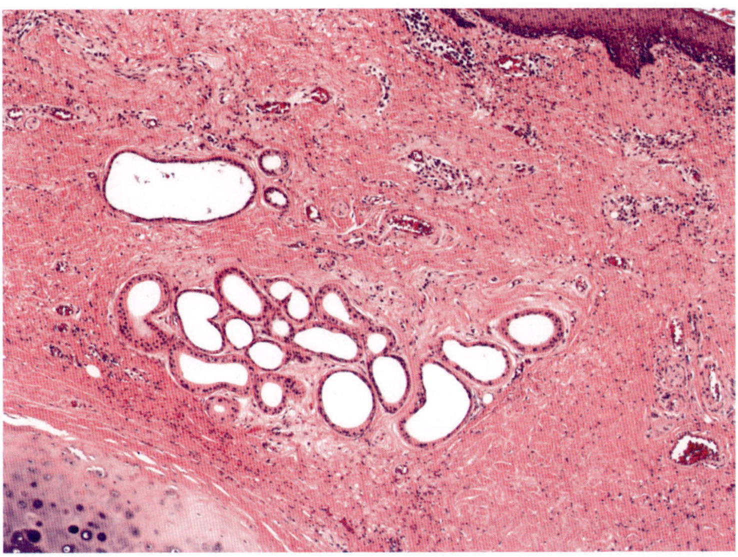

FIGURE 1.21 External auditory canal with ceruminous glands.

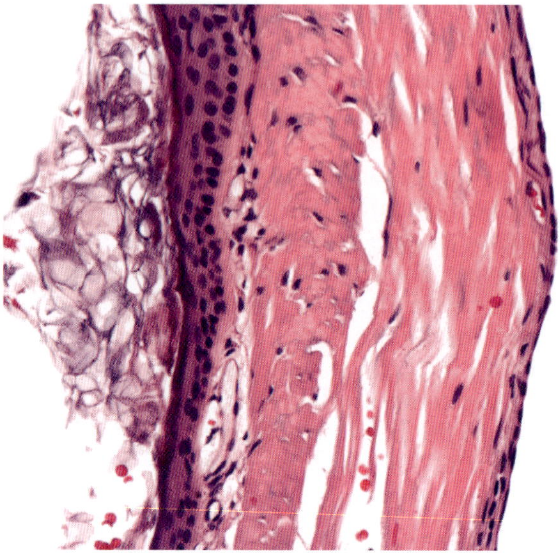

FIGURE 1.22 The tympanic membrane.

layer of spindled myoepithelial cells is also present. The glands empty via ducts into hair follicles.

The tympanic membrane separates the external ear from the middle ear. Externally, it is covered by keratinizing, stratified squamous epithelium; and internally, it is covered by a single layer of cuboidal cells (Fig. 1.22, eFig. 1.25). Underlying the epithelia are multiple layers of dense connective tissue.

The eustachian tube is lined by a single layer of pseudostratified, ciliated columnar cells with intermixed goblet cells. The tympanic cavity has a variable amount of respiratory epithelia admixed with a simple squamous and cuboidal lining. The simple cuboidal cells cover epitympanic recess, ossicles, and mastoid air cells. Underlying the epithelia of the middle ear is fibrous tissue with occasional small vessels and nerves. Seromucinous glands and lymphoid tissue (Gerlach tubular tonsil) are also present.

The histology of the inner ear is extremely complicated and a detailed description is beyond the scope of this text. The inner ear is surrounded by the otic capsule, which is composed predominately of dense, somewhat unique-appearing bone.[4,5] Its inner surface is lined by periosteum. Both the seventh and eighth cranial nerves involve this area and small paraganglia are present (jugular and tympanic paraganglia). The utricle and saccule are linked to the endolymphatic sac and duct which are lined by a single layer of cuboidal and tall, papillary epithelium, respectively. The cochlea and vestibular structures are not discussed here and are fortunately not often sampled by biopsy. A detailed description may be found elsewhere.[5]

REFERENCES

1. Balogh K. Mouth, nose, and paranasal sinuses. In: Sternberg SS, ed. *Histology for Pathologists*. 2nd ed. Philadelphia: Lippincott-Raven; 1997:367-389.
2. Mills SE, Gaffey MJ, Frierson HF. *Tumors of the upper aerodigestive tract and ear*. In: *Atlas of Tumor Pathology*. Vol 26. 3rd ed. Washington, DC: Armed Forces Institute of Pathology; 2000:1-19.
3. Mills SE, Fechner RE. Larynx and pharynx. In: Sternberg SS, ed. *Hisology for Pathologists*. 2nd ed. Philadelphia: Lippincott-Raven; 1997:391-403.
4. Mills SE, Gaffey MJ, Frierson HF. *Tumors of the upper aerodigestive tract and ear*. In: *Atlas of Tumor Pathology*. Vol 26. Washington, DC: Armed Forces Institute of Pathology; 2000:383-450.
5. Michaels L. The ear. In: Sternberg SS, ed. *Histology for Pathologists*. Philadelphia: Lippincott-Raven; 1997:337-366.

2

BENIGN SQUAMOUS PROLIFERATIONS AND NEOPLASMS

Most neoplasia of the upper aerodigestive tract shows squamous differentiation. Clinically, squamous lesions may be single or multifocal, benign, aggressive, or malignant. Risk factors for the diseases overlap, as do clinicopathologic features, and the definitive diagnosis of some lesions may be extremely difficult, especially with small biopsy specimens. This chapter discusses benign squamous proliferations and neoplasms as they occur throughout the upper aerodigestive tract with further discussion of some distinct clinicopathologic entities.

PAPILLOMAS

Unifocal and multifocal squamous papillomas occur throughout the upper aerodigestive tract, from the nasal vestibule, to the oral cavity, to the larynx. They can develop at any age, but often occur in children and young to middle-aged adults, possibly reflecting a relationship with exposure to human papillomavirus (HPV). Some lesions may be distinguished as condylomas or verruca when they are caused by HPV; however, such distinction is usually not necessary, and unequivocal infection is rarely demonstrated without ancillary testing. It should be noted that although koilocytic change may be helpful for identifying lesions induced by HPV, the appearance of an HPV-associated viral cytopathic effect is also not entirely specific. True HPV-induced lesions are often multiple and are more common in individuals infected with human immunodeficiency virus (HIV) or who are otherwise immunosuppressed. While most papillomas are not considered to be at risk for malignant transformation and do not show dysplastic changes, lesions in immunocompromised patients may show dysplasia and may be at increased risk for malignant transformation.

Grossly, these lesions are exophytic and may vary considerably in size. A rough, warty appearance may be noted. Histologically, the squamous epithelium is thickened and covers papillary cores of stromal tissue (Fig. 2.1, eFigs. 2.1 and 2.2).[1] Keratinization may be present

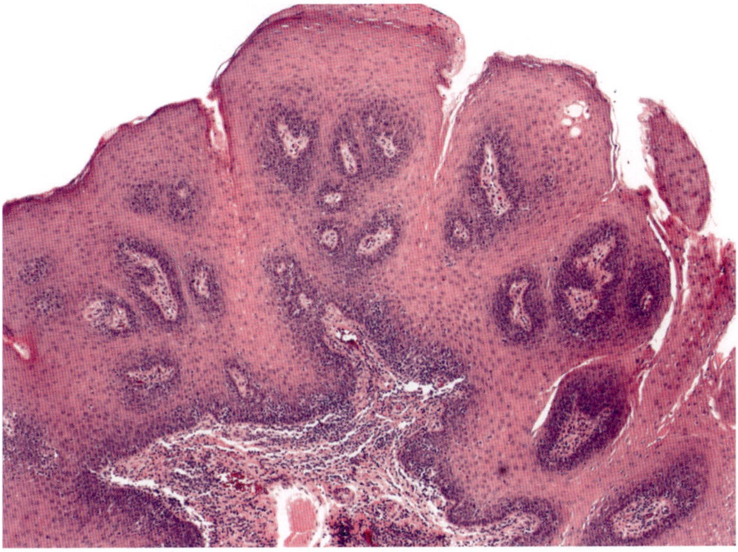

FIGURE 2.1 Squamous papilloma of the palate.

and the granular cell layer may appear thickened (Fig. 2.2, eFig. 2.3). The stratified squamous epithelium usually shows normal maturation with limited, if any, atypia. Mitotic figures should be located near the basal layer of the epithelium and some degree of chronic inflammation may be present, especially at the bases of the lesions within the stroma

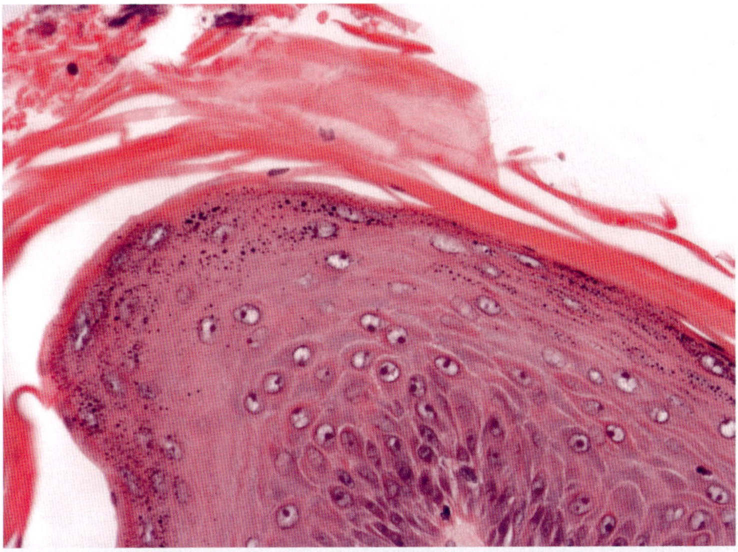

FIGURE 2.2 Keratinization and thickened granular cell layer in a squamous papilloma.

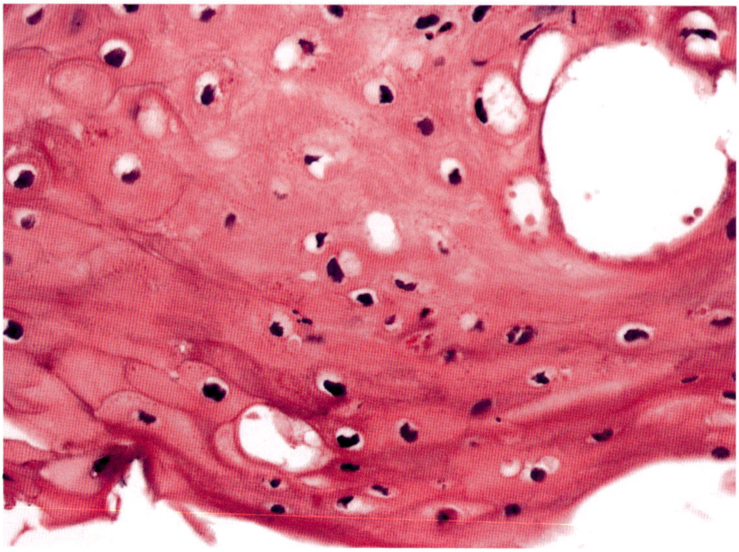

FIGURE 2.3 Koilocytes in a papilloma.

(eFig. 2.4). The stroma of papillomas of the nasal vestibule will contain skin appendages.[2] Many lesions have broader bases with more rounded surfaces and less keratinization and thus appear similar to condylomata of the cervix, replete with focal, apparent koilocytic change (Fig. 2.3, eFig. 2.5).

Benign squamous papillomas must be distinguished from malignant or potentially premalignant disease such as verrucous carcinoma or verrucous hyperplasia (see Chapters 3 and 4). Patients with verrucous carcinoma or verrucous hyperplasia are older and will usually have long histories of tobacco use. Verrucous carcinoma and verrucous hyperplasia generally do not appear as discrete polypoid masses; verrucous carcinoma is a destructive lesion which infiltrates the underlying stroma in a pushing manner. As mentioned, squamous papillomas of the upper aerodigestive tract appear less verrucoid than typical skin lesions and more like condylomata.

A particular lesion of the oral cavity, *focal epithelial hyperplasia*, arises more commonly in children and young adults and tends to be more common is certain geographic locations and in certain ethnicities.[3] These lesions are benign and regress as patients age. Numerous small, slightly raised, pink lesions are seen grossly which may become confluent. Histologically, the lesions have squamous hyperplasia, usually devoid of papillary architecture. Koilocytes are readily identified and the clumped chromatin may sometimes appear similar to mitotic figures (mitosoid bodies).

LARYNGEAL PAPILLOMAS AND PAPILLOMATOSIS

Squamous papillomas of the larynx are categorized according to their number (solitary or multiple) and the age of the patient affected (juvenile or adult).[4,5] Most laryngeal papillomatosis occurs in younger patients. The lesions usually are located in the region of the true vocal cords; however, they may be found throughout the larynx and even throughout the oropharynx and trachea.[4] They often recur after resection and may cause obstruction. The juvenile lesions and some of the adult lesions are etiologically related to infection of the mucosa with HPV types 6 and 11.[4] In cases of juvenile papillomatosis, it is thought that infection occurs at birth, whereas with adults, it is believed that the infection may occur at a later age.[4]

Grossly, the lesions are variably sized but are usually smaller than a centimeter in greatest dimension. Histologically, these lesions are characterized by a branched fibrovascular core, covered with maturing stratified squamous epithelium (Fig. 2.4, eFigs. 2.6 and 2.7).[4] Keratosis is generally not seen. Intraepithelial dysplasia is infrequent but has been noted, and severe or full-thickness dysplasia is very uncommon and should suggest a diagnosis of papillary carcinoma (Fig. 2.5, eFig. 2.8).[6] Koilocytic change may be seen. Rare cases of extremely well-differentiated squamous cell carcinomas arising in patients with laryngeal papillomatosis have been recorded.[7,8]

The differential diagnosis includes other squamoproliferative lesions especially squamous cell carcinoma, and some cases of laryngeal papillomas in older individuals may be very difficult to separate from papillary

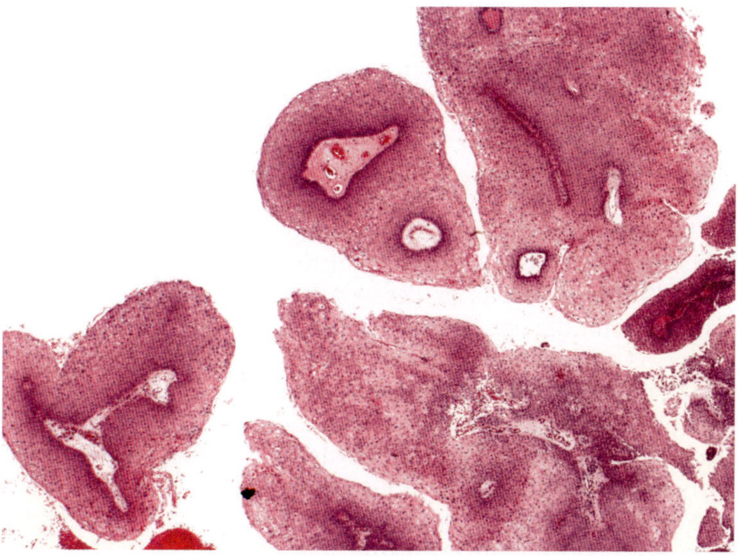

FIGURE 2.4 Laryngeal papillomas.

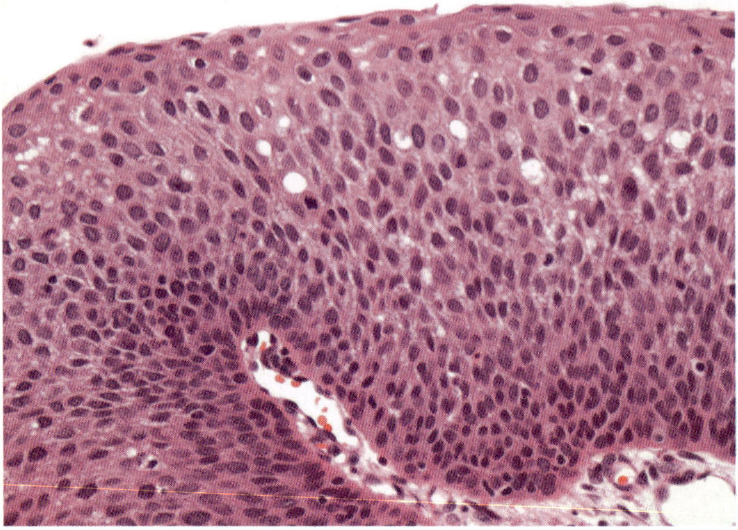

FIGURE 2.5 Mild to moderate squamous dysplasia in a laryngeal papilloma.

squamous cell carcinomas or verrucous carcinomas. In general, these other lesions are destructive or will show invasion; however, history may be unknown or unclear and invasion may be difficult to assess with small biopsies. Papillary squamous cell carcinoma should show full-thickness cytologic atypia; however, as was mentioned, laryngeal papillomas may also show cytologic atypia. For this reason, clinical follow-up and complete excision are recommended for any adult with a solitary papillary lesion that shows any degree of atypia. Verrucous carcinomas will not, by definition, show severe cytologic atypia and should show keratinization. They should not be diagnosed if the base of the lesion cannot be assessed on biopsy.

SINONASAL (SCHNEIDERIAN) PAPILLOMAS

Sinonasal or schneiderian papillomas arise almost exclusively within the nasal cavity and paranasal sinuses from the ectodermally derived ciliated columnar epithelium that lines these surfaces; they arise rarely at other sites such as the middle ear.[9,10] They occur in middle-aged patients and are at least twice as common in men.[10,11] They are classified according to their growth pattern (exophytic/fungiform vs. endophytic/inverted) and by their epithelial cell type (squamous vs. oncocytic/cylindrical cell), although some lesions may show combined features.[10–12] Most develop within the nasal cavity proper or maxillary sinus (Table 2.1).

Exophytic or *fungiform sinonasal papillomas* are polypoid growths that almost always originate from the nasal septum.[10,13] The patients are more often men who tend to be somewhat younger than those with other

TABLE 2.1 **Schneiderian Papillomas**

Lesion	Exophytic Papilloma	Inverted Papilloma	Oncocytic Papilloma
Clinical	More common in men who are younger than those with other schneiderian papillomas. The nasal septum usually involved.	Lateral nasal wall or paranasal sinuses. Occasionally associated with invasive squamous cell carcinomas.	Equally common in men and women. Lateral nasal wall or paranasal sinuses. Sometimes associated with squamous cell carcinoma or "mucoepidermoid carcinoma."
Histology	Exophytic. Squamous epithelium with occasional mucus-filled cysts. Dysplasia is uncommon. Generally not keratinized.	Like exophytic variety except with numerous endophytic invaginations. Atypia and dysplasia more frequent but still uncommon.	Endophytic and exophytic. Lined by oncocytic epithelium with numerous, intraepithelial mucinous cysts.

types of sinonasal papillomas. The lesions may be more often associated with detectable low-risk HPV than endophytic papillomas and are much less likely to be associated with malignancy.[14]

Grossly, these lesions are pink-tan, somewhat firm, and complex. Histologically, the lesions have numerous papillary fronds which are covered by a stratified squamous epithelium that may contain occasional ciliated and mucinous cells (Fig. 2.6, eFigs. 2.9 and 2.10).[10,11] Larger, cystic, mucus-filled spaces may also be seen throughout the epithelium (eFig. 2.11).[11] Nuclear and cytologic atypia are rarely present and mitotic figures are almost always located at or near the basal layer. Acute inflammation may be seen throughout the epithelium and "microabscesses" may be seen (eFig. 2.12). Keratinization is rarely present. The stroma often contains some degree of chronic inflammation.

The differential diagnosis for these lesions, either sampled by biopsy or resection, may sometimes include papillary squamous cell carcinoma. Papillary squamous cell carcinomas, as shall be discussed later, are covered with a dysplastic squamous epithelium that appears similar to high-grade intraepithelial lesions of the cervix. Papillary squamous cell carcinomas are often diffusely p16 immunoreactive and associated with high-risk HPV

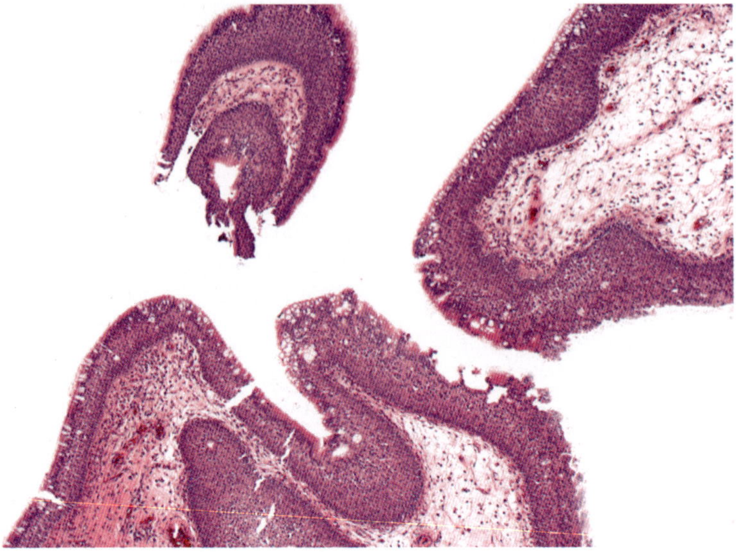

FIGURE 2.6 Fragments of an exophytic schneiderian papilloma.

that can be demonstrated by in situ hybridization.[15] Dermally derived papillomas of the nasal vestibule can be distinguished by their keratinization and lack of mucinous and ciliated cells.

Endophytic or *inverted sinonasal papillomas* are somewhat more common than the exophytic or fungiform variant. They most commonly involve the lateral nasal wall or the paranasal sinuses, either primarily or secondarily, but may involve any area of the nasal cavity including the septum.[10,16] They are almost always unilateral. Unlike fungiform or exophytic sinonasal papillomas, these lesions are associated with invasive squamous cell carcinoma in up to 5% to 10% of cases.[10] Rarely, they have been reported to be associated with other malignancies, such as mucoepidermoid carcinoma or even malignant melanoma or yolk sac tumor.[17] The lesions usually present as bulging, wrinkled masses with nasal obstruction and typically recur with inadequate surgery. Overall, approximately 10% of inverted nononcocytic papillomas are associated with low-risk HPV.[18] Schneiderian papillomas are rarely, if ever, associated with high-risk HPV. Approximately 90% of nononcocytic inverted lesions have *EGFR* mutations and these cases are not associated with low-risk HPV. Interestingly, the low-risk HPV–associated lesions appear to be more likely to recur and progress.

Histologically, the lesions show numerous twisting ducts within the stroma lined by a maturing, stratified squamous epithelium with acute inflammation, mucinous cells, and occasional mucinous cysts within the squamous epithelium (Fig. 2.7, eFigs. 2.13 and 2.14).[10,16] The squamous epithelium is often covered by a layer of columnar, ciliated cells. As many of the ducts are cut in cross section, the squamous epithelium will appear

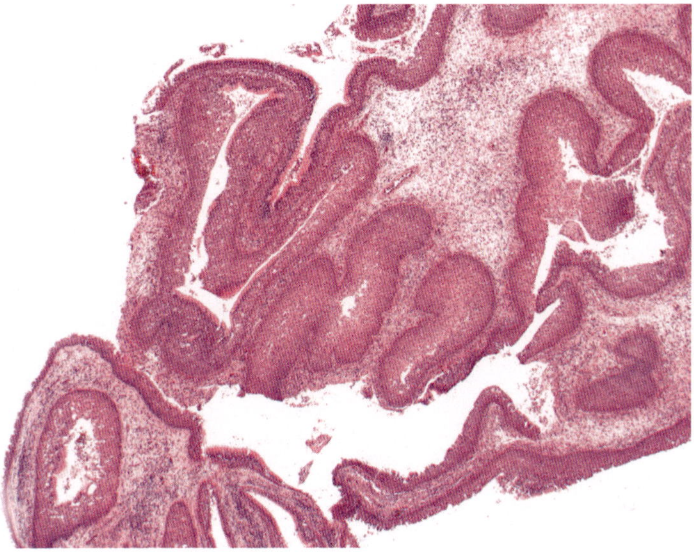

FIGURE 2.7 Schneiderian papilloma with endophytic growth.

nested with maturing cells toward the center of the nests. Even here, the surface generally still is covered by an intact ciliated or squamous epithelium (eFig. 2.15). Keratinization is usually absent and, if seen, is usually only present on the surface of the lesions. Nuclear atypia may be present but is usually limited and mitotic figures are generally located at the base of the epithelium. Stromal chronic inflammation is usually present to some degree.

Especially on small biopsies, these lesions may be difficult to distinguish from invasive squamous cell carcinomas. Certainly, underlying squamous cell carcinoma can never be entirely excluded on small biopsy. Inverted papillomas should not have marked atypia or atypical mitotic figures. Although the lesions may be locally aggressive, they should not have single-cell infiltration or irregular nests of squamous epithelium. Instead the nests should always have rounded and smooth contours.

Oncocytic schneiderian papillomas only constitute approximately 5% of all sinonasal papillomas.[10,19] These lesions are unilateral, usually involve the paranasal sinuses or lateral nasal cavity, and are both exophytic and endophytic.[10] They occur in slightly older patients, usually more than 50 years, and occur with equal incidence in men and women. Up to 20% of these neoplasms may be associated with invasive squamous cell carcinoma or "mucoepidermoid carcinoma" (Fig. 2.8, eFig. 2.16).[19–21] As with inverted papillomas, the neoplasms frequently recur after removal. These lesions have recently been shown to harbor *KRAS* mutations.[22]

These tumors are defined histologically as their epithelium is composed of cells with a more oncocytic than squamous appearance (Fig. 2.9, eFigs. 2.17 and 2.18).[10,19] Fibrovascular cores are covered by multiple

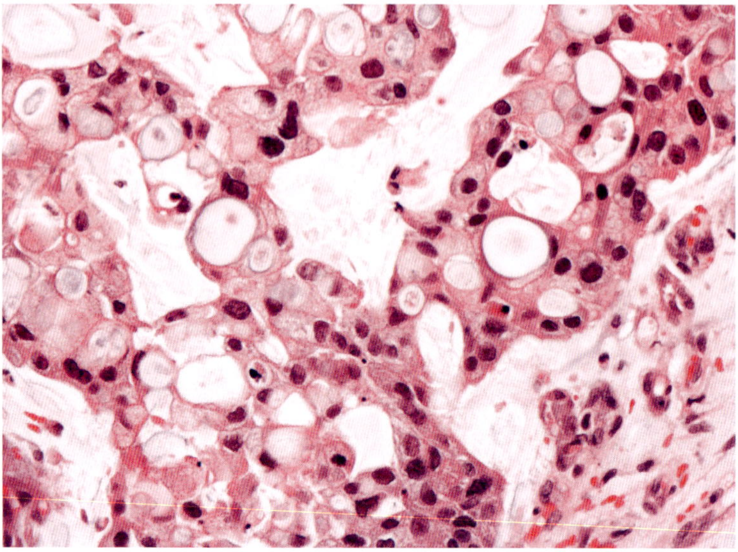

FIGURE 2.8 This invasive malignancy has features of mucoepidermoid carcinoma and was associated with an oncocytic schneiderian papilloma.

layers of large, distinct, somewhat columnar cells that have abundant, finely granular, eosinophilic cytoplasm. Cilia may sometimes be identified. The nuclei are uniform and mostly devoid of atypia. The underlying stroma will contain chronic inflammation and rounded nests and invaginations of neoplastic cells akin to those seen with inverted papillomas

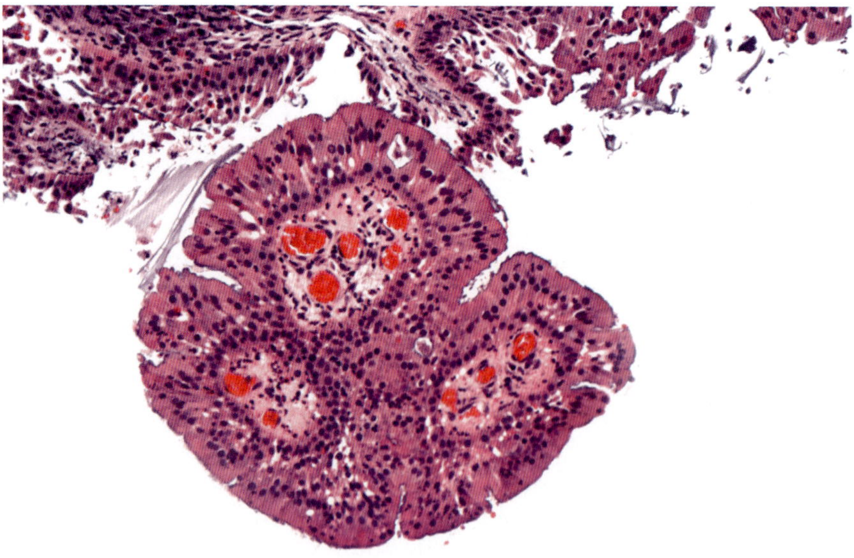

FIGURE 2.9 Oncocytic schneiderian papilloma.

except that the nests will be lined by oncocytes. Within the epithelium, numerous mucinous cells and small mucinous cysts are usually seen (eFig. 2.19).

NEOPLASTIC MIMICS

Aside from squamous neoplasms, there are a couple of squamous proliferations that mimic neoplasia of which all pathologists should be aware. These include pseudoepitheliomatous hyperplasia and necrotizing sialometaplasia and both may be seen throughout the upper aerodigestive tract (Table 2.2).

Pseudoepitheliomatous Hyperplasia

Pseudoepitheliomatous hyperplasia is a reactive hyperplasia of the squamous epithelium that can occur throughout the body. It may be associated with a wide variety of neoplastic or inflammatory conditions, but is especially noted with granular cell tumors.[23] Histologically, it is characterized

TABLE 2.2 Clinicopathologic Features of Mimics of Squamous Cell Carcinoma and Some Mimics

Lesion	Pseudoepitheliomatous Hyperplasia	Necrotizing Sialometaplasia	Squamous Cell Carcinoma
Clinical	May be seen throughout the upper aerodigestive tract and is associated with neoplastic or inflammatory lesions.	May be seen throughout the upper aerodigestive tract and is often related to previous therapy to the area.	May be seen throughout the upper aerodigestive tract.
Histology	Hyperplastic downgrowth of the squamous epithelium with irregular rete. Severe cytologic atypia and dyskeratosis should not be seen.	Squamous metaplasia and necrosis of the seromucinous glands. Retains a lobular architecture. May have some cytologic atypia. Should have intact myoepithelial layer.	Infiltrative, irregular nests of squamous cells devoid of a lobular architecture, usually with malignant cytologic atypia.

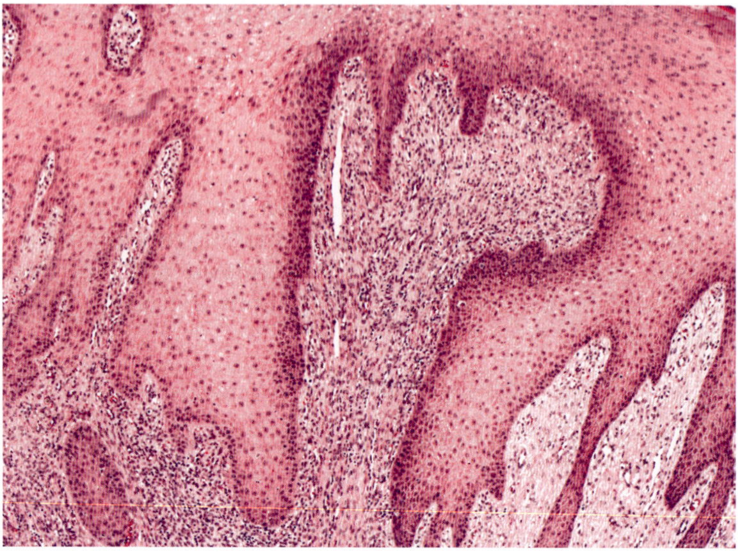

FIGURE 2.10 Pseudoepitheliomatous hyperplasia.

by downgrowth of the squamous epithelium into the underlying stroma, generally with quite elongated and jagged rete (Fig. 2.10, eFigs. 2.20 and 2.21). The bases of the lesions may sometimes be very complex and infiltrative in appearance. Although some mild architectural and cytologic disturbance may be present with focal abrupt keratinization and mild cytologic atypia, individual cell dyskeratosis and marked cytologic atypia should not be seen (eFig. 2.22). Occasional cases may be very difficult to distinguish from invasive, well-differentiated squamous cell carcinoma, especially as underlying lesions may not be sampled. Some authors have suggested the use of immunostains to p53 or other proteins in such cases; however, prudence is usually the best approach, and the diagnosis of invasive squamous cell carcinoma should only be made when other conditions can be definitely excluded.[23] Descriptive diagnoses, such as "atypical squamous proliferation," may be justified in some cases.

Necrotizing Sialometaplasia

Necrotizing sialometaplasia may involve any portion of the upper aerodigestive tract as it is a metaplastic condition of seromucinous or salivary glands.[24,25] It can develop spontaneously; however, it is most often seen following previous injury or therapy and may be secondary to vascular compromise. Thus, it is not an uncommon finding in patients with upper aerodigestive tract tumors who undergo radiation therapy prior to surgery. Histologically, it is characterized by a mix of necrotic seromucinous glands and glands which have undergone squamous metaplasia (Fig. 2.11, eFigs. 2.23 and 2.24). Abundant reactive changes and chronic inflammation

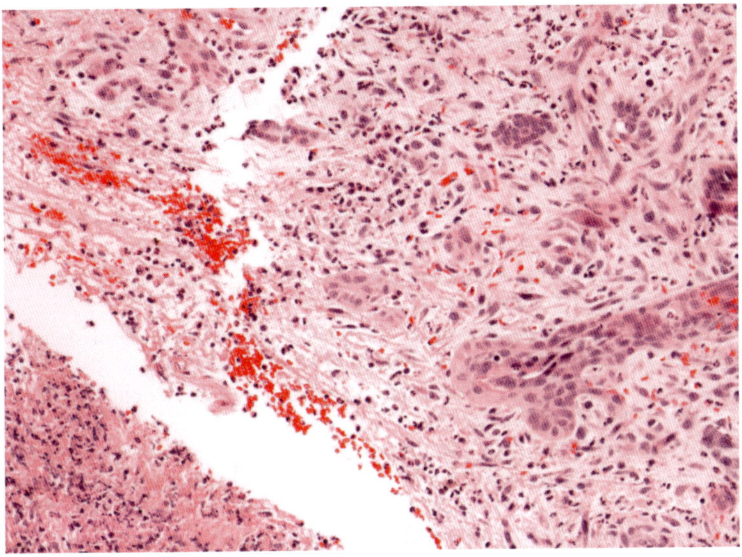

FIGURE 2.11 Necrotizing sialometaplasia.

may be present together with some degree of cytologic atypia. The nests of squamous epithelium maintain a lobular architecture, however, and nonmetaplastic seromucinous glands can often be identified within or at the periphery of these lesions. The lesions may be especially difficult to diagnose with small biopsy specimens or at the time of frozen section. As with pseudoepitheliomatous hyperplasia, prudence is recommended, and descriptive diagnoses should be used when definitive diagnoses cannot be rendered. p63 or smooth muscle actin immunostaining may be helpful with some cases as demonstration of a basal or myoepithelial layer would help to exclude an infiltrating squamous cell carcinoma or mucoepidermoid carcinoma.[26,27] Markers of neoplasia, such as p53 immunostain, are also potentially of use, as sialometaplasia will not show abnormal expression.

REFERENCES

1. Zunt SL, Tomich CE. Oral condyloma acuminatum. *J Dermatol Surg Oncol.* 1989;15:591-594.
2. Mills SE, Gaffey MJ, Frierson HF. *Tumors of the Upper Aerodigestive Tract and Ear.* Washington, DC: AFIP; 2000:21.
3. Carlos R, Sedano HO. Multifocal papilloma virus epithelial hyperplasia. *Oral Surg Oral Med Oral Pathol.* 1994;77:631-635.
4. Abramson AL, Steinberg BM, Winkler B. Laryngeal papillomatosis: clinical, histopathologic and molecular studies. *Laryngoscope.* 1987;97:678-685.
5. Doyle DJ, Gianoli GJ, Espinola T, Miller RH. Recurrent respiratory papillomatosis: juvenile versus adult forms. *Laryngoscope.* 1994;104:523-527.
6. Quick CA, Foucar E, Dehner LP. Frequency and significance of epithelial atypia in laryngeal papillomatosis. *Laryngoscope.* 1979;89:550-560.

7. Helmuth RA, Strate RW. Squamous carcinoma of the lung in a nonirradiated, non-smoking patient with juvenile laryngotracheal papillomatosis. *Am J Surg Pathol.* 1987;11:643-650.
8. Runckel D, Kessler S. Bronchogenic squamous carcinoma in nonirradiated juvenile laryngotracheal papillomatosis. *Am J Surg Pathol.* 1980;4:293-296.
9. Wenig BM. Schneiderian-type mucosal papillomas of the middle ear and mastoid. *Ann Otol Rhinol Laryngol.* 1996;105:226-233.
10. Hyams VJ. Papillomas of the nasal cavity and paranasal sinuses. A clinicopathological study of 315 cases. *Ann Otol Rhinol Laryngol.* 1971;80:192-206.
11. Ridolfi RL, Lieberman PH, Erlandson RA, Moore OS. Schneiderian papillomas: a clinicopathologic study of 30 cases. *Am J Surg Pathol.* 1977;1:43-53.
12. Snyder RN, Perzin KH. Papillomatosis of nasal cavity and paranasal sinuses (inverted papilloma, squamous papilloma). A clinicopathologic study. *Cancer.* 1972;30:668-690.
13. Christensen WN, Smith RR. Schneiderian papillomas: a clinicopathologic study of 67 cases. *Hum Pathol.* 1986;17:393-400.
14. Gaffey MJ, Frierson HF, Weiss LM, Barber CM, Baber GB, Stoler MH. Human papillomavirus and Epstein-Barr virus in sinonasal Schneiderian papillomas. An in situ hybridization and polymerase chain reaction study. *Am J Clin Pathol.* 1996;106:475-482.
15. Jo VY, Mills SE, Stoler MH, Stelow EB. Papillary squamous cell carcinoma of the head and neck: frequent association with human papillomavirus infection and invasive carcinoma. *Am J Surg Pathol.* 2009;33:1720-1724.
16. Kelly JH, Joseph M, Carroll E, et al. Inverted papilloma of the nasal septum. *Arch Otolaryngol.* 1980;106:767-771.
17. Manivel C, Wick MR, Dehner LP. Transitional (cylindric) cell carcinoma with endodermal sinus tumor-like features of the nasopharynx and paranasal sinuses. Clinicopathologic and immunohistochemical study of two cases. *Arch Pathol Lab Med.* 1986;110:198-202.
18. Udager AM, McHugh JB, Goudsmit CM, et al. Human papillomavirus (HPV) and somatic EGFR mutations are essential, mutually exclusive oncogenic mechanisms for inverted sinonasal papillomas and associated sinonasal squamous cell carcinomas. *Ann Oncol.* 2018;29:466-471.
19. Barnes L, Bedetti C. Oncocytic Schneiderian papilloma: a reappraisal of cylindrical cell papilloma of the sinonasal tract. *Hum Pathol.* 1984;15:344-351.
20. Ward BE, Fechner RE, Mills SE. Carcinoma arising in oncocytic Schneiderian papilloma. *Am J Surg Pathol.* 1990;14:364-369.
21. Kapadia SB, Barnes L, Pelzman K, Mirani N, Heffner DK, Bedetti C. Carcinoma ex oncocytic Schneiderian (cylindrical cell) papilloma. *Am J Otolaryngol.* 1993;14:332-338.
22. Udager AM, McHugh JB, Betz BL, et al. Activating KRAS mutations are characteristic of oncocytic sinonasal papilloma and associated sinonasal squamous cell carcinoma. *J Pathol.* 2016;239:394-398.
23. Zarovnaya E, Black C. Distinguishing pseudoepitheliomatous hyperplasia from squamous cell carcinoma in mucosal biopsy specimens from the head and neck. *Arch Pathol Lab Med.* 2005;129:1032-1036.
24. Abrams AM, Melrose RJ, Howell FV. Necrotizing sialometaplasia. A disease simulating malignancy. *Cancer.* 1973;32:130-135.
25. Fechner RE. Necrotizing sialometaplasia: a source of confusion with carcinoma of the palate. *Am J Clin Pathol.* 1977;67:315-317.
26. Carlson DL. Necrotizing sialometaplasia: a practical approach to the diagnosis. *Arch Pathol Lab Med.* 2009;133:692-698.
27. Rizkalla H, Toner M. Necrotizing sialometaplasia versus invasive carcinoma of the head and neck: the use of myoepithelial markers and keratin subtypes as an adjunct to diagnosis. *Histopathology.* 2007;51:184-189.

3

PRECURSOR LESIONS OF SQUAMOUS CELL CARCINOMA

Most anatomic pathologists are comfortable with the multihit model for the development of epithelial malignancy. As such, they are accustomed to diagnosing noninvasive premalignant neoplastic epithelial lesions at a number of sites. Perhaps the best-studied model for squamous cell carcinoma neogenesis is that for the development of squamous cell carcinoma of the uterine cervix, and most anatomic pathologists are comfortable diagnosing cervical squamous intraepithelial lesions.

There also is abundant evidence that squamous cell carcinoma of the upper aerodigestive tract develops through worsening intraepithelial neoplasia. Clinically, precursor lesions may appear white or red (or speckled) and are termed leukoplakia and erythroplakia. These clinical lesions do not correspond with definitive histologic features, although speckled and red lesions (erythroplakia) are more likely to show squamous dysplasia and be associated with concurrent squamous cell carcinoma or the eventual development of squamous cell carcinoma.[1–3] The data regarding the risk of these lesions progressing to malignancy are varied (Table 3.1), although worsening degrees of dysplasia are associated with greater risks in most studies.[3–18]

Unlike in the cervix, where high-risk human papillomavirus (HPV) infection causes the majority of intraepithelial lesions, there are a myriad of causes of upper aerodigestive tract squamous intraepithelial lesions, and HPV is involved in the development of the minority of cases.[19] The histologic features of most squamous intraepithelial neoplasia of the upper aerodigestive tract are thus not identical to those of the cervix, although obvious similarities exist. Undoubtedly, there is a complete spectrum of histologic changes that can be seen between the normal squamous epithelium of the upper aerodigestive tract and squamous cell carcinoma. How many lines one wishes to draw through this continuum is subjective. For the purpose of this chapter, we shall use the 2017 WHO classification systems for larynx and oral cavity (Table 3.2).[20]

TABLE 3.1 Risk for the Development of Squamous Cell Carcinoma of the Upper Aerodigestive Tract From Various Precursor Lesions

Study (Reference)	Location	Leukoplakia (Overall)	Dysplasia (Overall)	Mild Dysplasia	Moderate Dysplasia	Severe Dysplasia
3	Oral	45/257	8/22	–	–	–
4	Larynx	5/116	–	–	–	–
5	Oral	4%	–	–	–	–
6	Oral	11/248	–	–	–	–
7	Oral	7/117	–	–	–	–
8	Oral	1/117	–	–	–	–
9	Oral	–	9/68	1/13	3/43	5/12
10	Oral	0.13%	–	–	–	–
11	Oral	–	7/107	–	–	–
12	Oral	40/670	9/68	–	–	–
13	Larynx	3/92	–	–	–	–
14	Larynx	13/55	5/12	–	–	–
16	Oral	–	5/37	1/12	3/18	1/7
17	Oral	20/166	12/55	1/8	11/47	
18	Oral	11/311	–	–	–	–

WHO CLASSIFICATION SCHEME

The current WHO classification schemata use two histologic parameters for the diagnosis of squamous precursor lesions of the upper aerodigestive tract: architectural and cytologic atypia (Table 3.3). As was mentioned, although there are some similarities with squamous intraepithelial neoplasia of the cervix, the two are not usually identical. Indeed, evidence suggests that intraepithelial neoplasia of the upper aerodigestive tract may appear different dependent upon its etiology.[21] This is akin to squamous intraepithelial neoplasia of the vulva, where HPV-related lesions obtain a less differentiated appearance akin to lesions of the cervix, whereas other intraepithelial neoplasia may appear more differentiated (Fig. 3.1, eFig. 3.1).

Architectural disturbance is mostly considered a disturbance in cellular maturation. This is manifest histologically through lack of typical nuclear polarization, nonbasally located mitotic figures, dyskeratosis and abrupt, early keratinization. Unlike with cervical intraepithelial neoplasia, dyskeratotic cells are often very helpful for the diagnosis of squamous intraepithelial neoplasia of the upper aerodigestive tract and may be one of the few histologic clues of dysplasia. The identification of drop-shaped rete ridges can also be helpful, especially for the diagnosis of high-grade dysplastic lesions.

TABLE 3.2 **WHO Classification of Precursor Lesions of Squamous Cell Carcinoma**

WHO 2005	WHO Oral Cavity 2017	WHO Larynx 2017	Histology
Hyperplasia	**Mild dysplasia**	**Low-grade dysplasia**	Thickened epithelium due to increased cell numbers. Normal maturation with no cytologic atypia.
Mild dysplasia			Lack of cellular maturation within the lower one-third of the epithelium. Cytologic atypia, generally mild and confined to the lower one-third of the epithelium.
Moderate dysplasia	**Moderate dysplasia**	**High-grade dysplasia**	Architectural disturbance in the lower two-thirds of the squamous epithelium with moderate but not severe cytologic atypia.
Severe dysplasia	**Severe dysplasia**		Architectural disturbance extending into the upper one-third of the epithelium with severe cytologic atypia or severe cytologic atypia with any degree of architectural abnormality.
Carcinoma in situ			Full-thickness architectural disturbance with severe cytologic atypia.

Evaluation for cytologic atypia is also important for the assessment of squamous intraepithelial neoplasia. Atypical cytologic features include anisonucleosis and nuclear pleomorphism, anisocytosis and cytologic pleomorphism, increased nuclear size and increased nuclear to cytoplasmic ratios, nuclear hyperchromasia, prominent nucleoli, and atypical mitotic figures. The greater the degree of architectural disturbance or cytologic atypia is, the higher the grade of dysplasia.

Progressive molecular abnormalities have been shown to correlate with progressive histologic atypia and the risk of subsequent invasive squamous cell carcinoma. Worsening atypia correlates with aneuploidy, which has been shown to correlate with progression.[22,23] Loss of heterozygosity studies have shown that the losses at 3p and 9p are likely early

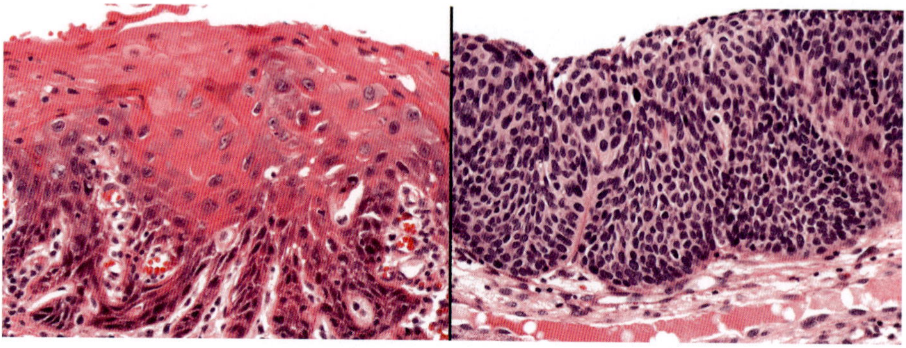

FIGURE 3.1 Squamous intraepithelial neoplasia of the upper aerodigestive tract. The left lesion is more differentiated and is p16 nonreactive, whereas the right lesion is undifferentiated and is p16 immunoreactive.

events in the development of squamous cell carcinoma of the upper aerodigestive tract and that such losses correlate with the risk for malignant transformation.[24] Furthermore, it has been shown that additional molecular abnormalities increase the risk even more. Much attention has also been paid to p53 mutations which are common in precursor lesions and are associated with increased risk for the development of invasive disease; however, other molecular markers, including but not limited to p16, p14, p12, p21, p27, MGMT, and retinoblastoma have been shown to be mutated or lost by other means to some degree in precursor lesions of the upper aerodigestive tract.[25–34] As with lesions of the cervix, high-grade intraepithelial lesions of the upper aerogestive tract associated with high-risk HPV will typically overexpress p16 and are less likely to have mutated p53.[35]

TABLE 3.3 Architectural and Cytologic Features of Dysplasia per the WHO[20]

Architectural Features of Dysplasia	Cytologic Features of Dysplasia
Irregular epithelial stratification	Anisonucleosis
Loss of nuclear polarity	Anisocytosis
Drop-shaped rete ridges	Nuclear pleomorphism
Increased number of mitotic figures	Cellular pleomorphism
Abnormally superficial mitoses	Increased nuclear to cytoplasmic ratios
Dyskeratosis	Increased nuclear size
Keratin pearls within the rete	Atypical mitotic figures
	Prominent nucleoli
	Nuclear hyperchromasia

Oral Cavity—Mild Dysplasia

Larynx—Low-Grade Dysplasia

Squamous hyperplasia is the most common cause of leukoplakia and is considered to be an epithelial precursor lesion by the WHO (Fig. 3.2, eFigs. 3.2 and 3.3). It is characterized by increased numbers of cells and often keratosis. The cellular proliferation may be located throughout the epithelium or appear somewhat localized to specific zones. These lesions should be devoid of architectural or cytologic atypia. Although considered to be a precursor lesion, the risk for the eventual development of squamous cell carcinoma in patients with these lesions is low. Within both the oral cavity and larynx, such lesions are considered forms of dysplasia. In the two-tiered system of the larynx, it is grouped within the category of low-grade dysplasia. In the oral cavity's three-tiered system, it falls within mild dysplasia. Lesions with minimal architectural and cytologic atypia (Fig. 3.3, eFigs. 3.4 and 3.5) are also categorized as such. Typically this mild atypia is characterized by basal cell hyperplasia with the cytologic atypia confined to the lower one-third of the epithelium.

Oral Cavity—Moderate Dysplasia and Severe Dysplasia

Larynx—High-Grade Dysplasia

Within the oral cavity, lesions showing a greater degree of architectural disturbance than mild dysplasia, with architectural changes extending into the middle one-third of the epithelium (Fig. 3.4, eFig. 3.6) are diagnosed

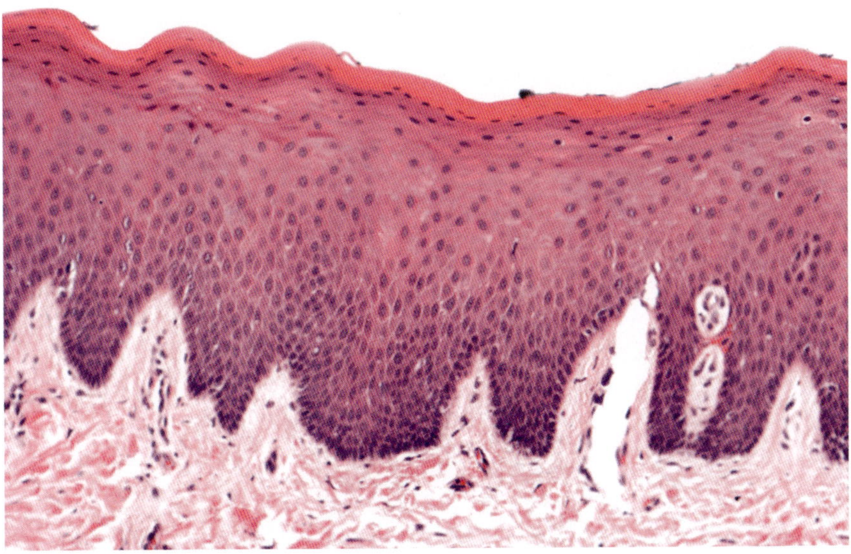

FIGURE 3.2 Squamous hyperplasia.

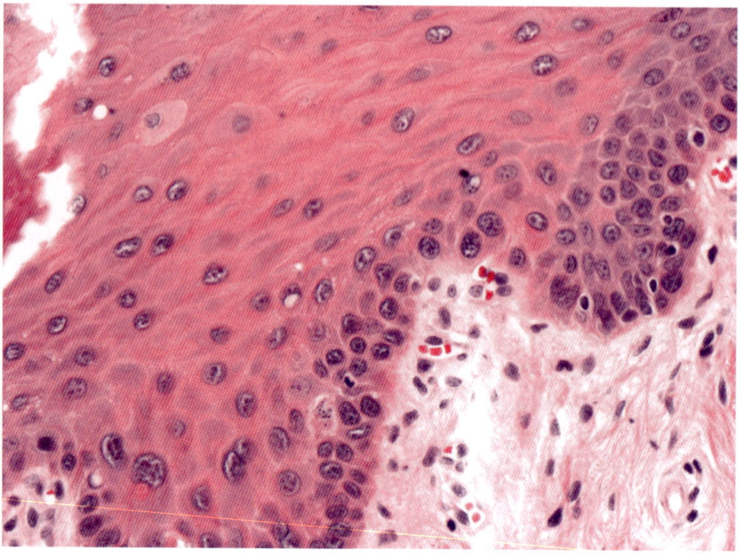

FIGURE 3.3 Mild dysplasia.

as moderate dysplasia. The atypia may also be more pronounced; however if it is severe, such lesions may be categorized as severe dysplasia. These lesions are defined as showing architectural disturbances that extend to more than two-thirds of the thickness of the squamous epithelium with marked cytologic atypia (Fig. 3.5, eFigs. 3.7 and 3.8). In the larynx, lesions showing more architectural and cytologic atypia than that of mild dysplasia

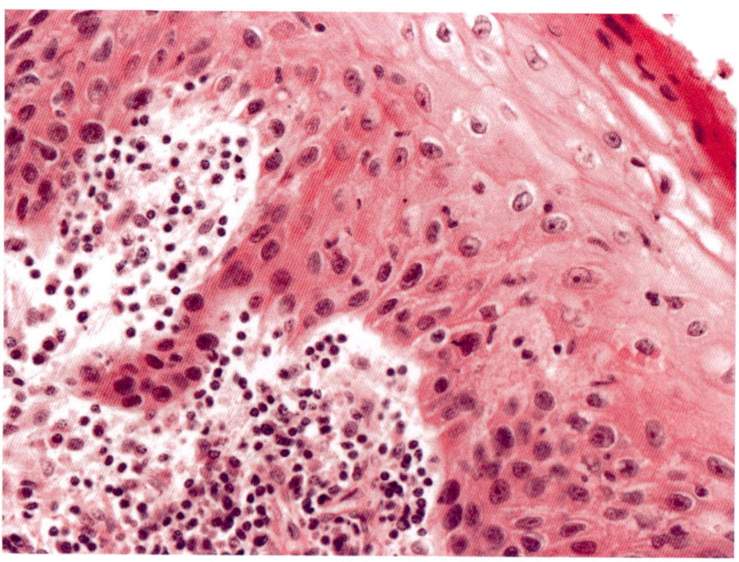

FIGURE 3.4 Moderate dysplasia.

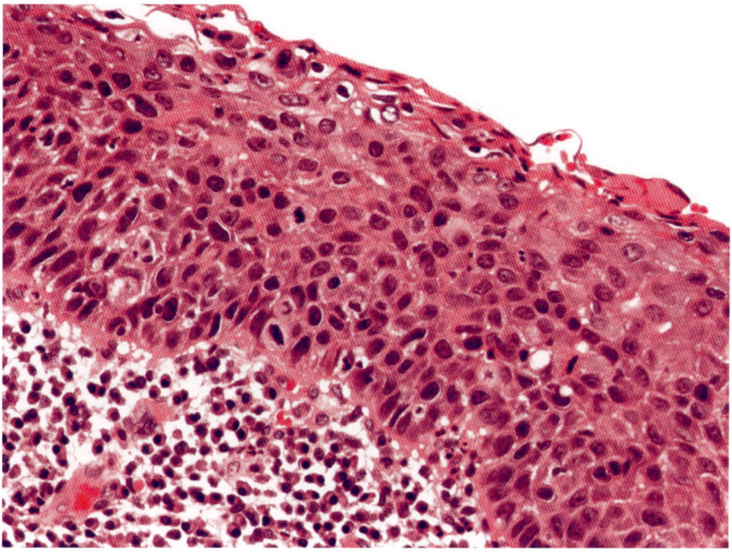

FIGURE 3.5 Severe dysplasia.

are diagnosed as high-grade dysplasia. Although the term "carcinoma in situ" is frowned on by some, the WHO does describe its use as acceptable for lesions showing full-thickness architectural disturbance and severe cytologic atypia (Fig. 3.6, eFigs. 3.9 and 3.10).

OTHER SPECIFIC PRECURSOR LESIONS

A number of other precursor lesions have been described which have been associated with the eventual development of squamous cell carcinoma and appear somewhat different for the conventional types of dysplasia.

Verrucous Hyperplasia

Proliferative verrucous leukoplakia is a clinical term used primarily for oral lesions.[36] The lesions appear white, may be multifocal, and appear exophytic as they progress. They arise in older individuals, are more common in women than men, and are less likely to be associated with smoking than other precursor lesions. They tend to involve the tongue and buccal mucosa.

Histologically, the lesions are characterized by verrucous hyperplasia with keratosis, squamous hyperplasia, and folding of the squamous epithelium (Fig. 3.7, eFig. 3.11). Unlike verrucous carcinoma (Table 3.4), these lesions are not yet invasive, and the bases of the lesions should not appear deeper than the surrounding normal squamous epithelium. Furthermore, these lesions may show cytologic atypia (eFig. 3.12), which should not be seen with verrucous carcinoma. Small biopsies can present obvious

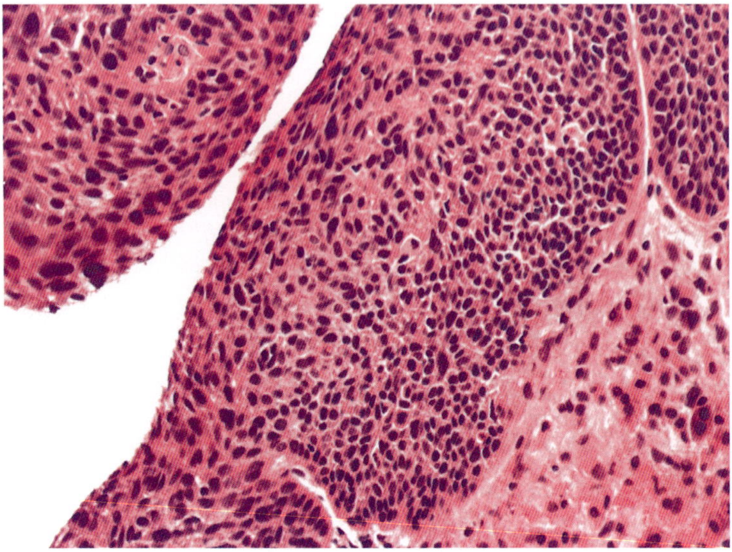

FIGURE 3.6 Squamous cell carcinoma in situ.

diagnostic difficulties as the bases of the lesions may not be visualized. With such cases, descriptors and qualified diagnoses should be considered with mention of the fact that the lesion's base is not visualized and invasion cannot be excluded.

Verrucous hyperplasia has a high recurrence rate and often eventually develops into invasive carcinoma, both verrucous carcinoma and

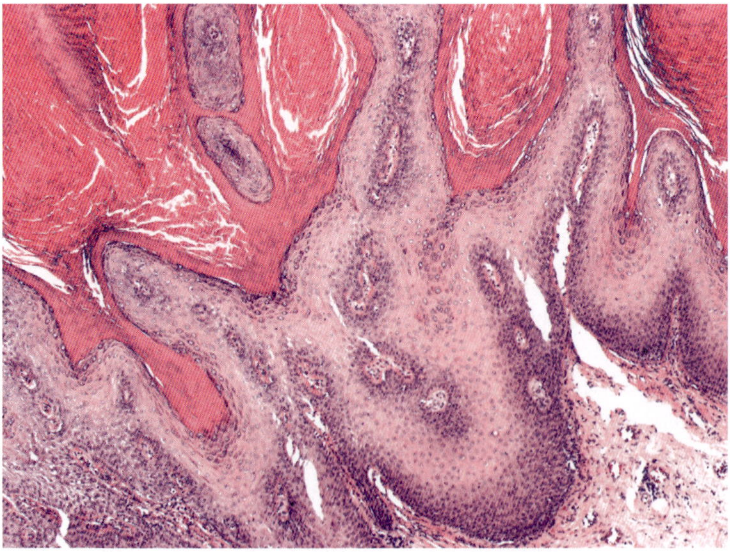

FIGURE 3.7 Verrucous hyperplasia.

TABLE 3.4 Verrucous Hyperplasia Versus Verrucous Carcinoma

Verrucous Hyperplasia	Verrucous Carcinoma
White, raised lesion. Should not be destructive.	Somewhat fungating. Destructive.
Base of lesion should not extend below the surrounding normal epithelium. Cytologic atypia may be present.	Circumscribed, pushing border of invasion, deeper than surrounding normal epithelium. Cytologic atypia should not be present.

conventional squamous cell carcinoma. Progression is related to the amount of cytologic atypia that is present.[16] It should again be stressed that proliferative verrucous leukoplakia and verrucous hyperplasia are considered different entities, one clinical and the other histologic.

Other Lesions

A number of disparate conditions associated with inflammation, atrophy, or genetic disease have been associated with the development of squamous cell carcinoma of the upper aerodigestive tract, especially of the mouth. These include syphilis, lichen planus, lupus, iron deficiency, and some hereditary defects in DNA repair.

An interesting precancerous condition occurs in patients who chew areca nuts either alone or in a mixture which sometimes contains tobacco (betel quid). The chewing can lead to a progressive histologic abnormality known as oral submucous fibrosis that is characterized by the deposition of fibrous, collagen bands immediately beneath the squamous epithelium (Fig. 3.8, eFig. 3.13). The epithelium also appears atrophic and dysplasia may be present.

ANCILLARY STUDIES

Ancillary studies are usually not very helpful for diagnosing precursor lesions, likely due to the heterogeneous molecular events that can lead to squamous cell carcinoma of the upper aerodigestive tract. Most methods involve the use of immunohistochemistry with antibodies directed toward proteins that are lost or gained secondary to genetic alterations in the development of squamous cell carcinoma. Immunostaining for p53 protein has often been touted as useful, as mutations of the gene are frequent and generally lead to an accumulation of defective protein.[25] Immunostaining for p16 protein appears to be helpful, especially with overexpression in high-risk HPV-related intraepithelial neoplasia. Alternatively, expression can be lost with gene promotor methylation with other squamous intraepithelial lesions.[32] Proliferation markers such as ki67 may also be helpful and substantial nuclear labeling above the

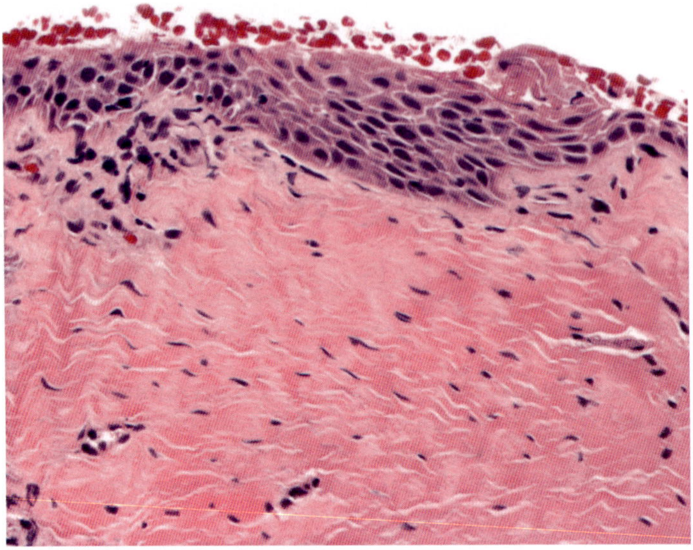

FIGURE 3.8 Oral submucosal fibrosis.

basal layer of the epithelium may be associated with intraepithelial neoplasia.[25,29,37] Immunostaining for the p21 protein, a target gene that can be activated by p53, may also be helpful, although results have been mixed.[29] Although some authors have attempted to use the expression of various keratins to assist in the diagnosis, the results have proven too mixed or inconsistent to be of much use.[25,30]

REFERENCES

1. Shafer WG, Waldron CA. Erythroplakia of the oral cavity. *Cancer*. 1975;36:1021-1028.
2. Mashberg A. Erythroplasia vs. leukoplasia in the diagnosis of early asymptomatic oral squamous carcinoma. *N Engl J Med*. 1977;297:109-110.
3. Silverman S Jr, Gorsky M, Lozada F. Oral leukoplakia and malignant transformation. A follow-up study of 257 patients. *Cancer*. 1984;53:563-568.
4. Norris CM, Peale AR. Keratosis of the larynx. *J Laryngol Otol*. 1963;77:635-647.
5. Einhorn J, Wersall J. Incidence of oral carcinoma in patients with leukoplakia of the oral mucosa. *Cancer*. 1967;20:2189-2193.
6. Pindborg JJ, Jolst O, Renstrup G, Roed-Petersen B. Studies in oral leukoplakia: a preliminary report on the period pervalence of malignant transformation in leukoplakia based on a follow-up study of 248 patients. *J Am Dent Assoc*. 1968;76:767-771.
7. Silverman S Jr. Observations on the clinical characteristics and natural history of oral leukoplakia. *J Am Dent Assoc*. 1968;76:772-777.
8. Mehta FS, Shroff BC, Gupta PC, Daftary DK. Oral leukoplakia in relation to tobacco habits. A ten-year follow-up study of Bombay policemen. *Oral Surg Oral Med Oral Pathol*. 1972;34:426-433.
9. Banoczy J, Csiba A. Occurrence of epithelial dysplasia in oral leukoplakia. Analysis and follow-up study of 12 cases. *Oral Surg Oral Med Oral Pathol*. 1976;42:766-774.

10. Silverman S, Bhargava K, Smith LW, Malaowalla AM. Malignant transformation and natural history of oral leukoplakia in 57,518 industrial workers of Gujarat, India. *Cancer*. 1976;38:1790-1795.
11. Pindborg JJ, Daftary DK, Mehta FS. A follow-up study of sixty-one oral dysplastic precancerous lesions in Indian villagers. *Oral Surg Oral Med Oral Pathol*. 1977;43:383-390.
12. Banoczy J. Follow-up studies in oral leukoplakia. *J Maxillofac Surg*. 1977;5:69-75.
13. Crissman JD. Laryngeal keratosis and subsequent carcinoma. *Head Neck Surg*. 1979;1:386-391.
14. Henry RC. The transformation of laryngeal leucoplakia to cancer. *J Laryngol Otol*. 1979;93:447-459.
15. Crissman JD, Zarbo RJ. Dysplasia, in situ carcinoma, and progression to invasive squamous cell carcinoma of the upper aerodigestive tract. *Am J Surg Pathol*. 1989;1(13 suppl):5-16.
16. Lumerman H, Freedman P, Kerpel S. Oral epithelial dysplasia and the development of invasive squamous cell carcinoma. *Oral Surg Oral Med Oral Pathol Oral Radiol Endod*. 1995;79:321-329.
17. Schepman KP, van der Meij EH, Smeele LE, van der Waal I. Malignant transformation of oral leukoplakia: a follow-up study of a hospital-based population of 166 patients with oral leukoplakia from The Netherlands. *Oral Oncol*. 1998;34:270-275.
18. Bromwich M. Retrospective study of the progression of oral premalignant lesions to squamous cell carcinoma: a South Wales experience. *J Otolaryngol*. 2002;31:150-156.
19. Stelow EB, Jo VY, Stoler MH, Mills SE. Human papillomavirus-associated squamous cell carcinoma of the upper aerodigestive tract. *Am J Surg Pathol*. 2010;34:e15-e24.
20. Gale N, Hille J, Jordan RC, Nadal A, Williams MD: Precursor lesions. In: El Nagger A, Chan JKC, Grandis DR, Takata T, Slootweg PJ, eds. *WHO Classification of Head and Neck Tumors*. Lyon: IARC Press; 2017:91-93.
21. Jo VY, O'Connor SM, Stoler MH, Stelow EB. Carcinoma in situ and p16 status of head and neck squamous cell carcinoma. *Mod Pathol*. 2010;23:274A-275A.
22. Crissman JD, Fu YS. Intraepithelial neoplasia of the larynx. A clinicopathologic study of six cases with DNA analysis. *Arch Otolaryngol Head Neck Surg*. 1986;112:522-528.
23. Hellquist H, Olofsson J, Grontoft O. Carcinoma in situ and severe dysplasia of the vocal cords. A clinicopathological and photometric investigation. *Acta Otolaryngol*. 1981;92:543-555.
24. Mao L, Lee JS, Fan YH, et al. Frequent microsatellite alterations at chromosomes 9p21 and 3p14 in oral premalignant lesions and their value in cancer risk assessment. *Nat Med*. 1996;2:682-685.
25. Coltrera MD, Zarbo RJ, Sakr WA, Gown AM. Markers for dysplasia of the upper aerodigestive tract. Suprabasal expression of PCNA, p53, and CK19 in alcohol-fixed, embedded tissue. *Am J Pathol*. 1992;141:817-825.
26. Girod SC, Kramer C, Knufermann R, Krueger GR. p53 expression in the carcinogenesis in the oral mucosa. *J Cell Biochem*. 1994;56:444-448.
27. Kudo Y, Takata T, Ogawa I, et al. Reduced expression of p27(Kip1) correlates with an early stage of cancer invasion in oral squamous cell carcinoma. *Cancer Lett*. 2000;151:217-222.
28. Shahnavaz SA, Bradley G, Regezi JA, et al. Patterns of CDKN2A gene loss in sequential oral epithelial dysplasias and carcinomas. *Cancer Res*. 2001;61:2371-2375.
29. Choi HR, Tucker SA, Huang Z, et al. Differential expressions of cyclin-dependent kinase inhibitors (p27 and p21) and their relation to p53 and Ki-67 in oral squamous tumorigenesis. *Int J Oncol*. 2003;22:409-414.
30. Farrar M, Sandison A, Peston D, Gailani M. Immunocytochemical analysis of AE1/AE3, CK 14, Ki-67 and p53 expression in benign, premalignant and malignant oral tissue to establish putative markers for progression of oral carcinoma. *Br J Biomed Sci*. 2004;61:117-124.

31. Viswanathan M, Tsuchida N, Shanmugam G. Promoter hypermethylation profile of tumor-associated genes p16, p15, hMLH1, MGMT and E-cadherin in oral squamous cell carcinoma. *Int J Cancer*. 2003;105:41-46.
32. Gologan O, Barnes EL, Hunt JL. Potential diagnostic use of p16INK4A, a new marker that correlates with dysplasia in oral squamoproliferative lesions. *Am J Surg Pathol*. 2005;29:792-796.
33. Kresty LA, Mallery SR, Knobloch TJ, et al. Alterations of p16(INK4a) and p14(ARF) in patients with severe oral epithelial dysplasia. *Cancer Res*. 2002;62:5295-5300.
34. Shintani S, Mihara M, Nakahara Y, et al. Expression of cell cycle control proteins in normal epithelium, premalignant and malignant lesions of oral cavity. *Oral Oncol*. 2002;38:235-243.
35. Chernock RD, Lewis JS Jr, Zhang Q, El-Mofty SK. Human papillomavirus-positive basaloid squamous cell carcinomas of the upper aerodigestive tract: a distinct clinicopathologic and molecular subtype of basaloid squamous cell carcinoma. *Hum Pathol*. 2010;41:1016-1023.
36. Silverman S Jr, Gorsky M. Proliferative verrucous leukoplakia: a follow-up study of 54 cases. *Oral Surg Oral Med Oral Pathol Oral Radiol Endod*. 1997;84:154-157.
37. Piattelli A, Rubini C, Fioroni M, Iezzi G, Santinelli A. Prevalence of p53, bcl-2, and Ki-67 immunoreactivity and of apoptosis in normal oral epithelium and in premalignant and malignant lesions of the oral cavity. *J Oral Maxillofac Surg*. 2002;60:532-540.

4

CONVENTIONAL SQUAMOUS CELL CARCINOMA

Conventional squamous cell carcinoma (SCC) is the most common malignant diagnosis made based on biopsy specimens from the upper aerodigestive tract. In fact, it may be the most common diagnosis of any type rendered on biopsy specimens from this area. This chapter will discuss the epidemiology and clinical aspects of the disease, the histologic features of conventional SCC, and some difficulties that can be faced with biopsy specimens. Specific variants of SCC that generally lead to more diagnostic difficulties are discussed in Chapter 5.

EPIDEMIOLOGY

SCC of the upper aerodigestive tract is a disease of older individuals, especially of men. A few notable exceptions occur (e.g., nonkeratinizing nasopharyngeal carcinoma); however, more than 90% of cancers of the oral cavity and pharynx and more than 95% of cancers of the larynx are diagnosed in patients older than 45 years.[1,2] According to the National Cancer Institute, slightly more than 53,000 cancers of the oral cavity and pharynx and nearly 12,500 cancers of the larynx will be diagnosed in the United States in 2019. They estimate that there will be approximately 11,000 deaths from oral and oropharyngeal cancers and approximately 3700 deaths from laryngeal cancers. Thus, the incidence of these cancers combined is similar to that of pancreatic cancer, whereas their mortality is similar to that of renal cell carcinoma.

Stage is the most important prognostic factor for conventional tumors not related to viral infection.[1,2] The overall 5-year relative survival rates for laryngeal and oral/pharyngeal cancers are about 60%, but are about 80% when the diseases were found to be localized. While a majority of laryngeal cancers are localized at the time of diagnosis, only a third of oral/pharyngeal cancers are.

SCC of the upper aerodigestive tract is strongly linked to the use of alcohol and tobacco products.[3–8] Indeed, using the two products together carries a relative risk for the development of these cancers of more than 20.[6] The risk is dose-related, and heavy users are much more likely to develop these malignancies than infrequent or occasional users.[8] Furthermore, the cessation of smoking is associated with a decreased risk for the development of these malignancies when compared to those who continue to smoke.

With regard to tobacco products, smoked tobacco is the major culprit.[6] Chewed tobacco, however, is also considered to be a risk factor, especially for the development of oral SCCs, although its role remains somewhat unclear, and it carries a significantly lower relative risk for the development of malignancy at all sites when compared to smoking.[9] Indeed, some have suggested that individuals should be encouraged to switch from smoked to chewed tobacco to reduce their risk for developing these malignancies.

In recent years, the incidence rate of tobacco product use has declined in the United States. Following this trend, there is now a well-established decline in the incidence rate of upper aerodigestive SCCs at sites most commonly related to the use of tobacco products (e.g., the larynx and oral cavity).

Other risk factors for SCC are both familial and environmental.[10–18] Although the data are somewhat unclear, some elucidation has been achieved based on studies of young patients with SCCs who have little or no history of exposure to alcohol or tobacco products. The better understood familial cancer syndromes, including Li-Fraumeni syndrome, Lynch syndrome, and familial atypical mole melanoma syndrome, with germline mutations of the genes encoding for the p53 protein, mismatch repair proteins, and the p16 protein all carry increased risk for the development of SCCs of the upper aerodigestive tract.[17–19] Some HLA types are also more prone to develop SCCs, particularly Epstein-Barr virus (EBV)-associated nasopharyngeal carcinomas.[10,20–22]

Aside from tobacco and alcohol use, environmental factors include both dietary and infectious factors. Although not commonly chewed in the United States, betel quid (a combination of a stimulant and alkaloid) has been associated with the development of oral SCC through the development of the precursor lesion, submucosal fibrosis (see Chapter 3).[13] Diets deficient in iron can lead to Plummer-Vinson syndrome (dysphagia, iron deficiency, and esophageal webs), which is associated with an increased risk for the development of hypopharyngeal SCC.[23] Finally, people with diets rich in fruits and vegetables may be at decreased risk for the development of SCC of the upper aerodigestive tract.[14]

EBV is believed to play a role in the development of some SCCs, namely with nonkeratinizing and undifferentiated SCCs.[24] These tumors almost always occur in the nasopharynx; however, they can occur anywhere throughout the upper aerodigestive tract. The exact role that EBV plays in the development of these tumors is unclear. EBV-associated tumors are discussed in more detail in Chapter 5.

High-risk human papillomavirus (HR-HPV) also plays an important role in the development of SCCs of the upper aerodigestive tract, especially in younger patients with no history of alcohol or tobacco abuse.[25–28] Our understanding of the role that HPV plays in the development of these tumors has progressed quickly over the past 20 years. We know that these tumors are most commonly located in the oropharynx (the palatine and lingual tonsils), although the tumors can occur throughout the entire tract. HPV-related SCCs are most commonly nonkeratinizing (see Chapter 5), although they may sometimes be keratinizing or associated with other variant morphologies. The tumors have better overall prognoses than SCCs secondary to tobacco and alcohol use and are more radiosensitive. While the incidence rate of laryngeal and oral SCCs has declined recently, there has been a surge in the incidence rate of oropharyngeal SSC, leading some to claim we now have an epidemic of HPV-related upper aerodigestive tract malignancy.[29]

CLINICAL

Patients who develop SCCs of the upper aerodigestive tract tend to be older and the disease is much more common in men. As noted above, exceptions include EBV-related tumors and tumors secondary to HR-HPV infection. Also, tumors with chromosomal rearrangement of the *nuclear protein of the testis* gene (NUT carcinomas) occur in patients of all ages (discussed in the Chapter 5).[30]

Patients' symptoms depend on the location of the tumor and stage of their disease. Most patients present with the nonspecific findings of a mass lesion, obstruction, pain, and bleeding. Laryngeal lesions are typically associated with hoarseness. Any tumor, especially those that develop in the nasopharynx and oropharynx, can present with metastases, for example, as a neck mass, without symptoms related to the primary tumor. More advanced tumors can present with symptoms secondary to distant metastases and with systemic complaints such as weight loss.

DIAGNOSIS

Although the diagnosis of some variants of SCC can be particularly challenging (see Chapter 5), the recognition of most conventional SCCs is routine. These are infiltrative tumors composed of irregular, often interconnected, and anastomosing nests of well-demarcated squamous cells that show varying degrees of intracellular and extracellular keratin formation (Fig. 4.1, eFig. 4.1). Increased differentiation is usually present toward the center of the nests with the most peripheral cells having a basaloid phenotype with scant basophilic cytoplasm (Fig. 4.2, eFig. 4.2). As the cells progress centrally within the nests, their cytoplasm tends to become more abundant and eosinophilic. Extracellular keratin, commonly intermixed with necrotic debris, is often identified at the centers of the nests (eFig. 4.3). This is not a firm rule and some degree of atypical maturation is usually seen with more peripheral cells having increased intracellular or

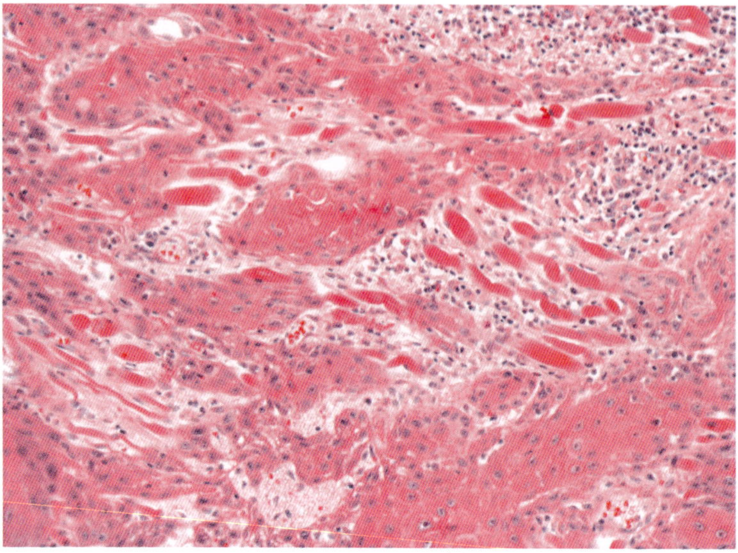

FIGURE 4.1 A squamous cell carcinoma with a typical pattern of infiltration.

extracellular keratinization and some central cells having a more basaloid phenotype. Furthermore, extracellular keratin formation may be seen anywhere throughout the nests and may even not be present. The squamous nests can vary considerably in size with some appearing large and cystic, resembling nonneoplastic keratinous cysts (eFig. 4.4). Single-cell

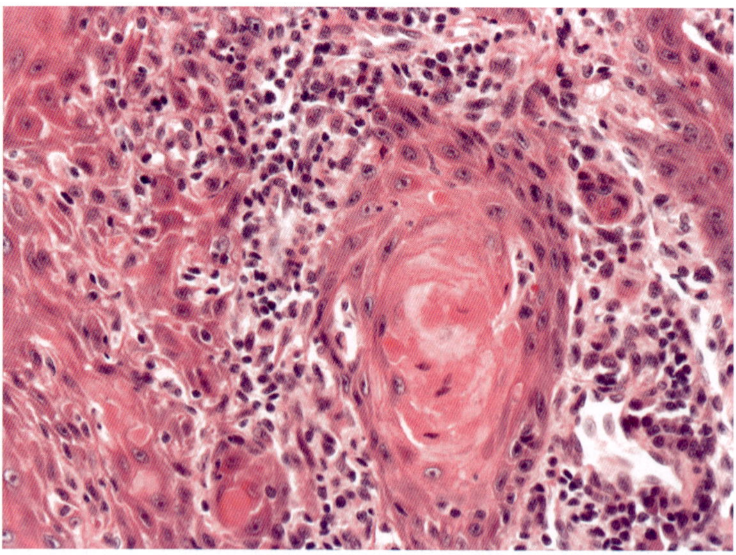

FIGURE 4.2 Maturing, keratinized squamous cells are present toward the center of the infiltrating nests.

infiltration may be present and can be very helpful for distinguishing non-neoplastic or noninvasive disease from invasive malignancy (eFig. 4.5). The surrounding stroma usually has some degree of chronic inflammation, often with stromal desmoplasia.

Cytologically, conventional SCCs have cells with varying degrees of differentiation and varying degrees of cytologic atypia. The smaller, basaloid cells have a more undifferentiated phenotype and can appear round with little cytoplasm. Larger cells will have more abundant eosinophilic to clear cytoplasm and typically have a more rigid, polygonal shape. These cells often show artifactual separation from one another and intercellular desmosomes can typically be identified between the neoplastic cells. Within the cytoplasm of the larger, differentiated cells, intracellular keratin formation and granules can sometimes be seen. The nuclei of the neoplastic cells show moderate to marked differences in shape and size with irregular contours and vesicular to granular, malignant-appearing chromatin. Prominent nucleoli are usually seen and mitotic figures, including atypical mitotic figures can usually be found. Necrosis of both individual tumor cells and of large portions of tumor is frequently seen with SCCs.

Immunohistochemistry is not commonly used for the diagnosis of conventional SCC. Neoplastic cells will be reactive with antibodies to pankeratins, and, specifically, with antibodies to CK 5/6, 8, 13, and 19. Immunoreactivity with antibodies to CK7 may be seen in some cases; however, immunoreactivity with antibodies to CK20 is almost never seen. Most cases are immunoreactive with antibodies to p63 and p40, and variable immunoreactivity can be seen with markers of molecular abnormalities such as p53, Cyclin D1, retinoblastoma protein, etc. The use of these molecular markers has been proposed by some to help distinguish neoplastic from nonneoplastic disease.

GRADING

Most pathologists grade biopsies of SCCs, and a variety of grading systems exist.[31–39] Nonetheless, grading is usually performed with a rather gestalt approach, and SCCs are classified as well-differentiated when they closely resemble nonneoplastic squamous epithelium and as poorly differentiated when their squamous differentiation is hard to appreciate. Much of what remains is then diagnosed as moderately differentiated. Scoring systems that combine histologic and macroscopic features do exist that attempt to objectify the diagnostic criteria.[39,40] We use a three-tiered system based on histologic and cytologic features.

Well-differentiated SCCs are those tumors that show both intracellular and extracellular keratinization with well-ordered maturation seen as one moves to the more central portions of the infiltrating nests (Fig. 4.3, eFigs. 4.6 and 4.7). The infiltrating nests of tumor cells are larger than those seen in less differentiated SCCs and can appear centrally cystic. Infiltrating small nests or single cells should not be seen. As ordered maturation is

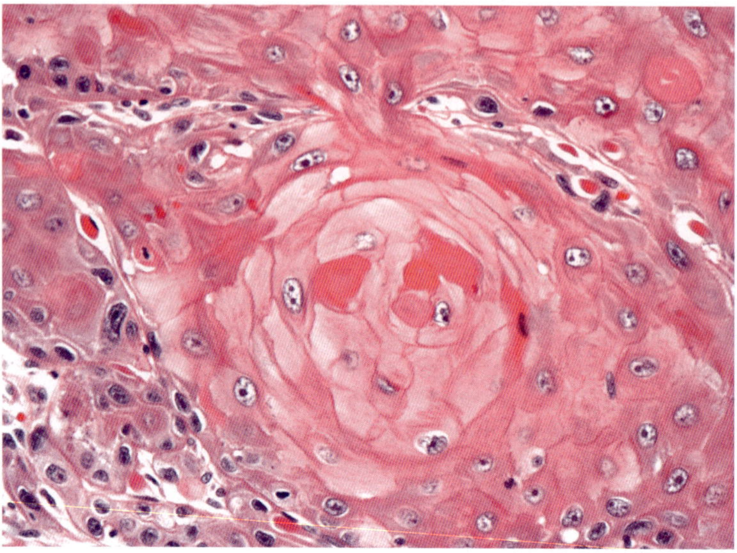

FIGURE 4.3 A well-differentiated squamous cell with abundant intracellular keratin.

present, relatively preserved nuclear to cytoplasmic ratios are usually seen. Nuclear atypia is usually only mild, and most nuclei mature to have vesicular chromatin. Mitotic figures can usually be found but generally number less than one per five high-powered fields and are located toward the periphery of the infiltrating islands of tumor cells.

Moderately differentiated SCCs usually show some degree of keratinization; however, it is less than that seen with well-differentiated SCCs (Figs. 4.4 and 4.5, eFigs. 4.8–4.10). It is also less ordered, and the less mature-appearing cells may show abrupt keratinization. The infiltrating nests of tumor cells are smaller, show more variation in size, and focally have a more cordlike pattern of infiltration. While many of the nuclei are mature, a significant number remain hyperchromatic and have more granular chromatin. Furthermore, more variation in nuclear size and shape is seen, and some nuclei will appear folded and irregular and have .six times the nuclear volume of surrounding neoplastic nuclei. Mitotic figures are more numerous and can be found throughout the squamous nests. More individual tumor cells undergo necrosis and necrotic debris is often seen within the central portions of the tumor nests.

Poorly differentiated SCCs show limited cellular keratinization and may show little or no extracellular keratin formation (Fig. 4.6, eFig. 4.11). Nests of tumor cells may be smaller, and individual tumor cell infiltration can be seen (Fig. 4.7, eFigs. 4.12 and 4.13). Conversely, some poorly differentiated tumors can display a sheetlike pattern of growth. Little maturation of the cells is seen, and the cells thus appear more monomorphic with centrally located cells showing little cytologic difference from those cells located toward the periphery of the infiltrating nests. Some cells can show

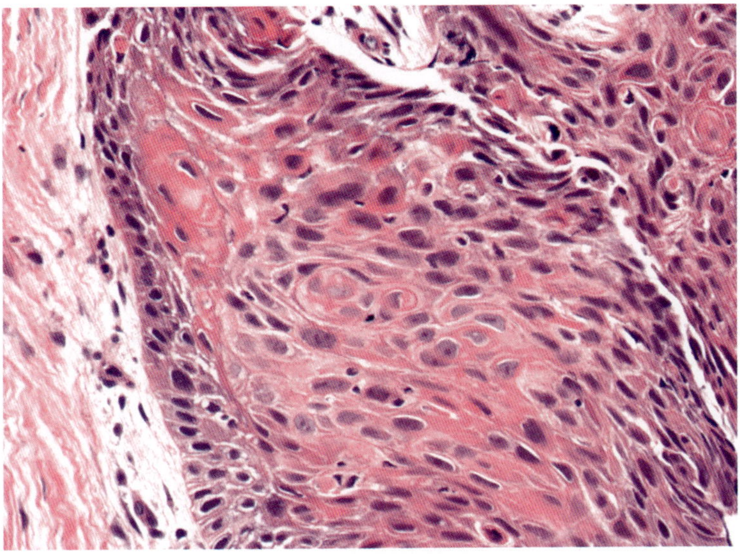

FIGURE 4.4 This moderately differentiated squamous cell carcinoma (SCC) has less organized maturation than a well-differentiated SCC.

marked nuclear pleomorphism. Most cells have granular and obviously malignant chromatin, and mitotic figures, both typical and atypical, are numerous. Many apoptotic figures can be seen, as can larger, more diffuse areas of necrosis.

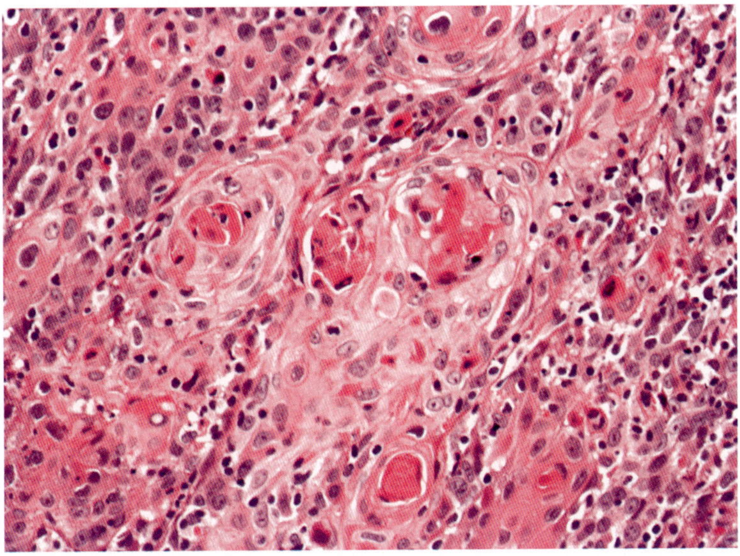

FIGURE 4.5 Occasional cells show abrupt keratinization in this moderately differentiated squamous cell carcinoma.

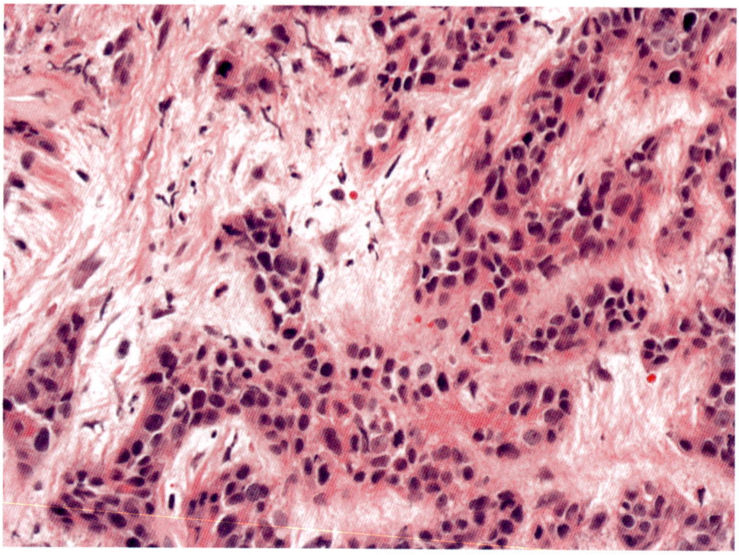

FIGURE 4.6 This poorly differentiated squamous cell carcinoma shows limited cellular maturation.

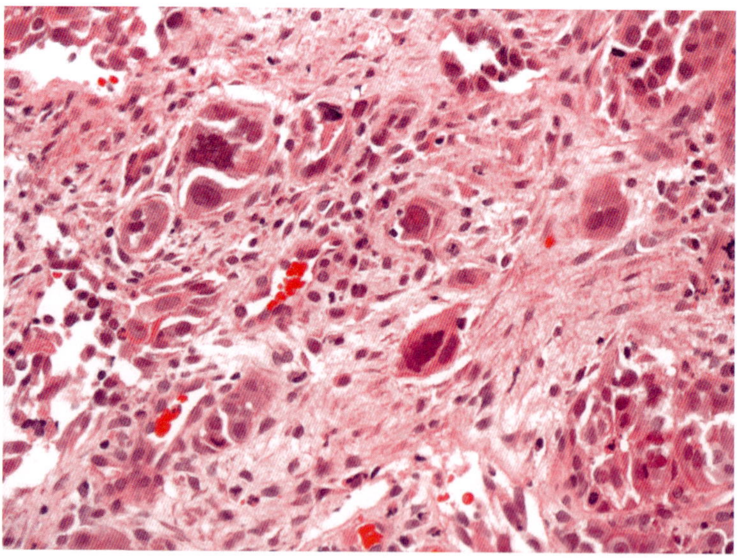

FIGURE 4.7 Single-cell infiltration is seen with this poorly differentiated squamous cell carcinoma.

PROBLEMS WITH DIAGNOSIS ON BIOPSY SPECIMEN

A number of problems can be encountered when considering the diagnosis of conventional SCC (Table 4.1). These are often related to the exophytic nature of many tumors, the superficial nature of most biopsies, and poor specimen orientation. In many instances, one can be very pressed to identify definitive invasive malignancy. Although we will go into some depth discussing how to distinguish invasive from noninvasive disease, we would like to preface this by stating that one should not be pressured into making a diagnosis of invasive malignancy with an insufficient specimen and should instead feel free to use nonspecific terminology such as "atypical squamous proliferation" with notes that discuss the limitations of the biopsy specimens and the differential diagnoses.

The most common diagnostic dilemma we face is the interpretation of fragmented, superficial biopsies of apparently exophytic mass lesions (Fig. 4.8). With these biopsies, one usually sees a thickened, stratified squamous epithelium with keratosis and parakeratosis. Epithelial atypia is usually seen, with changes of dysplasia as discussed in Chapter 3. (A similar dilemma is faced with the potential diagnosis of verrucous carcinoma on biopsy specimen; however here, by definition, little or no cytologic atypia is seen. This will be discussed in Chapter 5.) The squamous epithelium is folded with an intermixed, often inflamed stroma; however, in the areas where the border between the two can be best visualized, this interphase remains smooth and linear. In other words, no irregular margins to the nests of atypical epithelium are seen and, thus, the pathologist cannot make a definitive diagnosis of an invasive malignancy.

In such cases, the two biopsies, in and of themselves, are theoretically diagnostic of only dysplasia. Obviously, such an interpretation in the presence of a mass lesion would be problematic. With these lesions, when it is known that the patient has a mass or, as often happens, when no clinical history is provided, a descriptive diagnosis such as "atypical squamous proliferation" should be rendered. A note can then be provided stating the precise changes on the biopsy specimen and that invasive disease cannot be excluded. Re-biopsy or excision is then recommended as clinically

TABLE 4.1 Difficulties Faced With the Diagnosis of Conventional Squamous Cell Carcinoma
Superficial biopsies of exophytic masses
Complex, convoluted epithelium (e.g., tonsil)
Poor specimen orientation
Radiation changes
Necrotizing sialometaplasia
Pseudoepitheliomatous hyperplasia

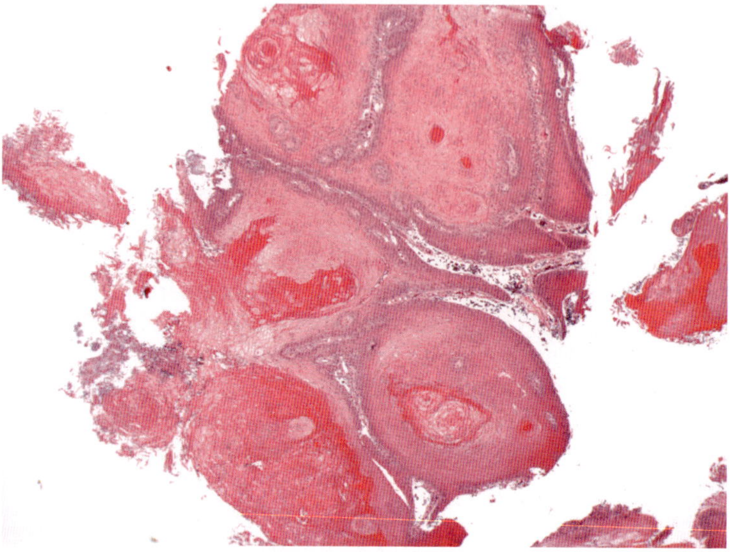

FIGURE 4.8 A sample from an extremely exophytic squamous cell carcinoma. Definitive invasion could not be identified.

indicated for a definitive diagnosis. The pathologist should not feel shy or inadequate when using such a diagnosis or that he is "hedging." Clinicians, especially otolaryngologists, should have enough understanding of these lesions to comprehend the difficulty faced by the pathologist, and they should be able to use such descriptive diagnoses with their clinical impressions to properly manage the patients.

Akin to this difficulty is the one faced with a poorly oriented specimen or with specimens from more convoluted structures such as the tonsils (Fig. 4.9, eFigs. 4.14–4.16). Indeed, these problems often occur together. With these biopsies, it is often apparent that the surface epithelium is not localized to the surface of the section, and islands of atypical squamous epithelium may be seen within central portions of the biopsy surrounded by stroma. Although the squamous epithelium may show changes diagnostic of dysplasia, the epithelial islands remain well-circumscribed with a smooth interphase between the epithelium and stroma. Furthermore, it can be difficult to judge maturation, as tangential cuts may be made entirely through the more basal portions of the epithelium.

With such cases, a diligent search through the entire specimen should be made for any better oriented fragments, smaller islands of epithelium with irregular contours, atypical single cells, and any areas where the smooth contours of the larger squamous epithelial islands are compromised (Fig. 4.10, eFig. 4.17). The identification of stromal desmoplasia may also be helpful. Often, at least microinvasive disease can be appreciated. As with the previous dilemma, pathologists may be forced in these situations to render descriptive diagnoses. Here, the danger often lies with

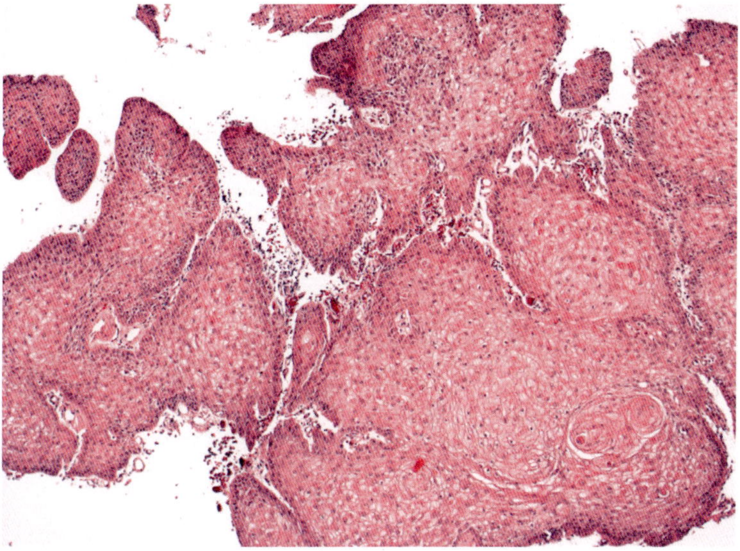

FIGURE 4.9 A poorly oriented sample from an exophytic squamous cell carcinoma.

overinterpretation and a possible false-positive diagnosis. In the absence of definitive invasion, descriptive diagnoses are assuredly preferred.

Radiation therapy remains a standard treatment modality for head and neck SCC. A pathologist will frequently receive biopsy specimens from irradiated upper aerodigestive tract mucosa either after or, sometimes, prior to resection (Figs. 4.11 and 4.12, eFigs. 4.18–4.21). As SCC

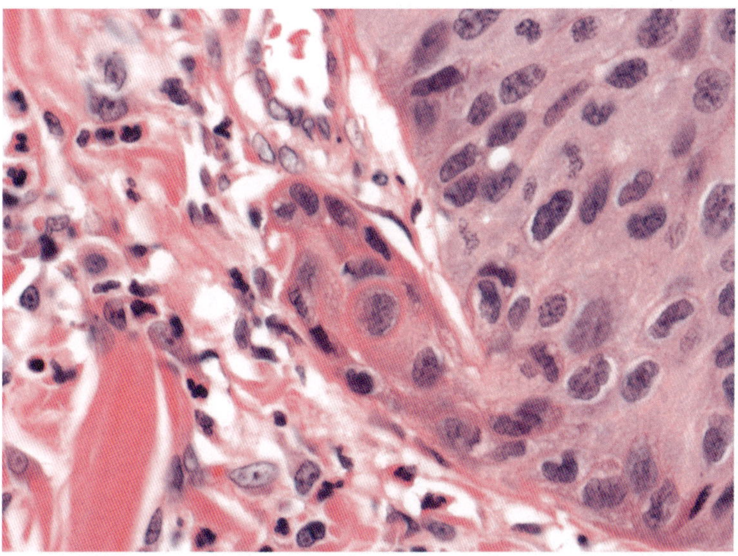

FIGURE 4.10 Squamous cell carcinoma with an irregular stromal-tumor interface.

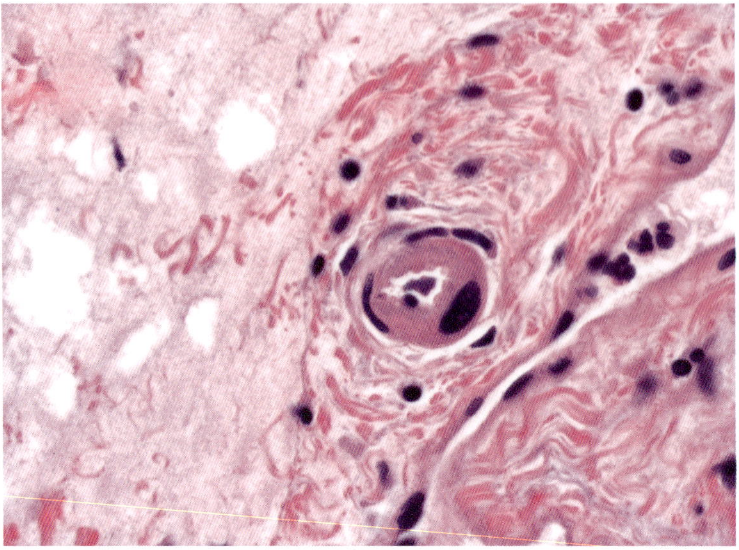

FIGURE 4.11 Radiation can induce atypia within endothelial cells.

of this area frequently recurs and is often multifocal, the pathologist must judge whether the biopsy is of cancer or of radiation change.

Radiation induces a number of cytologic changes including nuclear and cytologic atypia and nucleomegaly and cytomegaly with cytologic vacuolization. While the changes may appear somewhat localized, often to the vascular endothelium, they can be diffuse and be seen throughout

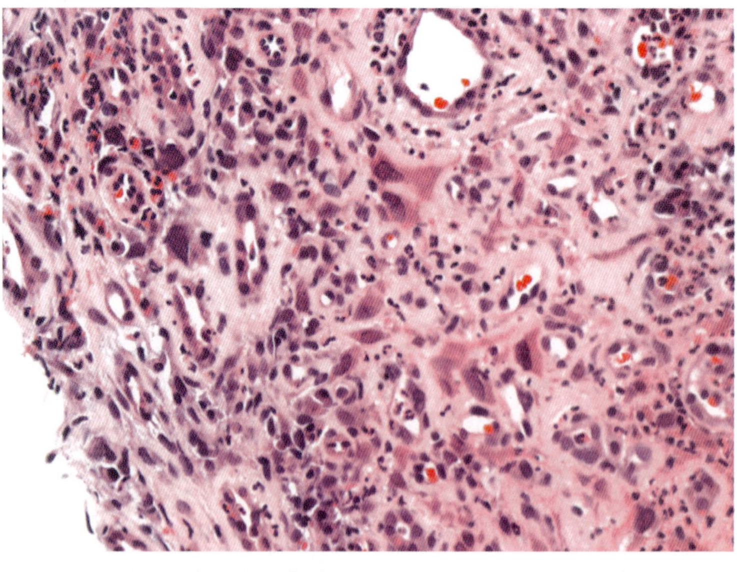

FIGURE 4.12 Stromal and endothelial atypia seen after radiation therapy.

the stroma and within surface epithelium and seromucinous glands.[41,42] Necrotizing sialometaplasia is often present, further complicating the interpretation of these specimens.

The atypia seen within the stroma may raise the question of a poorly differentiated or sarcomatoid carcinoma, especially as radiation has been reported to induce sarcomatoid change in preexistent SCCs. Often, the cytologic atypia seen with radiation change is more pronounced than that seen with sarcomatoid carcinomas, and it typically shows more variation between individual cells than in sarcomatoid carcinomas. Carcinomas, on the other hand, will have more mitotic activity and tend to show more nuclear enlargement relative to the cytologic changes. With small biopsy specimens, the distinction between these may be nearly impossible, especially at the time of frozen section. Immunostaining can be helpful, and immunoreactivity with antibodies to cytokeratins or p63/p40 would lead one to favor a diagnosis of carcinoma (eFig. 4.22).[42] Occasional cases must be diagnosed descriptively, often with notes that discuss the dilemma and state that one diagnosis is favored over the other.

Radiation changes within epithelial structures can also lead to interpretive difficulties, as the atypia induced within the epithelial cells is similar to that seen with the stromal cells. Here, the distinction between carcinoma and radiation change is assisted by the epithelial structures retaining their typical lobular architecture or being confined to the surface. This is also true for necrotizing sialometaplasia (as discussed in Chapter 2) which, although obviously squamous and atypical, should not appear to be truly infiltrative and will instead retain a lobular appearance.

One final difficulty that may be faced is the distinction between pseudoepitheliomatous hyperplasia and some well-differentiated SCCs that closely resemble this process. Most SCCs infiltrate the stroma as atypical nests of squamous cells; however, occasional cases will appear much more reticular in their infiltration pattern with anastomosing cords of squamous cells, similar to the deep components of pseudoepitheliomatous hyperplasia (Fig. 4.13, eFig. 4.23). In these cases, the identification of cytologic atypia is very helpful, as it is generally not seen to any significant degree with pseudoepitheliomatous hyperplasia. Furthermore, the reticular pattern of invasion with an SCC is usually seen with a more basaloid phenotype, with high nuclear to cytoplasmic ratios and numerous mitotic figures.

REPORTING

Aside from the problematic cases for which descriptive diagnoses are often needed, the reporting of SCC on biopsy specimen is rather mundane. The most important pathologic parameters (i.e., tumor size, depth of invasion, and margin status) for upper aerodigestive tract SCC cannot usually be assessed at the time of biopsy (Table 4.2).[39,43–48] Other information may be helpful, but its clinical utility is not fully understood and typically has been shown to have varying degrees of importance within the literature. Finally, even if

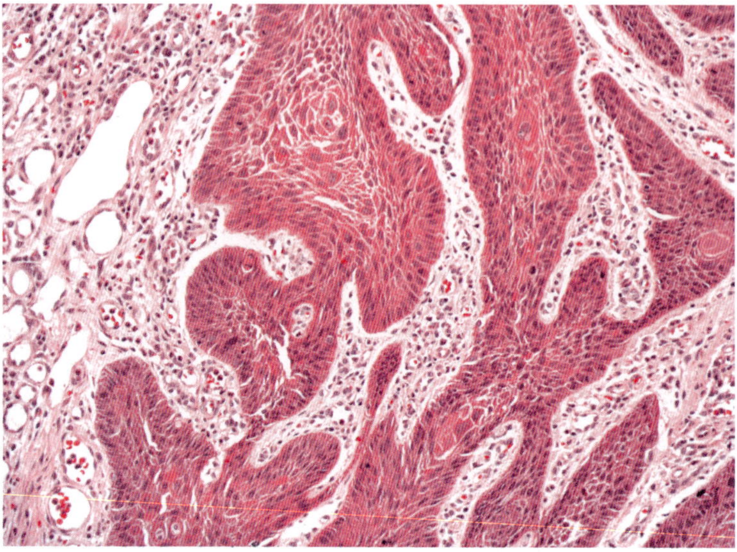

FIGURE 4.13 Anastomosing cords of squamous cells are seen at the infiltrating edge of this squamous cell carcinoma.

the factors have been shown to be predictive of local recurrence or overall survival, it is unclear if they need to be reported with biopsy specimens, as adequate reporting requires the assessment of the resected specimen.

Histologic grade is usually reported and most pathologists use a three-tiered system as previously discussed (i.e., well, moderately, and poorly differentiated SCC). Strict criteria for these interpretations are usually not applied, and the degree of interobserver agreement for these grades remains marginal. Furthermore, the vast majority of cases are interpreted as being "moderately differentiated." Finally, as only a small portion of the

TABLE 4.2 Features That Can and Cannot Be Assessed With Biopsy Specimens

Cannot Be Assessed	Can Be Assessed and Are Likely Important	Can Be Assessed and May Be Important
Size	Grade[a]	Inflammatory infiltrate
Depth of invasion	Lymphovascular invasion	Other molecular markers
Margin status	Perineural invasion	
Pattern of invasion	Variant histology and p16 immunohistochemistry	
Border configuration		

[a]Although the grade can obviously be assessed at biopsy, it may not correspond with the grade at resection. Also, the grade of the tumor at its infiltrative edge cannot be assessed at biopsy.

tumor is usually seen at biopsy, and as this is typically from near the surface of the tumor, many cases will actually be interpreted differently when the resection specimen is reviewed.[35] Some have reported grading of the tumor's infiltrating front is important; obviously, this cannot be reported on most biopsy specimens.[31,32,38]

The identification of either lymphovascular invasion or perineural spread is usually reported and probably indicates a worse prognosis, especially when the tumor is believed clinically to be localized (Fig. 4.14, eFig. 4.24).[40,43,49] Some have reported that the degree and type of inflammatory infiltrate have prognostic value and others have stated that the identification of specific molecular abnormalities may have some meaning. (Aside from p16 immunohistochemistry, see below, these tests are not routinely done at most institutions.)[40,50,51] Finally, the configuration of the tumor border (e.g., pushing) and the pattern of infiltration have been reported by some to have prognostic value. Again, these cannot generally be assessed on biopsy specimens.[32,40,44]

Many institutions perform p16 immunohistochemistry with all oropharyngeal SCCs. This is because HPV-related tumors are typically diffusely and strongly immunoreactive with the antibody, whereas most other SCCs have lost expression of the protein.[28] The data may be helpful for prognostication, as p16-immunoreactive tumors respond better to therapy than other SCCs of similar stage.[52] Immunohistochemistry can also be helpful for identifying the site of the primary tumor if only a metastasis is biopsied. p16-immunoreactive metastases are most often from oropharyngeal primaries.[53]

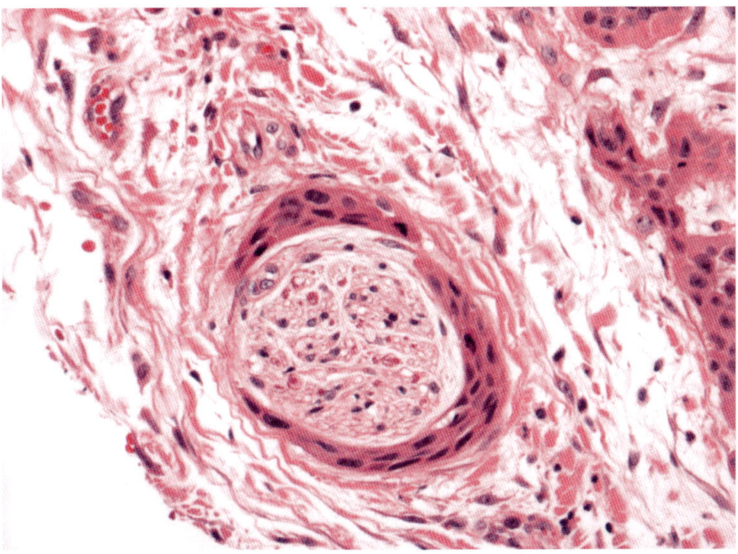

FIGURE 4.14 Perineural invasion is frequently identified with squamous cell carcinomas.

The identification of certain variants of SCC (to be discussed in Chapter 5) is important for a number of reasons. First, identifying them as SCCs rather than their mimics has prognostic importance and can lead to different treatments. Also, these tumors may behave differently than conventional SCCs (e.g., verrucous carcinoma) and may require different therapy.

TREATMENT

Treatment for conventional SCC depends on the site of involvement and the extent of disease. Some smaller tumors at particular sites (e.g., the glottis or tongue) or particular variants (e.g., verrucous carcinoma) may be excised, sometimes using a laser, without additional therapy. As many tumors present at high T stage, often with metastases to regional lymph nodes, multimodality therapy is usually used, combining radiation, surgery, and, with some tumors, chemotherapy.

REFERENCES

1. http://seer.cancer.gov/statfacts/html/oralcav.html.
2. http://seer.cancer.gov/statfacts/html/laryn.html.
3. Brugere J, Guenel P, Leclerc A, Rodriguez J. Differential effects of tobacco and alcohol in cancer of the larynx, pharynx, and mouth. *Cancer*. 1986;57:391-395.
4. Flanders WD, Rothman KJ. Interaction of alcohol and tobacco in laryngeal cancer. *Am J Epidemiol*. 1982;115:371-379.
5. Franceschi S, Bidoli E, Negri E, Barbone F, La Vecchia C. Alcohol and cancers of the upper aerodigestive tract in men and women. *Cancer Epidemiol Biomarkers Prev*. 1994;3:299-304.
6. Lewin F, Norell SE, Johansson H, et al. Smoking tobacco, oral snuff, and alcohol in the etiology of squamous cell carcinoma of the head and neck: a population-based case-referent study in Sweden. *Cancer*. 1998;82:1367-1375.
7. Tuyns AJ, Esteve J, Raymond L, et al. Cancer of the larynx/hypopharynx, tobacco and alcohol: IARC international case-control study in Turin and Varese (Italy), Zaragoza and Navarra (Spain), Geneva (Switzerland) and Calvados (France). *Int J Cancer*. 1988. 41:483-491.
8. Spitz MR, Fueger JJ, Goepfert H, Hong WK, Newell GR. Squamous cell carcinoma of the upper aerodigestive tract. A case comparison analysis. *Cancer*. 1988;61:203-208.
9. Winn DM, Blot WJ, Shy CM, Pickle LW, Toledo A, Fraumeni JF Jr. Snuff dipping and oral cancer among women in the southern United States, *N Engl J Med*. 1981. 304:745-749.
10. Coffin CM, Rich SS, Dehner LP. Familial aggregation of nasopharyngeal carcinoma and other malignancies. A clinicopathologic description. *Cancer*. 1991;68:1323-1328.
11. Llewellyn CD, Linklater K, Bell J, Johnson NW, Warnakulasuriya KA. Squamous cell carcinoma of the oral cavity in patients aged 45 years and under: a descriptive analysis of 116 cases diagnosed in the South East of England from 1990 to 1997. *Oral Oncol*. 2003;39:106-114.
12. Llewellyn CD, Linklater K, Bell J, Johnson NW, Warnakulasuriya S. An analysis of risk factors for oral cancer in young people: a case-control study. *Oral Oncol*. 2004;40: 304-313.

13. Sankaranarayanan R, Masuyer E, Swaminathan R, Ferlay J, Whelan S. Head and neck cancer: a global perspective on epidemiology and prognosis. *Anticancer Res.* 1998;18:4779-4786.
14. Winn DM, Ziegler RG, Pickle LW, Gridley G, Blot WJ, Hoover RN. Diet in the etiology of oral and pharyngeal cancer among women from the southern United States. *Cancer Res.* 1984;44:1216-1222.
15. Mork J, Moller B, Glattre E. Familial risk in head and neck squamous cell carcinoma diagnosed before the age of 45: a population-based study. *Oral Oncol.* 1999;35:360-367.
16. Suarez C, Rodrigo JP, Ferlito A, Cabanillas R, Shaha AR, Rinaldo A. Tumours of familial origin in the head and neck. *Oral Oncol.* 2006;42:965-978.
17. Yarbrough WG, Aprelikova O, Pei H, Olshan AF, Liu ET. Familial tumor syndrome associated with a germline nonfunctional p16INK4a allele. *J Natl Cancer Inst.* 1996;88:1489-1491.
18. Yu KK, Zanation AM, Moss JR, Yarbrough WG. Familial head and neck cancer: molecular analysis of a new clinical entity. *Laryngoscope.* 2002;112:1587-1593.
19. Trizna Z, Schantz SP. Hereditary and environmental factors associated with risk and progression of head and neck cancer. *Otolaryngol Clin North Am.* 1992;25: 1089-1103.
20. Hildesheim A, Apple RJ, Chen CJ, et al. Association of HLA class I and II alleles and extended haplotypes with nasopharyngeal carcinoma in Taiwan. *J Natl Cancer Inst.* 2002;94:1780-1789.
21. Simons MJ, Wee GB, Goh EH, et al. Immunogenetic aspects of nasopharyngeal carcinoma. IV. Increased risk in Chinese of nasopharyngeal carcinoma associated with a Chinese-related HLA profile (A2, Singapore 2). *J Natl Cancer Inst.* 1976;57:977-980.
22. Simons MJ, Wee GB, Day NE, Morris PJ, Shanmugaratnam K, De-The GB. Immunogenetic aspects of nasopharyngeal carcinoma: I. Differences in HL-A antigen profiles between patients and control groups. *Int J Cancer.* 1974;13:122-134.
23. Larsson LG, Sandstrom A, Westling P. Relationship of Plummer-Vinson disease to cancer of the upper alimentary tract in Sweden. *Cancer Res.* 1975;35:3308-3316.
24. Pattle SB, Farrell PJ. The role of Epstein-Barr virus in cancer,. *Expert Opin Biol Ther.* 2006;6:1193-1205.
25. Klussmann JP, Gultekin E, Weissenborn SJ, et al. Expression of p16 protein identifies a distinct entity of tonsillar carcinomas associated with human papillomavirus. *Am J Pathol.* 2003;162:747-753.
26. Klussmann JP, Weissenborn SJ, Wieland U, et al. Prevalence, distribution, and viral load of human papillomavirus 16 DNA in tonsillar carcinomas. *Cancer.* 2001;92:2875-2884.
27. Paz IB, Cook N, Odom-Maryon T, Xie Y, Wilczynski SP. Human papillomavirus (HPV) in head and neck cancer. An association of HPV 16 with squamous cell carcinoma of Waldeyer's tonsillar ring. *Cancer.* 1997;79:595-604.
28. Stelow EB, Jo VY, Stoler MH, Mills SE. Human papillomavirus-associated squamous cell carcinoma of the upper aerodigestive tract. *Am J Surg Pathol.* 2010;34:e15-e24.
29. Marur S, D'Souza G, Westra WH, Forastiere AA. HPV-associated head and neck cancer: a virus-related cancer epidemic. *Lancet Oncol.* 2010;11:781-789.
30. French CA, Kutok JL, Faquin WC, et al. Midline carcinoma of children and young adults with NUT rearrangement. *J Clin Oncol.* 2004;22:4135-4139.
31. Bryne M. Is the invasive front of an oral carcinoma the most important area for prognostication? *Oral Dis.* 1998;4:70-77.
32. Bryne M, Jenssen N, Boysen M. Histological grading in the deep invasive front of T1 and T2 glottic squamous cell carcinomas has high prognostic value. *Virchows Arch.* 1995;427:277-281.

33. Bryne M, Koppang HS, Lilleng R, Stene T, Bang G, Dabelsteen E. New malignancy grading is a better prognostic indicator than Broders' grading in oral squamous cell carcinomas. *J Oral Pathol Med.* 1989;18:432-437.
34. Bryne M, Nielsen K, Koppang HS, Dabelsteen E. Reproducibility of two malignancy grading systems with reportedly prognostic value for oral cancer patients. *J Oral Pathol Med.* 1991;20:369-372.
35. Chung CK, Stryker JA, Abt AB, Cunningham DE, Strauss M, Connor GH. Histologic grading in the clinical evaluation of laryngeal carcinoma. *Arch Otolaryngol.* 1980;106:623-624.
36. Roland NJ, Caslin AW, Nash J, Stell PM. Value of grading squamous cell carcinoma of the head and neck. *Head Neck.* 1992;14:224-229.
37. Rua S, Comino A, Fruttero A, et al. Relationship between histologic features, DNA flow cytometry, and clinical behavior of squamous cell carcinomas of the larynx. *Cancer.* 1991;67:141-149.
38. Sawair FA, Irwin CR, Gordon DJ, Leonard AG, Stephenson M, Napier SS. Invasive front grading: reliability and usefulness in the management of oral squamous cell carcinoma. *J Oral Pathol Med.* 2003;32:1-9.
39. Tralongo V, Rodolico V, Luciani A, Marra G, Daniele E. Prognostic factors in oral squamous cell carcinoma. A review of the literature,. *Anticancer Res.* 1999;19:3503-3510.
40. Martinez-Gimeno C, Rodriguez EM, Vila CN, Varela CL. Squamous cell carcinoma of the oral cavity: a clinicopathologic scoring system for evaluating risk of cervical lymph node metastasis. *Laryngoscope.* 1995;105:728-733.
41. Fajardo LF. The pathology of ionizing radiation as defined by morphologic patterns,. *Acta Oncol.* 2005;44:13-22.
42. Weidner N, Askin FB, Berthrong M, Hopkins MB, Kute TE, McGuirt FW. Bizarre (pseudomalignant) granulation-tissue reactions following ionizing-radiation exposure. A microscopic, immunohistochemical, and flow-cytometric study,. *Cancer.* 1987;59:1509-1514.
43. Brandwein-Gensler M, Teixeira MS, Lewis CM, et al. Oral squamous cell carcinoma: histologic risk assessment, but not margin status, is strongly predictive of local disease-free and overall survival. *Am J Surg Pathol.* 2005;29:167-178.
44. Bundgaard T, Rossen K, Henriksen SD, Charabi S, Sogaard H, Grau C. Histopathologic parameters in the evaluation of T1 squamous cell carcinomas of the oral cavity. *Head Neck.* 2002;24:656-660.
45. Garavello W, Ciardo A, Spreafico R, Gaini RM. Risk factors for distant metastases in head and neck squamous cell carcinoma. *Arch Otolaryngol Head Neck Surg.* 2006;132:762-766.
46. Gluckman JL, Pavelic ZP, Welkoborsky HJ, et al. Prognostic indicators for squamous cell carcinoma of the oral cavity: a clinicopathologic correlation. *Laryngoscope.* 1997;107:1239-1244.
47. Jacobs JR, Ahmad K, Casiano R, et al. Implications of positive surgical margins. *Laryngoscope.* 1993;103:64-68.
48. Po Wing Yuen A, Lam KY, Lam LK, et al. Prognostic factors of clinically stage I and II oral tongue carcinoma-A comparative study of stage, thickness, shape, growth pattern, invasive front malignancy grading, Martinez-Gimeno score, and pathologic features. *Head Neck.* 2002;24:513-520.
49. Frierson HF Jr, Cooper PH. Prognostic factors in squamous cell carcinoma of the lower lip. *Hum Pathol.* 1986;17:346-354.
50. Narayana A, Vaughan AT, Gunaratne S, Kathuria S, Walter SA, Reddy SP. Is p53 an independent prognostic factor in patients with laryngeal carcinoma? *Cancer.* 1998;82:286-291.

51. Suzuki H, Sugimura H, Hashimoto K. p16INK4A in oral squamous cell carcinomas–a correlation with biological behaviors: immunohistochemical and FISH analysis. *J Oral Maxillofac Surg*. 2006;64:1617-1623.
52. Lewis JS Jr, Thorstad WL, Chernock RD, et al. p16 positive oropharyngeal squamous cell carcinoma:an entity with a favorable prognosis regardless of tumor HPV status. *Am J Surg Pathol*. 2010;34:1088-1096.
53. Begum S, Gillison ML, Ansari-Lari MA, Shah K, Westra WH. Detection of human papillomavirus in cervical lymph nodes: a highly effective strategy for localizing site of tumor origin. *Clin Cancer Res*. 2003;9:6469-6475.

5

HISTOLOGIC AND ETIOLOGIC VARIANTS OF SQUAMOUS CELL CARCINOMA

Most squamous cell carcinomas (SCCs) of the upper aerodigestive tract are histologically *conventional type* and as such show, to some degree, a recapitulation of stratified squamous epithelium and are secondary to the use of tobacco products. Certain SCCs, however, of the upper aerodigestive tract have different growth patterns and histologic features. Not only can these tumors sometimes behave differently from conventional-type SCCs, but they can also present the pathologist with differential diagnoses that range from benign to malignant (Table 5.1). For example, verrucous carcinoma, a locally aggressive, nonmetastasizing variant of SCC, can be very difficult, if not impossible, to differentiate from benign disease on biopsy. In addition, variant histologies are sometimes associated with variant etiologies (e.g., high-risk human papillomavirus [HR-HPV] infection), which can affect the prognosis and treatment of the tumors (Table 5.2).

This chapter discusses the clinicopathologic features of the most common variants of SCC found in the upper aerodigestive tract. Verrucous carcinoma, papillary SCC, nonkeratinizing/basaloid SCC, spindle cell carcinoma, adenosquamous carcinoma, adenoid SCC, and undifferentiated carcinoma are all discussed along with their histologic mimics and methods for arriving at their correct diagnoses. It especially focuses on difficulties that are faced with small biopsy specimens. SCCs secondary to HR-HPV, Epstein-Barr virus (EBV), nuclear protein of the testis (*NUT*) translocations, and with SWI/SNF abnormalities (SMARCB1 and SMARCA4 deficiency) are also discussed (Table 5.3).

A short discussion of the molecular aspects of these neoplasms is also presented. As was discussed in the chapter describing precursor lesions, SCCs of the upper aerodigestive tract arise after a series of genetic events, although these currently appear complex and somewhat variable. It is unclear whether the lack of or acquisition of certain molecular abnormalities leads to the specific phenotypic and behavioral differences between these tumors. Data are currently mixed as to whether most histologic variants have specific abnormalities that would allow for their distinction from one another and conventional-type SCC.[1]

TABLE 5.1 Squamous Cell Carcinoma (SCC) Histologic Variants and Differential Diagnoses

Histologic Variant	Differential Diagnosis
Verrucous carcinoma	Verrucous vulgaris
	Verrucous hyperplasia
	Conventional-type SCC
	Papillary SCC
Papillary SCC	Benign squamous papilloma (e.g., laryngeal papilloma, sinonasal papilloma)
	Verrucous SCC
	Exophytic conventional-type SCC
Basaloid SCC	Adenoid cystic carcinoma
	Basal cell adenocarcinoma
	Other basaloid salivary gland-type neoplasms
	Adenosquamous carcinoma
	Small cell neuroendocrine carcinoma
Spindle cell carcinoma	Benign and malignant mesenchymal lesions
	Melanoma
Adenosquamous carcinoma	Mucoepidermoid carcinoma
	Adenoid SCC
	Basaloid SCC
Adenoid SCC	Vascular or other mesenchymal lesions
	Adenosquamous SCC or other glandular lesions
Undifferentiated carcinoma	Lymphoma
	Other undifferentiated neoplasms of the area (e.g., sinonasal undifferentiated carcinoma)

HISTOLOGIC VARIANTS

Verrucous Carcinoma

Verrucous carcinoma was first described and characterized as a distinct entity in 1948 by Lauren Ackerman and is sometimes referred to as "Ackerman tumor."[2] It may develop at different anatomic sites throughout the upper aerodigestive tract and body. When it involves the upper aerodigestive tract, it most commonly is located in the mouth, specifically at the buccal mucosa or gingiva, or the larynx.[3–13] These tumors occur in older individuals, usually in the seventh or eighth decade of life and, for oral lesions, are often related to the use of oral tobacco. Other etiologic

TABLE 5.2 Squamous Cell Carcinoma Histologic Variants and Their Etiologies

Variant	Etiology
Verrucous carcinoma	Tobacco and alcohol
Papillary squamous cell carcinoma	High-risk HPV Tobacco and alcohol
Basaloid squamous cell carcinoma	High-risk HPV Tobacco and alcohol
Spindle cell carcinoma	Tobacco and alcohol Radiation
Adenosquamous carcinoma	Tobacco and alcohol High-risk HPV (less common)
Adenoid squamous cell carcinoma	Radiation Tobacco and alcohol
Undifferentiated carcinoma	Epstein-Barr virus (nasopharynx) High-risk HPV (oropharynx) Chromosomal translocation (NC) Unique molecular abnormality (SDSC) Tobacco and alcohol

NC: NUT carcinoma.

SDSC: SMARCB1-deficient sinonasal carcinoma.

TABLE 5.3 Squamous Cell Carcinoma Etiologic Variants and Typical Histologies

Etiologic Variant	Histology
HR-HPV-related SCC	Mostly nonkeratinizing; may be consistent with basaloid or papillary SCC; other variants less common, especially outside of the oropharynx
EBV-related SCC	Undifferentiated with admixed lymphocytes; can grow as sheet or in a more trabecular/ribbonlike pattern
NUT carcinoma	Often undifferentiated, although "abrupt" keratinization can be seen; may be somewhat nested similar to infiltrating nonkeratinizing SCC
SMARCB1-deficient sinonasal carcinoma	Nonkeratinizing and may appear undifferentiated; cells may appear more eosinophilic and rhabdoid

factors include smoked tobacco, alcohol, and poor oral hygiene. What role, if any, HPV plays in the development of these lesions remains controversial despite extensive studies.[14,15] It does appear that if HPV has a role, it is limited, even in female, nonsmoking patients who develop oral tumors in association with proliferative verrucous leukoplakia. Most studies show that men are much more likely than women to be afflicted with these neoplasms.

The tumors grossly appear warty and fungating with ulcerations. Histologically, verrucous carcinomas are defined narrowly. They have a wartlike appearance with abundant keratosis and parakeratosis arising from a folded, thickened squamous epithelium (Fig. 5.1, eFigs. 5.1 and 5.2). This leads to the noted appearance of "church spires." The squamous cells mature toward the surface and only minimal cytologic atypia should be present (Fig. 5.2, eFigs. 5.3 and 5.4). That said, some of the squamous cells may undergo individual keratinization (dyskeratosis), and occasional squamous pearls may be seen within the squamous epithelium. Mitotic figures should be located within or near the basal epithelium. Nuclei have vesicular chromatin with small nucleoli. The bases of the tumors show downgrowth of broad tongues of mature, well-differentiated squamous epithelium that invade the underlying tissues with a circumscribed, pushing border (Fig. 5.3, eFigs. 5.5 and 5.6). Infiltrating irregular nests, typical of conventional-type SCC, should not be present. At the base of the tumors, a dense lymphoplasmacytic infiltrate may be present, as may occasional foreign body–type granulomas.

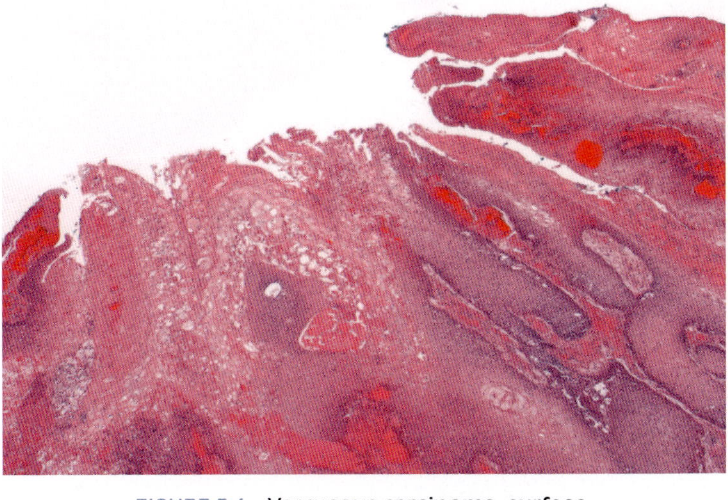

FIGURE 5.1 Verrucous carcinoma, surface.

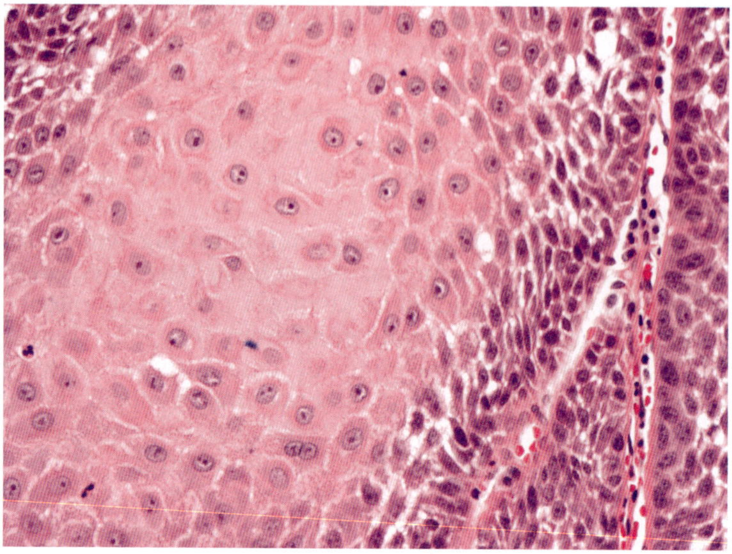

FIGURE 5.2 Verrucous carcinoma, maturing epithelium without atypia.

Although many SCCs will have *verrucoid* features, it has been noted that the diagnosis of verrucous carcinoma should only be made when tumors meet the strict histologic criteria listed above if the diagnosis is to have meaning. Tumors that are verrucoid, yet do not meet the strict criteria for the diagnosis of verrucous carcinoma, will generally behave in a

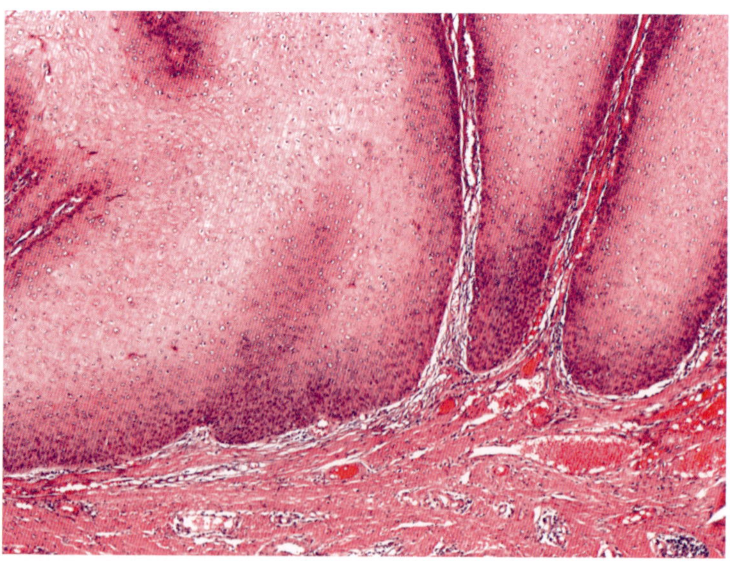

FIGURE 5.3 Verrucous carcinoma, base.

manner similar to more conventional-type SCCs. True verrucous carcinomas, however, have no metastatic potential. It is estimated that when strict criteria are applied, verrucous carcinomas represent less than 5% of oral and laryngeal tumors.

To diagnose verrucous carcinoma, ample sectioning of an excisional specimen and good sampling of the base of the lesion are needed. For this reason, an unequivocal diagnosis based upon a small biopsy is not warranted. Instead, qualified diagnoses such as *SCC with verrucoid features* or even *verrucoid lesion* should be considered, especially as benign diagnoses may sometimes feature in the differential diagnosis. Indeed, even today, most verrucous carcinomas are originally diagnosed as benign lesions on biopsy. The surgeon should be made aware of the diagnostic difficulty with these cases as clinical information often provides the information needed to guide subsequent therapy. Communication between the pathologist and surgeon is thus paramount. With final resection specimens we are loath to use the term "hybrid carcinoma" that others use for lesions that have features of verrucous carcinoma with focal infiltrating areas. It has been well known since the description of this tumor that some cases of upper aerodigestive tract conventional-type SCCs are deceptively bland and have some but not all of the required histologic features of verrucous carcinomas.

More aggressive yet benign forms of leukoplakia can have histologic features resembling verrucous carcinoma and are discussed in Chapter 3.[16,17] These lesions have been clinically termed "proliferative verrucous leukoplakia" and often histologically show *verrucous hyperplasia*. They may be differentiated from verrucous carcinoma both clinically and histologically. Clinically, these lesions tend to recur and often develop into invasive SCCs, both verrucous carcinoma and conventional-type SCC; however, they should not form destructive, mass lesions. Histologically, verrucous carcinoma will show features of invasion with much more acanthosis and larger tongues of squamous epithelium extending deeply into the stromal tissue. The epithelium of verrucous hyperplasia should not extend more deeply than adjacent uninvolved epithelium.[18]

Verrucous vulgaris has been reported in the larynx and may also enter into the differential diagnosis.[19] Like verrucous hyperplasia, these lesions should not invade the stroma. It has also been noted that the rete pegs tend to be thinner with verruca and that verruca have more prominent keratohyalin granules. Finally, papillary SCC is also occasionally mentioned as a differential consideration. The lesions are not very similar histologically and generally should not be confused (see below). Still, there appears to be some histologic overlap in phenotype, and some cases can show mixed features.

Immunohistochemistry has shown the accumulation of p53 protein in many of these tumors, and proliferation markers are often noted to be overexpressed when compared to benign epithelium (although not to the degree of more cytologically abnormal cases).[15,20] Retinoblastoma protein expression remains intact, and some growth factors, such as c-erb-3, have been shown to be overexpressed.[21] Loss of heterozygosity (LOH) studies investigating multiple microsatellite markers have shown that these tumors have fewer abnormalities than more poorly differentiated SCC variants such as basaloid SCC or spindle cell carcinoma and have an LOH incidence similar to that of well-differentiated conventional-type SCC.[1] The tumors frequently contain deletions at 9p, a region believed to be involved early in the development of upper aerodigestive tract SCC. Whether these tumors lack any specific genetic abnormalities that would explain their lack of metastatic potential has not conclusively been shown. While some have shown differences of LOH at 4q and 17p between verrucous SCC and conventional-type SCC, these differences were not confirmed with a study that compared verrucous carcinoma with only well-differentiated, conventional-type SCC. In our experience, verrucous carcinomas are not immunoreactive with antibodies to p16, nor do they contain HR-HPV by in situ hybridization.

Papillary Squamous Cell Carcinoma

Papillary SCC is an uncommon variant of SCC that may involve the upper aerodigestive tract.[22-29] The lesions occur most frequently in older male patients, like nearly all variants of SCC in this region. The lesions occur throughout the upper aerodigestive tract, but most often involve the larynx, oropharynx, and sinonasal tract. Because of their rarity, their pathogenesis remains unclear. Approximately half of the cases in a recent study were secondary to HR-HPV infection; these tumors most frequently involved the oropharynx or sinonasal tract.[29] Occasional cases have been reported in patients with previously diagnosed benign squamous papillomas.

Grossly, these lesions are largely exophytic and appear papillary or even warty, akin to verrucous carcinomas. These lesions are defined histologically and have a low-power appearance similar to sinonasal papillomas (Fig. 5.4, eFigs. 5.7 and 5.8). Numerous complex papillary and filiform structures extend in all planes, often rendering the assessment of true tissue invasion extremely difficult. The papillary fronds are covered with a stratified squamous epithelium, which has overt features of malignancy, replete with lack of maturation, increased nuclear to cytoplasmic ratios, nuclear irregularities, and numerous mitotic figures located throughout the entire thickness of the epithelium (Fig. 5.5, eFigs. 5.9 and 5.10). Koilocytic change is often noted (eFig. 5.11). The epithelial component thus appears similar to high-grade squamous intraepithelial lesions of the cervix. Intracellular keratinization or dyskeratosis may be present; however, surface keratosis is often not seen or may be only focal (Fig. 5.6, eFig. 5.12). The papillary fronds have fibrovascular cores that usually contain some degree of lymphoplasmacellular infiltrate, which then extends to the base of these lesions where it becomes denser.

The complex nature of these specimens can make the assessment of invasion difficult, especially when the invasive component remains papillary. Often, however, the invasive component will have infiltrating, irregular

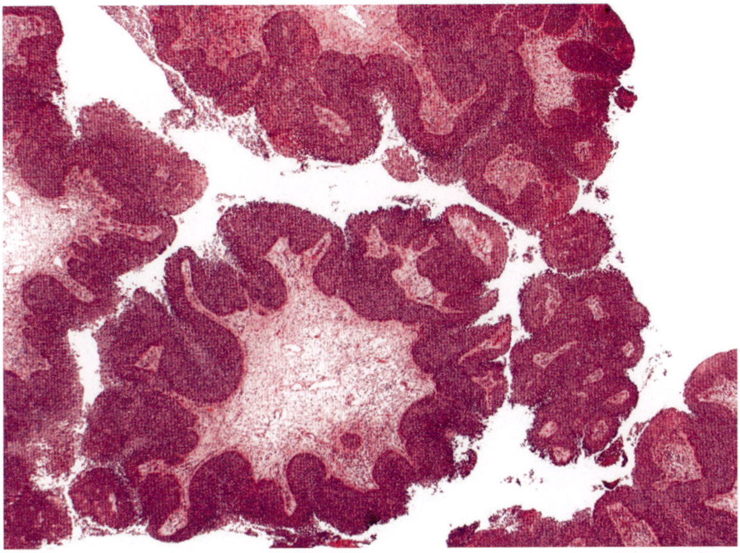

FIGURE 5.4 Papillary squamous cell carcinoma reminiscent of sinonasal papilloma.

nests of squamous epithelium morphologically identical to conventional-type SCC. As with verrucous carcinoma, invasion can almost never be excluded at biopsy, and, because of the complex and highly exophytic nature of the noninvasive component of these tumors, definitive invasion can rarely be diagnosed at biopsy. Resection specimens should be carefully

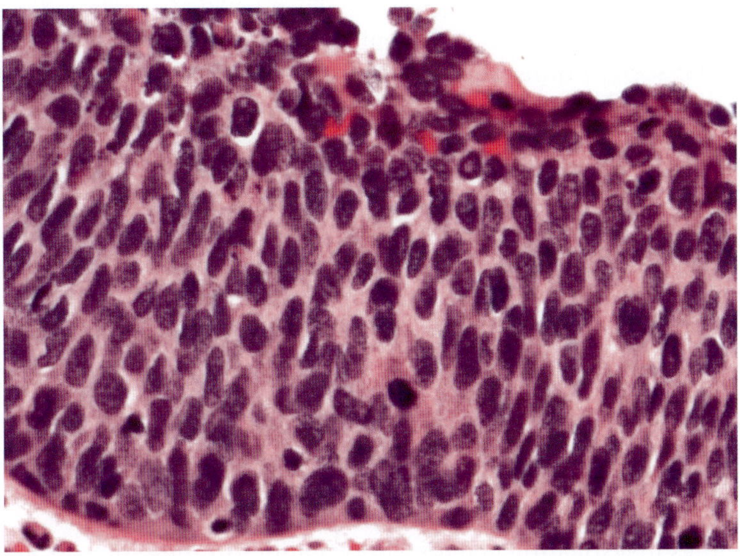

FIGURE 5.5 Full-thickness dysplasia in papillary squamous cell carcinoma.

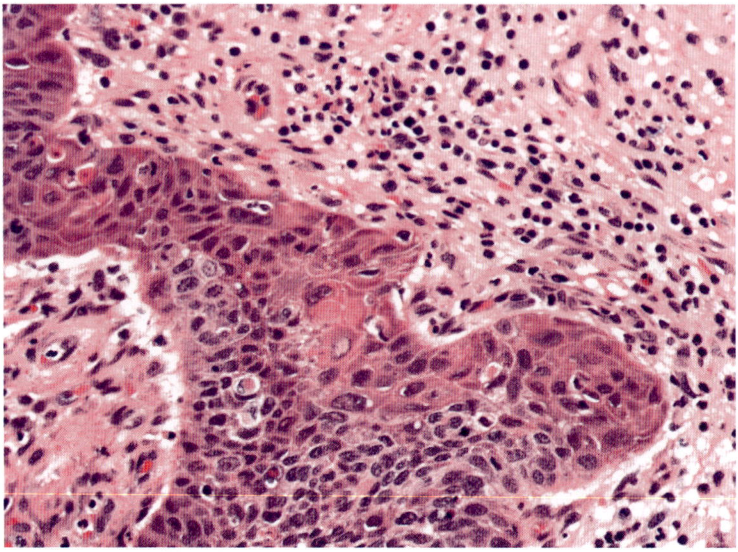

FIGURE 5.6 Intracellular keratinization at the base of a papillary squamous cell carcinoma.

assessed for invasion as invasive lesions tend to behave in a manner similar to conventional-type SCC of the upper aerodigestive tract. Lesions that lack invasion can be locally aggressive and difficult to fully resect, especially when they involve the sinonasal tract. Such lesions often eventually progress to invasive malignancies.

The most common differential to be considered with these lesions includes benign papillary lesions, especially *sinonasal* or *schneiderian papillomas*. The degree of epithelial atypia present in these lesions should not generally be seen in other squamous papillary lesions of the upper aerodigestive tract, and the diagnosis is usually not very difficult. Occasional sinonasal papillomas or laryngeal papillomas can show inflammation with cytologic atypia or even dysplasia with numerous mitotic figures, however, and methods for definitively distinguishing such lesions from noninvasive papillary carcinomas are lacking histologically. In general, papillary SCC should be a destruction lesion whereas laryngeal papillomas are not.

Distinguishing these lesions from verrucous carcinomas should not be difficult, although the two may grossly appear similar (Table 5.4). Thompson et al. have also argued that the lesions should be differentiated from a more garden-variety *exophytic* SCC.[25] They point out that true papillary SCC has a better prognosis than exophytic SCC. Histologically, it is more filiform and not as complex. The authors note that papillary SCCs appear more like stalks of celery cut on cross section and should not be complex and resemble a cut section of cauliflower.

Studies investigating genetic abnormalities in these tumors are somewhat limited due to the rarity of these neoplasms.[1,26] Overexpression of

TABLE 5.4 Verrucous Carcinoma Versus Papillary Squamous Cell Carcinoma

Verrucous Carcinoma	Papillary Squamous Cell Carcinoma
Clinical: Most common in older men in the mouth (buccal mucosa or gingival) or the larynx. Uncommon. Does not metastasize.	**Clinical:** Most common in older men in the larynx or sinonasal tract. Rare. May metastasize.
Pathology: Fungating and exophytic tumor. Well differentiated with little cytologic atypia. Folded, maturing, acanthotic epithelium infiltrating into adjacent tissue with a pushing border. Abundant surface keratinization.	**Pathology:** Extremely exophytic and friable. Filiform, papillary projections covered by an immature, cytologically atypical squamous epithelium. Invasion is hard to appreciate but may have a papillary or conventional-type growth. Surface keratinization is not present or rare.

p53 protein has been shown by immunohistochemistry. LOH studies have shown a similar incidence of genetic abnormalities between these tumors and verrucous carcinoma and well-differentiated conventional-type SCC. It is interesting to note that these tumors showed an increased LOH for a microsatellite marker on the long-arm of chromosome 11 when compared with other variants of SCC, although the finding was not statistically significant. Tumors secondary to HR-HPV infection are diffusely and strongly immunoreactive with antibodies to p16 (Fig. 5.7, eFig. 5.13).[29]

Nonkeratinizing Squamous Cell Carcinoma and Basaloid Squamous Cell Carcinoma

Some SCCs at various sites throughout the body retain a distinctly epidermoid phenotype while lacking cellular maturation and extracellular keratin formation (i.e., keratinization). The cells remain immature in appearance and resemble those of the basal layer of typical stratified squamous epithelium. For that reason, these tumors are termed "basaloid squamous cell carcinomas," although a variety of names have been used for these tumors when they occur at different sites in the body (e.g., cloacogenic carcinoma when they arise in the anus).[30–33] There has been and remains some confusion as to whether the terms "nonkeratinizing" and "basaloid" are synonymous. As the years have passed, we have come to use the term "basaloid" for a specific histology of nonkeratinizing SCC while acknowledging that there is a spectrum of histologic features for infiltrating nonkeratinizing SCCs (see below).

Basaloid SCCs of the upper aerodigestive tract, as originally described, occur in older individuals, usually in their seventh or eighth decades of life,

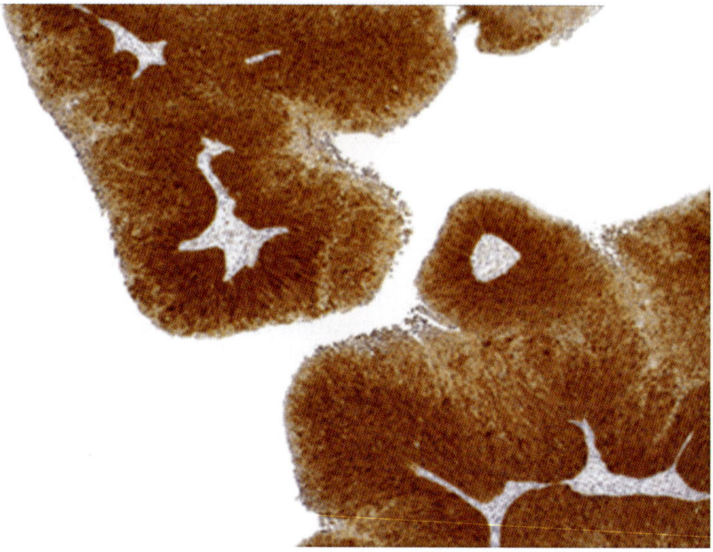

FIGURE 5.7 p16 immunoreactivity is sometimes seen with papillary squamous cell carcinoma and is associated with high-risk human papillomavirus infection.

and occur predominately in men. First reports of these tumors reported a strong association with tobacco and alcohol use; however, many cases that develop today are secondary to infection by HR-HPV and occur in younger patients than those first presented (many of these tumors we would simply diagnose as nonkeratinizing SCCs).[34–38] The tumors show a predilection for involvement of the base of tongue, hypopharynx, and supraglottic larynx but have been noted throughout the entire upper aerodigestive tract. Most patients present at a high stage with nodal metastases. Behavior for these tumors is related to HR-HPV status, with tumors harboring infection (especially those of the oropharynx) behaving better stage for stage than conventional SCCs, whereas those not secondary to HR-HPV infection behave the same or worse than other SCCs.[39]

The histology of basaloid SCC has been well described. The neoplasms are composed of variably sized nests and cords of basaloid cells (Fig. 5.8, eFigs. 5.14 and 5.15). Larger nests can have central comedoform necrosis (Fig. 5.9, eFig. 5.16). Nuclear palisading can sometimes be seen at the periphery of the nests. Focal cribriforming is often present and gland-like spaces are commonly identified (Fig. 5.10, eFigs. 5.17 and 5.18). The surrounding stroma can appear either hyalinized or somewhat myxoid and can be focally intimately intermixed with the basaloid cells. Adequate sectioning of most cases will reveal at least focal conventional-type SCC (Fig. 5.11, eFigs. 5.19 and 5.20). When overlying epithelium is present, an intimate relationship between it and the tumors can often be identified and high-grade dysplasia is usually seen. Cytologically, the cells have high nuclear to cytoplasmic ratios with dense, hyperchromatic nuclei. A

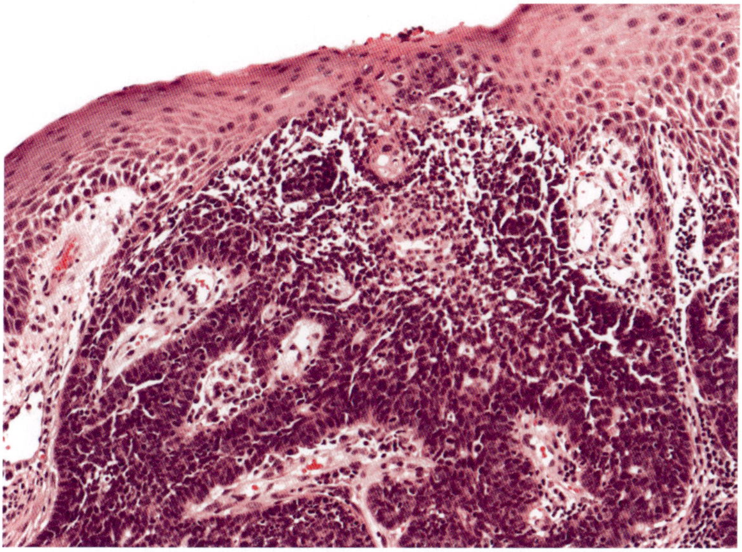

FIGURE 5.8 Basaloid squamous cell carcinoma.

moderate amount of cellular and nuclear size and shape variability is commonly present. Numerous mitotic figures and apoptotic bodies are often seen (Fig. 5.12, eFigs. 5.21 and 5.22).

When the majority of the features stated above are present, we use the diagnosis of "basaloid SCC." The is in contrast with the tumors that grow predominately as nests or islands of immature squamous cells but

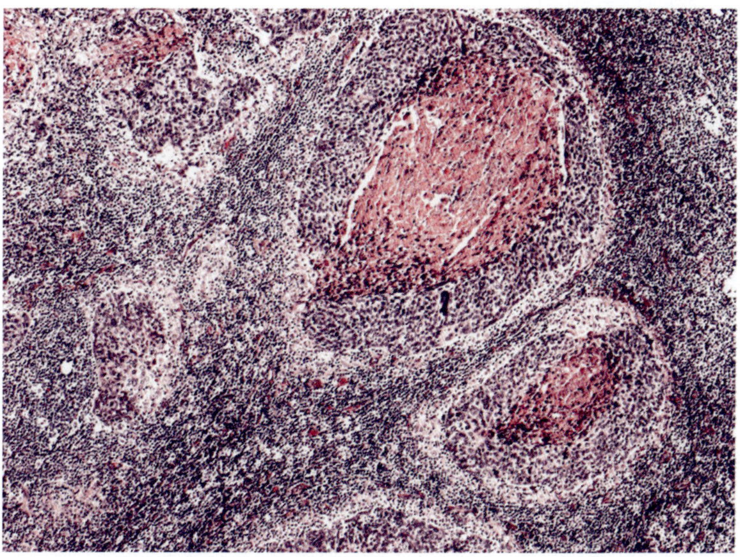

FIGURE 5.9 Basaloid squamous cell carcinoma with comedo necrosis.

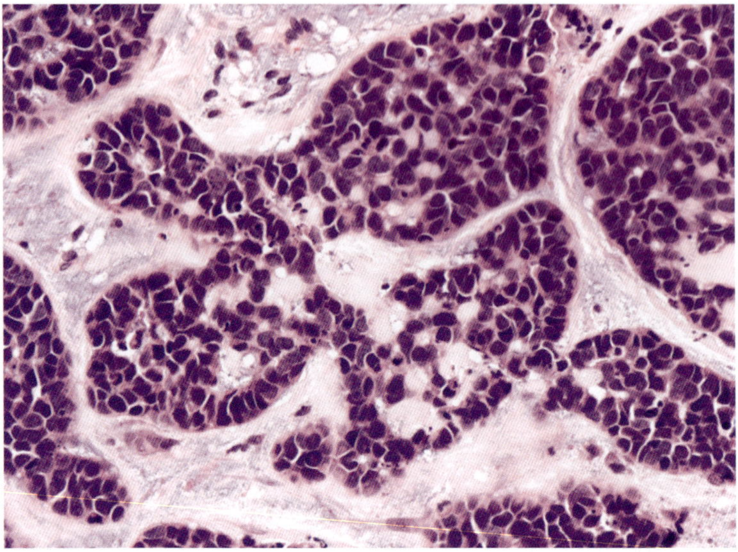

FIGURE 5.10 Basaloid squamous cell carcinoma with a cribriform architecture.

lack other features of basaloid SCC outlined above. For these tumors, we use the diagnosis of "nonkeratinizing SCC." In our experience, the vast majority of oropharyngeal and HR-HPV-related SCCs fall into this latter category. Indeed, basaloid SCC is now a diagnosis we use only seldom.

Correctly diagnosing basaloid and nonkeratinizing SCC can be challenging with small biopsies. The differential diagnosis may include adenoid

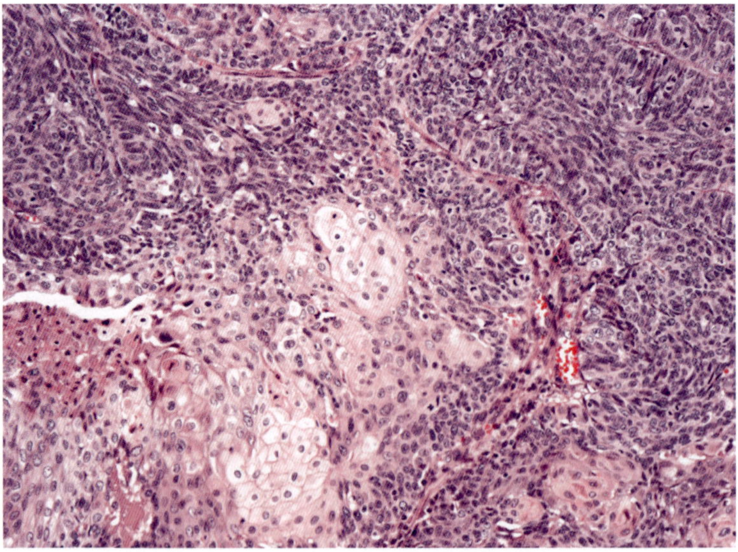

FIGURE 5.11 Focal keratinizing squamous cell carcinoma.

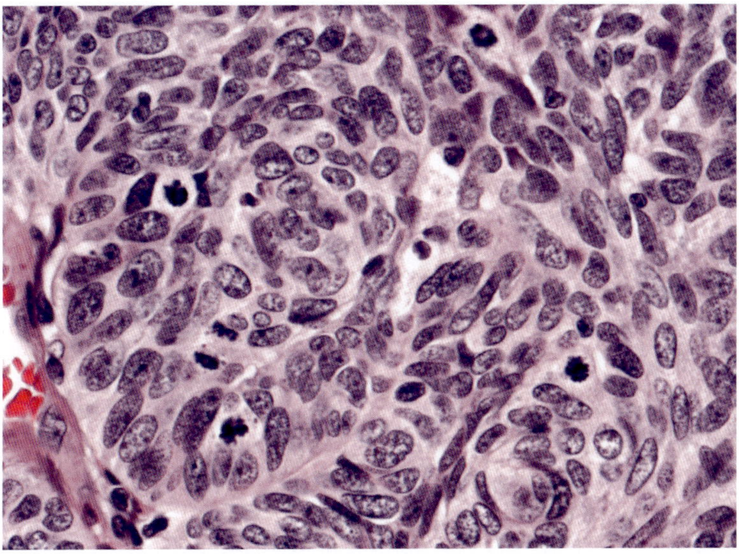

FIGURE 5.12 Basaloid squamous cell carcinoma, high-power image.

cystic carcinoma (ACC), small cell neuroendocrine carcinoma, and other rare basaloid neoplasms of the minor salivary glands, including basal cell adenocarcinoma. Distinguishing the tumors from salivary gland neoplasms, especially ACC, is sometimes difficult but is very important.

ACC is one of the most common malignancies of the minor salivary glands and will be discussed in the following chapter. While histologically some cases of basaloid SCC can resemble the cribriform or solid variant of ACC, there are both histologic and clinical differences that can help the pathologists distinguish these tumors (Table 5.5). Histologically, ACCs show less cytologic pleomorphism and fewer mitotic figures and should not contain areas of squamous differentiation or dysplasia of the surface epithelium. The presence of nodal metastases virtually excludes the diagnosis of ACC as this tumor rarely metastasizes to lymph nodes. A caveat of this stresses the importance of correct diagnosis at biopsy. A neck dissection is not warranted for patients prospectively diagnosed with ACC.

Basal cell adenocarcinoma is a malignant salivary gland–type neoplasm that arises most commonly in the major salivary glands although some smaller series of these tumors arising in the minor salivary glands have been reported.[40,41] The tumors are composed of nests of basaloid cells that may have nuclear and cytologic atypia and may show squamous metaplasia. The nests may be solid or contain multiple tubular profiles. Comedo-type necrosis has also been identified in these cases but is rare. Unlike ACCs, somewhere between 10% and 20% of these neoplasms will metastasize to regional lymph nodes. Basaloid SCCs share many of these features but should show more pleomorphism, overlying squamous dysplasia and conventional-type SCC focally. Cytokeratin 7 immunostaining may

TABLE 5.5 Basaloid Squamous Cell Carcinomas Versus Adenoid Cystic Carcinomas

Basaloid Squamous Cell Carcinoma	Adenoid Cystic Carcinoma
Clinical: Occurs mostly in older men with involvement of the supraglottic larynx and base of tongue. Nodal metastases are often present.	**Clinical:** Occurs equally in men and women and most commonly involves the subglottic larynx, palate, or retromolar area. Nodal metastases are almost never present.
Histology: Will have focal areas of obvious squamous differentiation and appears higher grade with prominent cytologic and nuclear atypia, numerous mitotic figures and individual cell and comedo-type necrosis. Surface squamous dysplasia is often seen.	**Histology:** Should not have areas of squamous differentiation and will lack cytologic and nuclear atypia. Mitotic figures and necrosis are not common. Dysplasia of the overlying squamous epithelium should not be seen.
Immunohistochemistry: Diffuse p63 immunoreactivity. Weak, focal immunoreactivity for CK7.	**Immunohistochemistry:** Positive for markers of myoepithelial differentiation. p63 immunoreactivity may be limited to nuclei at periphery of tumor nests. Strong and diffuse immunoreactivity for CK7.

be helpful as the rare cases of basal cell adenocarcinoma that have been stained have shown strong and diffuse reactivity, unlike basaloid SCCs.

On small biopsy, basaloid SCC can also resemble small cell neuroendocrine carcinoma. This problem is akin to that faced by pathologists when they deal with small, often crushed, bronchial biopsies. Small cell neuroendocrine carcinoma of the upper aerodigestive tract is extremely rare but can occur.[42] When it does, it most frequently involves the larynx. The presence of areas of squamous differentiation and surface dysplasia is suggestive of basaloid SCC. Large areas of geographic necrosis and identifiable Azzopardi effect are suggestive of small cell neuroendocrine carcinoma.

Immunohistochemistry has been shown in some cases to help differentiate basaloid SCC from other tumors, including ACC, although it only rarely presents a definitive answer in and of itself.[43–48] It is helpful with small biopsies, which may not show focal squamous differentiation. ACC should show myoepithelial differentiation and its neoplastic cells react with antibodies to muscle-specific actin and S-100. p63 staining of ACC shows staining of only peripheral nuclei located circumferentially around the nests of tumor cells (cribriform variant), whereas basaloid SCCs show diffuse nuclear staining throughout the entirety of the tumor nests (Fig. 5.13, eFig. 5.23). These features are less distinct for the solid variant of ACC. CK 7 may also be helpful as it has been noted to be strongly expressed in ACC but not basaloid SCC. Antibodies to CD117 react with most ACCs and demonstrate differential staining of tumor cells akin to p63 staining; however, a good percentage of basaloid SCCs will also show staining (eFig. 5.24). The solid pattern will show diffuse staining of all nuclei and shows significant overlap with the staining pattern of basaloid SCCs. Small cell neuroendocrine carcinomas should react with antibodies to endocrine markers such as CD56, chromogranin, and synaptophysin and will show characteristic punctate immunoreactivity with antibodies to cytokeratin. Some authors have noted that immunoreactivity for antibodies to cytokeratin 34βE12 is restricted to basaloid SCC. HR-HPV in situ hybridization may be helpful as salivary gland–type neoplasms (aside from very rare lesions in the sinonasal tract) should not harbor the virus (Fig. 5.14). p16 immunohistochemistry may also be helpful; however, the accumulation of the protein can sometimes be seen in salivary gland–type tumors and other malignancies including small cell carcinomas.[38] Molecular markers consistent with abnormalities seen in some salivary tumors (e.g., demonstration of MYB translocation by FISH (ACC) or nuclear accumulation of β-catenin by immunohistochemistry (basal cell adenoma/adenocarcinoma) may be useful for distinguishing some lesions.

p53 protein accumulation is frequently seen in cases of basaloid SCC, although it is less likely to accumulate in HR-HPV-related nonkeratinizing SCCs.[36,45] Basaloid SCCs are considered poorly differentiated and show genetic abnormalities similar to other poorly differentiated SCCs of

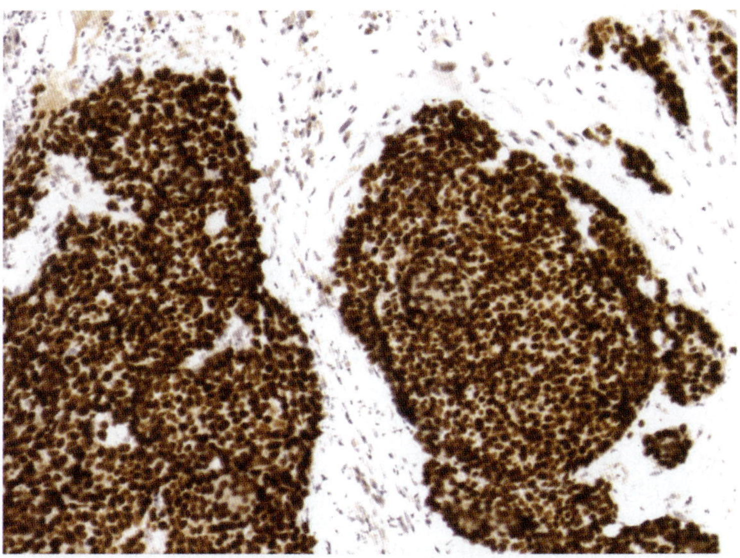

FIGURE 5.13 p63 immunostain of basaloid squamous cell carcinoma.

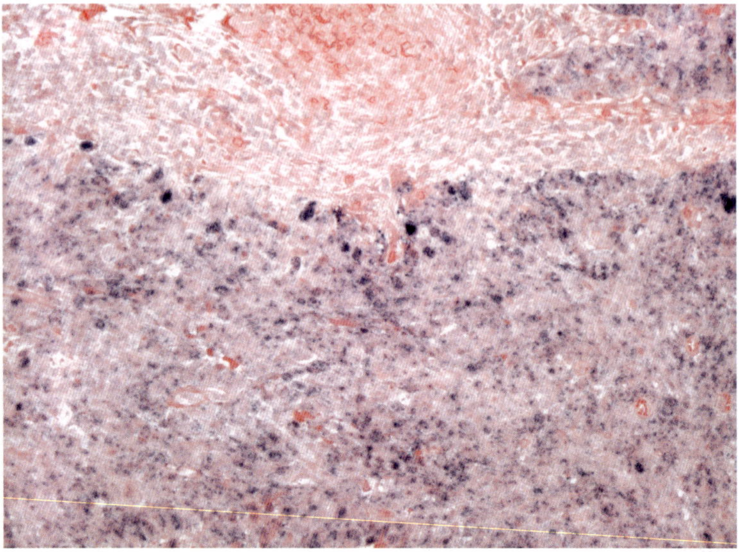

FIGURE 5.14 Many basaloid or nonkeratinizing squamous cell carcinomas are secondary to high-risk human papillomavirus infection, as demonstrated by in situ hybridization.

the upper aerodigestive tract. These tumors are more likely than other, better differentiated types of SCC to show abnormalities of 11q and 17p, areas which are believed to be involved later in the development of upper aerodigestive tract SCCs.[1] Differences of LOH frequency have been shown for certain microsatellite markers on chromosomes 9 and 11 compared to other variants of SCC.

Spindle Cell Carcinoma

Spindle cell carcinoma of the upper aerodigestive tract is a poorly differentiated variant of SCC.[49–54] It is so named because the majority of the neoplastic cells that form the neoplasm show a mesenchymal-like phenotype. The tumor occurs most frequently in older men who on average are in their seventh decade of life. It is related to alcohol abuse and the smoking of tobacco products. Rare tumors may arise from less aggressive types of SCC after exposure to radiation. These tumors most commonly present as an exophytic, polypoid masses in the larynx; however, they can arise anywhere in the upper aerodigestive tract and can appear flat. Because these tumors are most often polypoid and most frequently involve the glottis, they are frequently found at low stage.

Histologically, the tumors are often ulcerated, likely due to the polypoid nature of the lesions (Fig. 5.15, eFig. 5.25). When an overlying epithelial component is present, squamous dysplasia is sometimes noted. Although the mesenchymal component generally makes up the vast majority of the tumor, definitive squamous differentiation is usually seen, sometimes at

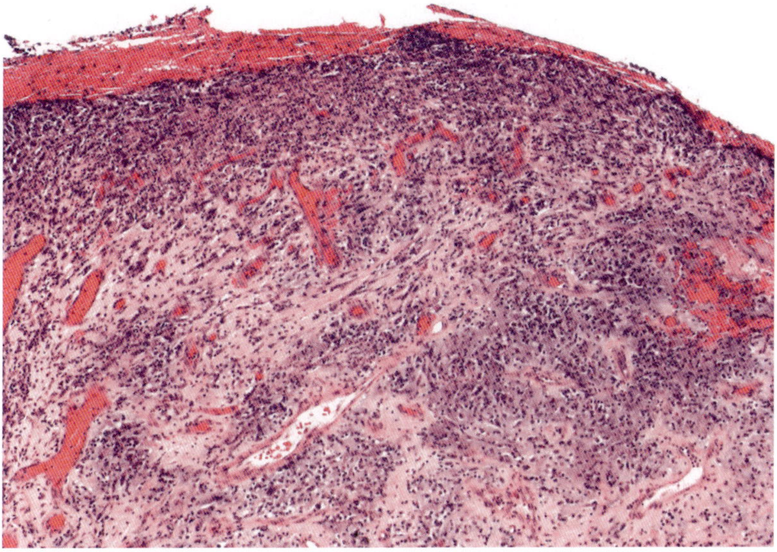

FIGURE 5.15 Ulcerated spindle cell carcinoma.

the advancing tumor front (Fig. 5.16, eFig. 5.26). This component has often been noted to "blend" into the mesenchymal component. In some tumors, the squamous component may be basaloid.[55] The mesenchymal component may have any of a variety of appearances and can show differentiation toward different mesenchymal phenotypes. The tumors are usually low to moderately cellular and, although obvious pleomorphism is

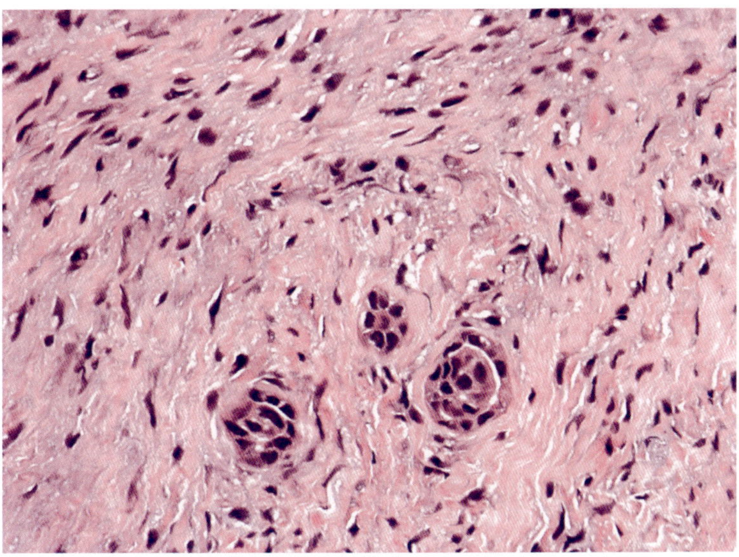

FIGURE 5.16 Occasional squamous nests are seen in this spindle cell carcinoma.

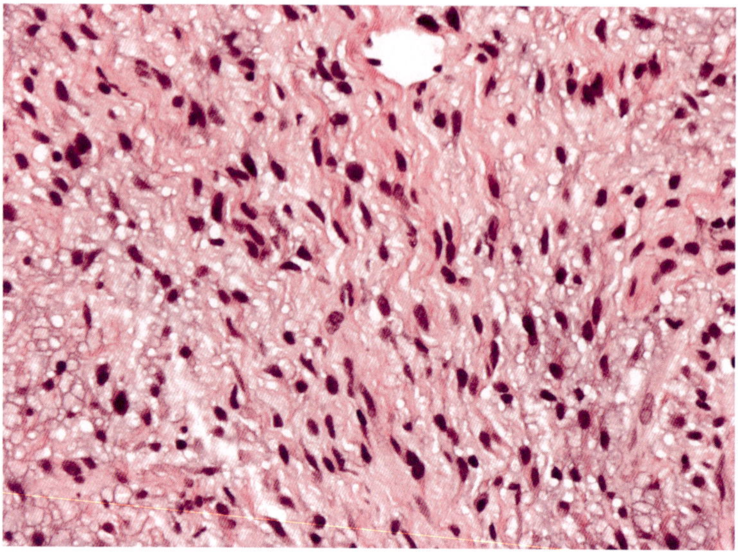

FIGURE 5.17 Spindle cell carcinoma, high power.

present, most tumors do not appear anaplastic (Figs. 5.17 and 5.18, eFigs. 5.27–5.30). Mitotic figures and atypical mitotic figures are usually found. The cellular arrangement may appear storiform, herringbone, fascicular, loose, or even hypocellular with intercellular, dense collagen. Giant cells can be present, as can cartilagenous or osseous metaplasia or malignant differentiation.

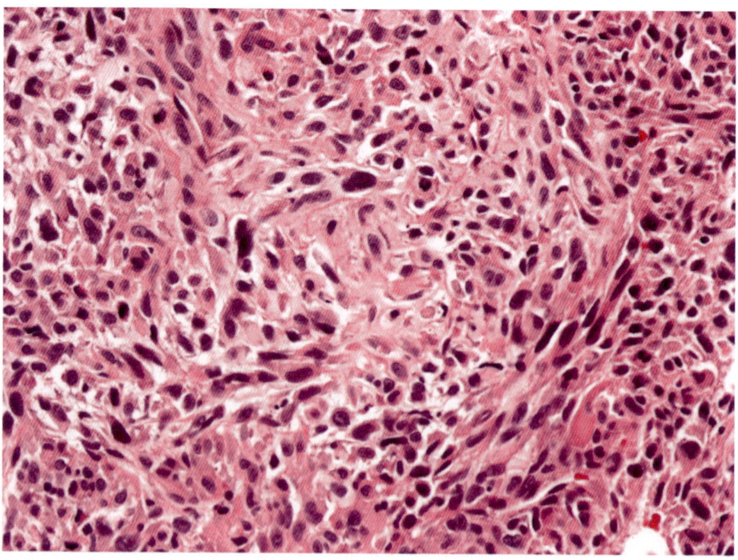

FIGURE 5.18 Spindle cell carcinoma, high power.

The differential diagnosis includes benign and malignant soft tissue neoplasms and malignant melanoma, and a definitive diagnosis can sometimes be difficult based upon histology alone, especially with small biopsies. In such cases immunohistochemistry can be very helpful. Many spindle cell carcinomas will react with antibodies to cytokeratin or other epithelial markers, and a pancytokeratin mixture or cocktail may be the most helpful immunostain to order (Fig. 5.19, eFig. 5.31).[51,52,54] Reactivity, however, tends to be focal. It should also be noted that an absence of keratin or other specific epithelial antigen expression should not dissuade the pathologist from making the diagnosis of spindle cell carcinoma as nearly a third of all cases do not react with antibodies to epithelial antigens. In such cases, a careful search should be made for histologic evidence of squamous differentiation. A caveat of this is that reactivity with antibodies to mesenchymal antigens does not rule out a spindle cell carcinoma (eFig. 5.32). Finally, immunostaining for p63 antigen may also be helpful in some cases as the antigen appears to be expressed in spindle cell carcinomas at a number of sites (Fig. 5.20, eFig. 5.33).[56]

Genetically, both the sarcomatoid and epithelial components of these tumors harbor similar mutations and have concordant ploidy.[52] p53 protein is overexpressed in both components and identical mutations can be found throughout the tumors.[57] The tumors are poorly differentiated and show LOH frequencies similar to other poorly differentiated SCCs of the upper aerodigestive tract.[1] A specific marker on the short arm of chromosome 4 was shown to be more commonly lost in these tumors compared to other SCC variants.

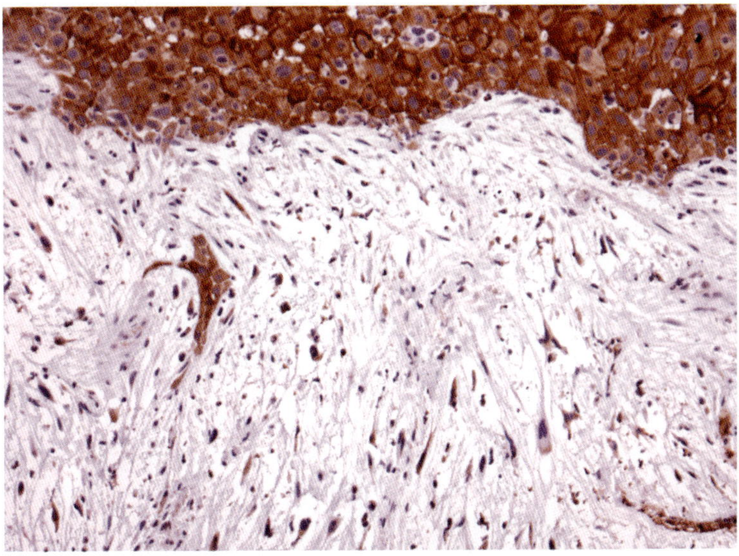

FIGURE 5.19 Cytokeratin immunostain of spindle cell carcinoma.

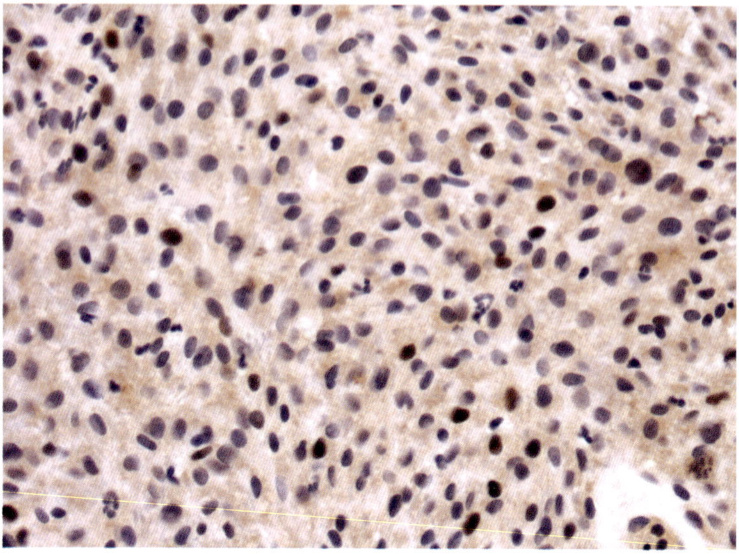

FIGURE 5.20 p63 immunostain of spindle cell carcinoma.

Adenosquamous Carcinoma

SCC of the upper aerodigestive tract will rarely show true glandular differentiation. After conventional-type SCC with entrapped benign glands, poorly differentiated mucoepidermoid carcinoma, and adenoid SCC are excluded, true adenosquamous carcinomas appear to be extremely rare.[58–61] They occur most frequently in older men and are related to alcohol and tobacco use. They can involve any site within the upper aerodigestive tract, but most commonly arise in the larynx and mouth. These tumors are aggressive, frequently metastasize early to lymph nodes, and often recur. Uncommonly, sinonasal or oropharyngeal tumors have been found to be secondary to HR-HPV infection.[62]

Histologically, the squamous component of adenosquamous carcinoma is usually predominant. Although the surface epithelium is often ulcerated, high-grade dysplasia can generally be identified (Fig. 5.21, eFig. 5.34). The lesions are thus believed to arise from the surface epithelium. (This is somewhat contrary to earlier opinions that favored the development of this neoplasm from seromucinous glands perhaps due to the identification of dysplastic epithelium extending into adjacent benign seromucinous glands.) The squamous component is usually moderately to poorly differentiated, will show areas of distinct keratinization, and may, as was mentioned, extend into surrounding benign seromucinous glands. Glandular differentiation is usually seen in the deepest areas of the tumors and usually appears ductular with occasional glands within glands (Fig. 5.22, eFigs. 5.35–5.37). Mucus-containing cells can often be seen histologically; however, glandular differentiation can also be shown

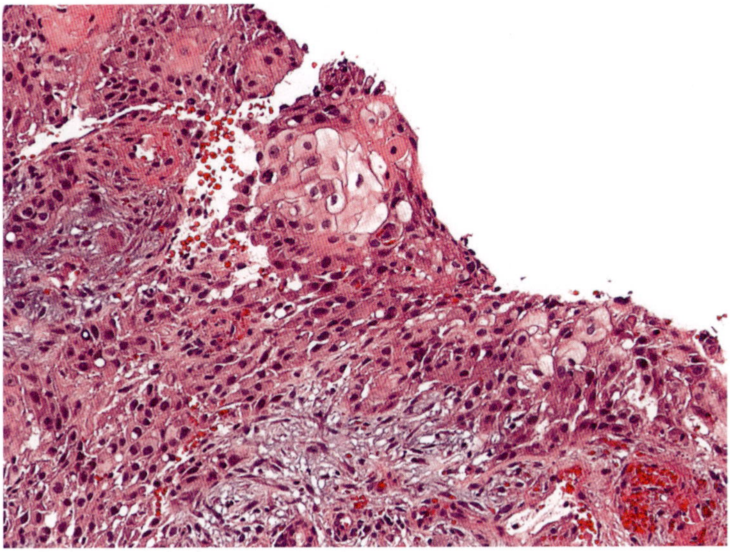

FIGURE 5.21 High-grade squamous dysplasia overlying an adenosquamous carcinoma.

histochemically with mucicarmine, PAS, or alcian blue stains and may be shown immunohistochemically with antibodies to CEA, CAM 5.2, or CK7 (Fig. 5.23, eFig. 5.38). It was noted by the authors of one series that the adenocarcinoma component "bore no resemblance to any distinctive salivary gland neoplasm." Cilia have been identified in rare cases of adenosquamous carcinoma secondary to HR-HPV infection.[63] A variable inflammatory component may be present.

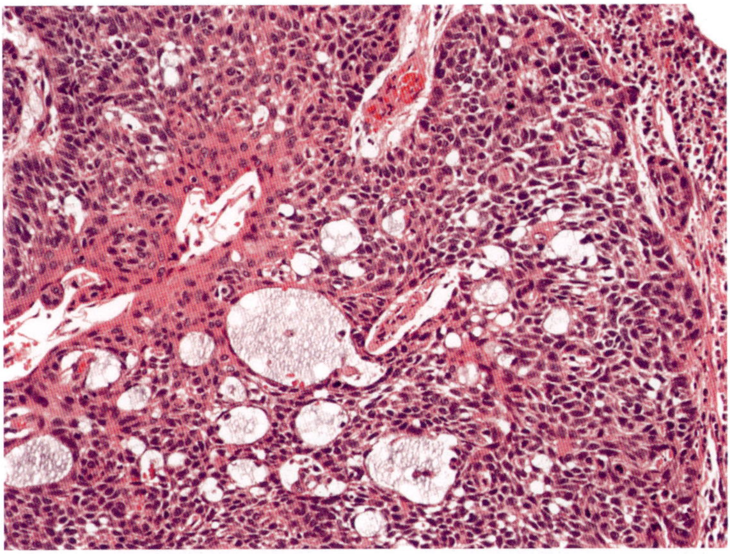

FIGURE 5.22 Adenosquamous carcinoma.

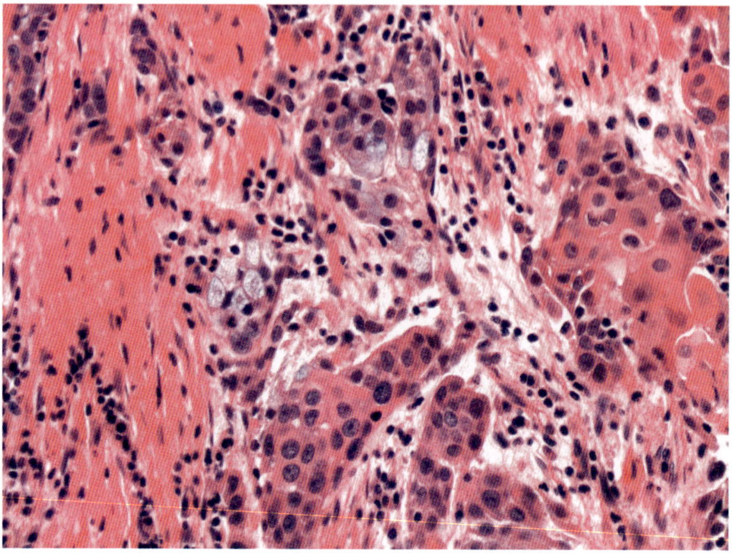

FIGURE 5.23 Intracytoplasmic mucus is seen with some adenosquamous carcinomas.

These tumors should be distinguished from mucoepidermoid carcinomas of the minor salivary glands, which have a better prognosis (Table 5.6). Unlike mucoepidermoid carcinomas, these tumors should show abnormalities of the surface epithelium. Adenosquamous carcinoma should show areas distinctly squamous with extracellular keratin formation and will show more nuclear atypia and mitotic activity than even high-grade

TABLE 5.6 Adenosquamous Carcinoma Versus Mucoepidermoid Carcinoma

Adenosquamous Carcinoma	Mucoepidermoid Carcinoma
Clinical: Occurs most frequently in older men and involves the larynx.	**Clinical:** Slightly more common in women. May occur at any age. Most often involves the parotid. When it involves minor salivary glands, it is most commonly found in the palate.
Histology: Tumors are composed primarily of moderately differentiated conventional-type squamous cell carcinoma. Extracellular keratinization is present. Surface epithelial dysplasia can be found. Glandular differentiation is usually focal.	**Histology:** Tumors are lobular and show mixed glandular and squamoid differentiation throughout. Surface dysplasia should not be seen. Intermediate-type cells can be found. Extracellular keratinization is usually not seen.

mucoepidermoid carcinomas. Mucoepidermoid carcinomas should appear more lobular, and glandular differentiation is usually seen throughout the tumor rather than predominately at the base. Unlike mucoepidermoid carcinomas, these tumors should not have chromosomal rearrangements of *MAML2*, and thus FISH may be helpful diagnostically in some cases.[64] Basaloid and adenoid SCCs may histologically appear glandular; however, true glandular differentiation cannot be demonstrated within these tumors.

Because of the rarity of these tumors, molecular findings are scant. Most tumors have been noted to be aneuploid by flow cytometry and most cases overexpress p53 protein by immunohistochemistry.

Adenoid Squamous Cell Carcinoma

Some invasive SCCs can show a high degree of acantholysis. Although individual cells retain their squamous differentiation, the overall histologic appearance of such tumors can appear either glandular or vascular in nature. This variant of SCC was first recognized in the skin by Lever but has been identified at most sites throughout the body, including the upper aerodigestive tract.[65–75] This morphologic pattern is most commonly seen near the lips at the vermillion border, when it has been identified here. Adenoid SCC of the skin and lips likely arises due to sun damage. Reports of this morphologic pattern at sites not exposed to sun are too few to determine an etiology although some have suggested that radiation exposure may play some role in the development of these tumors. In such cases, this morphologic pattern usually comprises a small portion of more conventional-type SCC.

Histologically, these tumors show alveolar or glandlike spaces lined by a single layer of acantholytic squamous cells (Fig. 5.24, eFigs. 5.39 and 5.40). Similar appearing discohesive cells often are present within the spaces with some necrotic debris and blood. The epithelial cells show a moderate to high degree of atypia with abundant, eosinophilic cytoplasm and both cytologic and nuclear atypia (Fig. 5.25, eFigs. 5.41 and 5.42). Lining the pseudoglandular spaces, the epithelial cells often have a hobnail appearance and numerous mitotic figures can be easily identified. Histologic and histochemical evidence of mucin should not be seen.

As was mentioned, this pattern is commonly seen in the presence of a more conventional-type of SCC, and in such cases does not create much of a diagnostic dilemma. There are a few difficulties that may arise with such cases, however. Small biopsies may sometimes only show the acantholytic, adenoid pattern, and benign and malignant glandular or vascular lesions may be considered. Also, although a larger resection specimen may show obvious conventional-type SCC, focal areas of an adenoid pattern may blend with reactive-appearing vascular areas of granulation tissue, rendering the true extent of the tumor difficult to assess. In all such cases, the degree of cytologic atypia should be greater than that of benign vascular or glandular lesions. If, however, the differential diagnosis includes a

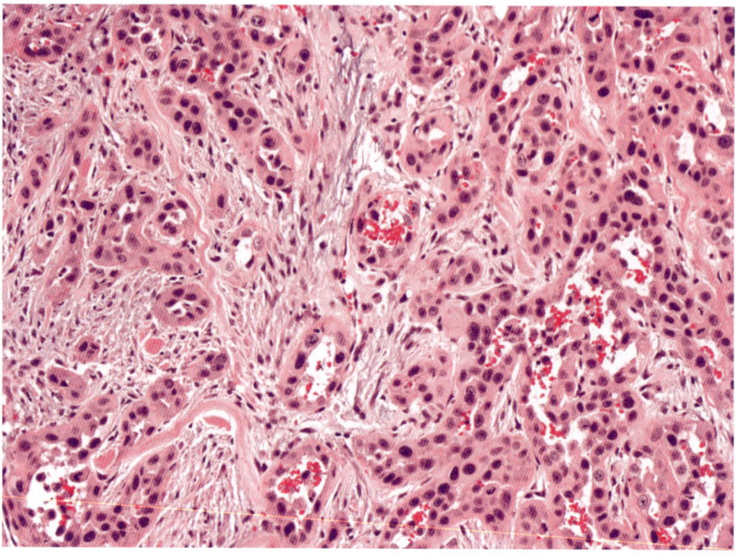

FIGURE 5.24 Adenoid squamous cell carcinoma.

malignant vascular lesion (e.g., angiosarcoma) or if the patient has received radiation therapy and the differential diagnosis includes benign radiation atypia, immunohistochemistry may be helpful. Adenoid SCCs will react diffusely and strongly with antibodies to cytokeratins, whereas benign and malignant vascular lesions will not (eFig. 5.43).[74] If these lesions are

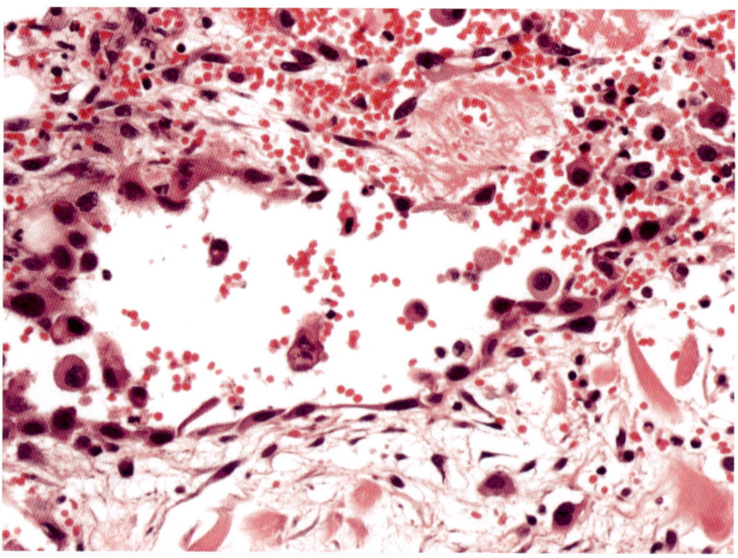

FIGURE 5.25 Adenoid squamous cell carcinoma, high power.

perceived as glandular, and a squamous component is also identified, mucoepidermoid carcinoma may enter the differential diagnosis. As was already mentioned, these lesions should show neither histochemical nor immunohistochemical evidence of glandular differentiation.

Undifferentiated Carcinoma

Undifferentiated carcinoma is a variant of upper aerodigestive tract nonkeratinizing SCC that shows little or no histologic evidence of squamous (or epithelial) differentiation.[76-81] The tumors are most often associated with variant etiologies. The majority occur in the nasopharynx and are associated with EBV. Today, however, a significant number are instead associated with HR-HPV and these lesions most often involve the oropharynx.[82] Other etiologies often associated with an undifferentiated phenotype include tumors having *NUTM1* translocations (NUT carcinomas) and tumors that have loss of INI1 expression (SMARCB1-deficient sinonasal carcinomas).[83-86] As the tumors are typically associated with variant etiologies, and as these etiologies appear to define distinct clinicopathologic entities, the clinical features of the tumors are discussed in more detail below. Because sinonasal undifferentiated carcinomas (SNUCs) often show some neuroendocrine differentiation and because they infrequently express p63 (in our hands), they are discussed in the chapter dealing with neuroendocrine tumors.[87]

By definition, these tumors appear histologically undifferentiated. As such, neoplastic cells grow in sheets with variable degrees of discohesion. The cells appear uniform and have indistinct cell borders. Nuclei are large and vesicular, frequently with prominent nucleoli. Cytologic and nuclear atypia, mitotic figures, and apoptotic cells are all present. A dense lymphoplasmacellular infiltrate is almost always present with EBV-associated tumors of the nasopharynx. It is frequently also seen with the undifferentiated oropharyngeal carcinomas that are secondary to HR-HPV infection. On the other hand, NUT carcinomas and SMARCB1-deficient sinonasal carcinomas are not usually associated with an inflammatory infiltrate.

EBV-associated carcinomas can show a number of growth patterns. When the malignant epithelial cells retain cohesion, they appear syncytial and grow as nests and cords among the inflammatory cells. This pattern in the nasopharynx is termed "differentiated, nonkeratinizing" (known previously as the *Regaud pattern*) as one usually suspects the tumor to be epithelial (Fig. 5.26, eFigs. 5.44 and 5.45). When the cells are less cohesive and the neoplastic cells grow as smaller nests or even single cells, the epithelial nature of these malignancies may be difficult to appreciate. Within the nasopharynx, this pattern of growth is now termed "undifferentiated" (previously referred to as the *Schmincke pattern*) (Fig. 5.27, eFigs. 5.46 and 5.47). HR-HPV-associated undifferentiated carcinomas show similar morphologies.[82]

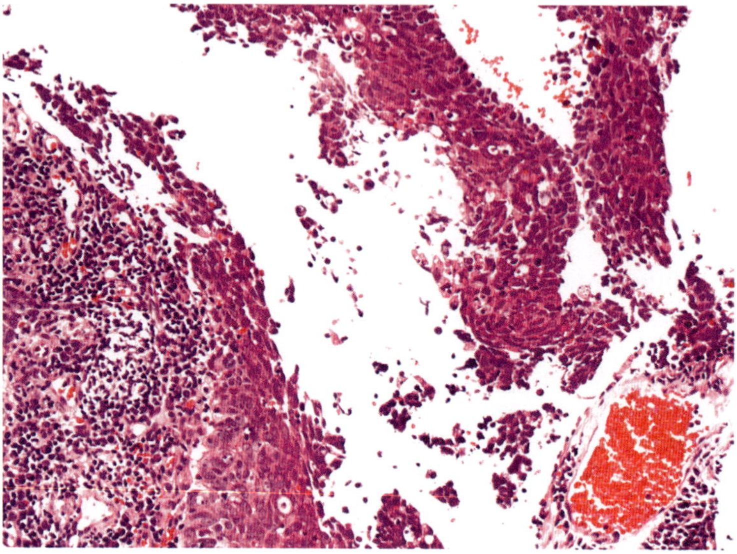

FIGURE 5.26 Undifferentiated carcinoma, Regaud pattern.

While NUT carcinomas are often undifferentiated, some squamous differentiation can often be identified histologically (Fig. 5.28, eFigs. 5.48 and 5.49).[85] Focally, this may be seen with islands of nonkeratinizing epithelioid cells with streaming nuclei. Rapid maturation or keratinization

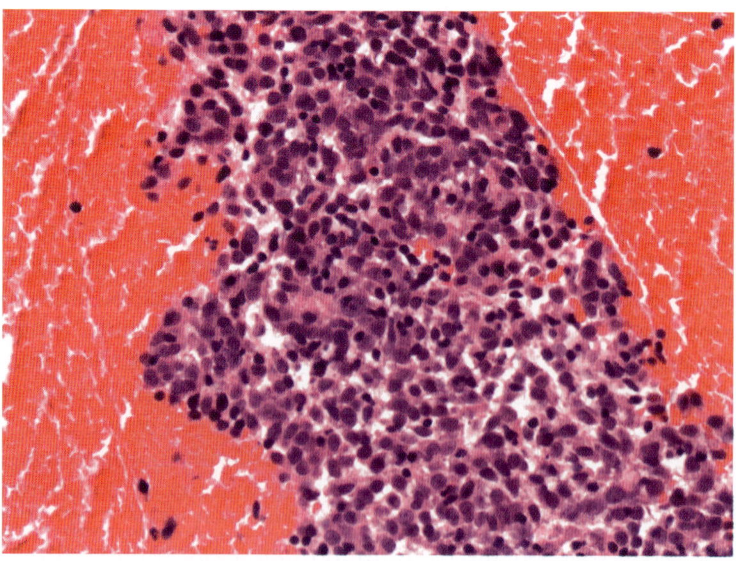

FIGURE 5.27 Undifferentiated carcinoma, Schmincke pattern.

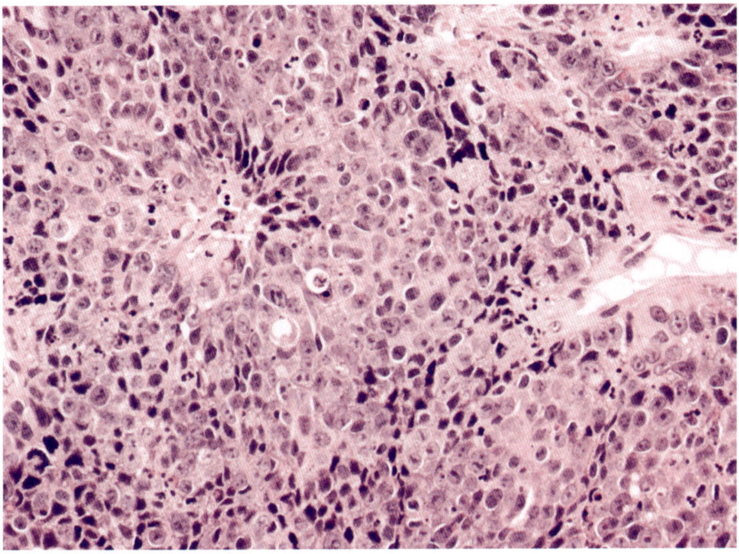

FIGURE 5.28 This undifferentiated carcinoma of the sinonasal tract harbored a translocation involving the nuclear protein of the testis (NUT) gene (NUT midline carcinoma).

can also be seen with very mature squamous cells or extracellular keratin, juxtaposed to undifferentiated, immature-appearing cells.

SMARCB1-deficient carcinomas may either appear more basaloid with a solid or nested and ribbonlike growth pattern or more eosinophilic, usually growing as sheets of neoplastic cells that have abundant eosinophilic cytoplasm and appear oncocytic or rhabdoid (Figs. 5.29 and 5.30; eFigs. 5.50–5.52).[86] Occasional tumors may have areas that are more glandular or sarcomatoid (eFig. 5.53). Some have even been demonstrated to show yolk sac differentiation, both histologically and by immunohistochemistry.[88] The tumors have been described as having a monotonous cytology with medium-sized round nuclei with dispersed chromatin and prominent nucleoli. Frequent mitotic figures and necrosis are seen. The tumors typically have infiltrative margins and cause some desmoplasia. Of note, conventional squamous dysplasia has not been described with these tumors.

Distinguishing undifferentiated carcinomas from lymphoma, although at one time difficult, has been made easy with immunohistochemistry.[89–91] It is now only a difficulty when one of the possible diagnoses is not considered. Most undifferentiated carcinomas, but not all, will react with antibodies directed against epithelial membrane antigen (EMA) or various cytokeratins (a cocktail is often best used in these cases) (Fig. 5.31, eFig. 5.54). The neoplastic cells should not react with antibodies to leukocyte common antigen, CD15 or CD30, unlike the various lymphomas that may be considered in the differential diagnosis. We have seen

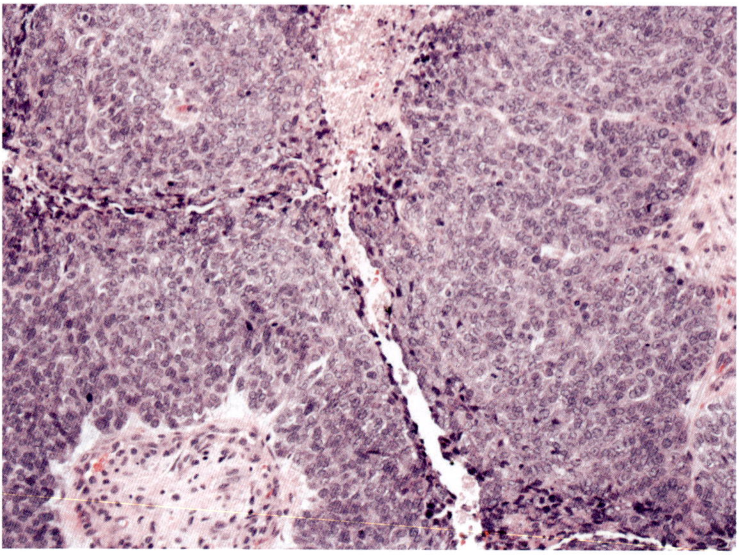

FIGURE 5.29 SMARCB1-deficient sinonasal carcinoma displaying a more basophilic cytology.

rare nasopharyngeal EBV-associated undifferentiated carcinomas that lack EMA and cytokeratin immunoreactivity. In such cases, in situ hybridization for EBV-encoded RNA and lack of immunoreactivity for lymphoid antigens may be sufficient for the correct diagnosis.[92]

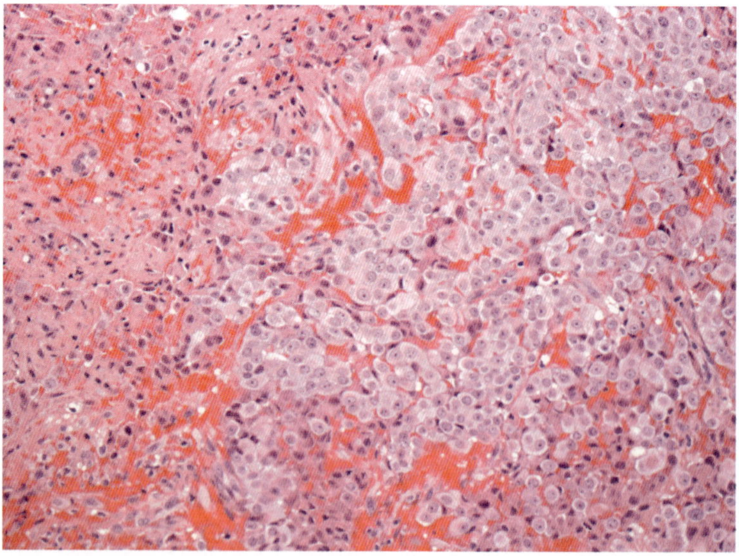

FIGURE 5.30 SMARCB1-deficient sinonasal carcinoma showing a more eosinophilic cytology.

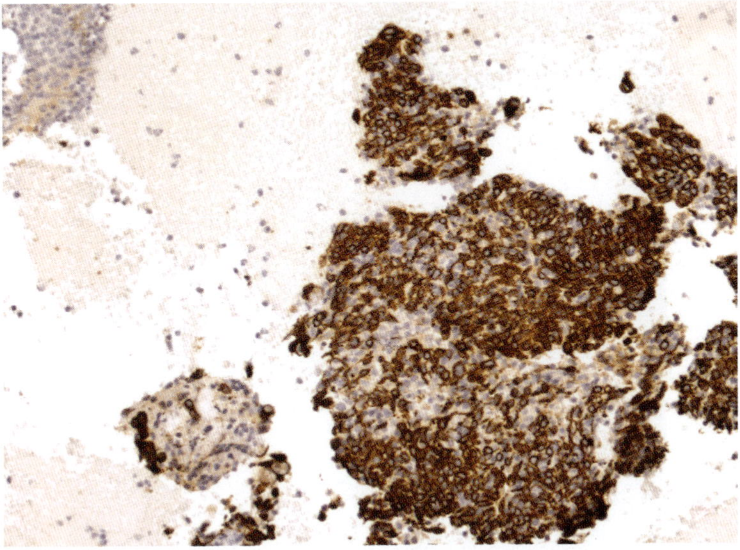

FIGURE 5.31 Undifferentiated carcinoma, cytokeratin immunostain.

Distinguishing these tumors from one another and from other undifferentiated carcinomas such as SNUC is important due to the vast differences in prognoses. For example, SNUCs are almost uniformly lethal and require very aggressive therapy.[93] This typically can be done with methods that specifically address the etiology, such as in situ hybridization for EBV or HR-HPV (Fig. 5.32, eFigs. 5.55 and 5.56) or

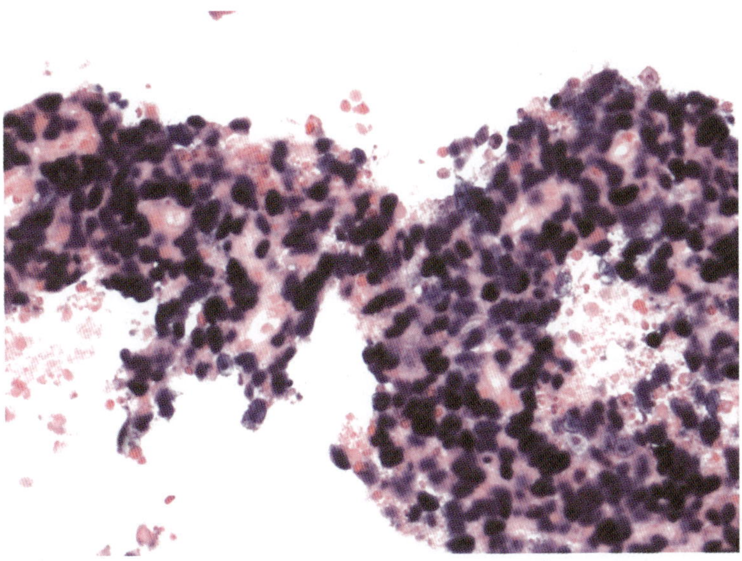

FIGURE 5.32 Undifferentiated carcinoma, in situ hybridization for Epstein-Barr virus.

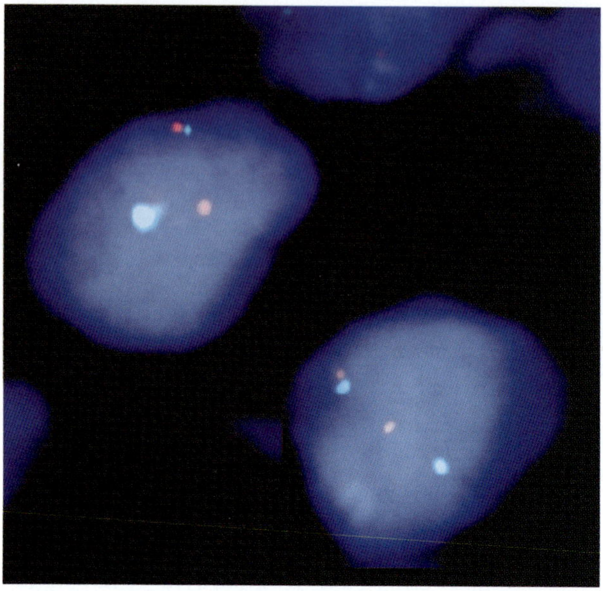

FIGURE 5.33 Nuclear protein of the testis (NUT) midline carcinoma showing broken NUT gene by fluorescent in situ hybridization.

using break-apart probes to identify the broken *NUTM1* gene (Fig. 5.33, eFig. 5.57). Immunohistochemistry can be helpful, but is not always specific. For example, while p16 overexpression is typically seen with HR-HPV-related SCCs and not with EBV-associated SCCs, we have seen overexpression in some NUT carcinomas. The NUT protein itself has been found to be overexpressed only in NUT carcinomas.[94] Finally, we have also noted that p63 immunoreactivity is typically seen with NUT carcinomas and EBV- and HPV-associated SCCs but not in most SNUCs.[87]

ETIOLOGIC VARIANTS

High-Risk Human Papillomavirus–Associated Squamous Cell Carcinoma

While smoking-related carcinomas, including those of the upper aerodigestive tract, have declined in incidence, upper aerodigestive tract SCCs secondary to HR-HPV have increased in incidence over the past few decades.[34,35,37,82,95–107] Indeed, the changes have been significant enough that some have referred to this as an "epidemic." These tumors occur in men more than women, in patients who are younger than those who develop tobacco-related tumors, and usually involve the oropharynx, although any sight of the upper aerodigestive tract can be affected. Oropharyngeal tumors have been shown to be related to oral intercourse. The tumors often present with neck lymph node metastases and the gross identification of a tumor may be difficult for the otolaryngologist. For this reason, a proportion of tumors are identified with so-called blind biopsies of the upper aerodigestive tract, similar to what occurs with some cases of EBV-associated nasopharyngeal carcinomas. Oropharyngeal tumors, stage for stage, have a better prognosis than SCCs related to tobacco use. For this reason, all oropharyngeal SCCs should be tested for HR-HPV (or for a surrogate marker).

The bulk HR-HPV-associated SCCs of the upper aerodigestive tract have a nonkeratinizing phenotype, that, when infiltrative, can overlap significantly with what has been termed "basaloid" SCC (see above). Here it should be noted that true infiltration may be difficult to identify, especially within complex tonsilar architecture. Nonetheless, a tumor that appears "in situ" within the oropharynx is almost certainly invasive regardless of its appearance. Some of these tumors, especially of the oropharynx and sinonasal tract, can grow as exophytic lesions and have a phenotype of papillary SCC. Again, even though definite invasion may be difficult to identify, it is likely always present. A subset of SCCs with other histologies, including typical keratinizing SCCs, adenosquamous carcinoma, undifferentiated carcinoma, and spindle cell carcinomas (as well as adenocarcinomas and neuroendocrine carcinomas), have been shown to be secondary to the virus.[36,62,82,108–110] Such tumors most often involve the oropharynx or sinonasal tract.

As mentioned, because of the relatively good prognosis for oropharyngeal SCCs secondary to HR-HPV, all oropharyngeal SCCs should be tested for the virus. It has, however, been shown that with oropharyngeal tumors p16 immunohistochemistry is roughly equivalent to RNA in situ hybridization techniques and is likely superior to DNA in situ hybridization techniques.[111] Thus, diffuse, blocklike staining with antibodies to p16 is considered sufficient for identifying an oropharyngeal SCC as HR-HPV-associated. Outside of the oropharynx this is not true. While p16 still is a very sensitive marker for HR-HPV-associated tumors, other testing, such as RNA-based in situ hybridization, should be used to definitively consider the tumor related to HR-HPV.

Epstein-Barr Virus–Associated Squamous Cell Carcinoma

These are typically nasopharyngeal malignancies that present most commonly in men and show a bimodal age distribution, peaking in both the second and sixth decades of life. They are much more common in East Asia, especially China, than in the United States, and both genetic and environmental factors are believed to play a role in its development. EBV can be demonstrated by a variety of molecular methods in most tumors of the nasopharynx.[112–114] Although undoubtedly involved in the onconeogenesis of these tumors, its exact role remains somewhat unclear.

Nasopharyngeal tumors most commonly arise near the opening of the eustachian tube at the fossa of Rosenmüller. The tumors are aggressive and generally present with cervical metastases, which may be bilateral at the time of diagnosis. The tumors may be grossly difficult for the otolaryngologist to identify, yet blind biopsies near the fossa of Rosenmüller often are diagnostic. As described above, the majority of these tumors appear undifferentiated (see above). In situ hybridization methods such as EBER ISH should be used to identify these tumors. Of note, EBV-associated SCCs do not show the typical strong blocklike staining with antibodies to p16 seen with HR-HPV-associated SCCs.

NUT Carcinoma

Rare carcinomas of the head and neck are associated with chromosomal rearrangement of nuclear protein of the testis (NUT) gene. Most rearrangements occur with the gene BRD4, although other partner genes (such as BRD3) have been identified. These tumors have been designated as "NUT carcinomas." The tumors almost always arise in the sinonasal tract, but rare lesions have been reported at other sites in the upper aerodigestive tract and within the salivary glands. These tumors frequently present in children, although they have been identified in patients of all ages.[83,85] These tumors typically present with nonspecific symptoms secondary to mass effect. They have a terrible prognosis.

NUT carcinomas are often relatively undifferentiated, composed of sheets of malignant somewhat monomorphic-appearing cells. In our experience, the tumors were most often diagnosed previously as SNUCs, given their appearance and typical site of presentation. Some tumors may appear more similar to nonkeratinizing SCCs with nests and ribbons of tumor cells within a desmoplastic stroma. Keratinization can sometimes be present, and when seen it may be closely juxtaposed to more undifferentiated tumor. This has been referred to as abrupt keratinization and, although nonspecific, should raise one's concern for this entity. The tumors are almost always immunoreactive with antibodies to p63, even when no definite squamous differentiation can be appreciated histologically. Diagnosis rests on the identification of NUT protein expression by immunohistochemistry or NUTM1 translocation by FISH.

SMARCB1-Deficient Sinonasal Carcinoma

Various tumors throughout the body have been shown to have loss of expression of SMARCB1 (INI1) (e.g., medullary carcinoma of the kidney, epithelioid sarcoma). The protein is a portion of the SWI/SNF complex and as such plays a role in chromatin remodeling and transcription. Other proteins of the complex are much less commonly lost, but rare SMARCA4 loss has been described. Tumors occur slightly more commonly in men and over a broad age range. They typically involve the paranasal sinuses, often with nasal and/or skull base involvement. Most patients die of disease in spite of treatment between 1 and 2 years after diagnosis. The histology of these tumors is discussed above in more detail. As stated, the tumors may appear more basaloid or eosinophilic with rhabdoid cells often present. The tumors usually express p63 by immunohistochemistry and, by definition,

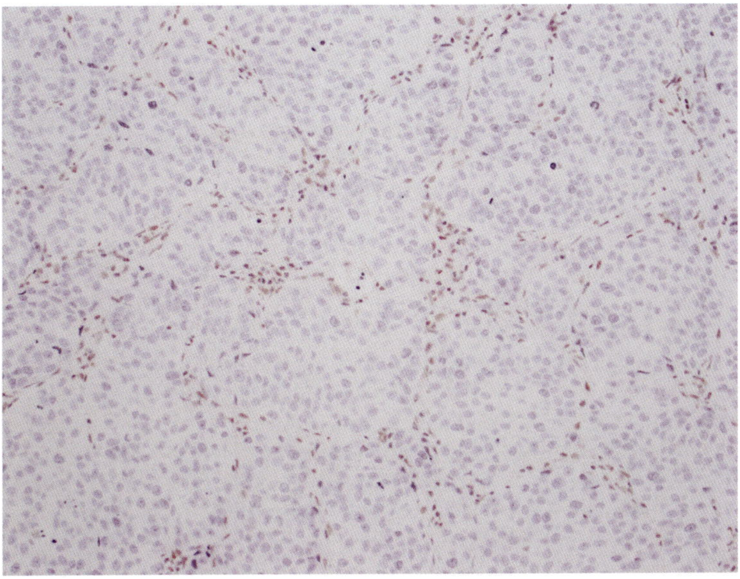

FIGURE 5.34 **SMARCB1/INI1 loss by immunohistochemistry.**

show SMARCB1 (or SMARCA4) loss (Fig. 5.34, eFig. 5.58). It should be noted, however, that not all SMARCB1-deficient sinonasal carcinomas express p63, and the diagnosis should be considered with any undifferentiated carcinoma. As noted above, some of these tumors even show yolk sac differentiation both histologically and by immunohistochemistry (e.g., α-fetoprotein and glypican-3).[88]

CONCLUSION

Knowledge of the histologic variants of upper aerodigestive tract SCC is important as it allows the pathologist to consider the correct differential diagnoses when atypical lesions are identified. As a whole, the lesions arise in a patient cohort similar to that of conventional-type SCC and will behave more akin to conventional-type SCC than to other neoplasms that must be considered in the differential diagnosis. The lesions do sometimes behave in unique fashions, such as is the case for verrucous carcinoma, and the correct diagnosis can provide valuable prognostic information and help to guide surgical treatment.

REFERENCES

1. Choi HR, Roberts DB, Johnigan RH, et al. Molecular and clinicopathologic comparisons of head and neck squamous carcinoma variants: common and distinctive features of biological significance. *Am J Surg Pathol*. 2004;28:1299-1310.
2. Ackerman LV. Verrucous carcinoma of the oral cavity. *Surgery*. 1948;23:670-678.

3. Kraus FT, Perezmesa C. Verrucous carcinoma. Clinical and pathologic study of 105 cases involving oral cavity, larynx and genitalia. *Cancer*. 1966;19:26-38.
4. Fonts EA, Greenlaw RH, Rush BF, Rovin S. Verrucous squamous cell carcinoma of the oral cavity. *Cancer*. 1969;23:152-160.
5. Ferlito A, Recher G. Ackerman's tumor (verrucous carcinoma) of the larynx: a clinicopathologic study of 77 cases. *Cancer*. 1980;46:1617-1630.
6. McCoy JM, Waldron CA. Verrucous carcinoma of the oral cavity. A review of forty-nine cases. *Oral Surg Oral Med Oral Pathol*. 1981;52:623-629.
7. Batsakis JG, Hybels R, Crissman JD, Rice DH. The pathology of head and neck tumors: verrucous carcinoma, Part 15. *Head Neck Surg*. 1982;5:29-38.
8. McDonald JS, Crissman JD, Gluckman JL. Verrucous carcinoma of the oral cavity. *Head Neck Surg*. 1982;5:22-28.
9. Medina JE, Dichtel W, Luna MA. Verrucous-squamous carcinomas of the oral cavity. A clinicopathologic study of 104 cases. *Arch Otolaryngol*. 1984;110:437-440.
10. Rajendran R, Varghese I, Sugathan CK, Vijayakumar T. Ackerman's tumour (verrucous carcinoma) of the oral cavity: a clinico-epidemiologic study of 426 cases. *Aust Dent J*. 1988;33:295-298.
11. Maurizi M, Cadoni G, Ottaviani F, Rabitti C, Almadori G. Verrucous squamous cell carcinoma of the larynx: diagnostic and therapeutic considerations. *Eur Arch Otorhinolaryngol*. 1996;253:130-135.
12. Orvidas LJ, Olsen KD, Lewis JE, Suman VJ. Verrucous carcinoma of the larynx: a review of 53 patients. *Head Neck*. 1998;20:197-203.
13. McCaffrey TV, Witte M, Ferguson MT. Verrucous carcinoma of the larynx. *Ann Otol Rhinol Laryngol*. 1998;107:391-395.
14. Fliss DM, Noble-Topham SE, McLachlin M, et al. Laryngeal verrucous carcinoma: a clinicopathologic study and detection of human papillomavirus using polymerase chain reaction. *Laryngoscope*. 1994;104:146-152.
15. Lopez-Amado M, Garcia-Caballero T, Lozano-Ramirez A, Labella-Caballero T. Human papillomavirus and p53 oncoprotein in verrucous carcinoma of the larynx. *J Laryngol Otol*. 1996;110:742-747.
16. Murrah VA, Batsakis JG. Proliferative verrucous leukoplakia and verrucous hyperplasia. *Ann Otol Rhinol Laryngol*. 1994;103:660-663.
17. Batsakis JG, Suarez P, el-Naggar AK. Proliferative verrucous leukoplakia and its related lesions. *Oral Oncol*. 1999;35:354-359.
18. Shear M, Pindborg JJ. Verrucous hyperplasia of the oral mucosa. *Cancer*. 1980;46:1855-1862.
19. Fechner RE, Mills SE. Verruca vulgaris of the larynx: a distinctive lesion of probable viral origin confused with verrucous carcinoma. *Am J Surg Pathol*. 1982;6:357-362.
20. Gimenez-Conti IB, Collet AM, Lanfranchi H, et al. p53, Rb, and cyclin D1 expression in human oral verrucous carcinomas. *Cancer*. 1996;78:17-23.
21. Sakurai K, Urade M, Takahashi Y, et al. Increased expression of c-erbB-3 protein and proliferating cell nuclear antigen during development of verrucous carcinoma of the oral mucosa. *Cancer*. 2000;89:2597-2605.
22. Crissman JD, Kessis T, Shah KV, et al. Squamous papillary neoplasia of the adult upper aerodigestive tract. *Hum Pathol*. 1988;19:1387-1396.
23. Judd R, Zaki SR, Coffield LM, Evatt BL. Human papillomavirus type 6 detected by the polymerase chain reaction in invasive sinonasal papillary squamous cell carcinoma. *Arch Pathol Lab Med*. 1991;115:1150-1153.
24. Ferlito A, Devaney KO, Rinaldo A, Putzi MJ. Papillary squamous cell carcinoma versus verrucous squamous cell carcinoma of the head and neck. *Ann Otol Rhinol Laryngol*. 1999;108:318-322.

25. Thompson LD, Wenig BM, Heffner DK, Gnepp DR. Exophytic and papillary squamous cell carcinomas of the larynx: a clinicopathologic series of 104 cases. *Otolaryngol Head Neck Surg*. 1999;120:718-724.

26. Suarez PA, Adler-Storthz K, Luna MA, El-Naggar AK, Abdul-Karim FW, Batsakis JG. Papillary squamous cell carcinomas of the upper aerodigestive tract: a clinicopathologic and molecular study. *Head Neck*. 2000;22:360-368.

27. Ereno C, Lopez JI, Sanchez JM, Bilbao FJ. Papillary squamous cell carcinoma of the larynx. *J Laryngol Otol*. 2001;115:164-166.

28. Ferrer MJ, Estelles E, Villanueva A, Lopez R. Papillary squamous cell carcinoma of the oropharynx. *Eur Arch Otorhinolaryngol*. 2003;260:444-445.

29. Jo VY, Mills SE, Stoler MH, Stelow EB. Papillary squamous cell carcinoma of the head and neck: frequent association with human papillomavirus infection and invasive carcinoma. *Am J Surg Pathol*. 2009;33:1720-1724.

30. Banks ER, Frierson HF Jr, Mills SE, George E, Zarbo RJ, Swanson PE. Basaloid squamous cell carcinoma of the head and neck. A clinicopathologic and immunohistochemical study of 40 cases. *Am J Surg Pathol*. 1992;16:939-946.

31. Barnes L, Ferlito A, Altavilla G, MacMillan C, Rinaldo A, Doglioni C. Basaloid squamous cell carcinoma of the head and neck: clinicopathological features and differential diagnosis. *Ann Otol Rhinol Laryngol*. 1996;105:75-82.

32. Ferlito A, Altavilla G, Rinaldo A, Doglioni C. Basaloid squamous cell carcinoma of the larynx and hypopharynx. *Ann Otol Rhinol Laryngol*. 1997;106:1024-1035.

33. Coletta RD, Cotrim P, Almeida OP, Alves VA, Wakamatsu A, Vargas PA. Basaloid squamous carcinoma of oral cavity: a histologic and immunohistochemical study. *Oral Oncol*. 2002;38:723-729.

34. El-Mofty SK, Patil S. Human papillomavirus (HPV)-related oropharyngeal nonkeratinizing squamous cell carcinoma: characterization of a distinct phenotype. *Oral Surg Oral Med Oral Pathol Oral Radiol Endod*. 2006;101:339-345.

35. Begum S, Westra WH. Basaloid squamous cell carcinoma of the head and neck is a mixed variant that can be further resolved by HPV status. *Am J Surg Pathol*. 2008;32:1044-1050.

36. Chernock RD, Lewis JS Jr, Zhang Q, El-Mofty SK. Human papillomavirus-positive basaloid squamous cell carcinomas of the upper aerodigestive tract: a distinct clinicopathologic and molecular subtype of basaloid squamous cell carcinoma. *Hum Pathol*. 2010;41:1016-1023.

37. Laco J, Vosmikova H, Novakova V, et al. The role of high-risk human papillomavirus infection in oral and oropharyngeal squamous cell carcinoma in non-smoking and non-drinking patients: a clinicopathological and molecular study of 46 cases. *Virchows Arch*. 2011;458:179-187.

38. Stelow EB, Jo VY, Stoler MH, Mills SE. Human papillomavirus-associated squamous cell carcinoma of the upper aerodigestive tract. *Am J Surg Pathol*. 2010;34:e15-e24.

39. Thariat J, Badoual C, Faure C, Butori C, Marcy PY, Righini CA. Basaloid squamous cell carcinoma of the head and neck: role of HPV and implication in treatment and prognosis. *J Clin Pathol*. 2010;63:857-866.

40. Fonseca I, Soares J. Basal cell adenocarcinoma of minor salivary and seromucous glands of the head and neck region. *Semin Diagn Pathol*. 1996;13:128-137.

41. Jayakrishnan A, Elmalah I, Hussain K, Odell EW. Basal cell adenocarcinoma in minor salivary glands. *Histopathology*. 2003;42:610-614.

42. Mills SE, Cooper PH, Garland TA, Johns ME. Small cell undifferentiated carcinoma of the larynx. Report of two patients and review of 13 additional cases. *Cancer*. 1983;51:116-120.

43. Klijanienko J, el-Naggar A, Ponzio-Prion A, Marandas P, Micheau C, Caillaud JM. Basaloid squamous carcinoma of the head and neck. Immunohistochemical comparison with adenoid cystic carcinoma and squamous cell carcinoma. *Arch Otolaryngol Head Neck Surg.* 1993;119:887-890.
44. Morice WG, Ferreiro JA. Distinction of basaloid squamous cell carcinoma from adenoid cystic and small cell undifferentiated carcinoma by immunohistochemistry. *Hum Pathol.* 1998;29:609-612.
45. Tsubochi H, Suzuki T, Suzuki S, et al. Immunohistochemical study of basaloid squamous cell carcinoma, adenoid cystic and mucoepidermoid carcinoma in the upper aerodigestive tract. *Anticancer Res.* 2000;20:1205-1211.
46. Mino M, Pilch BZ, Faquin WC. Expression of KIT (CD117) in neoplasms of the head and neck: an ancillary marker for adenoid cystic carcinoma. *Mod Pathol.* 2003;16:1224-1231.
47. Nikitakis NG, Tosios KI, Papanikolaou VS, Rivera H, Papanicolaou SI, Ioffe OB. Immunohistochemical expression of cytokeratins 7 and 20 in malignant salivary gland tumors. *Mod Pathol.* 2004;17:407-415.
48. Emanuel P, Wang B, Wu M, Burstein DE. p63 Immunohistochemistry in the distinction of adenoid cystic carcinoma from basaloid squamous cell carcinoma. *Mod Pathol.* 2005;18:645-650.
49. Leventon GS, Evans HL. Sarcomatoid squamous cell carcinoma of the mucous membranes of the head and neck: a clinicopathologic study of 20 cases. *Cancer.* 1981;48:994-1003.
50. Zarbo RJ, Crissman JD, Venkat H, Weiss MA. Spindle-cell carcinoma of the upper aerodigestive tract mucosa. An immunohistologic and ultrastructural study of 18 biphasic tumors and comparison with seven monophasic spindle-cell tumors. *Am J Surg Pathol.* 1986;10:741-753.
51. Ellis GL, Langloss JM, Heffner DK, Hyams VJ. Spindle-cell carcinoma of the aerodigestive tract. An immunohistochemical analysis of 21 cases. *Am J Surg Pathol.* 1987;11:335-342.
52. Lewis JE, Olsen KD, Sebo TJ. Spindle cell carcinoma of the larynx: review of 26 cases including DNA content and immunohistochemistry. *Hum Pathol.* 1997;28:664-673.
53. Olsen KD, Lewis JE, Suman VJ. Spindle cell carcinoma of the larynx and hypopharynx. *Otolaryngol Head Neck Surg.* 1997;116:47-52.
54. Thompson LD, Wieneke JA, Miettinen M, Heffner DK. Spindle cell (sarcomatoid) carcinomas of the larynx: a clinicopathologic study of 187 cases. *Am J Surg Pathol.* 2002;26:153-170.
55. Altrabulsi B, Carrizo F, Luna MA. Spindle basaloid squamous carcinoma of the upper aerodigestive tract: immunohistochemical and clinicopathological study of three cases. *Ann Diagn Pathol.* 2006;10:149-153.
56. Lewis JS, Ritter JH, El-Mofty S. Alternative epithelial markers in sarcomatoid carcinomas of the head and neck, lung, and bladder-p63, MOC-31, and TTF-1. *Mod Pathol.* 2005;18:1471-1481.
57. Ansari-Lari MA, Hoque MO, Califano J, Westra WH. Immunohistochemical p53 expression patterns in sarcomatoid carcinomas of the upper respiratory tract. *Am J Surg Pathol.* 2002;26:1024-1031.
58. Gerughty RM, Hennigar GR, Brown FM. Adenosquamous carcinoma of the nasal, oral and laryngeal cavities. A clinicopathologic survey of ten cases. *Cancer.* 1968;22:1140-1155.
59. Damiani JM, Damiani KK, Hauck K, Hyams VJ. Mucoepidermoid-adenosquamous carcinoma of the larynx and hypopharynx: a report of 21 cases and a review of the literature. *Otolaryngol Head Neck Surg.* 1981;89:235-243.

60. Keelawat S, Liu CZ, Roehm PC, Barnes L. Adenosquamous carcinoma of the upper aerodigestive tract: a clinicopathologic study of 12 cases and review of the literature. *Am J Otolaryngol.* 2002;23:160-168.

61. Alos L, Castillo M, Nadal A, et al. Adenosquamous carcinoma of the head and neck: criteria for diagnosis in a study of 12 cases. *Histopathology.* 2004;44:570-579.

62. Masand RP, El-Mofty SK, Ma XJ, Luo Y, Flanagan JJ, Lewis JS, Jr. Adenosquamous carcinoma of the head and neck: relationship to human papillomavirus and review of the literature. *Head Neck Pathol.* 2011;5(2):108-116.

63. Radkay-Gonzalez L, Faquin W, McHugh JB, Lewis JS Jr, Tuluc M, Seethala RR. Ciliated adenosquamous carcinoma: expanding the phenotypic diversity of human papillomavirus-associated tumors. *Head Neck Pathol.* 2016;10:167-175.

64. Seethala RR, Dacic S, Cieply K, Kelly LM, Nikiforova MN. A reappraisal of the MECT1/MAML2 translocation in salivary mucoepidermoid carcinomas. *Am J Surg Pathol.* 2010;34:1106-1121.

65. Lever WF. Adenoacanthoma of sweat glands: carcinoma of sweat glands with glandular and epidermal elements. *Arch Dermatol Syph.* 1947;56:157-171.

66. Johnson WC, Helwig EB. Adenoid squamous cell carcinoma (adenoacanthoma). A clinicopathologic study of 155 patients. *Cancer.* 1966;19:1639-1650.

67. Jacoway JR, Nelson JF, Boyers RC. Adenoid squamous-cell carcinoma (adenocanthoma) of the oral labial mucosa. A clinicopathologic study of fifteen cases. *Oral Surg Oral Med Oral Pathol.* 1971;32:444-449.

68. Weitzner S. Adenoid squamous-cell carcinoma of vermilion mucosa of lower lip. *Oral Surg Oral Med Oral Pathol.* 1974;37:589-593.

69. Takagi M, Sakota Y, Takayama S, Ishikawa G. Adenoid squamous cell carcinoma of the oral mucosa: report of two autopsy cases. *Cancer.* 1977;40:2250-2255.

70. Zaatari GS, Santoianni RA. Adenoid squamous cell carcinoma of the nasopharynx and neck region. *Arch Pathol Lab Med.* 1986;110:542-546.

71. Batsakis JG, Huser J. Squamous carcinomas with glandlike (adenoid) features. *Ann Otol Rhinol Laryngol.* 1990;99:87-88.

72. Nappi O, Wick MR, Pettinato G, Ghiselli RW, Swanson PE. Pseudovascular adenoid squamous cell carcinoma of the skin. A neoplasm that may be mistaken for angiosarcoma. *Am J Surg Pathol.* 1992;16:429-438.

73. Jones AC, Freedman PD, Kerpel SM. Oral adenoid squamous cell carcinoma: a report of three cases and review of the literature. *J Oral Maxillofac Surg.* 1993;51:676-681.

74. Ritter JH, Mills SE, Nappi O, Wick MR. Angiosarcoma-like neoplasms of epithelial organs: true endothelial tumors or variants of carcinoma?. *Semin Diagn Pathol.* 1995;12:270-282.

75. Ferlito A, Devaney KO, Rinaldo A, Milroy CM, Carbone A. Mucosal adenoid squamous cell carcinoma of the head and neck. *Ann Otol Rhinol Laryngol.* 1996;105:409-413.

76. Hara HJ. Cancer of the nasopharynx. Review of the literature. Report of 72 cases. *Laryngoscope.* 1969;79:1315-1329.

77. Perez CA, Ackerman LV, Mill WB, Ogura JH, Powers WE. Cancer of the nasopharynx. Factors influencing prognosis. *Cancer.* 1969;24:1-17.

78. Giffler RF, Gillespie JJ, Ayala AG, Newland JR. Lymphoepithelioma in cervical lymph nodes of children and young adults. *Am J Surg Pathol.* 1977;1:293-302.

79. Shanmugaratnam K, Chan SH, de-The G, et al. Histopathology of nasopharyngeal carcinoma: correlations with epidemiology, survival rates and other biological characteristics. *Cancer.* 1979;44:1029-1044.

80. Carbone A, Micheau C. Pitfalls in microscopic diagnosis of undifferentiated carcinoma of nasopharyngeal type (lymphoepithelioma). *Cancer.* 1982;50:1344-1351.

81. Wei WI, Sham JS. Nasopharyngeal carcinoma. *Lancet.* 2005;365:2041-2054.

82. Singhi AD, Stelow EB, Mills SE, Westra WH. Lymphoepithelial-like carcinoma of the oropharynx: a morphologic variant of HPV-related head and neck carcinoma. *Am J Surg Pathol*. 2010;34:800-805.
83. Stelow EB. A review of NUT midline carcinoma. *Head Neck Pathol*. 2011;5:31-35.
84. Stelow EB, Bellizzi AM, Taneja K, et al. NUT rearrangement in undifferentiated carcinomas of the upper aerodigestive tract. *Am J Surg Pathol*. 2008;32:828-834.
85. Stelow EB, French CA. Carcinomas of the upper aerodigestive tract with rearrangement of the nuclear protein of the testis (NUT) gene (NUT midline carcinomas). *Adv Anat Pathol*. 2009;16:92-96.
86. Agaimy A, Hartmann A, Antonescu CR, et al. SMARCB1 (INI-1)-deficient sinonasal carcinoma: a series of 39 cases expanding the morphologic and clinicopathologic spectrum of a recently described entity. *Am J Surg Pathol*. 2017;41:458-471.
87. Bourne TD, Bellizzi AM, Stelow EB, et al. p63 Expression in olfactory neuroblastoma and other small cell tumors of the sinonasal tract. *Am J Clin Pathol*. 2008;130:213-218.
88. Zamecnik M, Rychnovsky J, Syrovatka J. Sinonasal SMARCB1 (INI1) deficient carcinoma with yolk sac tumor differentiation: report of a case and comparison with INI1 expression in gonadal germ cell tumors. *Int J Surg Pathol*. 2018;26:245-249.
89. Madri JA, Barwick KW. An immunohistochemical study of nasopharyngeal neoplasms using keratin antibodies: epithelial versus nonepithelial neoplasms. *Am J Surg Pathol*. 1982;6:143-149.
90. Lauder I, Holland D, Mason DY, Gowland G, Cunliffe WJ. Identification of large cell undifferentiated tumours in lymph nodes using leucocyte common and keratin antibodies. *Histopathology*. 1984;8:259-272.
91. Shi SR, Goodman ML, Bhan AK, Pilch BZ, Chen LB, Sun TT. Immunohistochemical study of nasopharyngeal carcinoma using monoclonal keratin antibodies. *Am J Pathol*. 1984;117:53-63.
92. Chao TY, Chow KC, Chang JY, et al. Expression of Epstein-Barr virus-encoded RNAs as a marker for metastatic undifferentiated nasopharyngeal carcinoma. *Cancer*. 1996;78:24-29.
93. Cerilli LA, Holst VA, Brandwein MS, Stoler MH, Mills SE. Sinonasal undifferentiated carcinoma: immunohistochemical profile and lack of EBV association. *Am J Surg Pathol*. 2001;25:156-163.
94. Haack H, Johnson LA, Fry CJ, et al. Diagnosis of NUT midline carcinoma using a NUT-specific monoclonal antibody. *Am J Surg Pathol*. 2009;33:984-991.
95. Brandsma JL, Abramson AL. Association of papillomavirus with cancers of the head and neck. *Arch Otolaryngol Head Neck Surg*. 1989;115:621-625.
96. Brandsma JL, Steinberg BM, Abramson AL, Winkler B. Presence of human papillomavirus type 16 related sequences in verrucous carcinoma of the larynx. *Cancer Res*. 1986;46:2185-2188.
97. Chaturvedi AK, Engels EA, Anderson WF, Gillison ML. Incidence trends for human papillomavirus-related and -unrelated oral squamous cell carcinomas in the United States. *J Clin Oncol*. 2008;26:612-619.
98. Chernock RD, El-Mofty SK, Thorstad WL, Parvin CA, Lewis JS Jr. HPV-related nonkeratinizing squamous cell carcinoma of the oropharynx: utility of microscopic features in predicting patient outcome. *Head Neck Pathol*. 2009;3:186-194.
99. Cobo F, Talavera P, Concha A. Review article: relationship of human papillomavirus with papillary squamous cell carcinoma of the upper aerodigestive tract: a review. *Int J Surg Pathol*. 2008;16:127-136.
100. D'Souza G, Kreimer AR, Viscidi R, et al. Case-control study of human papillomavirus and oropharyngeal cancer. *N Engl J Med*. 2007;356:1944-1956.
101. El-Mofty SK. HPV-related squamous cell carcinoma variants in the head and neck. *Head Neck Pathol*. 2012;1(6 suppl):S55-S62.

102. El-Mofty SK, Lu DW. Prevalence of high-risk human papillomavirus DNA in nonkeratinizing (cylindrical cell) carcinoma of the sinonasal tract: a distinct clinicopathologic and molecular disease entity. *Am J Surg Pathol.* 2005;29:1367-1372.
103. El-Mofty SK, Lu DW. Prevalence of human papillomavirus type 16 DNA in squamous cell carcinoma of the palatine tonsil, and not the oral cavity, in young patients: a distinct clinicopathologic and molecular disease entity. *Am J Surg Pathol.* 2003;27:1463-1470.
104. Ernster JA, Sciotto CG, O'Brien MM, et al. Rising incidence of oropharyngeal cancer and the role of oncogenic human papilloma virus. *Laryngoscope.* 2007;117:2115-2128.
105. Fakhry C, Westra WH, Li S, et al. Improved survival of patients with human papillomavirus-positive head and neck squamous cell carcinoma in a prospective clinical trial. *J Natl Cancer Inst.* 2008;100:261-269.
106. Gillison ML, Koch WM, Capone RB, et al. Evidence for a causal association between human papillomavirus and a subset of head and neck cancers. *J Natl Cancer Inst.* 2000;92:709-720.
107. Jo VY, Mills SE, Stoler MH, Stelow EB. Papillary squamous cell carcinoma of the head and neck: frequent association with human papillomavirus infection and invasive carcinoma. *Am J Surg Pathol.* 2009;33(11):1720-1724.
108. Watson RF, Chernock RD, Wang X, et al. Spindle cell carcinomas of the head and neck rarely harbor transcriptionally-active human papillomavirus. *Head Neck Pathol.* 2013;7:250-257.
109. Kraft S, Faquin WC, Krane JF. HPV-associated neuroendocrine carcinoma of the oropharynx: a rare new entity with potentially aggressive clinical behavior. *Am J Surg Pathol.* 2012;36:321-330.
110. Thompson ED, Stelow EB, Mills SE, Westra WH, Bishop JA. Large cell neuroendocrine carcinoma of the head and neck: a clinicopathologic series of 10 cases with an emphasis on HPV status. *Am J Surg Pathol.* 2016;40:471-478.
111. Lewis JS Jr, Beadle B, Bishop JA, et al. Human papillomavirus testing in head and neck carcinomas: guideline from the college of American pathologists. *Arch Pathol Lab Med.* 2018;142:559-597.
112. Weiss LM, Movahed LA, Butler AE, et al. Analysis of lymphoepithelioma and lymphoepithelioma-like carcinomas for Epstein-Barr viral genomes by in situ hybridization. *Am J Surg Pathol.* 1989;13:625-631.
113. Iezzoni JC, Gaffey MJ, Weiss LM. The role of Epstein-Barr virus in lymphoepithelioma-like carcinomas. *Am J Clin Pathol.* 1995;103:308-315.
114. Young LS, Murray PG. Epstein-Barr virus and oncogenesis: from latent genes to tumours. *Oncogene.* 2003;22:5108-5121.

6

SALIVARY GLAND–TYPE NEOPLASMS

Salivary gland–type neoplasms can develop throughout the entire upper aerodigestive tract, likely because seromucinous glands underlie the epithelium throughout these structures. Although these neoplasms occur with different frequencies than they do in the major salivary glands, most of the vast variety of neoplasms that can involve the major salivary glands have been described involving the upper aerodgestive tract (Table 6.1).[1] While the oral cavity is the most common site of involvement, the neoplasms may be found throughout the entire tract and will need to be considered in differential diagnoses with biopsies from all sites.

The diagnosis of salivary gland–type neoplasms by small biopsy may be difficult, especially as many specific diagnoses require the histologic examination of the entire tumor. Furthermore, these tumors have a predilection for histologic heterogeneity and can show overlapping features. Nonetheless, many tumors can be given a definitive diagnosis on biopsy specimen allowing for proper therapy. For example, myoepithelioma can be distinguished from melanoma with immunohistochemistry, and adenoid cystic carcinoma can often be distinguished from basaloid squamous cell carcinoma based on histology alone.

BENIGN NEOPLASMS

Benign salivary gland–type tumors of the upper aerodigestive tract appear to be somewhat more common than their malignant counterparts; however, they comprise a smaller proportion of the total number of neoplasms than they do in the major salivary glands.[2–5] Many are pleomorphic adenomas; however, other types of adenomas and cystic or papillary neoplasms of the ducts also occur.

Pleomorphic Adenoma

Overall, pleomorphic adenoma or mixed tumor is the most common neoplasm of the seromucinous glands of the upper aerodigestive tract.[3,5] These tumors may develop in patients of any age and are somewhat more

TABLE 6.1 2017 WHO Classification of Epithelial Tumors of the Salivary Glands

Malignant Epithelial Tumors	Benign Epithelial Tumors
Acinic cell carcinoma	Pleomorphic adenoma
Mucoepidermoid carcinoma	Myoepithelioma
Adenoid cystic carcinoma	Basal cell adenoma
Polymorphous (low-grade) adenocarcinoma	Warthin tumor
Epithelial-myoepithelial carcinoma	Oncocytoma
Clear cell carcinoma	Canalicular adenoma
Basal cell adenocarcinoma	Sebaceous adenoma
Sebaceous adenocarcinoma	Lymphadenoma
Undifferentiated carcinoma	Sebaceous and nonsebaceous
Intraductal carcinoma	Ductal papillomas
(Mammary analogue) secretory carcinoma	Sialadenoma papilliferum
Oncocytic carcinoma	Cystadenoma
Salivary duct carcinoma	
Adenocarcinoma, not otherwise specified	
Myoepithelial carcinoma	
Carcinoma ex pleomorphic adenoma	
Carcinosarcoma	
Squamous cell carcinoma	
Small and large cell neuroendocrine carcinoma	
Lymphoepithelial carcinoma	
Sialoblastoma	

common in women. Within the upper aerodigestive tract, the tumors most commonly develop in the palate, likely secondary to the large number of seromucinous glands present at this site.

Grossly, the tumors are firm and appear circumscribed. They may be noted to be mobile; however, they can involve adjacent bone, as space for growth is limited throughout the upper aerodigestive tract.[6] Unlike their counterparts in the major salivary glands, these tumors rarely will have well-developed capsules. They should, however, remain without infiltrative margins (eFig. 6.1).[5,6]

Pleomorphic adenomas are especially known for their histologic heterogeneity and will display both epithelial and mesenchymal components.[3,5,6] The epithelial components show both true epithelial and myoepithelial differentiation. Architecturally, the epithelial cells often form

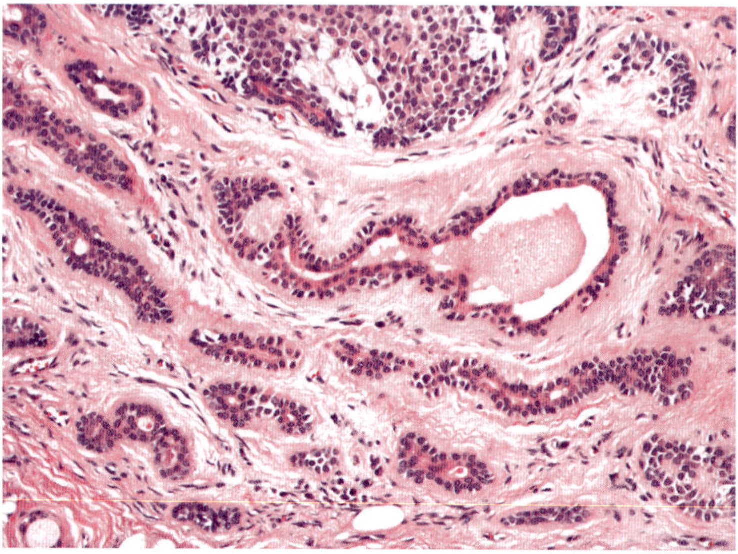

FIGURE 6.1 Glandular structures and groups of myoepithelial cells are usually seen with pleomorphic adenomas.

glandular structures with lumens (Fig. 6.1; eFig. 6.2). The architecture, however, can be complex and numerous anastomosing trabeculae, small tubular glands, nests, and single epithelioid cells can be present (eFig. 6.3). The epithelial cells may be columnar, cuboidal, squamous, plasmacytoid, oncocytoid, basaloid, clear, or spindled (eFig. 6.4). Most tumors have more than one epithelial cell type scattered throughout the lesion. The stromal elements may by myxoid, hyaline, chondroid, or even osseous (Fig. 6.2; eFig. 6.5). Both the mesenchymal and epithelial elements generally show bland cytology, and mitotic figures are rare. Pleomorphic adenomas of the seromucinous glands typically show a more cellular, myoepithelial phenotype than their counterparts in the major salivary glands and have less stromal elements.[5] Furthermore, in our experience, they often contain more prominent squamous differentiation.

The differential diagnosis for these lesions may include other salivary gland–type adenomas and malignancies such as polymorphous (low-grade) adenocarcinoma, adenoid cystic carcinoma, and, occasionally, mucoepidermoid carcinoma when a prominent squamous component is seen. The distinction between these neoplasms and other adenomas on biopsy is somewhat academic; however, even distinguishing them from malignancies is not always necessary as complete excision is recommended for all these lesions. This is the case as the benign tumors may recur without compete excision and even sometimes develop into or concomitantly harbor malignancies (carcinoma ex pleomorphic adenoma).

The immunohistochemical profile of pleomorphic adenomas depends somewhat on the dominant phenotype of the tumor, i.e., whether the

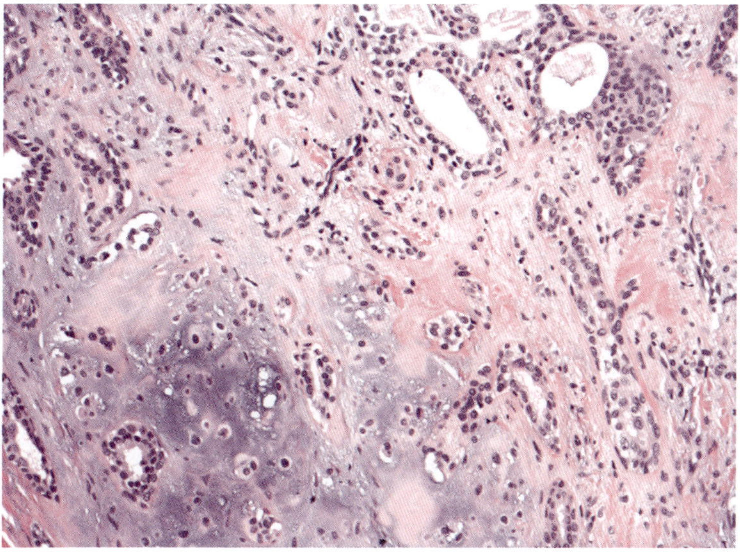

FIGURE 6.2 The stromal components of pleomorphic adenomas of the upper aerodigestive tract are less abundant than in pleomorphic adenomas of the major salivary glands.

tumor shows mostly epithelial, myoepithelial, or mesenchymal differentiation.[7] Most of the epithelial components will express various cytokeratins and show variable degrees of myoepithelial differentiation with expression of smooth muscle actin (SMA), calponin, S100, and glial fibrillary acidic protein (GFAP), CD10 and p63 (eFig. 6.6).[6–9]

Many pleomorphic adenomas have been shown to harbor karyotypic abnormalities with frequent abnormalities involving 8q12 and the long arm of chromosome 12.[10,11] These abnormalities correspond with the PLAG1 and HMGA2 genes, respectively, two genes involved in transcription.[12–14] Both proteins can be shown to be overexpressed in some pleomorphic adenomas by immunohistochemistry.

The distinction between pleomorphic adenomas and polymorphous (low-grade) adenocarcinomas or even adenoid cystic carcinomas can be difficult on biopsy, especially when the particular pleomorphic adenoma is very cellular. The identification of a mesenchymal component would be indicative of a pleomorphic adenoma whereas the identification of perineural invasion or infiltration of surrounding tissues would be indicative of a polymorphous (low-grade) adenocarcinoma or adenoid cystic carcinoma. Pleomorphic adenomas almost always behave in a benign fashion and rarely recur.[6,15]

Other Adenomas

Other benign salivary gland–type epithelial tumors also may develop throughout the upper aerodigestive tract. These primarily include myoepitheliomas and canalicular adenomas; however, basal cell adenomas and sebaceous adenomas also have been described. One should note that malignancy is usually determined by overall infiltration with these neoplasms and that the unequivocal diagnosis of benignancy cannot always be made based on small biopsies.

Canalicular adenomas most often involve the upper lip.[16–18] They are usually solitary and multilobulated. They are rarely larger than 2 cm and are usually described as painless. The tumors are circumscribed but most do not have capsules. Microscopically, long rows or columns of cuboidal to columnar epithelial cells interweave throughout the tumors and lead to a "beaded" canalicular pattern (Fig. 6.3; eFig. 6.7). Cellular atypia and mitotic figures are rare (eFig. 6.8). The entrapped stroma is pink and often contains many small capillaries. Epithelial antigen expression can be detected by immunohistochemistry as can the expression of S100 protein and SOX10.[19] Other markers of myoepithelial differentiation such as actins or p63 are not expressed.[20] After excision, the tumors rarely recur.

Myoepitheliomas resemble pleomorphic adenomas grossly and clinically but microscopically lack epithelial architecture and a significant mesenchymal component (other than myxoid stroma) (Fig. 6.4).[21–23] In other words, they are composed entirely of myoepithelial cells. The myoepithelial cells can show a variety of histologic appearances but are usually categorized as epithelioid, spindled, plasmacytoid (rhabdoid), or clear cell (Fig. 6.5; eFigs. 6.9–6.11). The tumors can have a variable cellularity, and some tumors may have a prominent myxoid background. Immunohistochemically, the cells express cytokeratins and will show some degree of myogenous or basal differentiation that can be demonstrated with antibodies to SMA, calponin, S100, SOX10, GFAP, p40, or p63, although more specific markers of myogenous differentiation are

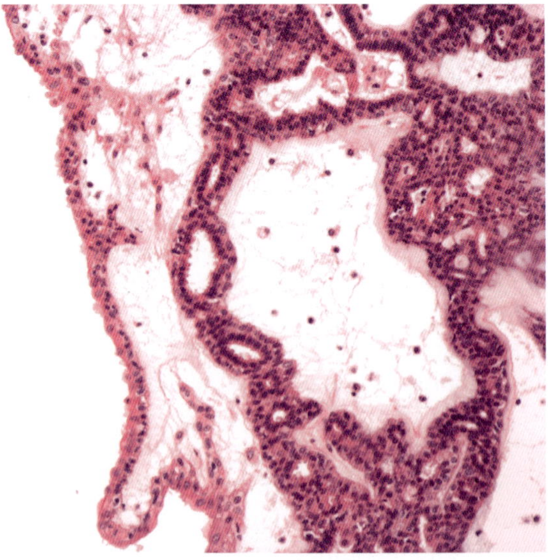

FIGURE 6.3 Ribbons of bland cuboidal cells are seen with this canalicular adenoma.

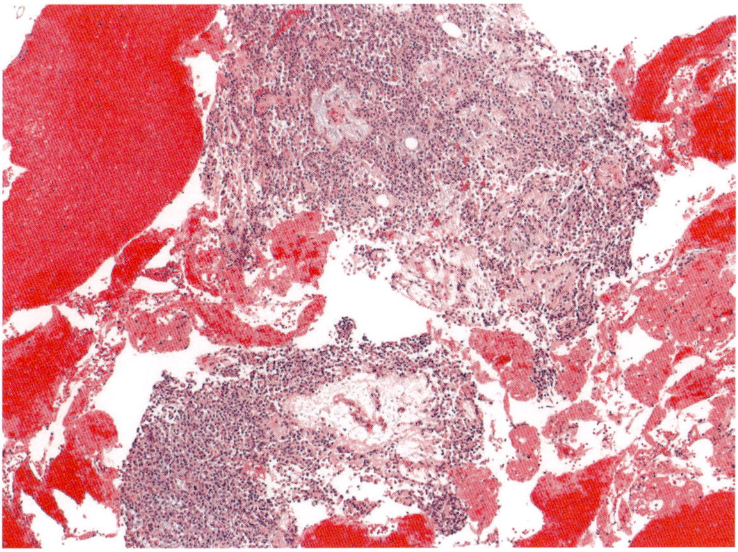

FIGURE 6.4 Fragments of a myoepithelioma seen on biopsy. Infiltration cannot be excluded with such a sample.

sometimes not seen, especially with the plasmacytoid variant (Fig. 6.6; eFigs. 6.12–6.14).[8,22–26] A minority of tumors have been shown to harbor EWSR1 translocation similar to soft tissue myoepithliomas and clear cell carcinomas.[27] Surgical resection should attempt to achieve free margins and the tumors only rarely recur.[21,23]

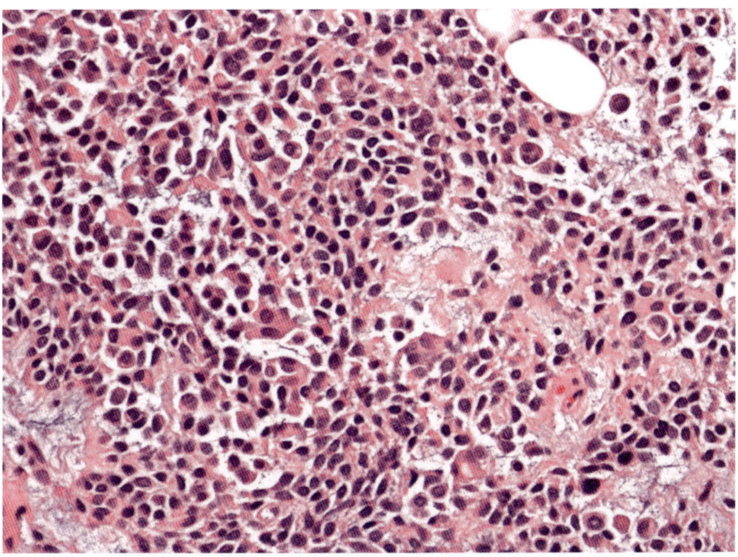

FIGURE 6.5 Myoepitheliomas are typically composed of plasmacytoid, monomorphic cells.

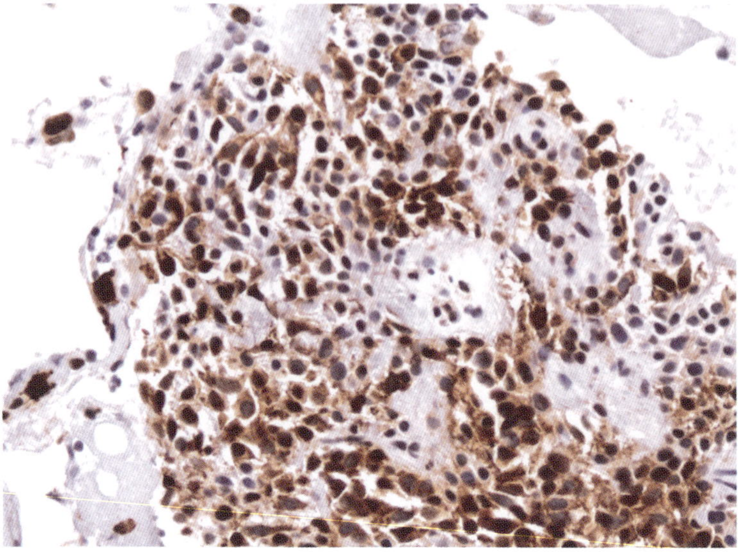

FIGURE 6.6 Strong immunoreactivity with antibodies to S100 protein was seen with this myoepithelioma myoepitheliomas.

The differential diagnosis for myoepitheliomas depends on the histologic phenotype. The plasmacytoid variant must be distinguished from melanoma and plasmacytoma, which can be done by showing epithelial or myogenous differentiation. Antibodies more specific for melanoma or plasmacytoma antigens such as HMB-45 or CD138, respectively, may also be helpful. Spindle cell myoepitheliomas have a broad differential diagnosis including numerous mesenchymal tumors (e.g., nodular fasciitis, schwannoma, neurofibroma, solitary fibrous tumor, melanoma, etc). Antibodies to epithelial antigens or p63 may be helpful, as may antibodies more specific to some of the mesenchymal tumors in the differential diagnosis (e.g., CD34 for solitary fibrous tumors). Finally, clear cell myoepitheliomas must be differentiated from other clear cell tumors (see below). To distinguish myoepithelioma from myoepithelial carcinoma, one must rely on both cytologic features and growth pattern (see below).

Many reported cases of *basal cell adenoma* of the upper aerodigestive tract appear to have been canalicular adenomas and some authors consider canalicular adenoma simply to be a variant of basal cell adenoma.[28,29] Indeed, in reviewing the literature, it is actually difficult to calculate the number of basal cell adenomas that involved the upper aerodigestive tract that did not have a canalicular pattern. It appears that even if basal cell adenomas are distinguished from canalicular adenomas, basal cell adenomas still most frequently involve the lip when they involve the upper aerodigestive tract.[6]

Grossly, basal cell adenomas are well circumscribed.[30] Histologically, they are composed of basaloid cells that grow as somewhat organoid nests (the solid pattern), trabeculae, and tubules (Fig. 6.7; eFigs.

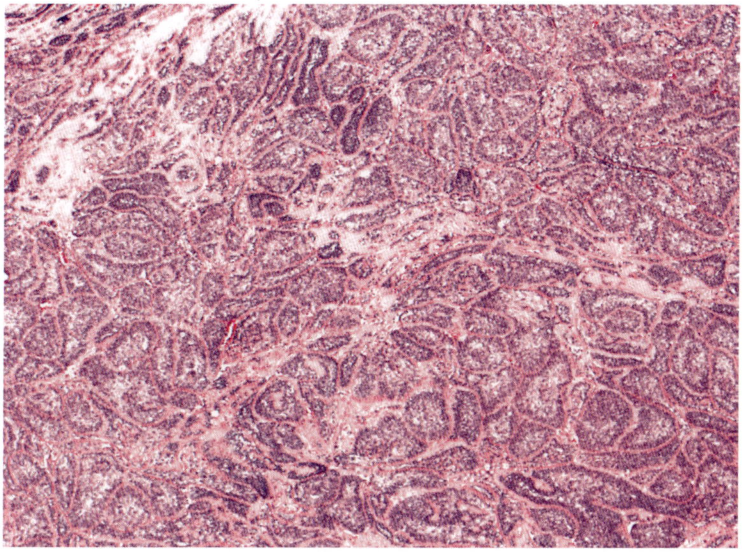

FIGURE 6.7 Organoid nests of basaloid cells are seen with basal cell adenomas.

6.15 and 6.16).[6,30–33] A variable amount of moderately cellular stroma is present between the aggregates of basaloid cells. The basaloid cells themselves are bland cytologically and have scant cytoplasm (Fig. 6.8). Nuclear palisading is usually noted at the periphery of the epithelial structures, and some cells may have more abundant, eosinophilic cytoplasm and show overt squamous differentiation. Lumens may be seen within the epithelial nests and trabeculae and are often lined by columnar ductal cells. Some cases may have hyaline material surrounding the groups of basaloid cells (membranous-type or dermal analogue tumor). Immunohistochemically, all the cells will show immunoreactivity with antibodies to keratins; however, cells lining the apparent lumina stain most intensely.[34] Conversely, antibodies to S100 protein, SMA, and p63 highlight the peripheral cells that are juxtaposed to the connective tissues (eFig. 6.17). p63 will also highlight areas of squamous differentiation. c-kit expression can be seen with both basal cell adenomas and adenocarcinomas.[35] Immunostaining with antibodies to beta-catenin will show nuclear localization in most basal cell adenomas as the tumors often harbor *CTNNB1* mutations.[36]

Basal cell adenomas must be distinguished from other basaloid neoplasms such as basaloid squamous cell carcinomas, basal cell adenocarcinomas, and adenoid cystic carcinomas. Basaloid squamous cell carcinomas are high-grade, infiltrative malignancies with numerous mitotic figures and severe cytologic atypia. Basal cell adenocarcinomas are primarily distinguished from adenomas by their infiltrative borders, and thus the two cannot usually be distinguished on small biopsy. Adenoid cystic carcinomas

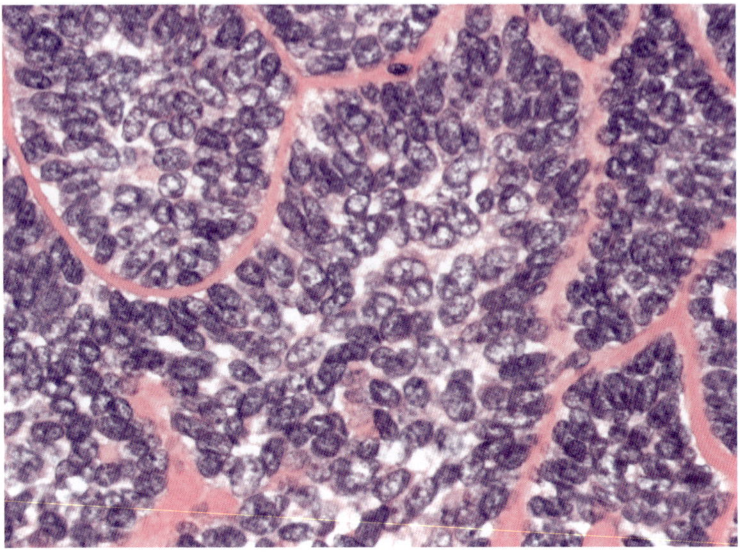

FIGURE 6.8 Basal cell adenomas are composed of bland cells with oval nuclei and vesicular chromatin.

are infiltrative, typically have perineural invasion, and many have higher grade cytology. Furthermore, a cribriform growth pattern is not often seen with basal cell adenomas. Aside from the membranous type, basal cell adenomas do very well and almost never recur after adequate resection.[6]

Papillomas

Papillary neoplasms of the salivary glands that cannot better be classified as other salivary gland–type neoplasms occur predominately within the seromucinous glands of the upper aerodigestive tract. These include inverted papillomas, intraductal papillomas, and the rare sialadenoma papilliferum.[37] These lesions are all benign and do not develop into malignancies.

Inverted papillomas occur most frequently in the mouth either at the lip or beneath the buccal mucosa.[37,38] These lesions present as nodules or swellings that typically measure approximately 1 cm in size. Grossly, they appear well circumscribed. Microscopically, these tumors appear to involve a large duct that may be seen to be in continuity with the surface epithelium (eFig. 6.18). The duct is filled and expanded by a papillary proliferation of predominately squamous epithelium with scattered mucous cells that is frequently covered by columnar cells (eFig. 6.19). This squamous epithelium shows maturation without atypia and usually does not keratinize (Fig. 6.9). True infiltration of the stroma should not be seen and if identified should raise the question of a malignancy.

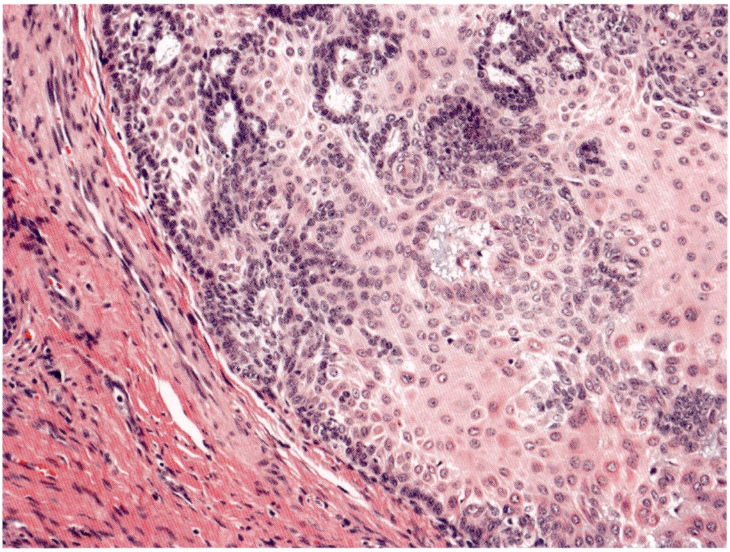

FIGURE 6.9 Inverted papillomas are well circumscribed and composed of maturing, stratified squamous epithelium.

Intraductal papillomas also most frequently involve the lip or buccal mucosa.[37] The lesions present as swellings or nodules and usually measure about 1 cm in size. Microscopic examination shows a large duct lumen distended by arborizing papillae that are lined by a single layer of cuboidal to columnar epithelium with occasional mucous cells, all devoid of cytologic atypia.

Sialadenoma papilliferum is extremely rare and most often involves the palate of middle-aged to older individuals.[37,39] The lesions usually appear somewhat verrucoid or papillary grossly. The papillary structures are covered at the tips by a thickened and often keratotic squamous epithelium (Fig. 6.10). Lining the sides of these papillae and separating one from another is ductal epithelium that is often two cells thick (eFigs. 6.20 and 6.21). These epithelial cells may appear somewhat oncocytic and can show tufting. The ducts extend into the stroma and branch. Some degree of chronic inflammation is usually noted within the stroma. Tumors frequently have *BRAF*V600E or *HRAS* mutations except in cases where the ductal components appear oncocytic.[40]

Other Benign Neoplasms

Cystadenomas represent between 5% and 10% of benign salivary gland–type neoplasms of the upper aerodigestinve tract and often involve the lips, buccal mucosa, and palate.[5] The age range of patients with these lesions is large, and about twice as many occur in women. Nodular and cystic spaces can be seen on cut section.[6,41] Histologically, the cysts are lined by a cuboidal or columnar epithelium (Fig. 6.11; eFig. 6.22). Mucinous,

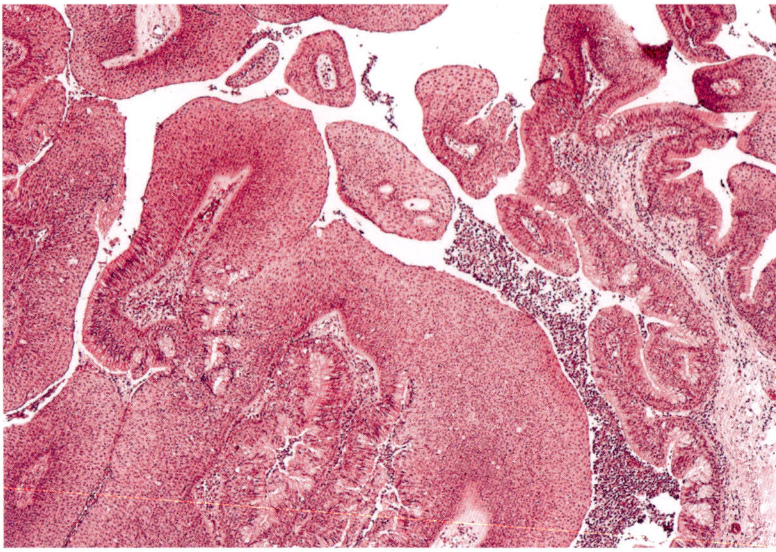

FIGURE 6.10 Numerous papillae lined by a stratified squamous epithelium are seen with this sialadenoma papilliferum.

oncocytic and squamous epithelia have all been described. The cytologically bland epithelium varies in thickness and papilla can often be found. Some cystadenomas have been noted to involve the larynx. Here, they have been noted to have a bland oncocytic epithelium often with papillae.[42,43]

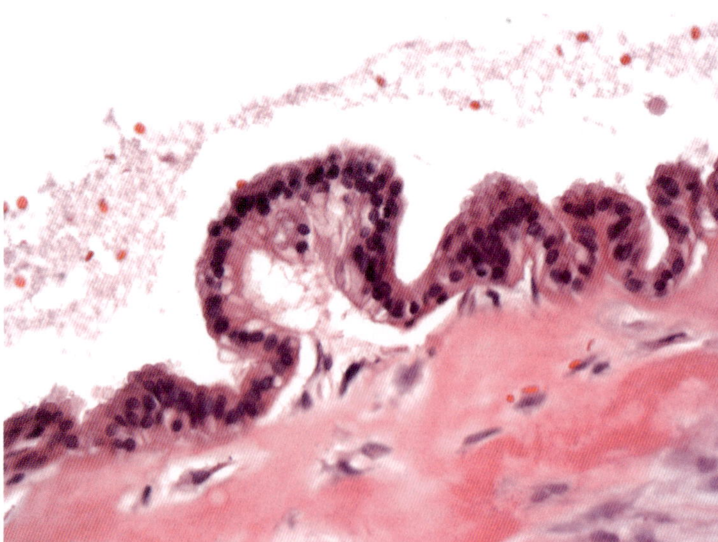

FIGURE 6.11 Cystadenomas typically have bland, mucinous epithelial cells.

Other benign salivary gland–type tumors described in the upper aerodigestive tract include *sebaceous adenomas* and oncocytic proliferations, including *oncocytomas*.[44,45] Lesion similar in appearance to *Warthin tumors* have been described also here.[46] These tumors share the histologic features of those tumors described in the major salivary glands.

MALIGNANT NEOPLASMS

Malignant salivary gland–type tumors occur in the upper aerodigestive tract somewhat less frequently than benign neoplasms.[5,44] As with benign tumors, these lesions most often develop in the palate, where there is a great abundance of seromucinous glands. The malignancies occur with a somewhat different frequency than they do in the major salivary glands with adenoid cystic carcinomas, mucoepidermoid carcinomas, and polymorphous (low-grade) adenocarcinomas predominating. Some tumors that occur here, such as polymorphous (low-grade) adenocarcinomas and clear cell carcinomas, rarely occur in the major salivary glands. The tumors show histologic overlap with one another, with benign salivary gland–type neoplasms, and with other malignancies. A specific diagnosis may be difficult or impossible with small biopsies. Some methods for distinguishing the neoplasms are discussed.

Adenoid Cystic Carcinoma

Adenoid cystic carcinoma is usually listed as the second most common malignant salivary gland–type neoplasm of the seromucinous glands of the upper aerodigestive tract.[44] They occur anywhere throughout the tract but most often involve the palate.[5,47,48] They show no sex predilection and may involve patients of any age, although they usually present in middle-aged or older patients. The tumors are often painful, possibly because they frequently show perineural invasion. Patients with adenoid cystic carcinomas do rather poorly and are at a very high (up to 85%) risk for recurrence.[49] Although the disease is somewhat indolent, it is almost always deadly, and up to 90% of patients die within 15 years of their diagnosis. Adenoid cystic carcinomas also often metastasize to distant locations, especially the lung, unlike most other salivary gland malignancies.

Grossly, the tumors may appear deceptively circumscribed while they are, in fact, quite infiltrative. Microscopically, the tumors show three characteristic growth patterns: cribriform, tubular, and solid (Fig. 6.12).[47,48] Most tumors show some mixture of these patterns. The cribriform pattern is the most common and is characterized by nests and larger islands of epithelioid cells, which contain numerous punched out circular spaces. These spaces may contain a basophilic, somewhat frothy material or dense eosinophilic material (Fig. 6.13; eFigs. 6.23 and 6.24). The frothy basophilic material may also be seen within the surrounding stroma. The stroma may appear hyalinized and can resemble the eosinophilic material

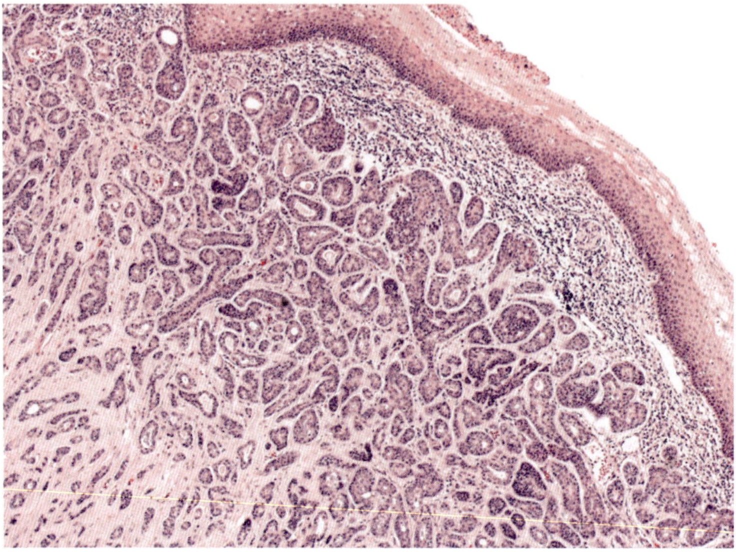

FIGURE 6.12 Adenoid cystic carcinomas are composed of nests and tubules of basaloid cells.

found within the cystic spaces that is believed to be basal lamina. The individual neoplastic cells are small with angulated nuclei (eFig. 6.25). Cytoplasm is usually scant and may vary from basophilic to eosinophilic to clear. Small nucleoli may be present, and apoptotic and mitotic figures are

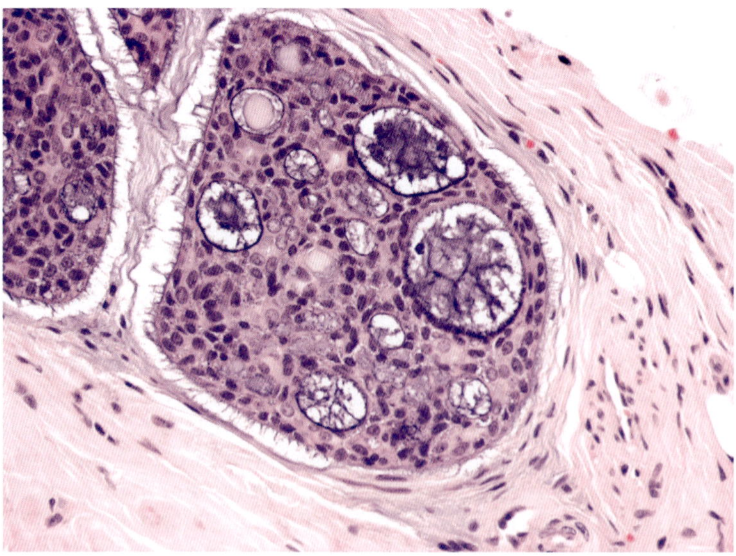

FIGURE 6.13 Adenoid cystic carcinomas often have a cribriform architecture with frothy basophilic or dense eosinophilic material within the cystic spaces.

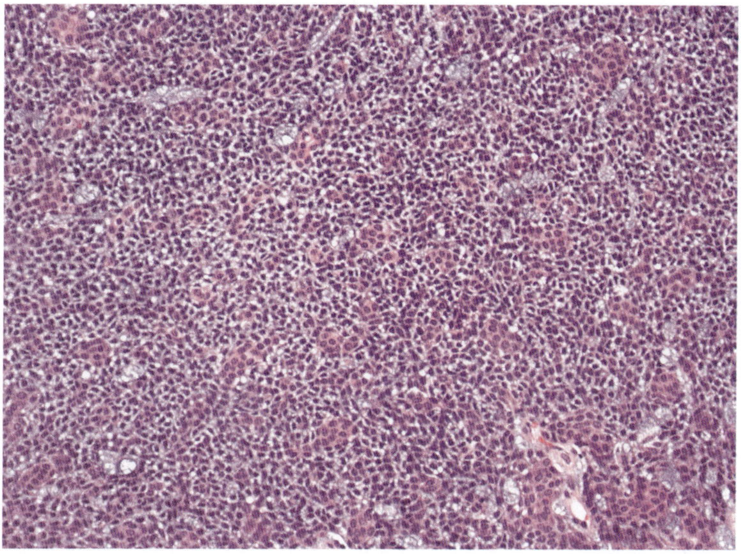

FIGURE 6.14 Some adenoid cystic carcinomas have a solid architecture.

usually infrequent. Rare ductal structures may be seen with all histologic patterns and are lined by epithelial cells. The tubular pattern of growth often is composed of cells that tend to show more distinct epithelial or myoepithelial differentiation, and the tubules will contain the same materials noted previously. Finally, the solid pattern is composed of variably sized nests of basaloid cells with no or very few cystic spaces (Fig. 6.14). This pattern is considered to be higher grade than the others, and apoptotic figures, mitotic figures, and even comedo-type necrosis may be seen (some tumors that have been described as such may actually be other tumors, however, e.g., basaloid squamous cell carcinoma and salivary duct carcinoma).[47] All patterns typically infiltrate the surrounding stroma and perineural invasion can almost always be identified (Fig. 6.15; eFig. 6.26).

The grading of adenoid cystic carcinomas is probably of no use with biopsy, although it may be important at resection.[50] Some studies, however, have shown that tumors with any solid components (grade 2) or with more than 30% solid component (grade 3) are associated with higher mortality rates.[51] We believe that grading may be of limited use and that many reports discussing its predictive value predate the widespread recognition of polymorphous (low-grade) adenocarcinoma and basaloid squamous cell carcinoma.

Adenoid cystic carcinomas rarely undergo high-grade transformation or "dedifferentiation." Of the 17 cases reported in two larger series, 11 originated in the upper aerodigestive tract, most often in the sinonasal area.[52,53] For such a diagnosis, a conventional component of adenoid cystic carcinoma must be present with a high-grade carcinoma. The high-grade component typically lacks the biphasic differentiation seen with conventional

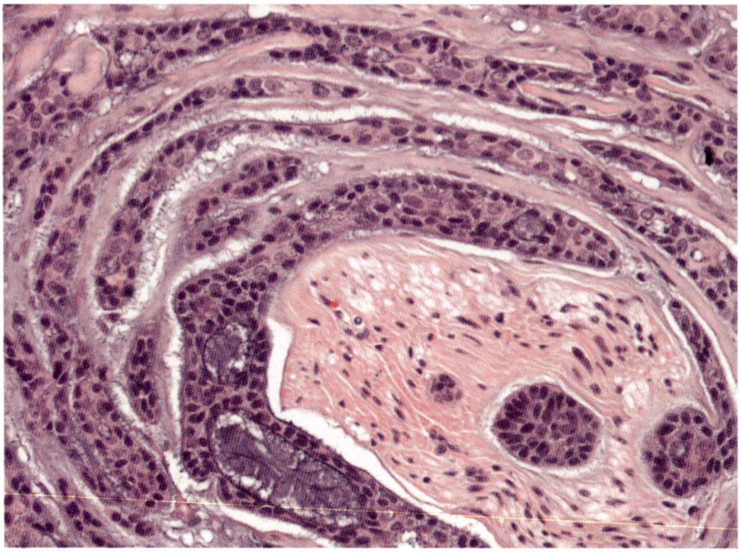

FIGURE 6.15 Perineural invasion is almost always seen with adenoid cystic carcinomas.

adenoid cystic carcinoma and can show squamous differentiation (Fig. 6.16). This can be demonstrated with immunohistochemistry as myoepithelial staining is typically lost. The high-grade component most frequently grows as solid sheets or nests, although cribriform, and micropapillary

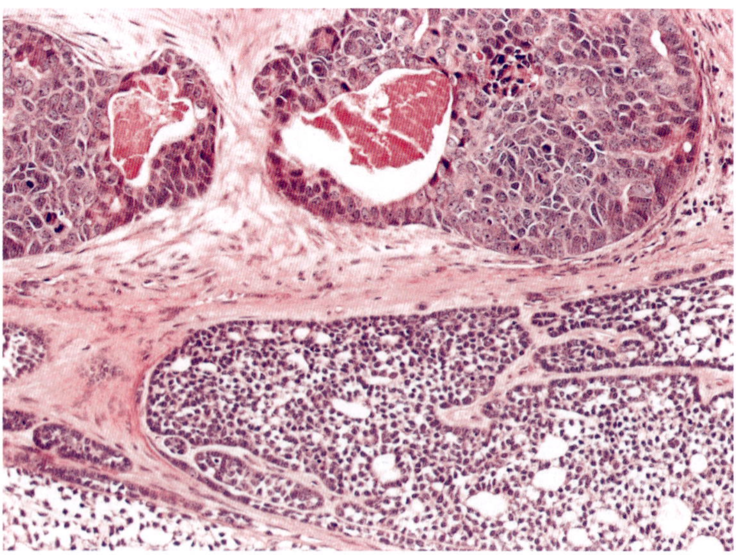

FIGURE 6.16 Areas of conventional cribriform adenoid cystic carcinoma (bottom) contrast with the transformed high-grade carcinoma (top).

growth has been described. Individual cells are enlarged and pleomorphic with atypical nuclei that have vesicular chromatin and prominent nucleoli. Numerous mitotic figures are present with necrosis, including comedoform necrosis within the large nests of neoplastic cells. Unlike with conventional adenoid cystic carcinoma, lymph node metastases develop in half the cases showing high-grade transformation; thus, some suggest lymph node dissections may be warranted for these patients.

By immunohistochemistry, neoplastic cells show myoepithelial and epithelial differentiation and react with antibodies to p63, S100, SMA, and pancytokeratin.[20,54,55] The staining patterns reflect the differentiation of the various cells with the peripheral cells (those juxtaposed to the stroma) showing mostly myoepithelial differentiation (eFigs. 6.27 and 6.28). Some cells within the solid and cribriform nests also show myoepithelial differentiation including those surrounding the apparent ducts. Other ducts, however, have a more epithelial phenotype and do not express myogenous antigens. The trabecular components show a much more obvious biphenotypic differentiation with the outer cells showing a myoepithelial phenotype and the inner cells showing an epithelial phenotype. The tumors are sometimes strongly immunoreactive for antibodies to c-kit (expressed by the more epithelial cells) which may be useful for distinguishing the tumors from other neoplasms, especially polymorphous (low-grade) adenocarcinomas (Fig. 6.17).[35,56] Solid patterns have been noted to show more diffuse immunoreactivity. This antibody cannot be used outside of histologic context, however, and we do not believe that it provides for definitive distinction of salivary gland–type tumors in and of itself.

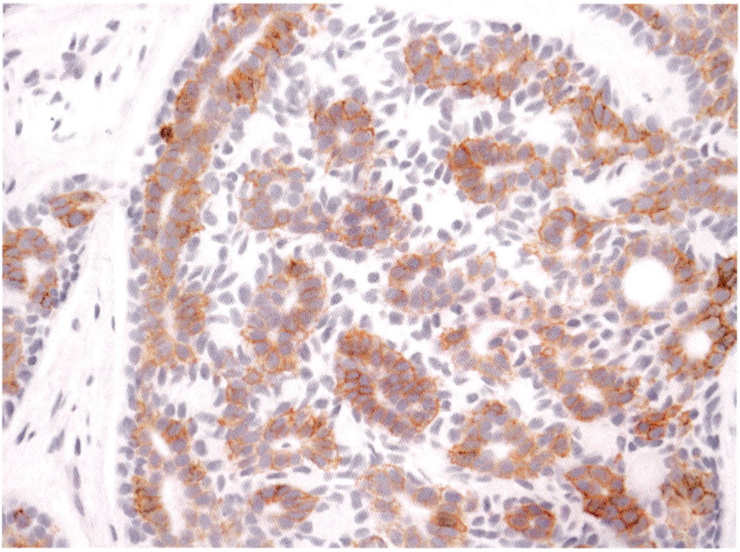

FIGURE 6.17 c-kit immunoreactivity is usually limited to the more epithelial cells in adenoid cystic carcinoma.

Approximately two-thirds of adenoid cystic carcinomas have been shown to have a recurrent cytogenetic abnormality, the t(6;9) (q22-23;p23-24) that juxtaopposes the *MYB* and *NFIB* genes.[57–60] This results in the expression of the MYB-NFIB fusion protein which can be demonstrated with immunohistochemistry in more than 80% of adenoid cystic carcinomas (including those apparently lacking the translocation) using antibodies to MYB. Unfortunately, other tumors in the differential diagnosis also stain positive, including most basaloid squamous cell carcinomas.[59] Although the tumors are often strongly reactive with antibodies to c-kit, molecular abnormalities of its gene have not been noted and the tumors have not been found to be responsive to tyrosine kinase inhibitors.[61]

The differential diagnosis for adenoid cystic carcinoma can be extensive and includes other salivary gland and basaloid neoplasms (Table 6.2). On biopsy, the most important distinction is with basaloid squamous cell carcinoma (as discussed in Chapter 5). This is because preoperative radiation and neck dissection may be employed with basaloid squamous cell carcinoma but should not be used with most adenoid cystic carcinomas. Although much time is spent with biopsies trying to distinguish adenoid cystic carcinomas from polymorphous (low-grade) adenocarcinomas, it may not always be necessary. The distinction will be discussed, however, below. Adenoid cystic carcinoma must also be distinguished from HPV-related multiphenotypic sinonasal carcinoma.[62] These tumors occur in the sinonasal tract and can appear morphologically and immunohistochemically similar to adenoid cystic carcinomas. The tumors, however, show a wider spectrum of growth (see below), p16 expression and HR-HPV infection.

Polymorphous (Low-Grade) Adenocarcinoma

Polymorphous (low-grade) adenocarcinoma occurs almost exclusively in the seromucinous glands of the upper aerodigestive tract, most commonly in the palate.[63] It occurs over a broad age range, most often in older individuals. The tumors develop more frequently in women and blacks. These lesions usually present as painless masses or "swellings." Unlike adenoid cystic carcinomas, polymorphous (low-grade) adenocarcinomas are not very aggressive. Up to one-third of patients may have recurrences, and

TABLE 6.2 **Differential Diagnosis of Adenoid Cystic Carcinoma**
Polymorphous (low-grade) adenocarcinoma
Pleomorphic adenoma
Basal cell adenoma/adenocarcinoma
Epithelial-myoepithelial carcinoma
Basaloid squamous cell carcinoma

unlike patients with adenoid cystic carcinomas, some may develop lymph node metastases (usually solitary).[64] Reports of mortality have varied from very low (<1%) to nearly 15%.[63,64] Rarely, these tumors have been noted to transform into high-grade carcinomas.[65,66]

Grossly, polymorphous (low-grade) adenocarcinoma is indistinct and is usually described as yellow to tan, firm and circumscribed.[63,64,67] Consistent with its appellation, these tumors show various growth patterns microscopically throughout individual lesions. These patterns include solid, trabecular, ductal, cribriform, tubular, and cystic formations sometimes with intracystic papillae (Figs. 6.18 and 6.19; eFigs. 6.29–6.31). Concentric whirling around a nidus, often a nerve, is characteristically seen. Although the tumors appear grossly circumscribed, they frequently infiltrate surrounding seromucinous glands and stromal tissues, and perineural invasion is commonly seen (eFig. 6.32). Individual tumor cells are monomorphic, round to polygonal, and usually have a scant to moderate amount of eosinophilic cytoplasm although more oncocytic cells, clear cells, and mucin-containing cells may sometimes be seen (Fig. 6.20; eFig. 6.33). The nuclei are bland, round to oval with vesicular chromatin, and usually have inconspicuous nucleoli. Mitotic figures and necrosis are rare. These tumors are not usually associated with abundant stroma, although focal hyaline or myxoid stroma may be seen.

It can be difficult to distinguish polymorphous (low-grade) adenocarcinoma from other salivary gland–type neoplasms especially on small biopsy. Many pleomorphic adenomas will be stroma poor and show growth patterns similar to polymorphous (low-grade) adenocarcinoma. Infiltration

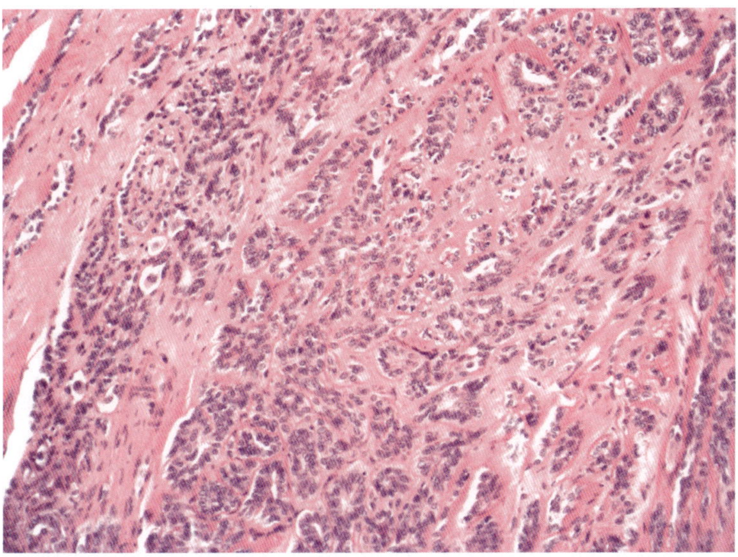

FIGURE 6.18 This polymorphous (low-grade) adenocarcinoma has a prominent tubular pattern.

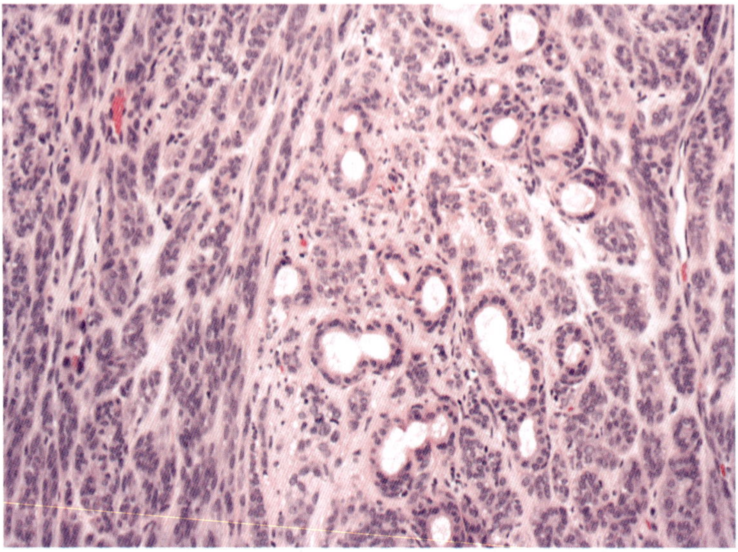

FIGURE 6.19 The tubules seen with polymorphous (low-grade) adenocarcinomas can appear similar to those of adenoid cystic carcinomas.

of the surrounding stromal tissue or perineural invasion should not be seen with pleomorphic adenomas, however. As this may not be seen on smaller biopsy specimens, some cases may require less definitive diagnoses with some discussion of the differential diagnosis.

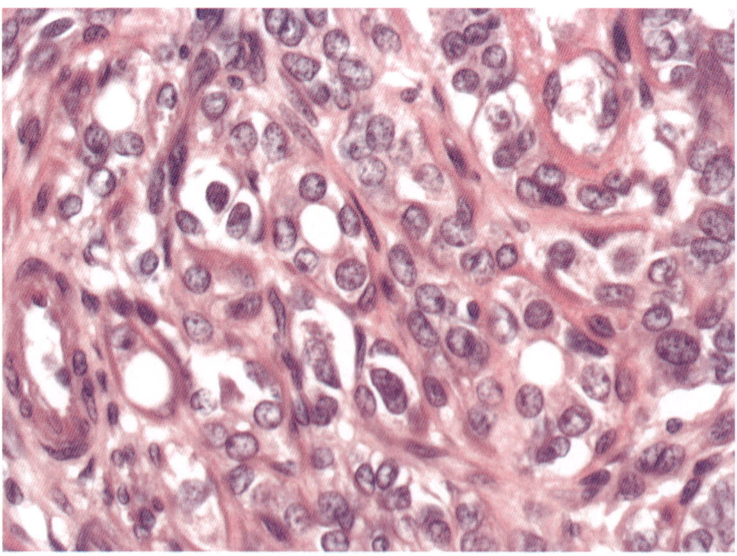

FIGURE 6.20 The nuclei of polymorhous (low-grade) adenocarcinomas are usually larger and more oval than those of adneoid cystic carcinomas. Their chromatin is also more open and vesicular.

Polymorphous (low-grade) adenocarcinomas can also be particularly difficult to distinguish from adenoid cystic carcinomas, especially those which have predominately tubular growth patterns (Table 6.3). Polymorphous (low-grade) adenocarcinomas usually show more heterogeneity in their growth patterns and cytologic features while adenoid cystic carcinomas tend to have smaller and more angulated nuclei. The identification of mitotic figures can also be helpful as polymorphous (low-grade) adenocarcinomas should have virtually none, whereas a few mitotic figures can be seen with adenoid cystic carcinomas (this can also be demonstrated by immunostaining for proliferative activity and polymorphous [low-grade] adenocarcinomas usually have mib-1/ki67 staining indices of less than 5%). Immunohistochemistry may be helpful here as adenoid cystic carcinomas have been shown much more likely to stain with antibodies to c-kit (eFig. 6.34).[35,56] Negative staining, however, is not particularly helpful. The staining pattern for polymorphous (low-grade) adenocarcinomas with other antibodies showed marked overlap with adenoid cystic carcinomas and epithelial, and myoepithelial differentiation is frequently identified with antibodies to keratins, S100 protein, p63, and SMA (eFig. 6.35).[8,68,69] That said, the typical biphasic staining seen with many adnoid cystic carcinomas is usually not seen with polymorphous (low-grade) adenocarcinomas. Occasional authors have noted that staining with antibodies to vimentin may be helpful as polymorphous (low-grade) adenocarcinomas show immunoreactivity whereas adenoid cystic carcinomas do not.[68,70]

A tumor similar to polymorphous (low-grade) carcinoma (indeed, it is unclear if it is its own tumor) has recently been described affecting the minor salivary glands, typically the tongue.[71] The authors have termed it "cribriform adenocarcinoma." Of the 23 described in one series, 14 involved the tongue and the others all involved other locations within the mouth. The tumors were much more aggressive than typical polymorphous (low-grade) adenocarcinomas, and more than 60% had lymph node metastases at presentation. Histologically, the tumors were covered by intact squamous epithelium and had infiltrative borders. The tumor cells grew as solid, cribriform, microcystic, and tubular structures (Fig. 6.21). Tumor cells had a moderate to abundant amount of clear to eosinophilic cytoplasm. The nuclei frequently overlapped with mild atypia and had vesicular chromatin that often appeared "cleared out" similar to the nuclei of papillary thyroid carcinoma. Immunohistochemical results were similar to those seen with typical polymorphous (low-grade) adenocarcinomas with a few caveats. These tumors were more likely to show immunoreactivity with antibodies to c-kit and were frequently immunoreactive with antibodies to p16 (although testing for human papillomavirus was consistently negative). While polymorphous (low-grade) adenocarcinomas have been shown to have frequent PRKD1 mutations, cribriform adenocarcinomas have frequent translocations involving PRKD1-3.[72,73]

TABLE 6.3 Adenoid Cystic Carcinoma vs Polymorphous (Low-Grade) Adenocarcinoma

	ACC	PLGA
Clinical	Involves both the major salivary glands and upper aerodigestive tract	Almost exclusively involves the upper aerodigestive tract, especially the palate More common in women and blacks
Architecture	Solid, cribriform, or tubular Infiltrative Perineural invasion is common	Solid, trabecular, ductal, cribriform, tubular, cystic, and papillary Infiltrative Perineural invasion is common
Cytology	Small, monomorphic cells with scant eosinophilic cytoplasm Smaller, more angulated, hyperchromatic nuclei Occasional mitotic figures can be present	Small cells with scant cytoplasms and sometimes larger cells with more abundant eosinophilic cytoplasm Round to oval nuclei with open chromatin Mitotic figures are uncommon
IHC	Variable reactivity with antibodies to myoepithelial and epithelial antigens Can show reactivity with antibodies to c-kit in solid or epithelial components No vimentin immunoreactivity	Variable reactivity with antibodies to myoepithelial and epithelial antigens but staining is not biphasic Mostly does not show reactivity with antibodies to c-kit Vimentin immunoreactivity
Behavior	Aggressive Almost always recurs Almost never metastasizes to lymph nodes Frequently metastasizes to lungs Often results in the death of the patient	Not aggressive Can recur Can metastasize to lymph nodes Rarely metastasizes distally Rarely results in the death of the patient

ACC, adenoid cystic carcinoma; IHC, immunohistochemistry; PLGA, polymorphous (low-grade) adenocarcinoma.

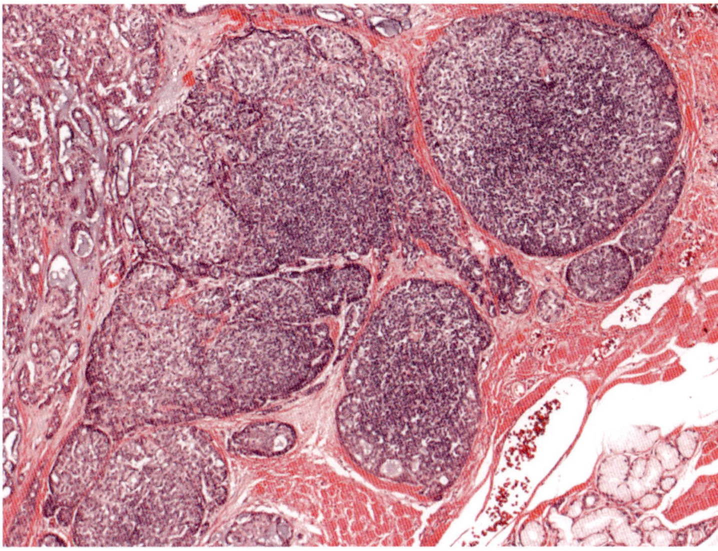

FIGURE 6.21 Solid nests of this "cirbriform adencarcinoma" of the tongue infiltrate the stromal tissues.

Mucoepidermoid Carcinoma

Mucoepidermoid carcinoma is notorious for affecting individuals of any age and is the most common salivary gland malignancy in both children and adults. Although it is slightly more common in the major salivary glands, it still represents a significant portion of salivary gland–type neoplasms that involve the seromucinous glands the upper aerodigestive tract. As with other salivary gland–type neoplasms, mucoepidermoid carcinomas most frequently involve the mouth, specifically the palate.[74–76] The tumors for the most part behave well, and less than 15% of patients have recurrences or metastases; fewer than 5% to 10% of patients will die from their tumors.[74,77] More than 60% of mucoepidermoid carcinomas have the t(11;19)(q21;p13), that creates an MECT1/MAML2 fusion protein.[78,79] The frequency of the translocation is higher in lower grade tumors.

Mucoepidermoid carcinomas are noncircumscribed and invasive.[75,76] They show varying proportions of mucous, basaloid, squamous, intermediate, oncocytic, and clear cells which themselves show varying degrees of differentiation (Figs. 6.22–6.25; eFigs. 6.36–6.40).[74,75] The tumors grow as solid and/or cystic masses. Mucous cells are simply epithelial cells that contain mucin and have pale, eosinophilic foamy cytoplasm. These can appear somewhat like goblet cells or even signet ring cells. Intermediate cells are smaller cells with more basophilic cytoplasm. Squamoid (or epidermoid) cells are larger than intermediate cells and have more abundant and eosinophilic cytoplasm. These cells are often round or ovoid but can

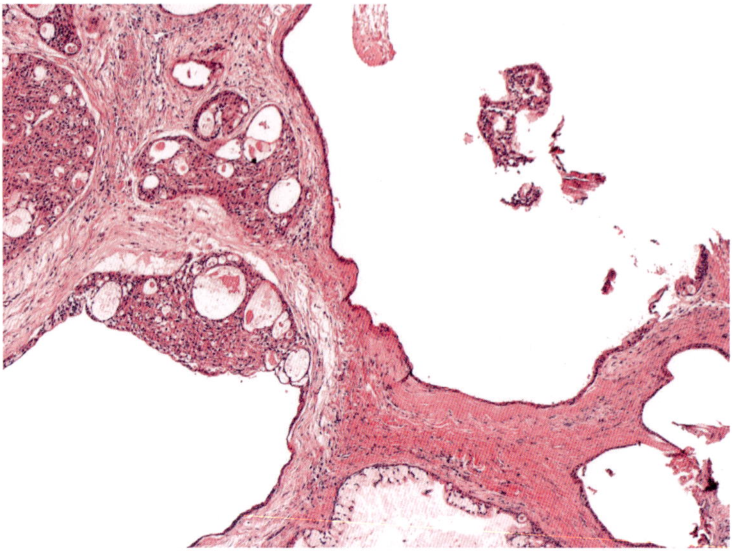

FIGURE 6.22 Low-grade mucoepidermoid carcinomas are cystic with mucinous and epidermoid cells easily seen at low power.

become polygonal and more obviously squamoid in appearance. Clear cells are large and polygonal and resemble squamous cells but for their clear cytoplasm. Mucus can be demonstrated within the mucus cells or within cystic spaces with histochemical staining. Clear cells, however, do

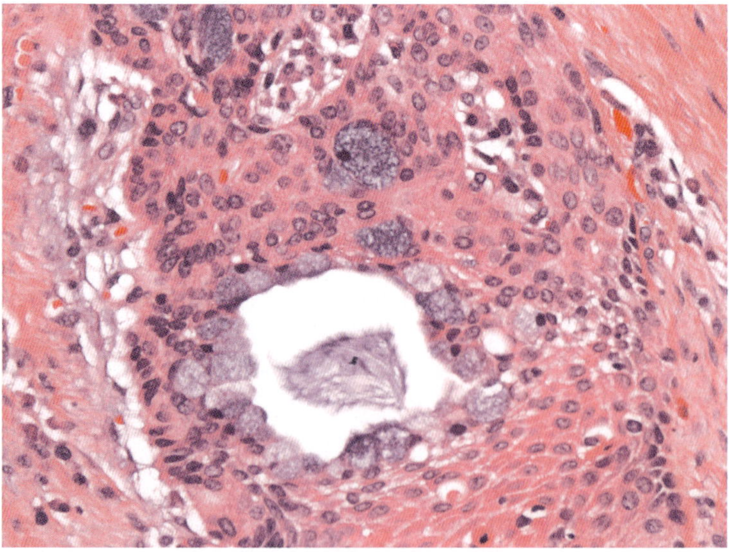

FIGURE 6.23 Mucinous and epidermoid cells are intimately intermixed in mucoepidermoid carcinomas.

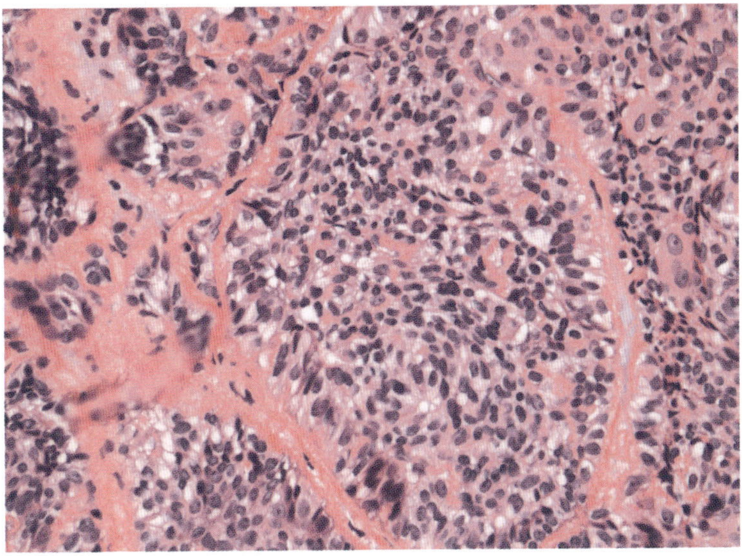

FIGURE 6.24 This solid area in a mucoepidermoid carcinoma has numerous transitional cells.

not contain mucus but instead contain glycogen. Although cytologic atypia and mitotic activity are uncommon, both may be occasionally seen and generally denote a higher grade tumor.

A number of grading systems for mucoepidermoid carcinomas have been proposed that take into account growth pattern (solid vs. cystic) and histologic characteristics (proportions of cell types, mitotic rate, cellular

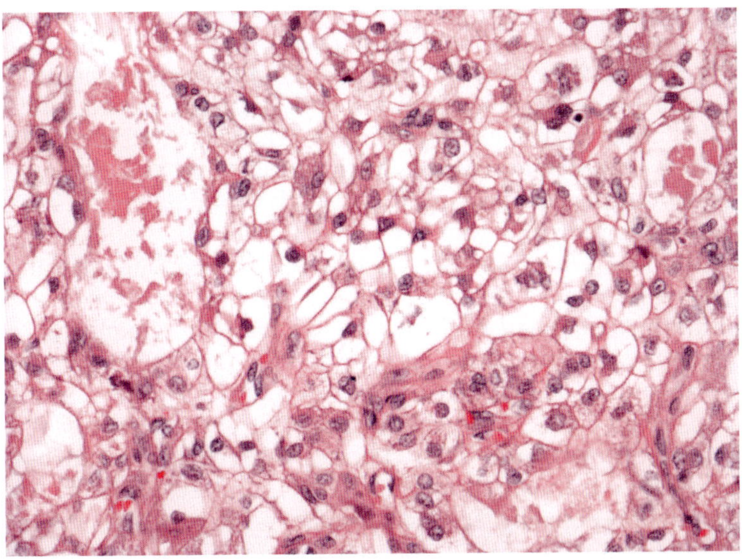

FIGURE 6.25 Clear cells are frequently seen in mucoepidermoid carcinomas.

TABLE 6.4 Grading of Mucoepidermoid Carcinoma

	Characteristic Features	Defining Features
Grade 1	Prominent goblet cell component Cyst formation Intermediate cells may be prominent Circumscribed growth pattern	Lack of grade 3 defining features Lack of aggressive invasion
Grade 2	Intermediate cells predominate over mucinous cells Mostly solid Squamous cell may be seen	Aggressive invasion pattern Lack of grade 3 defining features
Grade 3	Squamous cells predominate Mostly solid	Necrosis Perineural spread Vascular invasion Bony invasion >4 mitotic figures/10 hpf High-grade nuclear pleomorphism

Scoring System: Intracystic component <25%; tumor front invades in small nests or islands; pronounced nuclear atypia; angiolymphatic invasion; bony invasion; >4 mitotic figures/10 hpf; perineural spread; necrosis.

Grade 1, no features; grade 2, one feature; grade 3, two or more features.

anaplasia, vascular invasion, neural invasion, and the pattern of infiltration).[74,80,81] A somewhat recently proposed grading system has been shown to have better reproducibility than others with good predictability (Table 6.4).[81] With most grading systems, low-grade mucoepidermoid carcinomas, when completely excised, have virtually no risk for recurrence. Higher grade tumors can carry up to a 63% risk for cervical metastases and roughly the same mortality rate.[74]

The tumors must be distinguished from adenosqamous carcinomas (see Chapter 5) as those tumors have a much worse prognosis. Immunohistochemistry is rarely needed for diagnostic reasons. Histochemistry can sometimes be used to demonstrate intracellular and extracellular mucins (e.g., periodic acid–Schiff [PAS], mucicarmine, etc.) (Fig. 6.26; eFig. 6.41). Mucoepidermoid carcinomas do not express myoepithelial antigens and such staining may be helpful in cases with abundant clear cells in which other salivary gland–type tumors with myoepithelial phenotypes may be considered.[82,83] Interestingly, immunoreactivity with antibodies to MUC1 and HER-2/neu has been associated with higher grade tumors.[84,85]

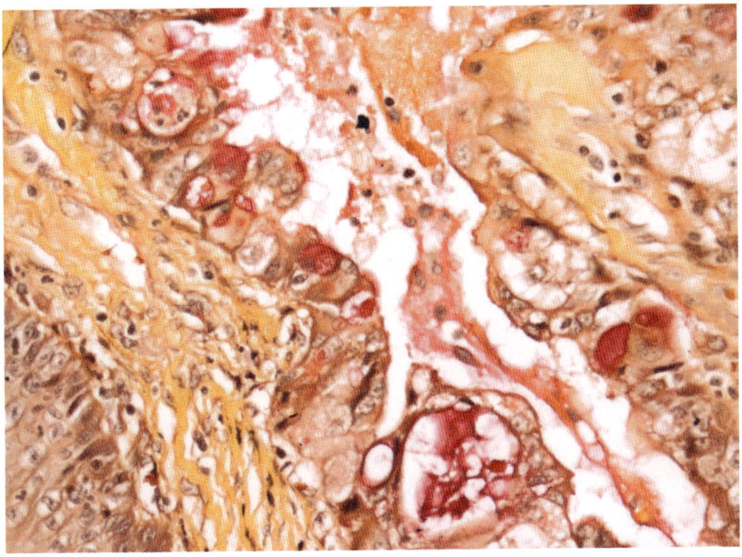

FIGURE 6.26 A mucicarmine stain can be used to highlight intracellular mucin.

Acinic Cell Carcinoma

Outside of the major salivary glands, particularly the parotid gland, acinic cell carcinomas are relatively uncommon, and they represent between 1 and 10% of salivary gland–type malignancies of the upper aerodigestive tract.[86-89] The tumors develop over a wide age range and occur slightly more often in women. Although they occur throughout the tract, they have most often been noted in the mouth and have primarily involved the lips, buccal mucosa, and palate. The tumors recur approximately one-third of the time; however, patients rarely die from disease.

Acinic cell carcinomas usually present as swellings or nodules and are noted to be circumscribed and rubbery.[86-89] Cystic change is sometimes noted. They can display a wide range of architectural patterns including solid, cystic, papillary-cystic, and follicular patterns (Figs. 6.27 and 6.28; eFigs. 6.42 and 6.43). Most of the neoplastic cells should have acinic or serous differentiation and be polyhedral with abundant granular basophilic cytoplasm and small, hyperchromatic nuclei (Fig. 6.29; eFigs. 6.44 and 6.45). Vacuolated, clear, and ductal cells are also sometimes noted. Features of a high-grade malignancy such as necrosis, anaplasia, and increased mitotic activity should not be seen in conventional acinic cell carcinomas; however, dedifferentiation has been described.[90] Also, focal atypia, characterized by hypercellularity, nuclear enlargement, and prominent nucleoli, can sometimes be seen and correlates with an increased risk for recurrence.[89]

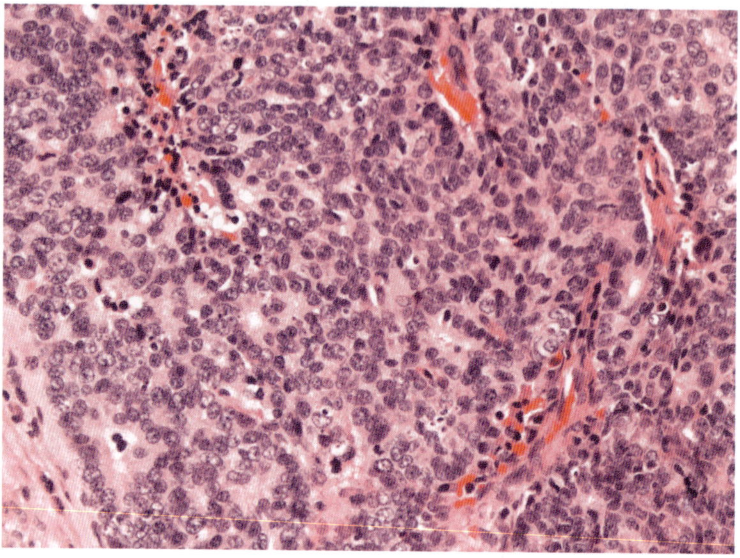

FIGURE 6.27 Acinic cell carcinomas are usually solid and obviously form acini.

The acinic cells contain PAS-positive diastase-resistant granules.[89] By immunohistochemistry, the acinic cells are immunoreactive with antibodies to cytokeratins and DOG1.[91,92] Myoepithelial antigens are not expressed although most tumors do express SOX10.[25,55] Only a small percentage of cases will react with antibodies to amylase.[93] Loss of heterozygosity studies

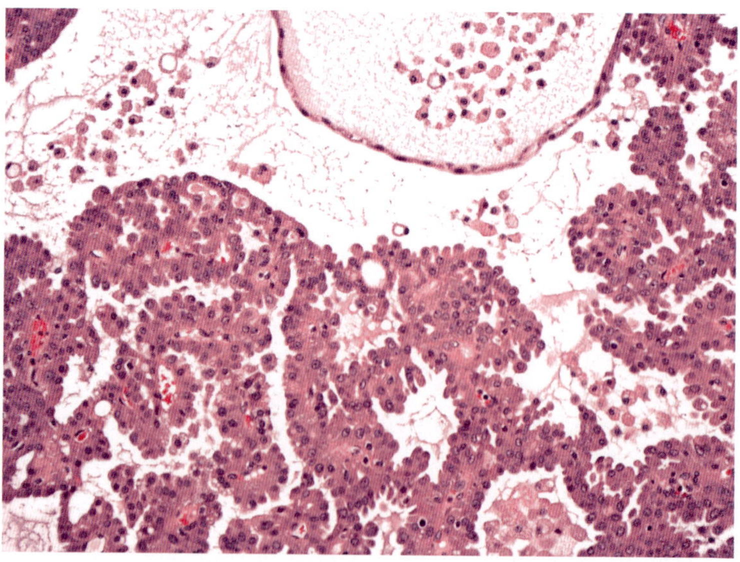

FIGURE 6.28 Some acinic cell carcinomas are papillary and cystic.

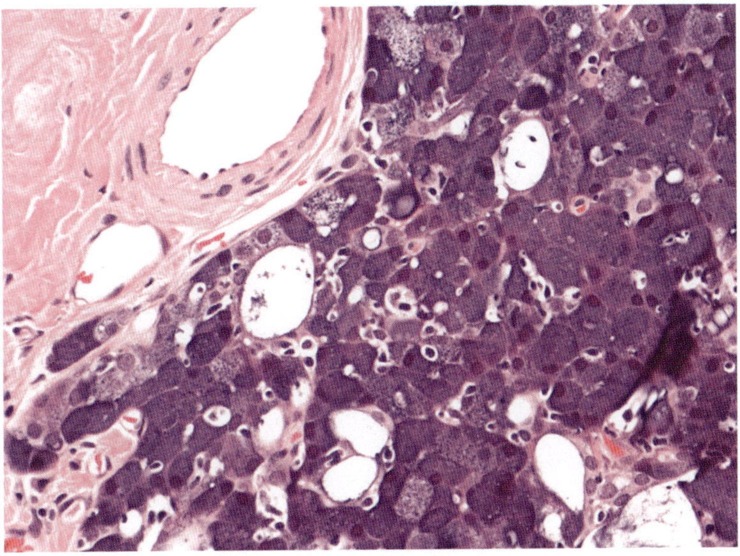

FIGURE 6.29 Large, polygonal cells with abundant granular, basophilic cytoplasm are seen in acinic cell carcinomas.

have shown losses at 4p15-16, 6p25-qter, and 17p11.[94] Tumors frequently show *NR4A3* rearrangements and uncommonly show *HTN3-MSANTD3* translocations.[95,96] (Mammary analogue) secretory carcinoma, a tumor often previously classified as acinic cell carcinoma, is discussed below.

(Mammary Analogue) Secretory Carcinoma

(Mammary analogue) secretory carcinoma is a salivary gland malignancy characterized by a t(12;15) (p13;q25) that juxtaposes the *ETV6* and *NTRK3* genes, similar to that seen in breast secretory carcinomas.[97,98] Of the 16 cases reported in a large series, three involved the upper aerodigestive tract, all within the mouth. The tumors occurred about equally in both sexes and over a broad age range.[98] Nearly half of the patients with follow-up developed metastases or recurrent disease.

Histologically, the tumors are circumscribed or lobulated with intervening fibrous septa (Fig. 6.30). They are composed of microcystic, tubular, and solid structures (Fig. 6.31). Neoplastic cells have pink granular or vacuolated cytoplasm with low-grade nuclei that have vesicular chromatin and small, sometimes distinct nucleoli. Necrosis, prominent atypia, and serous acinar differentiation are not seen. Neoplastic cells are immunoreactive with antibodies to CK7, S100, GCDFP-15 (most cases), and mammaglobin. Myoepithelial differentiation is not seen and tumors do not express DOG1.[92]

Epithelial-Myoepithelial Carcinoma

Epithelial-myoepithelial carcinomas are rare biphasic malignancies.[99–101] Overall, about 25% of these malignancies involve the upper aerodigestive tract, frequently in the sinonasal area or mouth. As with many salivary

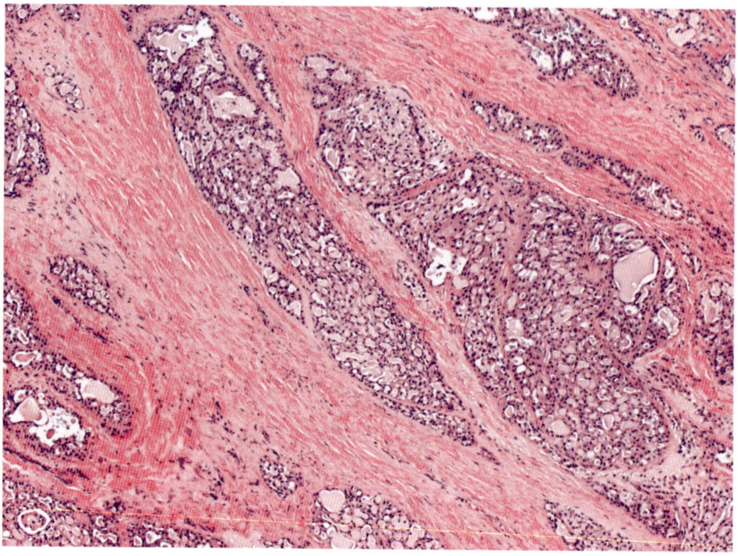

FIGURE 6.30 Fibrous bands separate lobules of tumor in this (mammary analogue) secretory carcinoma.

gland–type tumors, the age range of the patients is wide; however, most patients are older and the mean age is about 60 years. There is a female predominance. Although about one-third of the tumors have been noted to recur, less than 10% of patients have died of disease.[99,101]

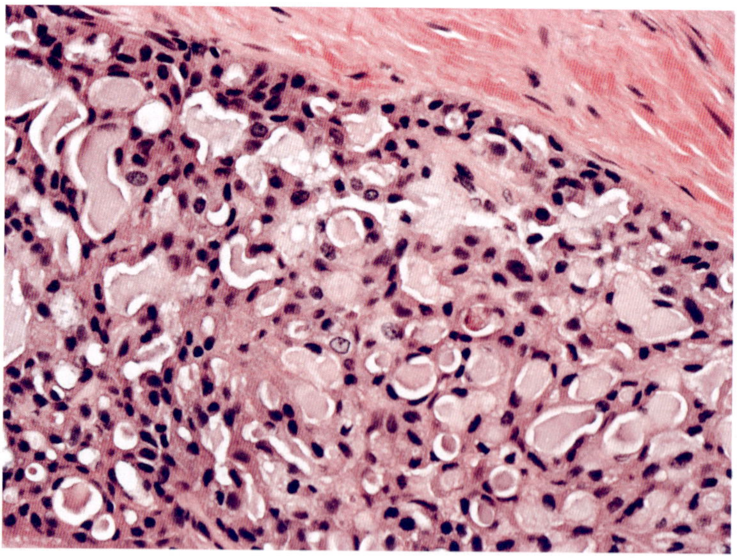

FIGURE 6.31 Smalls cysts and tubules surrounded by mildly atypical epithelial cells are characteristic of (mammary analogue) secretory carcinoma.

Grossly, tumors are nodular or infiltrative, and some are even noted to be completely encapsulated.[99,100] Histologically, the tumors have a classic biphasic appearance with tubules and trabeculae lined by an outer layer of myoepithelial cells and an inner layer of epithelial cells (Fig. 6.32; eFigs. 6.46 and 6.47). Solid areas are present, and these are almost always composed of myoepithelial cells, sometimes with marked atypia ("anaplasia") (eFig. 6.48). Although most myoepithelial cells will have clear cytoplasm, they have also been noted to have amphophilic cytoplasm or to appear oncocytic. The epithelial cells are usually noted to be lightly eosinophilic and to appear reminiscent of intercalated ducts. The epithelial cells have also been noted to be have clear cytoplasm or to appear oncocytic or mucinous. Squamous and sebaceous differentiation has also been noted. Most cases have only mild nuclear atypia, although severe nuclear atypia has been noted in both the myoepithelial and epithelial components (Fig. 6.33; eFig. 6.49). About one-third of cases have perineural invasion, and approximately 10% exhibit angiolymphatic invasion. Calcifications and necrosis can also be seen. The tumors have rarely been noted to "dedifferentiate," and in such cases, mitotic activity is noted to be much increased.

Immunohistochemistry can be used to highlight the epithelial and myoepithelial components of these tumors.[99,100] The epithelial cells will almost universally show strong and diffuse immunoreactivity with antibodies to keratins which often also lightly stain the myoepithelial cells (Fig. 6.34; eFig. 6.50). Antibodies to p63, S100, SMA, and vimentin have

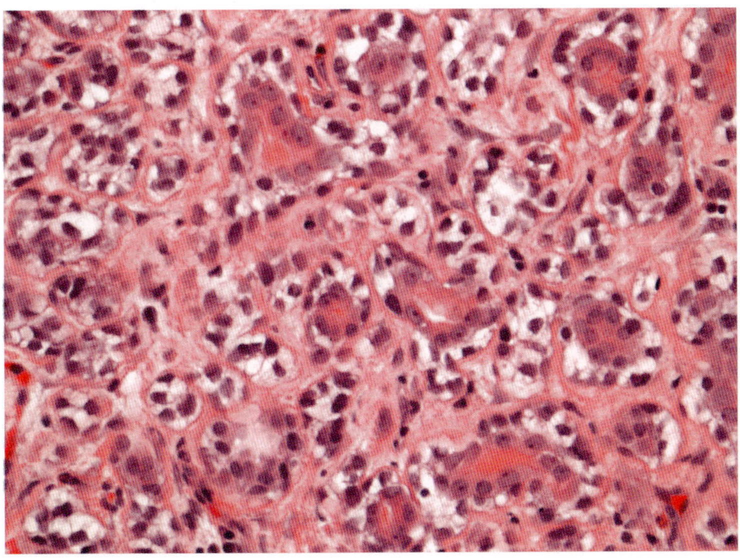

FIGURE 6.32 The epithelial and myoepithelial cells are readily identified in this epithelial-myoepithelial carcinoma.

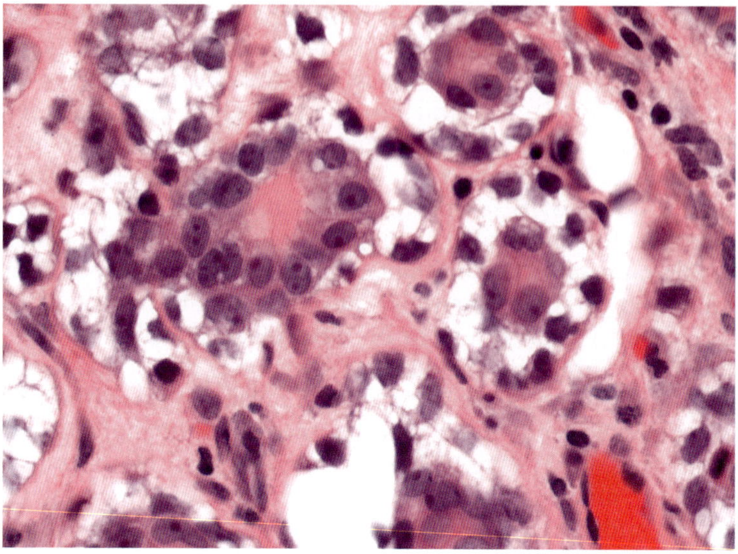

FIGURE 6.33 Only mild cellular and nuclear atypia is seen in this epithelial-myoepithelial carcinoma.

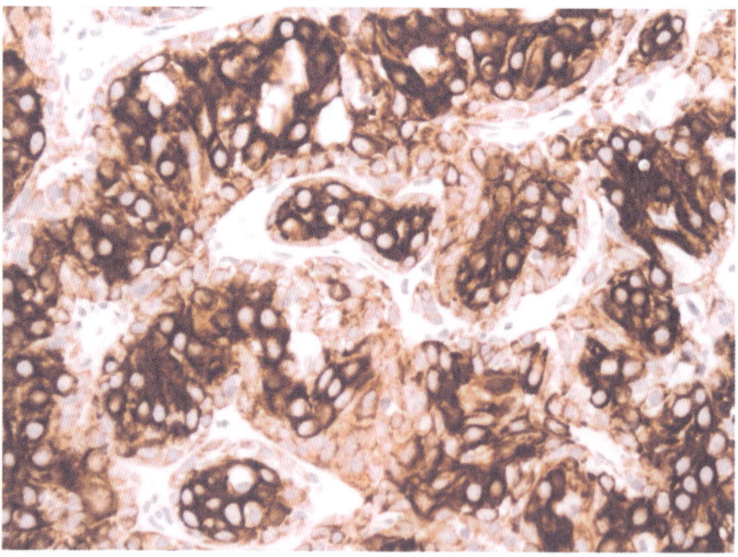

FIGURE 6.34 Both the epithelial and myoepithelial cells will be immunoreactive with antibodies to cytokratins, although the myoepithelial cells usually stain more weakly.

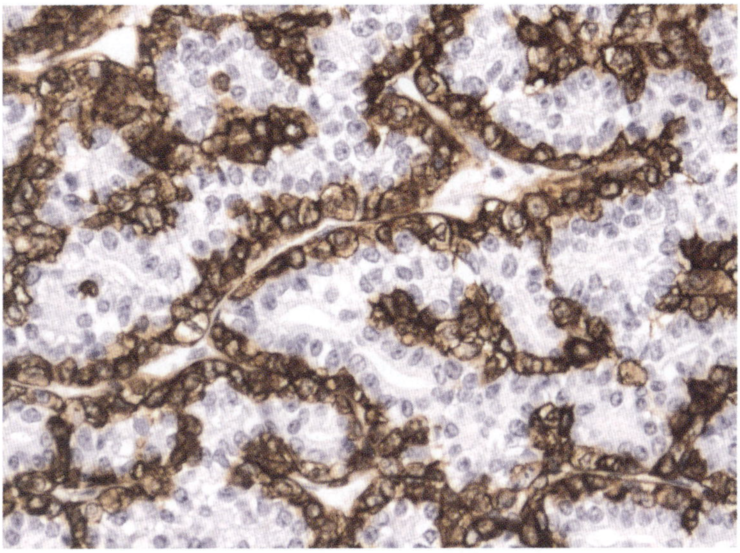

FIGURE 6.35 The myoepithleial cells of this epithelial-myoepithelial carcinoma are nicely highlighted with a smooth muscle actin (SMA) immunostain.

been noted to demonstrate the myoepithelial components well (Fig. 6.35; eFigs. 6.51 and 6.52). Immunoreactivity with antibodies to c-kit has been noted in up to 70% of cases and is localized to the epithelial cells (eFig. 6.53).[99]

(Hyalinizing) Clear Cell Carcinoma

Many tumors involving the upper aerodigestive tract, especially salivary gland–type tumors, can show clear cell change (Table 6.5).[102–104] Such neoplasms can usually be distinguished from one another by a thorough search throughout the lesion for more conventional areas. Occasionally, immunohistochemistry can help; however, indefinite diagnoses may sometimes be required with small biopsies.

TABLE 6.5 **Salivary Gland–Type Tumors That May Have a Clear Cell Morphology**
Clear cell carcinoma
Epithelial-myoepithelial carcinoma
Clear cell myoepithelioma/myoepithelial carcinoma
Acinic cell carcinoma
Oncocytoma
Mucoepidermoid carcinoma

Hyalinizing clear cell carcinoma is a clear cell malignancy that has been distinguished from other salivary gland carcinomas.[105] It is considered to be a low-grade malignancy that behaves indolently even after metastasis. These lesions arise most commonly at the base of the tongue; however, they can be found throughout the upper aerodigestive tract and even rarely in the major salivary glands. The tumors are generally found in older individuals, most often women.

Grossly, these tumors have been described as firm and gray-white and are usually smaller than 3 cm in size.[105] The tumors have infiltrative borders that may be appreciated grossly or microscopically. They are composed of round to polygonal cells that have clear cytoplasm although occasional cells will have granular and eosinophilic cytoplasm (Fig. 6.36; eFigs. 6.54 and 6.55). The nuclei have irregular, indented contours with finely granular to coarse chromatin. Nucleoli are often noted; however, they are not prominent. Mitotic figures and necrosis are usually not seen. The neoplastic cells grow in trabeculae, cords, and nests which are separated and encircled by fibrous bands. Focally, the stroma may appear more myxoid and loose.

As was mentioned, many tumors may have clear cells. The most frequent differential diagnoses considered with these tumors are epithelial-myoepithelial carcinoma and myoepithelioma or myoepithelial carcinoma.[103] Unlike epithelial-myoepithelial carcinoma, hyalinizing clear cell carcinoma will not appear biphasic. Neoplastic cells fail to react with antibodies to SMA, MSA, and S-100 but do frequently show immunoreactivity with antibodies to p63. They will react with antibodies to

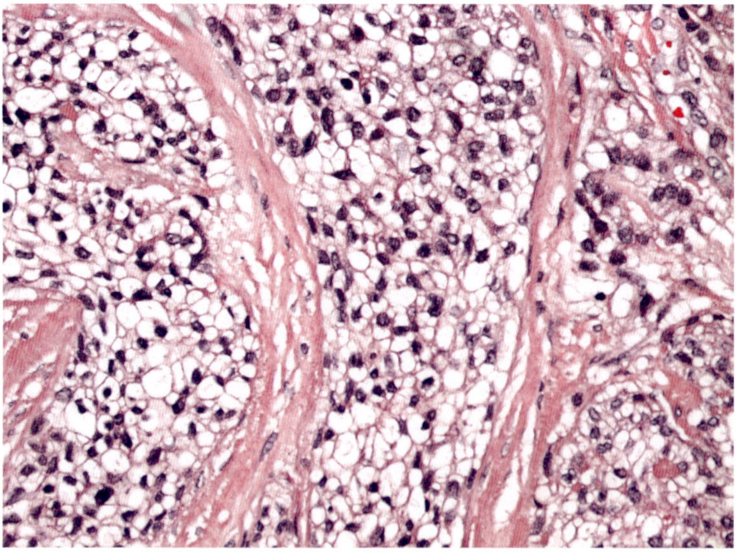

FIGURE 6.36 Islands of clear cells separated by fibrous bands are characteristically seen in hyalinizing clear cell carcinomas.

cytokeratins and do contain PAS-positive material that is diastase sensitive (glycogen).[105] Others have shown mucin positivity in some cases.

It has been shown that more than 80% of these tumors harbor translocations involving *EWSR1*, almost always partnering with *ATF1*.[106] This is especially interesting as the same translocation has been identified in many of the so-called "soft tissue myoepithelial tumors." Furthermore, nearly identical translocations have also been identified in clear cell sarcomas and angiomatoid fibrous histiocytoma.

MICROSECRETORY ADENOCARCINOMA

Microsecretory adenocarcinoma is a recently described morphologically and genetically distinct salivary gland tumor (described after the most recent WHO classification system).[107] Of the five cases described, one arose in the parotid gland and four in the oral cavity (palate and buccal surface). Patients ranged in age from 21 to 80 years. Tumors measured between 0.8 and 2.2 cm in greatest dimensions and were painless. All tumors were found to harbor a novel *MEF2C-SS18* fusion. The prognosis for these tumors is unknown at this time.

Microsecreotry adenocarcinoma is nonencapsulated but well circumscribed. Perineural and angiolymphatic invasion have not been seen with the tumors. The tumors are composed of microcysts, tubules, and cords lined by flattened and attenuated epithelial cells with eosinophilic to clear cytoplasm (Fig. 6.37; eFig. 6.56). Pale, basophilic secretions

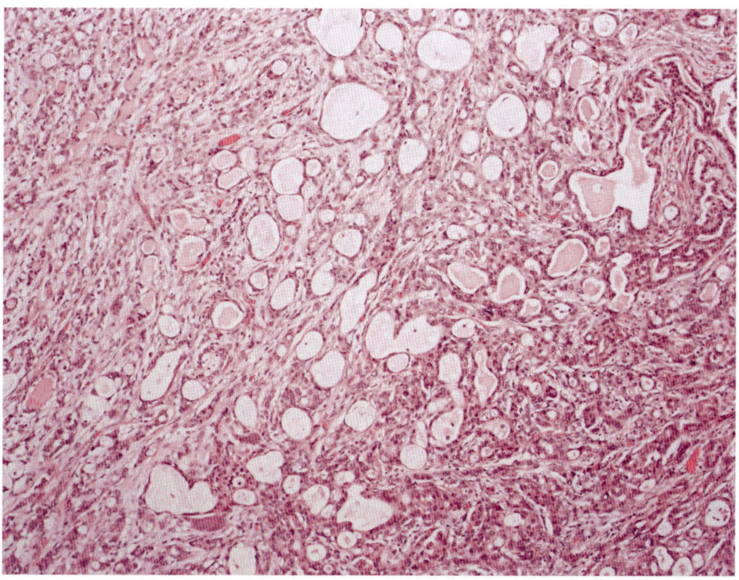

FIGURE 6.37 Microsecretory carcinoma is composed of numerous cords and microcysts.

are present within the tubules and microcysts. The stroma appears myxoid to sclerotic. Mitotic activity is rare and necrosis is not present. Tumor cells express S100 and p63 but do not express p40, SMA, calponin, and mammaglobin.

CARCINOMA EX PLEOMORPHIC ADENOMA

Epithelial malignancies can develop in pleomorphic adenomas or benign mixed tumors and, as such, are termed carcinomas ex pleomorphic adenomas. These tumors represent perhaps 5% to 15% of all salivary gland malignancies and less than 10% of salivary gland–type malignancies of the seromucinous glands.[108–111] Some have estimated that up to 25% of benign mixed tumors would eventually develop into malignancies if left untreated.[111] These malignancies occur in patients older than those with pleomorphic adenomas and present more frequently in men. Molecular and cytogenetic data confirm that these neoplasms typically develop sequentially as the malignancies often contain typical chromosomal rearrangements seen in pleomorphic adenomas (e.g., rearrangement of the *PLAG1* gene) with additional loss of heterozygosity of multiple tumor suppressor genes.[111,112] Clinically, the tumors are sometimes noted to be painful, likely secondary to perineural invasion. Even with multimodality treatment, up to 50% of patients have died from their disease in some studies.

Grossly, carcinomas ex pleomorphic adenomas are larger than typical pleomorphic adenomas and typically appear infiltrative.[110,111] Residual pleomorphic adenoma can often be grossly identified, and some tumors may appear circumscribed and encapsulated with only focal areas of infiltration.[109] The histologic appearance can vary greatly and virtually all differentiated salivary gland–type malignancies have been noted to arise from pleomorphic adenomas.[109–111] That said, most of these carcinomas will be classified as adenocarcinomas, not otherwise specified, or as salivary duct carcinomas and will frequently show perineural and vascular invasion together with abundant necrosis (Figs. 6.38 and 6.39; eFigs. 6.57–6.59). On biopsy, either the malignant or the benign component may be solely sampled, and thus, the correct diagnosis is usually made only at resection. Indeed, the risks for both a concurrent or subsequent malignancy are what necessitate resection of tumors diagnosed as pleomorphic adenomas on biopsy.

Salivary Duct Carcinoma

Salivary duct carcinomas are rare high-grade malignancies (as opposed to the so-called “low-grade salivary duct carcinoma”).[113–117] They are slightly more common in men and develop in older individuals with patients often in their seventh decades of life. Although primarily arising in the parotid gland, approximately 10% of salivary duct carcinomas develop in the seromucinous glands of the upper aerodigestive tract. Patients with these malignancies do poorly and local recurrence and distant metastases are common. The mean survival time is between 3 and 5 years.

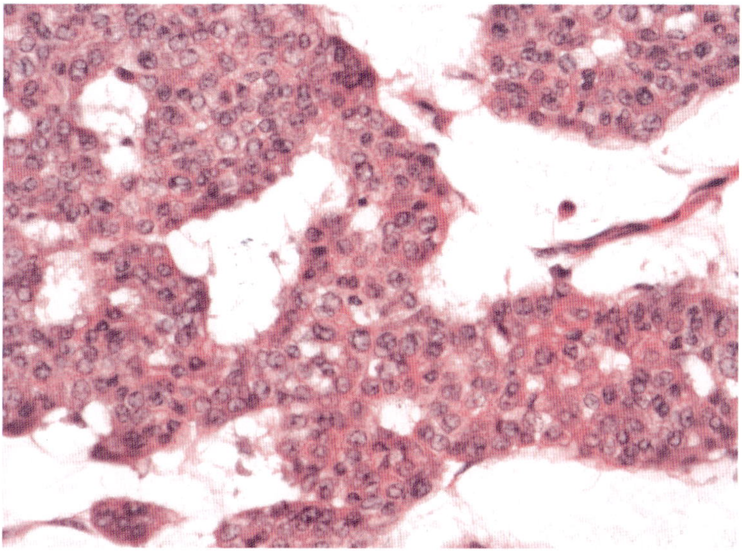

FIGURE 6.38 This low-grade adenocarcinoma was associated with a pleomorphic adenoma.

Grossly, the lesions are poorly circumscribed and have been described as firm and gritty.[113–116] Histologically, they are notable for their marked similarity to mammary ductal carcinoma, especially ductal carcinoma in situ with comedo-type necrosis (Fig. 6.40; eFigs. 6.60 and 6.61).

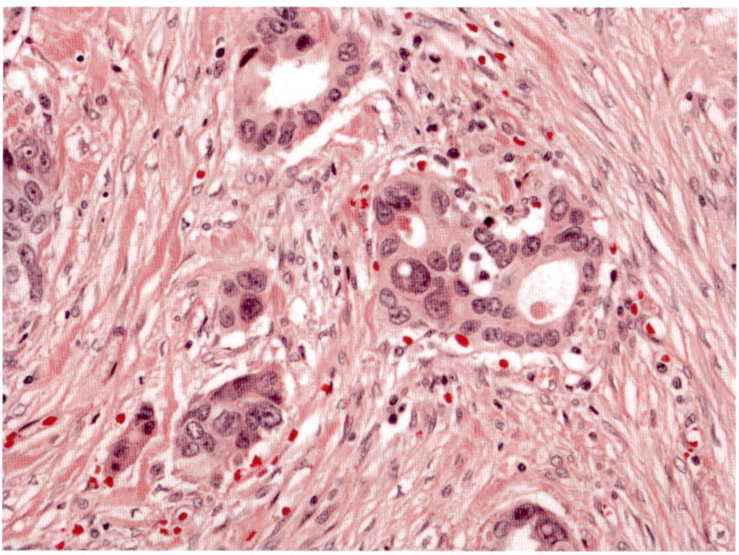

FIGURE 6.39 This adenocarcinoma appears higher grade and was also associated with a pleomorphic adenoma.

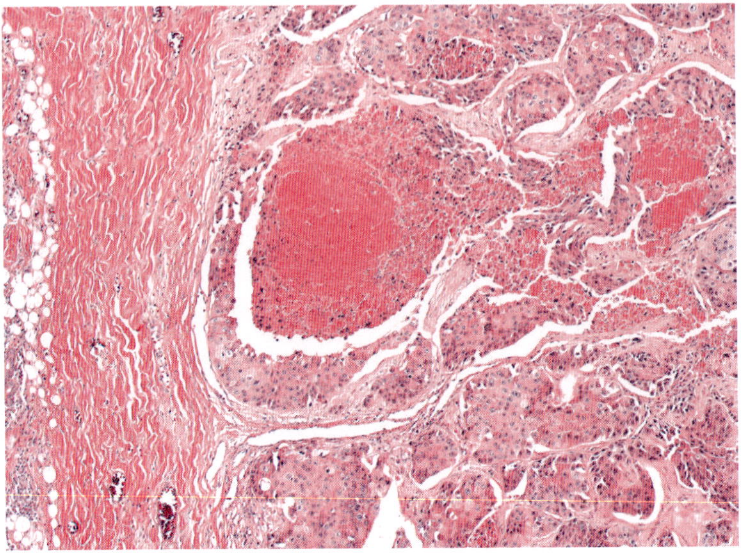

FIGURE 6.40 Comedoform necrosis is generally seen with salivary duct carcinomas.

Well-circumscribed large nests of tumor cells are present that often have central necrosis. Areas appearing more infiltrative are also usually seen, with smaller nests and glands and even single cells set in a densely sclerotic stroma (Fig. 6.41; eFigs. 6.62 and 6.63). The tumor cells are large and polygonal and usually have abundant eosinophilic, apocrine-like cytoplasm. The nuclei are large, atypical, and pleomorphic with vesicular chromatin and prominent nucleoli. Mitotic figures, necrosis, and perineural invasion can all be seen.

Immunohistochemistry is not generally needed for the diagnosis of salivary duct carcinoma. Tumors show immunoreactivity with antibodies to keratins and have been shown, interestingly, to be immunoreactive with antibodies to GCDFP-15.[114] Almost all salivary duct carcinomas fail to express estrogen and progesterone receptors, although some will show intense immunoreactivity with antibodies to HER-2/neu, some with gene ampification.[113,118] Androgen receptors have also been shown to be expressed.[119]

Myoepithelial carcinoma

Myoepithelial carcinomas are rare and may present throughout the upper aerodigestive tract.[23,120,121] They occur in older individuals, and a sex predilection has not been noted. They may arise de novo but are often noted in association with a benign tumor, either a conventional pleomorphic adenoma or a myoepithelioma. More than half of patients with myoepithelial carcinomas will develop recurrences and nearly half will develop metastases. Almost a third of patients have been noted to die of the disease.

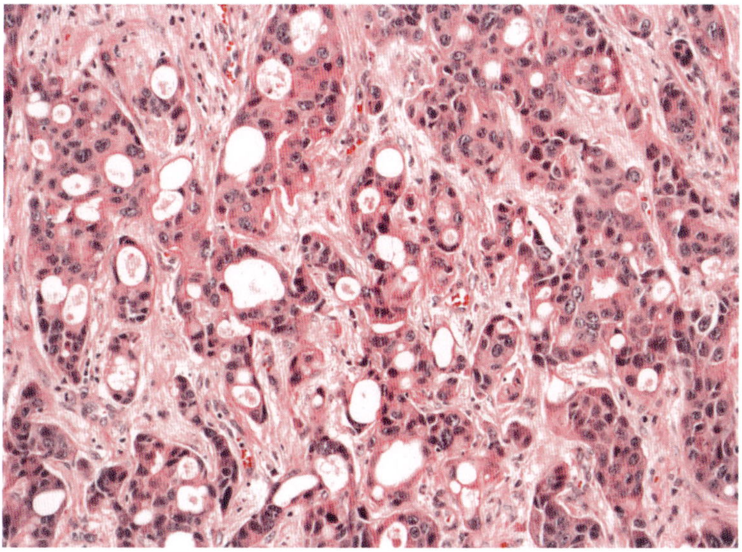

FIGURE 6.41 The infiltrating glands seen with salivary duct carcinomas appear similar to those seen with infiltrating ductal carcinomas of the breast.

The tumors are frequently noted to be multinodular.[23,120,121] Unlike the benign tumors that they are sometimes associated with, myoepithelial carcinomas are clearly infiltrative into surrounding tissues, and bony invasion is often noted when the tumors are located in the palate. The tumor cells show the same phenotypes as seen in myoepithelioma and epithelioid, clear, spindled, and plasmacytoid variants may be seen (Figs. 6.42 and 6.43; eFigs. 6.64–6.66). Nearly one half of the cases will show high-grade cytology with enlarged nuclei, nuclear pleomorphism, chromatin clumping, prominent nucleoli, and nuclear membrane irregularities. Necrosis, increased numbers of mitotic figures and perineural invasion are all frequently present. A little more than half of the cases will instead show bland cytologic features similar to those of myoepithlioma. A myxoid or hyalinized stroma is common. The immunohistochemical staining pattern is similar to that of myoepithelioma with nearly all tumors showing immunoreactivity with antibodies to keratins and most showing immunoreactivity with antibodies to S100, SOX10, SMA, p40, p63, or calponin (Fig. 6.44; eFig. 6.67).[23,25,26,120,121] As with myoepitheliomas, a subset of myoepithelial carcinomas have been shown to harbor *EWSR1* rearrangements.[27]

Basal Cell Adenocarcinomas

Basal cell adenocarcinomas occur much more frequently in the major salivary glands, but they have been noted in the upper aerodigestive tract.[122–124] The tumors histologically resemble basal cell adenomas (see above); however, tumor necrosis (often comedo-type), cellular atypia, and increased mitotic figures can be seen. The two tumors are primarily distinguished

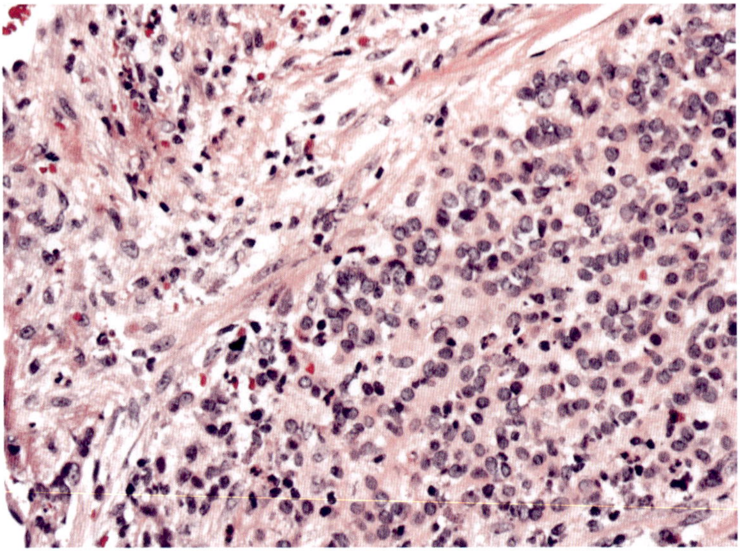

FIGURE 6.42 This myoepithelial carcinoma had a low-grade cytology similar to that seen with myoepitheliomas.

from one another by their growth patterns and thus are usually not distinguishable on small biopsy (Fig. 6.45). Basal cell adenocarcinomas have strands or islands of tumor cells extending into adjacent structures and can show perineural or intravascular invasion. The tumors recur approximately

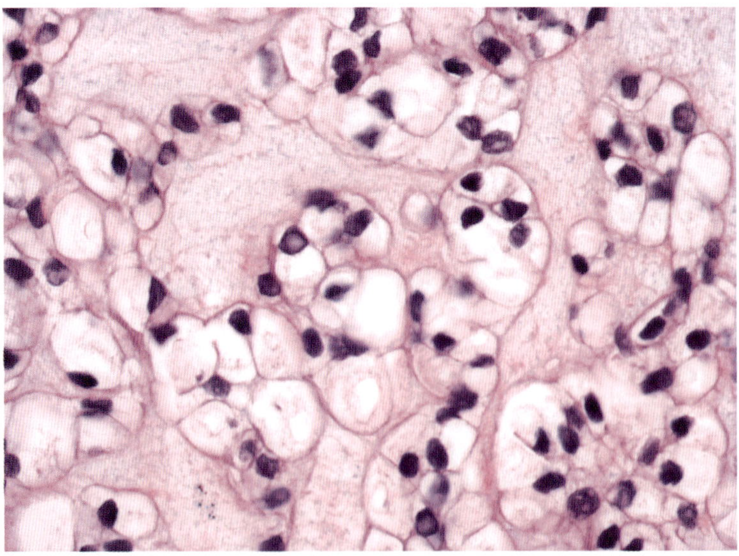

FIGURE 6.43 Like myoepitheliomas, myoepithelial carcinomas can be composed of clear cells.

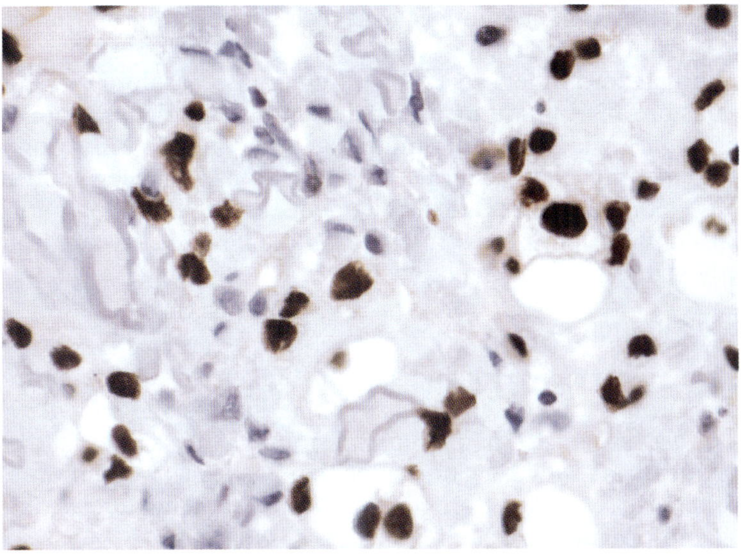

FIGURE 6.44 This clear cell myoepithelial carcinoma shows immunoreactivity with antibodies to p63.

one-third of the time and can metastasize to regional lymph nodes. Immunohistochemical results are similar to those of basal cell adenoma and the tumors will express CD117.[34] They will also show beta-catenin nuclear localization by immunohistochemistry due to CTNNB1 mutations.[36]

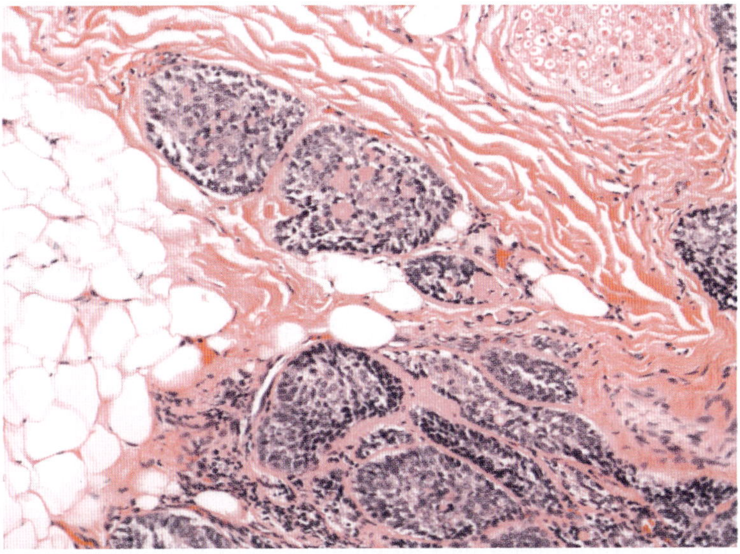

FIGURE 6.45 Basal cell adenocarcinomas have a similar histology to basal cell adenomas except that they will infiltrate surrounding tissues.

As with basal cell adenomas, basal cell adenocarcinomas must be distinguished from other basaloid neoplasms, especially basaloid squamous cell carcinomas and adenoid cystic carcinomas. Basaloid squamous cell carcinomas are high-grade malignancies and show higher grade cytology with more cytologic atypia and mitotic activity. The identification of overlying squamous dysplasia can also be helpful, as it is seen with basaloid squamous cell carcinomas. Basal cell adenocarcinomas show more prominent palisading of peripheral nuclei than adenoid cystic carcinomas and frequently have squamous metaplasia.[123]

Other Malignancies

A number of other salivary gland–type malignancies can arise throughout the upper aerodigestive tract. The use of the diagnosis of *adenocarcinoma, not otherwise specified* to diagnose lesions in the upper aerodigestive tract specifically as salivary gland–type neoplasms is uncommon. As these lesions likely represent a heterogeneous group of malignancies, the overall meaning and prognosis of such a diagnosis is unclear.

Cystadenocarcinomas are rare tumors that, when they do arise, often involve the mouth.[125] They are now considered a variant of adenocarcinoma, not otherwise specified, as they may represent a heterogeneous group of tumors that are currently indistinguishable from other nonspecific adenocarcinomas. The tumors are noted to be multicystic, grossly. Histologically, the lesions infiltrate surrounding tissues and induce a desmoplastic response. The cysts show variable morphology and range greatly in diameter. Papillae are seen within the cysts that can vary in complexity. The cysts and papillae are lined by a cuboidal epithelium with eosinophilic cytoplasm and uniform, hyperchromatic nuclei. Occasional cases have larger or columnar cells with more cytologic atypia. Perineural invasion is frequently seen. Focal cyst rupture and chronic inflammation are common. Fewer than 10% of patients will develop metastases or recurrent tumor.

HPV-related multiphenotypic sinonasal carcinoma is a tumor difficult to categorize and will be discussed here as it shows a salivary gland/seromucinous gland phenotype in spite of being secondary to HR-HPV.[62] The tumors by definition arise in the sinonasal tract. A slight majority involve only the nasal cavity whereas the maxillary sinus ethmoids are the most common sinuses involved. A slight majority of reported patients with the tumors have been women, and patient ages have ranged from 28 to 90 years. Epistaxis and obstruction are the most common presenting symptoms. Although local recurrences have been noted in 36% of cases, only 5% of patients have developed metastases. Death secondary to disease has not been noted.

Tumors are cellular and composed of sheets and nests of tumor cells separated by fibrous bands (Fig. 6. 46). Cribriform and tubular architectures similar to those seen with adenoid cystic carcinoma are frequently noted (Fig. 6.47). Single cell growth with spindled cells associated

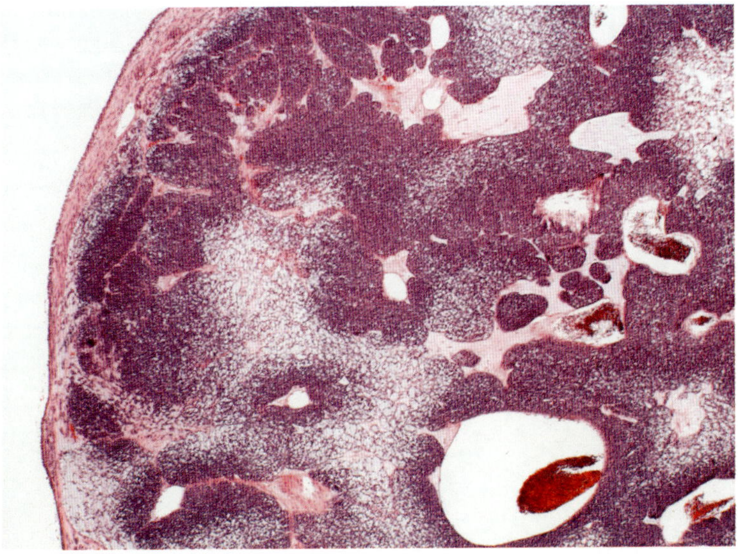

FIGURE 6.46 A low-power view of a cellular multiphenotypic HPV-related sinonasal carcinoma.

closely associated with the epithelial components is frequently seen somewhat reminiscent of a malignant mixed tumor. Indeed, occasional cases appear focal sarcomatous with malignant appearing chondroid or osseous material. Within the epithelial portions of the tumors, more eosinophilic

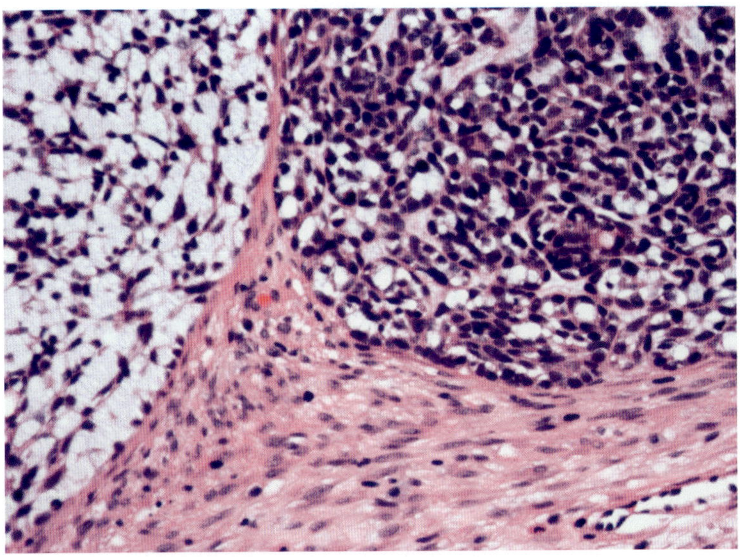

FIGURE 6.47 HPV-related multiphenotypic sinonasal carcinoma may have areas somewhat reminiscent of adenoid cystic carcinoma.

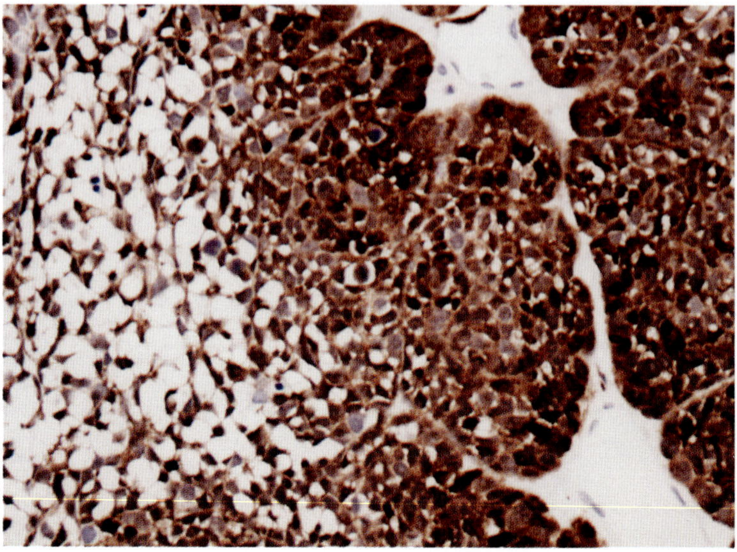

FIGURE 6.48 Diffuse p16 expression is seen with this case of HPV-related multiphenotypic sinonasal carcinoma.

ductal cells may be present, further lending the tumors a biphasic appearance. Unlike with typical salivary gland tumors, surface squamous dysplasia is usually seen (eFig. 6.68). Most cases show necrosis and mitotic activity, and cytologic pleomorphism are usually much greater than what is seen with a typical salivary gland tumor.

Tumor cells express keratins and immunohistochemical staining with keratin cocktails of antibodies often highlight the neoplastic cells differentially, further demonstrating the bi- or multiphenotypic nature of the tumor. p63 and p40 are expressed in most cells but may be absent in the more ductal-appearing cells. c-kit, SMA, S100, and calponin are also frequently expressed, frequently in a differential pattern. Diffuse expression of p16 is always seen as the tumors are secondary to HR-HPV infection (Fig. 6.48). Interestingly, most cases are secondary to HPV-type 33.

REFERENCES

1. WHO classification of tumours of salivary glands. In: El-Naggar AK, Chan JKC, Grandis JR, Takata T, Slootweg PJ, eds. *WHO Classification of Head and Neck Tumours*. Lyon: IARC Press; 2017:160.
2. Jansisyanont P, Blanchaert RH Jr, Ord RA. Intraoral minor salivary gland neoplasm: a single institution experience of 80 cases. *Int J Oral Maxillofac Surg*. 2002;31:257-261.
3. Regezi JA, Lloyd RV, Zarbo RJ, McClatchey KD. Minor salivary gland tumors. A histologic and immunohistochemical study. *Cancer*. 1985;55:108-115.
4. Toida M, Shimokawa K, Makita H, et al. Intraoral minor salivary gland tumors: a clinicopathological study of 82 cases. *Int J Oral Maxillofac Surg*. 2005;34:528-532.

5. Waldron CA, el-Mofty SK, Gnepp DR. Tumors of the intraoral minor salivary glands: a demographic and histologic study of 426 cases. *Oral Surg Oral Med Oral Pathol.* 1988;66:323-333.
6. Ellis GL, Auclair PL. *Benign epithelial neoplasms.* In: *Tumors of the Salivary Glands.* 3rd ed. Washington, D.C.: Armed Forces Institute of Pathology; 1996:39-153.
7. Erlandson RA, Cardon-Cardo C, Higgins PJ. Histogenesis of benign pleomorphic adenoma (mixed tumor) of the major salivary glands. An ultrastructural and immunohistochemical study. *Am J Surg Pathol.* 1984;8:803-820.
8. Bilal H, Handra-Luca A, Bertrand JC, Fouret PJ. P63 is expressed in basal and myoepithelial cells of human normal and tumor salivary gland tissues. *J Histochem Cytochem.* 2003;51:133-139.
9. Eveson JE, Kusafuka K, Stenman G, Nagao T. Pleomorphic adenoma. In: Barnes L, Eveson JW, Reichart P, Sidransky D, eds. *Pathology and Genetics of Tumours of the Head and Neck.* Lyon: IARP Press; 2005:254-258.
10. Bullerdiek J, Wobst G, Meyer-Bolte K, et al. Cytogenetic subtyping of 220 salivary gland pleomorphic adenomas: correlation to occurrence, histological subtype, and in vitro cellular behavior. *Cancer Genet Cytogenet.* 1993;65:27-31.
11. Sandros J, Stenman G, Mark J. Cytogenetic and molecular observations in human and experimental salivary gland tumors. *Cancer Genet Cytogenet.* 1990;44:153-167.
12. Geurts JM, Schoenmakers EF, Roijer E, Astrom AK, Stenman G, van de Ven WJ. Identification of NFIB as recurrent translocation partner gene of HMGIC in pleomorphic adenomas. *Oncogene.* 1998;16:865-872.
13. Kas K, Voz ML, Roijer E, et al. Promoter swapping between the genes for a novel zinc finger protein and beta-catenin in pleiomorphic adenomas with t(3;8)(p21;q12) translocations. *Nat Genet.* 1997;15:170-174.
14. Voz ML, Astrom AK, Kas K, Mark J, Stenman G, Van de Ven WJ. The recurrent translocation t(5;8)(p13;q12) in pleomorphic adenomas results in upregulation of PLAG1 gene expression under control of the LIFR promoter. *Oncogene.* 1998;16:1409-1416.
15. Hickman RE, Cawson RA, Duffy SW. The prognosis of specific types of salivary gland tumors. *Cancer.* 1984;54:1620-1624.
16. Nelson JF, Jacoway JR. Monomorphic adenoma (canalicular type). Report of 29 cases. *Cancer.* 1973;31:1511-1513.
17. Daley TD, Gardner DG, Smout MS. Canalicular adenoma: not a basal cell adenoma. *Oral Surg Oral Med Oral Pathol.* 1984;57:181-188.
18. Thompson LD, Bauer JL, Chiosea S, et al. Canalicular adenoma: a clinicopathologic and immunohistochemical analysis of 67 cases with a review of the literature. *Head Neck Pathol.* 2015;9:181-195.
19. Ferreiro JA. Immunohistochemical analysis of salivary gland canalicular adenoma. *Oral Surg Oral Med Oral Pathol.* 1994;78:761-765.
20. Edwards PC, Bhuiya T, Kelsch RD. Assessment of p63 expression in the salivary gland neoplasms adenoid cystic carcinoma, polymorphous low-grade adenocarcinoma, and basal cell and canalicular adenomas. *Oral Surg Oral Med Oral Pathol Oral Radiol Endod.* 2004;97:613-619.
21. Sciubba JJ, Brannon RB. Myoepithelioma of salivary glands: report of 23 cases. *Cancer.* 1982;49:562-572.
22. Simpson RH, Jones H, Beasley P. Benign myoepithelioma of the salivary glands: a true entity? *Histopathology.* 1995;27:1-9.
23. Alos L, Cardesa A, Bombi JA, Mallofre C, Cuchi A, Traserra J. Myoepithelial tumors of salivary glands: a clinicopathologic, immunohistochemical, ultrastructural, and flow-cytometric study. *Semin Diagn Pathol.* 1996;13:138-147.

24. Franquemont DW, Mills SE. Plasmacytoid monomorphic adenoma of salivary glands. Absence of myogenous differentiation and comparison to spindle cell myoepithelioma. *Am J Surg Pathol.* 1993;17:146-153.
25. Ohtomo R, Mori T, Shibata S, et al. SOX10 is a novel marker of acinus and intercalated duct differentiation in salivary gland tumors: a clue to the histogenesis for tumor diagnosis. *Mod Pathol.* 2013;26:1041-1050.
26. Owosho AA, Aguilar CE, Seethala RR. Comparison of p63 and p40 (DeltaNp63) as basal, squamoid, and myoepithelial markers in salivary gland tumors. *Appl Immunohistochem Mol Morphol.* 2016;24:501-508.
27. Ni H, Zhao PY, Wang XT, et al. EWSR1 rearrangement is present in a subset of myoepithelial tumors of salivary glands with variable morphology and does not correlate with clinical behavior. *Ann Diagn Pathol.* 2017;28:19-23.
28. Christ TF, Crocker D. Basal cell adenoma of minor salivary gland origin. *Cancer.* 1972;30:214-219.
29. Fantasia JE, Neville BW. Basal cell adenomas of the minor salivary glands. A clinicopathologic study of seventeen new cases and a review of the literature. *Oral Surg Oral Med Oral Pathol.* 1980;50:433-440.
30. Mintz GA, Abrams AM, Melrose RJ. Monomorphic adenomas of the major and minor salivary glands. Report of twenty-one cases and review of the literature. *Oral Surg Oral Med Oral Pathol.* 1982;53:375-386.
31. Batsakis JG. Basal cell adenoma of the parotid gland. *Cancer.* 1972;29:226-230.
32. Batsakis JG, Luna MA, el-Naggar AK. Basaloid monomorphic adenomas. *Ann Otol Rhinol Laryngol.* 1991;100:687-690.
33. Gardner DG, Daley TD. The use of the terms monomorphic adenoma, basal cell adenoma, and canalicular adenoma as applied to salivary gland tumors. *Oral Surg Oral Med Oral Pathol.* 1983;56:608-615.
34. Williams SB, Ellis GL, Auclair PL. Immunohistochemical analysis of basal cell adenocarcinoma. *Oral Surg Oral Med Oral Pathol.* 1993;75:64-69.
35. Mino M, Pilch BZ, Faquin WC. Expression of KIT (CD117) in neoplasms of the head and neck: an ancillary marker for adenoid cystic carcinoma. *Mod Pathol.* 2003;16:1224-1231.
36. Jo VY, Sholl LM, Krane JF. Distinctive patterns of CTNNB1 (β-catenin) alterations in salivary gland basal cell adenoma and basal cell adenocarcinoma. *Am J Surg Pathol.* 2016;40:1143-1150.
37. Brannon RB, Sciubba JJ, Giulani M. Ductal papillomas of salivary gland origin: A report of 19 cases and a review of the literature. *Oral Surg Oral Med Oral Pathol Oral Radiol Endod.* 2001;92:68-77.
38. White DK, Miller AS, McDaniel RK, Rothman BN. Inverted ductal papilloma: a distinctive lesion of minor salivary gland. *Cancer.* 1982;49:519-524.
39. Abrams AM, Finck FM. Sialadenoma papilliferum. A previously unreported salivary gland tumor. *Cancer.* 1969;24:1057-1063.
40. Hsieh MS, Bishop JA, Wang YP, et al. Salivary sialadenoma papilliferum consists of two morphologically, immunophenotypically, and genetically distinct subtypes. *Head Neck Pathol.* 2019.
41. Wilson DF, MacEntee MI. Papillary cystadenoma of ectopic minor salivary gland origin. *Oral Surg Oral Med Oral Pathol.* 1974;37:915-918.
42. Yamase HT, Putman HC III. Oncocytic papillary cystadenomatosis of the larynx: a clinicopathologic entity. *Cancer.* 1979;44:2306-2311.
43. Gallagher JC, Puzon BQ. Oncocytic lesions of the larynx. *Ann Otol Rhinol Laryngol.* 1969;78:307-318.

44. Yih WY, Kratochvil FJ, Stewart JC. Intraoral minor salivary gland neoplasms: review of 213 cases. *J Oral Maxillofac Surg*. 2005;63:805-810.
45. Gnepp DR, Brannon R. Sebaceous neoplasms of salivary gland origin. Report of 21 cases. *Cancer*. 1984;53:2155-2170.
46. Hart MN, Andrews JL. Papillary cystadenoma lymphomatosum arising in the oral cavity. *Oral Surg Oral Med Oral Pathol*. 1968;26:588-591.
47. Nascimento AG, Amaral AL, Prado LA, Kligerman J, Silveira TR. Adenoid cystic carcinoma of salivary glands. A study of 61 cases with clinicopathologic correlation. *Cancer*. 1986;57:312-319.
48. Perzin KH, Gullane P, Clairmont AC. Adenoid cystic carcinomas arising in salivary glands: a correlation of histologic features and clinical course. *Cancer*. 1978;42:265-282.
49. Ellis GL, Auclair PL. *Malignant Epithelial Neoplasms*. In: *Tumors of the Salivary Glands*. Washington, D.C.: Armed Forces Institute of Pathology; 1996:155-373.
50. Zarbo RJ. Salivary gland neoplasia: a review for the practicing pathologist. *Mod Pathol*. 2002;15:298-323.
51. Szanto PA, Luna MA, Tortoledo ME, White RA. Histologic grading of adenoid cystic carcinoma of the salivary glands. *Cancer*. 1984;54:1062-1069.
52. Seethala RR, Hunt JL, Baloch ZW, Livolsi VA, Leon Barnes E. Adenoid cystic carcinoma with high-grade transformation: a report of 11 cases and a review of the literature. *Am J Surg Pathol*. 2007;31:1683-1694.
53. Nagao T, Gaffey TA, Serizawa H, et al. Dedifferentiated adenoid cystic carcinoma: a clinicopathologic study of 6 cases. *Mod Pathol*. 2003;16:1265-1272.
54. Azumi N, Battifora H. The cellular composition of adenoid cystic carcinoma. An immunohistochemical study. *Cancer*. 1987;60:1589-1598.
55. Prasad AR, Savera AT, Gown AM, Zarbo RJ. The myoepithelial immunophenotype in 135 benign and malignant salivary gland tumors other than pleomorphic adenoma. *Arch Pathol Lab Med*. 1999;123:801-806.
56. Penner CR, Folpe AL, Budnick SD. C-kit expression distinguishes salivary gland adenoid cystic carcinoma from polymorphous low-grade adenocarcinoma. *Mod Pathol*. 2002;15:687-691.
57. Nordkvist A, Mark J, Gustafsson H, Bang G, Stenman G. Non-random chromosome rearrangements in adenoid cystic carcinoma of the salivary glands. *Genes Chromosomes Cancer*. 1994;10:115-121.
58. Stallmach I, Zenklusen P, Komminoth P, et al. Loss of heterozygosity at chromosome 6q23-25 correlates with clinical and histologic parameters in salivary gland adenoid cystic carcinoma. *Virchows Arch*. 2002;440:77-84.
59. Brill LB II, Kanner WA, Fehr A, et al. Analysis of MYB expression and MYB-NFIB gene fusions in adenoid cystic carcinoma and other salivary neoplasms. *Mod Pathol*. 2011;24:1169-1176.
60. West RB, Kong C, Clarke N, et al. MYB expression and translocation in adenoid cystic carcinomas and other salivary gland tumors with clinicopathologic correlation. *Am J Surg Pathol*. 2011;35:92-99.
61. Holst VA, Marshall CE, Moskaluk CA, Frierson HF Jr. KIT protein expression and analysis of c-kit gene mutation in adenoid cystic carcinoma. *Mod Pathol*. 1999;12:956-960.
62. Bishop JA, Andreasen S, Hang JF, et al. HPV-related multiphenotypic sinonasal carcinoma: an expanded series of 49 cases of the tumor formerly known as HPV-related carcinoma with adenoid cystic carcinoma-like features. *Am J Surg Pathol*. 2017;41:1690-1701.
63. Castle JT, Thompson LD, Frommelt RA, Wenig BM, Kessler HP. Polymorphous low grade adenocarcinoma: a clinicopathologic study of 164 cases. *Cancer*. 1999;86:207-219.

64. Evans HL, Luna MA. Polymorphous low-grade adenocarcinoma: a study of 40 cases with long-term follow up and an evaluation of the importance of papillary areas. *Am J Surg Pathol.* 2000;24:1319-1328.
65. Pelkey TJ, Mills SE. Histologic transformation of polymorphous low-grade adenocarcinoma of salivary gland. *Am J Clin Pathol.* 1999;111:785-791.
66. Simpson RH, Pereira EM, Ribeiro AC, Abdulkadir A, Reis-Filho JS. Polymorphous low-grade adenocarcinoma of the salivary glands with transformation to high-grade carcinoma. *Histopathology.* 2002;41:250-259.
67. Evans HL, Batsakis JG. Polymorphous low-grade adenocarcinoma of minor salivary glands. A study of 14 cases of a distinctive neoplasm. *Cancer.* 1984;53:935-942.
68. Simpson RH, Clarke TJ, Sarsfield PT, Gluckman PG, Babajews AV. Polymorphous low-grade adenocarcinoma of the salivary glands: a clinicopathological comparison with adenoid cystic carcinoma. *Histopathology.* 1991;19:121-129.
69. Gnepp DR, Chen JC, Warren C. Polymorphous low-grade adenocarcinoma of minor salivary gland. An immunohistochemical and clinicopathologic study. *Am J Surg Pathol.* 1988;12:461-468.
70. Darling MR, Schneider JW, Phillips VM. Polymorphous low-grade adenocarcinoma and adenoid cystic carcinoma: a review and comparison of immunohistochemical markers. *Oral Oncol.* 2002;38:641-645.
71. Skalova A, Sima R, Kaspirkova-Nemcova J, et al. Cribriform adenocarcinoma of minor salivary gland origin principally affecting the tongue: characterization of new entity. *Am J Surg Pathol.* 2011;35:1168-1176.
72. Weinreb I, Piscuoglio S, Martelotto LG, et al. Hotspot activating PRKD1 somatic mutations in polymorphous low-grade adenocarcinomas of the salivary glands. *Nat Genet.* 2014;46:1166-1169.
73. Weinreb I, Zhang L, Tirunagari LM, et al. Novel PRKD gene rearrangements and variant fusions in cribriform adenocarcinoma of salivary gland origin. *Genes Chromosomes Cancer.* 2014;53:845-856.
74. Auclair PL, Goode RK, Ellis GL. Mucoepidermoid carcinoma of intraoral salivary glands. Evaluation and application of grading criteria in 143 cases. *Cancer.* 1992;69:2021-2030.
75. Evans HL. Mucoepidermoid carcinoma of salivary glands: a study of 69 cases with special attention to histologic grading. *Am J Clin Pathol.* 1984;81:696-701.
76. Accetta PA, Gray GF Jr, Hunter RM, Rosenfeld L. Mucoepidermoid carcinoma of salivary glands. *Arch Pathol Lab Med.* 1984;108:321-325.
77. Hamper K, Schimmelpenning H, Caselitz J, et al. Mucoepidermoid tumors of the salivary glands. Correlation of cytophotometrical data and prognosis. *Cancer.* 1989;63:708-717.
78. Tonon G, Modi S, Wu L, et al. t(11;19)(q21;p13) translocation in mucoepidermoid carcinoma creates a novel fusion product that disrupts a Notch signaling pathway. *Nat Genet.* 2003;33:208-213.
79. Seethala RR, Dacic S, Cieply K, Kelly LM, Nikiforova MN. A reappraisal of the MECT1/MAML2 translocation in salivary mucoepidermoid carcinomas. *Am J Surg Pathol.* 2010;34:1106-1121.
80. Healey WV, Perzin KH, Smith L. Mucoepidermoid carcinoma of salivary gland origin. Classification, clinical-pathologic correlation, and results of treatment. *Cancer.* 1970;26:368-388.
81. Brandwein MS, Ivanov K, Wallace DI, et al. Mucoepidermoid carcinoma: a clinicopathologic study of 80 patients with special reference to histological grading. *Am J Surg Pathol.* 2001;25:835-845.
82. Regezi JA, Zarbo RJ, Batsakis JG. Immunoprofile of mucoepidermoid carcinomas of minor salivary glands. *Oral Surg Oral Med Oral Pathol.* 1991;71:189-192.

83. Loyola AM, de Sousa SO, Araujo NS, Araujo VC. Study of minor salivary gland mucoepidermoid carcinoma differentiation based on immunohistochemical expression of cytokeratins, vimentin and muscle-specific actin. *Oral Oncol.* 1998;34:112-118.
84. Nguyen LH, Black MJ, Hier M, Chauvin P, Rochon L. HER2/neu and Ki-67 as prognostic indicators in mucoepidermoid carcinoma of salivary glands. *J Otolaryngol.* 2003;32:328-331.
85. Alos L, Lujan B, Castillo M, et al. Expression of membrane-bound mucins (MUC1 and MUC4) and secreted mucins (MUC2, MUC5AC, MUC5B, MUC6 and MUC7) in mucoepidermoid carcinomas of salivary glands. *Am J Surg Pathol.* 2005;29:806-813.
86. Abrams AM, Melrose RJ. Acinic cell tumors of minor salivary gland origin. *Oral Surg Oral Med Oral Pathol.* 1978;46:220-233.
87. Perzin KH, LiVolsi VA. Acinic cell carcinomas arising in salivary glands: a clinicopathologic study. *Cancer.* 1979;44:1434-1457.
88. Spiro RH, Huvos AG, Strong EW. Acinic cell carcinoma of salivary origin. A clinicopathologic study of 67 cases. *Cancer.* 1978;41:924-935.
89. Lewis JE, Olsen KD, Weiland LH. Acinic cell carcinoma. Clinicopathologic review. *Cancer.* 1991;67:172-179.
90. Stanley RJ, Weiland LH, Olsen KD, Pearson BW. Dedifferentiated acinic cell (acinous) carcinoma of the parotid gland. *Otolaryngol Head Neck Surg.* 1988;98:155-161.
91. Nikitakis NG, Tosios KI, Papanikolaou VS, Rivera H, Papanicolaou SI, Ioffe OB. Immunohistochemical expression of cytokeratins 7 and 20 in malignant salivary gland tumors. *Mod Pathol.* 2004;17:407-415.
92. Chenevert J, Duvvuri U, Chiosea S, et al. DOG1: a novel marker of salivary acinar and intercalated duct differentiation. *Mod Pathol.* 2012;25:919-929.
93. Childers EL, Ellis GL, Auclair PL. An immunohistochemical analysis of anti-amylase antibody reactivity in acinic cell adenocarcinoma. *Oral Surg Oral Med Oral Pathol Oral Radiol Endod.* 1996;81:691-694.
94. el-Naggar AK, Abdul-Karim FW, Hurr K, Callender D, Luna MA, Batsakis JG. Genetic alterations in acinic cell carcinoma of the parotid gland determined by microsatellite analysis. *Cancer Genet Cytogenet.* 1998;102:19-24.
95. Andreasen S, Varma S, Barasch N, et al. The HTN3-MSANTD3 Fusion gene defines a subset of acinic cell carcinoma of the salivary gland. *Am J Surg Pathol.* 2019;43:489-496.
96. Haller F, Bieg M, Will R, et al. Enhancer hijacking activates oncogenic transcription factor NR4A3 in acinic cell carcinomas of the salivary glands. *Nat Commun.* 2019;10:368.
97. Griffith C, Seethala R, Chiosea SI. Mammary analogue secretory carcinoma: a new twist to the diagnostic dilemma of zymogen granule poor acinic cell carcinoma. *Virchows Arch.* 2011;459:117-118.
98. Skalova A, Vanecek T, Sima R, et al. Mammary analogue secretory carcinoma of salivary glands, containing the ETV6-NTRK3 fusion gene: a hitherto undescribed salivary gland tumor entity. *Am J Surg Pathol.* 2010;34:599-608.
99. Seethala RR, Leon Barnes E, Hunt JL. Epithelial-myoepithelial carcinoma: a review of the clinicopathologic spectrum and immunophenotypic characteristics in 61 tumors of the salivary glands and upper aerodigestive tract. *Am J Surg Pathol.* 2007;31:44-57.
100. Fonseca I, Soares J. Epithelial-myoepithelial carcinoma of the salivary glands. A study of 22 cases. *Virchows Arch A Pathol Anat Histopathol.* 1993;422:389-396.
101. Batsakis JG, el-Naggar AK, Luna MA. Epithelial-myoepithelial carcinoma of salivary glands. *Ann Otol Rhinol Laryngol.* 1992;101:540-542.
102. Maiorano E, Altini M, Favia G. Clear cell tumors of the salivary glands, jaws, and oral mucosa. *Semin Diagn Pathol.* 1997;14:203-212.

103. Wang B, Brandwein M, Gordon R, Robinson R, Urken M, Zarbo RJ. Primary salivary clear cell tumors–a diagnostic approach: a clinicopathologic and immunohistochemical study of 20 patients with clear cell carcinoma, clear cell myoepithelial carcinoma, and epithelial-myoepithelial carcinoma. *Arch Pathol Lab Med.* 2002;126:676-685.
104. Ellis GL. Clear cell neoplasms in salivary glands: clearly a diagnostic challenge. *Ann Diagn Pathol.* 1998;2:61-78.
105. Milchgrub S, Gnepp DR, Vuitch F, Delgado R, Albores-Saavedra J. Hyalinizing clear cell carcinoma of salivary gland. *Am J Surg Pathol.* 1994;18:74-82.
106. Antonescu CR, Katabi N, Zhang L, et al. EWSR1-ATF1 fusion is a novel and consistent finding in hyalinizing clear-cell carcinoma of salivary gland. *Genes Chromosomes Cancer.* 2011;50:559-570.
107. Bishop JA, Weinreb I, Swanson D, et al. Microsecretory adenocarcinoma: a novel salivary gland tumor characterized by a recurrent MEF2C-SS18 fusion. *Am J Surg Pathol.* 2019;43:1023-1032.
108. Nagao K, Matsuzaki O, Saiga H, et al. Histopathologic studies on carcinoma in pleomorphic adenoma of the parotid gland. *Cancer.* 1981;48:113-121.
109. Spiro RH, Huvos AG, Strong EW. Malignant mixed tumor of salivary origin: a clinicopathologic study of 146 cases. *Cancer.* 1977;39:388-396.
110. LiVolsi VA, Perzin KH. Malignant mixed tumors arising in salivary glands. I. Carcinomas arising in benign mixed tumors: a clinicopathologic study. *Cancer.* 1977;39:2209-2230.
111. Lewis JE, Olsen KD, Sebo TJ. Carcinoma ex pleomorphic adenoma: pathologic analysis of 73 cases. *Hum Pathol.* 2001;32:596-604.
112. Martins C, Fonseca I, Roque L, et al. PLAG1 gene alterations in salivary gland pleomorphic adenoma and carcinoma ex-pleomorphic adenoma: a combined study using chromosome banding, in situ hybridization and immunocytochemistry. *Mod Pathol.* 2005;18:1048-1055.
113. Jaehne M, Roeser K, Jaekel T, Schepers JD, Albert N, Loning T. Clinical and immunohistologic typing of salivary duct carcinoma: a report of 50 cases. *Cancer.* 2005;103:2526-2533.
114. Lewis JE, McKinney BC, Weiland LH, Ferreiro JA, Olsen KD. Salivary duct carcinoma. Clinicopathologic and immunohistochemical review of 26 cases. *Cancer.* 1996;77:223-230.
115. Garland TA, Innes DJ Jr, Fechner RE. Salivary duct carcinoma: an analysis of four cases with review of literature. *Am J Clin Pathol.* 1984;81:436-441.
116. van Heerden WF, Raubenheimer EJ, Swart TJ, Boy SC. Intraoral salivary duct carcinoma: a report of 5 cases. *J Oral Maxillofac Surg.* 2003;61:126-131.
117. Brandwein MS, Jagirdar J, Patil J, Biller H, Kaneko M. Salivary duct carcinoma (cribriform salivary carcinoma of excretory ducts). A clinicopathologic and immunohistochemical study of 12 cases. *Cancer.* 1990;65:2307-2314.
118. Williams MD, Roberts DB, Kies MS, Mao L, Weber RS, El-Naggar AK. Genetic and expression analysis of HER-2 and EGFR genes in salivary duct carcinoma: empirical and therapeutic significance. *Clin Cancer Res.* 2010;16:2266-2274.
119. Nasser SM, Faquin WC, Dayal Y. Expression of androgen, estrogen, and progesterone receptors in salivary gland tumors. Frequent expression of androgen receptor in a subset of malignant salivary gland tumors. *Am J Clin Pathol.* 2003;119:801-806.
120. Savera AT, Sloman A, Huvos AG, Klimstra DS. Myoepithelial carcinoma of the salivary glands: a clinicopathologic study of 25 patients. *Am J Surg Pathol.* 2000;24:761-774.
121. Di Palma S, Guzzo M. Malignant myoepithelioma of salivary glands: clinicopathological features of ten cases. *Virchows Arch A Pathol Anat Histopathol.* 1993;423:389-396.
122. Ellis GL, Wiscovitch JG. Basal cell adenocarcinomas of the major salivary glands. *Oral Surg Oral Med Oral Pathol.* 1990;69:461-469.

123. Fonseca I, Soares J. Basal cell adenocarcinoma of minor salivary and seromucous glands of the head and neck region. *Semin Diagn Pathol*. 1996;13:128-137.

124. Jayakrishnan A, Elmalah I, Hussain K, Odell EW. Basal cell adenocarcinoma in minor salivary glands. *Histopathology*. 2003;42:610-614.

125. Foss RD, Ellis GL, Auclair PL. Salivary gland cystadenocarcinomas. A clinicopathologic study of 57 cases. *Am J Surg Pathol*. 1996;20:1440-1447.

7

ADENOCARCINOMAS, OTHER THAN THOSE THAT CAN BE CLASSIFIED AS SALIVARY GLAND–TYPE

Most glandular malignancies of the upper aerodigestive tract can best be classified as salivary gland–type malignancies (Table 7.1). A notable exception occurs in the sinonasal region, where a significant percentage of adenocarcinomas have an intestinal phenotype, and other low- and high-grade nonintestinal-type adenocarcinomas also appear distinct from traditional salivary gland–type malignancies. On small biopsy, the distinction between these tumors is not always easy. Nonetheless, the higher grade or worse behaving adenocarcinomas, e.g., the intestinal-type adenocarcinomas and adenoid cystic carcinomas, are usually readily distinguished from the lower grade, better-behaved tumors.

SINONASAL INTESTINAL-TYPE ADENOCARCINOMA

Sinonasal intestinal-type adenocarcinomas comprise a distinct clinicopathologic entity.[1] The tumors most frequently involve the ethmoid sinuses and nasal cavity; however, they may be found within the other sinuses as well.[2–4] They arise mostly in adult men over a wide age range, although most are diagnosed in the fifth and sixth decades of life. Occasional series that have attempted to report only cases not secondary to environmental exposures have shown no sex predilection, however.[1] The tumors are noteworthy for their increased prevalence in persons exposed to hardwood and other dusts, although the risks for such exposure do not appear to be the same throughout the world.[2–7] Sinonasal intestinal-type adenocarcinomas have much higher recurrent rates than lower grade adenocarcinomas and accordingly worse prognoses; between 50% and 83% of patients survive 5 years after their diagnoses.[8] Most tumors do not show the abnormalities typical of colorectal adenocarcinomas such as *BRAF* or *RAS* mutations, abnormalities of *wnt*-signaling pathway or mismatch repair protein loss,

TABLE 7.1 Adenocarcinomas of the Upper Aerodigestive Tract
Salivary gland–type malignancies
Non–salivary gland–type adenocarcinomas
Intestinal-type adenocarcinomas
Nonintestinal-type adenocarcinomas
Low-grade sinonasal adenocarcinomas (papillary, tubulopapillary, seromucous, clear cell/"renal-cell like," etc.; including some with *ETV6* translocations)
Nasopharyngeal papillary adenocarcinomas
High-grade adenocarcinomas (including some related to HR-HPV, some arising with enteric duplication cysts or oncocytic schneiderian papillomas, some with INI1 loss, etc.)

and resultant microsatellite instability.[9–12] Comparative genomic hybridization studies have consistently shown gains at 7q, 8q, and 20q with losses at 5q, 17p, and 18q.[13,14]

Grossly, sinonasal intestinal-type adenocarcinomas have been described as papillary and friable and range in color from white-tan to red-purple.[1,15] Microscopically, the tumors show an intestinal phenotype that can vary greatly with some tumors appearing akin to normal small intestinal epithelium (authors have even described an apparent muscularis mucosae), while others can be poorly differentiated and have a signet ring phenotype (Table 7.2; Figs. 7.1–7.3, eFigs. 7.1 and 7.2).[15–17] Most tumors (70%–80%) have a *papillary-tubular cylinder cell* pattern akin to that seen with most colorectal adenocarcinomas. These usually show papillae or villi that spread across the surface and fold into the stroma. Numerous tubular structures can then be seen on cut surface that infiltrate the underlying stroma, some of which will have intratubular papillary growths. These tumors can produce a variable amount of mucus, and solid and cribriform areas can be seen. The neoplastic cells are tall and columnar with oval, hyperchromatic nuclei that appear stratified. A variable number of goblet cells, Paneth cells, and enterochromaffin cells can also be seen. These tumors can be graded as well-differentiated, moderately differentiated, and

TABLE 7.2 Histologic Types of Sinonasal Intestinal-type Adenocarcinomas
Papillary-tubular cylinder cell (grades 1–3)
Alveolar-goblet cell
Signet-ring

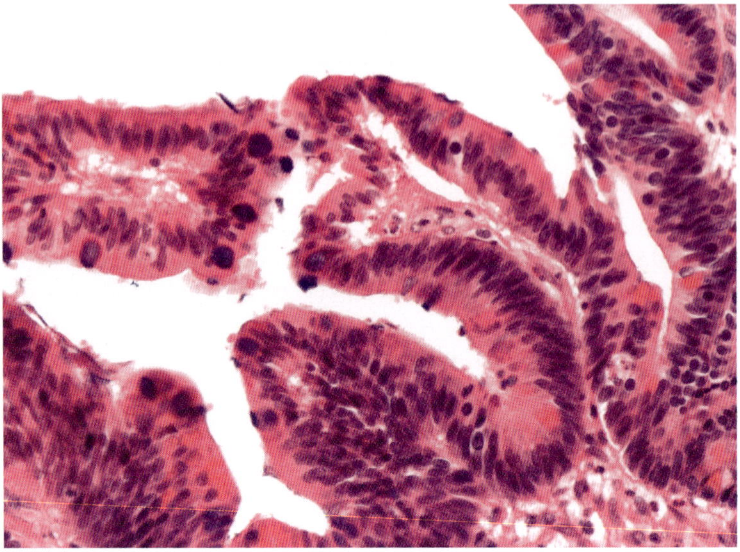

FIGURE 7.1 Sinonasal intestinal-type adenocarcinoma showing a typical papillary pattern.

poorly differentiated much like colorectal adenocarcinomas are graded. Another histologic pattern that may be seen has been termed the *alveolar goblet cell* pattern. This pattern is characterized by numerous mucus-filled cavities. These cavities are separated by thin septa of fibrous tissue and

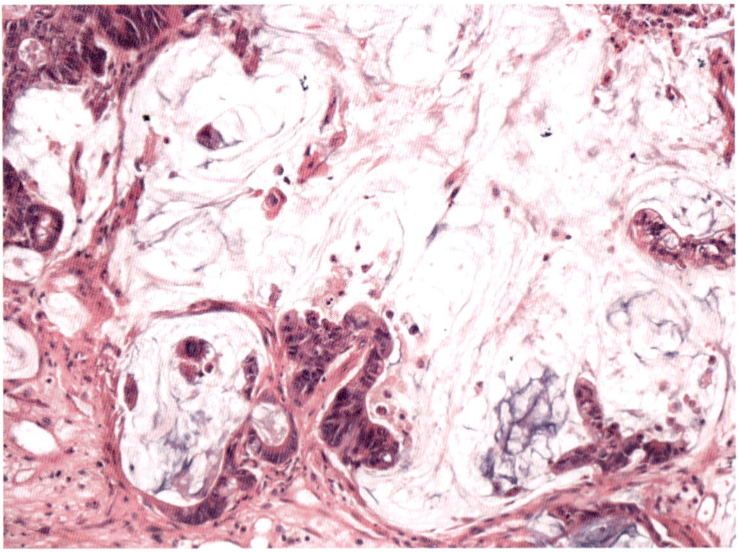

FIGURE 7.2 Sinonasal intestinal-type adenocarcinoma with abundant mucus production.

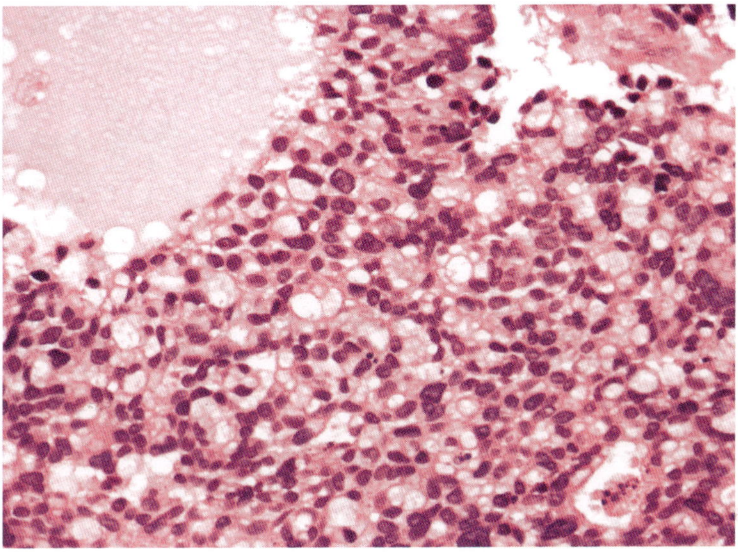

FIGURE 7.3 Sinonasal intestinal-type adenocarcinoma showing a signet-ring pattern.

have mucinous epithelial cells either lining the spaces or floating within the cavities. Finally, less than 5% of these tumors will show a signet-ring morphology akin to that seen throughout the enteric tract.

The subclassification of sinonasal intestinal-type adenocarcinomas and the grading of the most common pattern, the papillary-tubular type, have been shown to be predictive of overall survival with the lower grade papillary tubular variants showing the longest survival and highest survival rate at 5 years.[16,18,19] Because the tumors are so rare, and because a limited number of therapeutic options are available, subtyping and grading are often not performed. It is unlikely that either is necessary with small biopsies.

Immunohistochemically, sinonasal intestinal-type adenocarcinomas show a marked resemblance to true colorectal adenocarcinomas and most tumors will react with antibodies to CK20, CDX2, SATB2, and MUC2 (Fig. 7.4, eFigs. 7.3–7.5).[12,20–23] This allows them to be distinguished from other sinonasal adenocarcinomas. Unlike true colorectal adenocarcinomas, sinonasal intestinal-type adenocarcinomas show greater immunoreactivity with antibodies to neuroendocrine antigens such as NSE and chromogranin, whereas they are less likely to show immunoreactivity with antibodies to carcinoembryonic antigen.[24]

OTHER ADENOCARCINOMAS

The WHO currently classifies nonintestinal-type adenocarcinomas of the sinonasal tract as low grade and high grade. Most are of lower grade cytologically and carry with their diagnosis a much better prognosis than the

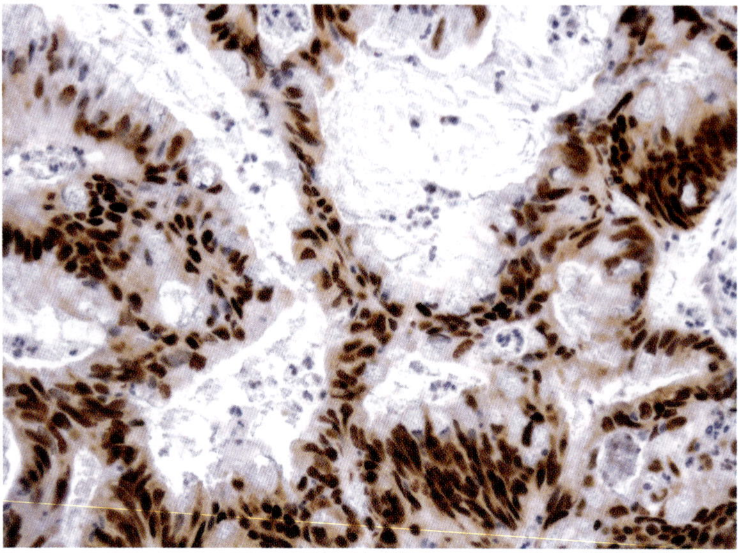

FIGURE 7.4 CDX-2 expression in a sinonasal intestinal-type adenocarcinoma demonstrated by immunostain.

intestinal-type adenocarcinomas.[25,26] A low-grade papillary adenocarcinoma of the nasopharynx is also discussed here.

Low-grade adenocarcinomas have been described involving the nasal cavity and/or paranasal sinuses (i.e., low-grade sinonasal adenocarcinoma [SNAC]).[25–34] Patient ages have varied greatly, with median ages ranging from 37 to 54 years. The tumors occur equally in both sexes and present with nonspecific symptoms such as obstruction or epistaxis. The tumors generally behave in a benign fashion, only occasionally recurring.[30]

Grossly, these tumors have been described as papillary or nodular and friable.[26] Histologically, they have been described as having the features of very well-differentiated adenocarcinomas. Papillae are often noted, especially with tumors of the nasopharynx (Fig. 7.5, eFig. 7.6).[27] Infiltrating glands are crowded, small, and uniform in most cases, but occasionally have been noted to be cystically dilated and to have papillary formations (Fig. 7.6, eFig. 7.7). The papilla and glands are lined by a single row of bland cuboidal to columnar mucinous cells with marked uniformity and only rare mitotic figures (Fig. 7.7). Mild to moderate anisonucleosis may sometimes be noted and nuclei are occasionally noted to lose their basal polarity. Rarely, calcispherules are identified (eFig. 7.8).

A tubulopapillary variant has been described that differs from the other descriptions of low-grade adenocarcinomas in that some of the neoplastic epithelial cells contained intraepithelial mucus and the tumors

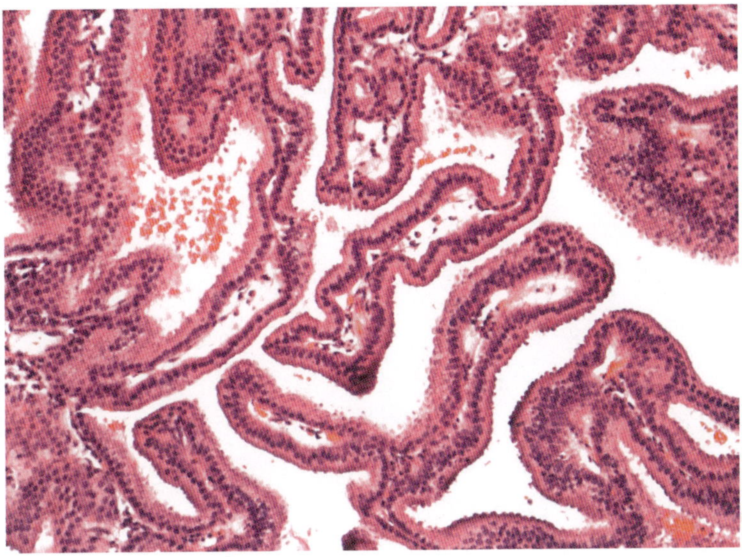

FIGURE 7.5 A low-grade adenocarcinoma with a prominent papillary architecture.

were not noted to ever have cystically dilated glands.[32,34] Furthermore, the also-described "seromucous adenocarcinoma" also shares most of the previously described features of other low-grade adenocarcinomas other than that it lacks the typical papillary architecture of the other tumors.[35]

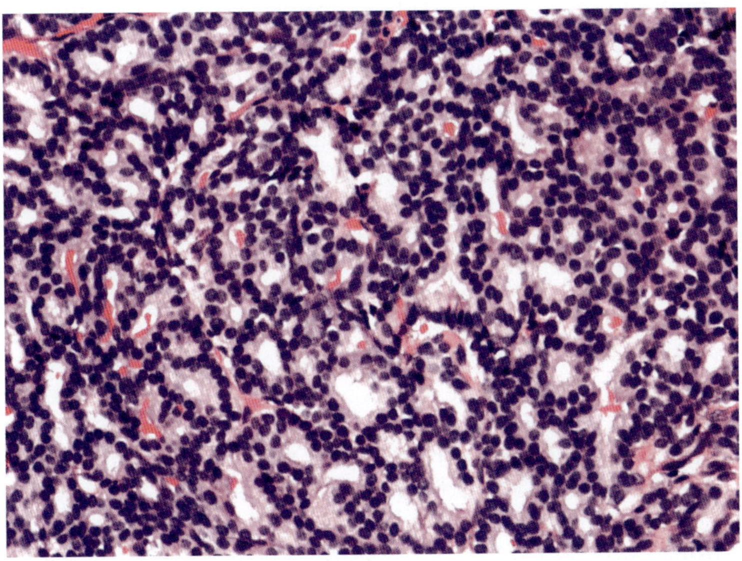

FIGURE 7.6 Tubules are back to back in this low-grade adenocarcinoma.

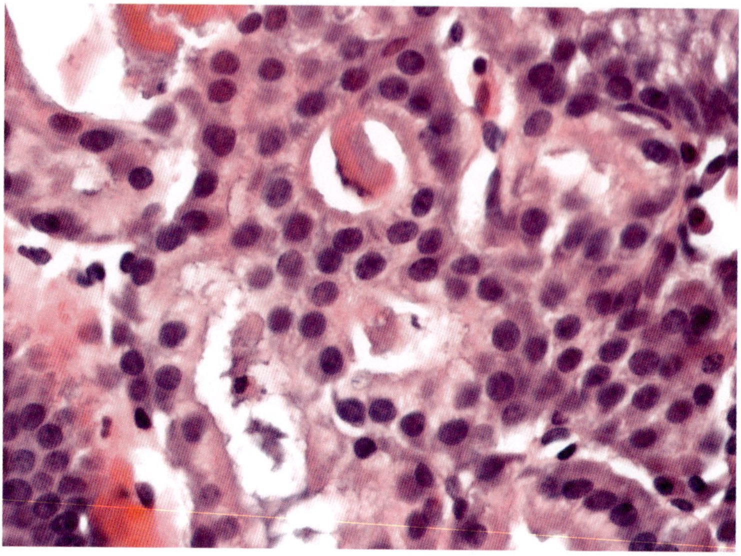

FIGURE 7.7 The tubules are lined by a cytologically bland layer of cuboidal cells.

Histochemical stains can be used to show the mucinous nature of these tumors. By immunohistochemistry, the tumors express epithelial antigens and CK7 but do not express markers of intestinal differentiation such as CK20, MUC2, and CDX2.[21–23] The tumors can be distinguished from many salivary gland–type neoplasms as they do not express myoepithelial markers.[32,35] Furthermore, unlike polymorphous (low-grade) adenocarcinomas, these tumors do not generally show perineural invasion.

Low-grade SNACs also need to be distinguished from respiratory epithelioid and seromucinous hamartomas (REAHs).[30,36,37] REAHs should be polypoid and covered by a schneiderian-type epithelium, sometimes with squamous metaplasia. Seromucinous glands can be increased in number but should retain a lobular pattern. We have seen cases of an apparent REAH with a low-grade adenocarcinoma (seromucous adenocarcinoma).[30] The overgrowth of the REAH by the adenocarcinoma was obvious, with a loss of lobular architecture and back-to-back proliferation of tubules. That said, others may have also called these tumors seromucinous hamartomas.[37]

Recently, some low-grade SNACs have been shown to harbor *ETV6* translocations, with either *NTRK3* or *RET*.[38,39] The tumors do not histologically resemble secretory carcinoma of the salivary glands and do not express mammaglobin. They do typically express CK7, DOG1, GCDFP-15, and SOX10. β-Catenin mutations have also been described in a subset of these tumors.[40]

Uncommonly, some low-grade SNACs may be composed of clear cells and resemble renal cell carcinoma (so-called renal cell–like adenocarcinoma) (eFig. 7.9).[41–43] These tumors appear to be more common in women and occur over a broad age range. They typically express S100, CK7, SOX10, and CAIX. PAX8, RCC, and vimentin expression is usually not seen. As with other low-grade SNACs, these tumors rarely recur and do not metastasize.

Nasopharyngeal papillary adenocarcinoma is a rare gland-forming malignancy of the nasopharynx occurring in patients of any age.[26–28] No sex predilection has been noted. Patients typically present with obstruction although middle ear infections and hearing problems can also be present. Tumors grossly appear exophytic and papillary and have been noted to be gritty on cut section. Histologically, the tumors have arborizing papillary lined by a single layer of cuboidal to columnar epithelial cells that have a moderate amount of eosinophilic cytoplasm and round to oval nuclei with nuclear membrane irregularities and vesicular chromatin, similar to those seen with papillary thyroid carcinoma. Tubular glands and infiltration are often present and occasional psammomatoid calcification can be seen. The tumors express cytokeratin and many express S100. Some have been shown to express TTF1 but not thyroglobulin.[27,28]

Sinonasal nonintestinal-type *high-grade adenocarcinomas* are a poorly characterized group of tumors. These are adenocarcinomas that cannot be better diagnosed as a specific salivary gland–type adenocarcinoma, do not have an intestinal phenotype, and have moderate to marked cytologic pleomorphism, high mitotic activity, and necrosis.[25,42,44] They have been described almost exclusively in the sinonasal tract. The majority of sinonasal high-grade adenocarcinomas have occurred in men and the tumors have developed in patients ranging in age from 15 to 83 years. Most have involved both the nasal cavities and paranasal sinuses at presentation. Symptoms have included obstruction and facial mass. In spite of aggressive therapy, more than half of the people with these tumors have died of disease.[25,33]

The histology of these tumors has been variable.[42,44] Some are reminiscent of the blastomatous component of teratocarcinosarcoma or of pulmonary blastomas and have solid and trabecular growth with occasional small cystic spaces, and are composed of neoplastic cells that have a small amount of amphiphilic cytoplasm (Fig. 7.8). Occasional cases are more nested and composed of larger cells, with more abundant eosinophilic cytoplasm (somewhat akin to salivary duct carcinoma) (Fig. 7.9). Many cases will have focal areas of solid growth with areas that are akin to those of sinonasal undifferentiated carcinoma. We and others have noted that some cases may appear akin to high-grade mucoepidermoid carcinomas and be associated with oncocytic schneiderian papillomas (eFig. 7.10).[42,45–47] Most cases, by definition, have marked cytologic and nuclear pleomorphism, abundant mitotic activity, and necrosis. Tumors generally

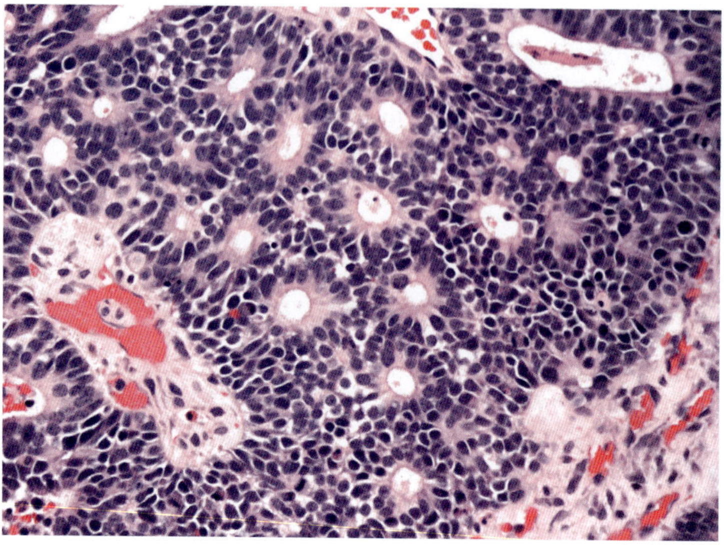

FIGURE 7.8 This high-grade sinonasal adenocarcinoma has numerous small cystlike spaces.

lack CDX2 and CK20 immunoreactivity.[42] Diffuse, strong CK7 immunoreactivity has been seen in nearly half of cases. S100, p63, and neuroendocrine antigen immunoreactivity is only rarely seen. Some tumors that are more undifferentiated, sometimes with clear cells, or even yolk-sac differentiation have been shown to be SMARCB1/INI1-deficient.[48]

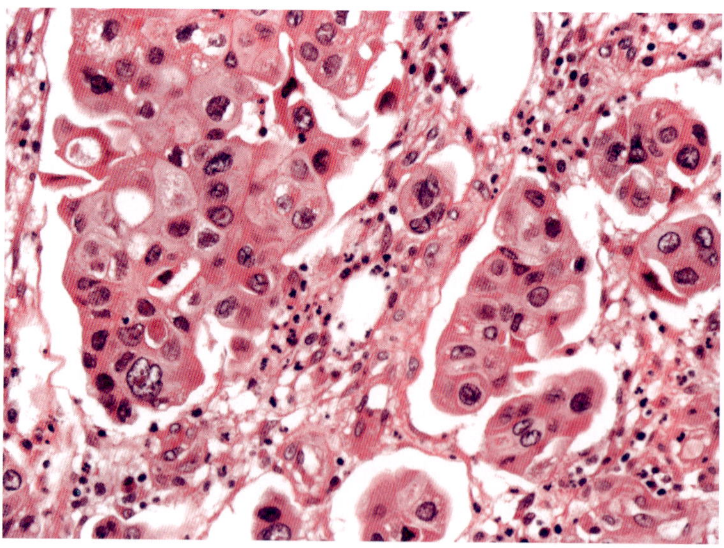

FIGURE 7.9 This sinonasal adenocarcinoma has nested, high-grade cells with abundant eosinophilic cytoplasm.

High-grade nonintestinal sinonasal adenocarcinomas should be distinguished from low-grade nonintestinal sinonasal adenocarcinomas because of their marked difference in prognosis. Low-grade lesions should be predominately papillary or tubular unlike high-grade lesions which are frequently solid or trabecular. Although focal cytologic atypia is sometimes seen with low-grade lesions, abundant mitotic figures or tumor necrosis is seen with high-grade lesions.

High-grade nonintestinal adenocarcinomas should also be distinguished from intestinal-type adenocarcinomas. Most sinonasal intestinal-type adenocarcinomas are gland forming and the tumors frequently produce extracellular mucus. Immunohistochemistry may be helpful, especially with small biopsies. Intestinal-type sinonasal adenocarcinomas frequently are immunoreactive with antibodies to CK20, CDX-2, and MUC2, whereas high-grade, nonintestinal adenocarcinomas rarely are immunoreactive with these antibodies.

Sinonasal undifferentiated carcinoma is sometimes considered in one's differential. For a diagnosis of SNUC, no or very, very limited glandular differentiation should be seen by routine histology. As mentioned above, some tumors will be deficient of SMARCB1/INI1. These tumors are best classified as sinonasal SMARCB1-deficient carcinomas. Finally, the distinction of these tumors from high-grade salivary duct carcinoma can be very difficult and, indeed, may be semantic. Some tumors appear akin to salivary duct carcinomas with infiltrating islands of pleomorphic glandular cells, sometimes with abundant eosinophilic cytoplasm. Furthermore, within the current WHO classification system of salivary gland tumors is the diagnosis "adenocarcinoma, not otherwise specified," a wastepaper basket diagnosis that could easily be made to include these tumors.

Recently, primary lingual adenocarcinomas with a colonic phenotype were described.[49] These tumors were immunoreactive with antibodies to CK20 and CDX-2. A case of adenocarcinoma associated with a lingual enteric duplication cyst has also been described.[50] We have encountered tongue lesions that have an intestinal appearance, two of which were associated with apparent benign duplication cysts.[44] The single case tested was immunoreactive with antibodies to CDX-2.

We have seen occasional high-grade adenocarcinomas of the base of tongue, tonsil, or sinonasal tract that express p16 and contain high-risk types of human papillomavirus by in situ hybridization (Fig. 7.10). Some of these have had limited p63 immunoreactivity and may perhaps be best classified as adenosquamous carcinomas, although they differ from the typical adenosquamous carcinomas that have obvious intracellular mucin accumulation.[51] The tumors typically have had a trabecular and cystic growth, lined focally with tall columnar cells. They have been immunoreactive with antibodies to CK7 and some with antibodies to neuroendocrine antigens.

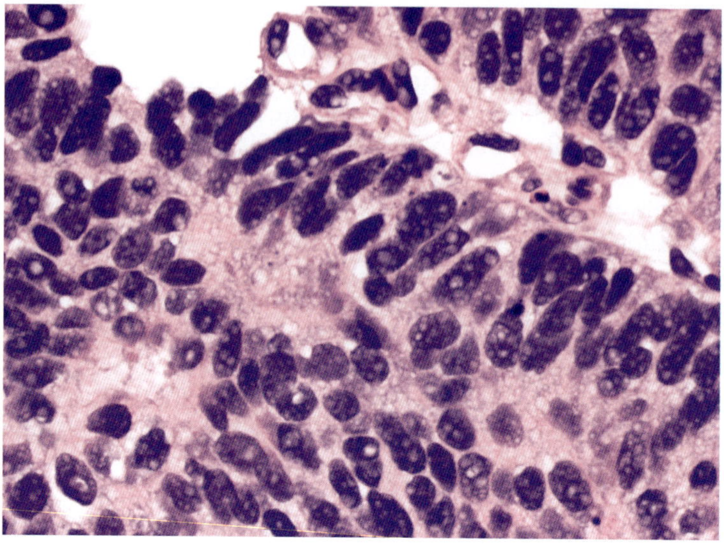

FIGURE 7.10 A high-grade adenocarcinoma of the sinonasal tract that was associated with high-risk human papillomavirus.

REFERENCES

1. Barnes L. Intestinal-type adenocarcinoma of the nasal cavity and paranasal sinuses. *Am J Surg Pathol*. 1986;10:192-202.
2. Ironside P, Matthews J. Adenocarcinoma of the nose and paranasal sinuses in woodworkers in the state of Victoria, Australia. *Cancer*. 1975;36:1115-1124.
3. Hadfield EH, Macbeth RG. Adenocarcinoma of ethmoids in furniture workers. *Ann Otol Rhinol Laryngol*. 1971;80:699-703.
4. Klintenberg C, Olofsson J, Hellquist H, Sokjer H. Adenocarcinoma of the ethmoid sinuses. A review of 28 cases with special reference to wood dust exposure. *Cancer*. 1984;54:482-488.
5. Imbus HR, Dyson WL. A review of nasal cancer in furniture manufacturing and woodworking in North Carolina, the United States, and other countries. *J Occup Med*. 1987;29:734-740.
6. Acheson ED, Cowdell RH, Hadfield E, Macbeth RG. Nasal cancer in woodworkers in the furniture industry. *Br Med J*. 1968;2:587-596.
7. Hadfield EH. A study of adenocarcinoma of the paranasal sinuses in woodworkers in the furniture industry. *Ann R Coll Surg Engl*. 1970;46:301-319.
8. Rampinelli V, Ferrari M, Nicolai P. Intestinal-type adenocarcinoma of the sinonasal tract: an update. *Curr Opin Otolaryngol Head Neck Surg*. 2018;26:115-121.
9. Perez-Ordonez B, Huynh NN, Berean KW, Jordan RC. Expression of mismatch repair proteins, beta catenin, and E cadherin in intestinal-type sinonasal adenocarcinoma. *J Clin Pathol*. 2004;57:1080-1083.
10. Yom SS, Rashid A, Rosenthal DI, et al. Genetic analysis of sinonasal adenocarcinoma phenotypes: distinct alterations of histogenetic significance. *Mod Pathol*. 2005;18:315-319.
11. Franchi A, Innocenti DR, Palomba A, et al. Low prevalence of K-RAS, EGF-R and BRAF mutations in sinonasal adenocarcinomas. Implications for anti-EGFR treatments. *Pathol Oncol Res*. 2014;20:571-579.

12. Skalova A, Sar A, Laco J, et al. The role of SATB2 as a diagnostic marker of sinonasal intestinal-type adenocarcinoma. *Appl Immunohistochem Mol Morphol*. 2018;26:140-146.
13. Korinth D, Pacyna-Gengelbach M, Deutschmann N, et al. Chromosomal imbalances in wood dust-related adenocarcinomas of the inner nose and their associations with pathological parameters. *J Pathol*. 2005;207:207-215.
14. Ariza M, Llorente JL, Alvarez-Marcas C, et al. Comparative genomic hybridization in primary sinonasal adenocarcinomas. *Cancer*. 2004;100:335-341.
15. Sanchez-Casis G, Devine KD, Weiland LH. Nasal adenocarcinomas that closely simulate colonic carcinomas. *Cancer*. 1971;28:714-720.
16. Kleinsasser O, Schroeder HG. Adenocarcinomas of the inner nose after exposure to wood dust. Morphological findings and relationships between histopathology and clinical behavior in 79 cases. *Arch Otorhinolaryngol*. 1988;245:1-15.
17. Mills SE, Fechner RE, Cantrell RW. Aggressive sinonasal lesion resembling normal intestinal mucosa. *Am J Surg Pathol*. 1982;6:803-809.
18. Franchi A, Gallo O, Santucci M. Clinical relevance of the histological classification of sinonasal intestinal-type adenocarcinomas. *Hum Pathol*. 1999;30:1140-1145.
19. Franquemont DW, Fechner RE, Mills SE. Histologic classification of sinonasal intestinal-type adenocarcinoma. *Am J Surg Pathol*. 1991;15:368-375.
20. Choi HR, Sturgis EM, Rashid A, et al. Sinonasal adenocarcinoma: evidence for histogenetic divergence of the enteric and nonenteric phenotypes. *Hum Pathol*. 2003;34:1101-1107.
21. Franchi A, Massi D, Palomba A, Biancalani M, Santucci M. CDX-2, cytokeratin 7 and cytokeratin 20 immunohistochemical expression in the differential diagnosis of primary adenocarcinomas of the sinonasal tract. *Virchows Arch*. 2004;445:63-67.
22. Cathro HP, Mills SE. Immunophenotypic differences between intestinal-type and low-grade papillary sinonasal adenocarcinomas: an immunohistochemical study of 22 cases utilizing CDX2 and MUC2. *Am J Surg Pathol*. 2004;28:1026-1032.
23. Kennedy MT, Jordan RC, Berean KW, Perez-Ordonez B. Expression pattern of CK7, CK20, CDX-2, and villin in intestinal-type sinonasal adenocarcinoma. *J Clin Pathol*. 2004;57:932-937.
24. McKinney CD, Mills SE, Franquemont DW. Sinonasal intestinal-type adenocarcinoma: immunohistochemical profile and comparison with colonic adenocarcinoma. *Mod Pathol*. 1995;8:421-426.
25. Heffner DK, Hyams VJ, Hauck KW, Lingeman C. Low-grade adenocarcinoma of the nasal cavity and paranasal sinuses. *Cancer*. 1982;50:312-322.
26. Wenig BM, Hyams VJ, Heffner DK. Nasopharyngeal papillary adenocarcinoma. A clinicopathologic study of a low-grade carcinoma. *Am J Surg Pathol*. 1988;12:946-953.
27. Pineda-Daboin K, Neto A, Ochoa-Perez V, Luna MA. Nasopharyngeal adenocarcinomas: a clinicopathologic study of 44 cases including immunohistochemical features of 18 papillary phenotypes. *Ann Diagn Pathol*. 2006;10:215-221.
28. Zeizafoun N, Elmberger G, Wenig BM: Thyroid transcription factor (TTF-1) immunoreactivity in low-grade nasopharyngeal papillary adenocarcinomas (LGNPPA): a report of three cases. *Mod Pathol*. 2007;20:231-232A.
29. Franchi A, Palomba A, Massi D, et al. Low-grade salivary type tubulo-papillary adenocarcinoma of the sinonasal tract. *Histopathology*. 2006;48:881-884.
30. Jo VY, Mills SE, Cathro HP, Carlson DL, Stelow EB. Low-grade sinonasal adenocarcinomas: the association with and distinction from respiratory epithelial adenomatoid hamartomas and other glandular lesions. *Am J Surg Pathol*. 2009;33(3):401-408.
31. Kleinsasser O. Terminal tubulus adenocarcinoma of the nasal seromucous glands. A specific entity. *Arch Otorhinolaryngol*. 1985;241:183-93.
32. Luna MA. Sinonasal tubulopapillary low-grade adenocarcinoma: a specific diagnosis or just another seromucous adenocarcinoma?. *Adv Anat Pathol*. 2005;12:109-115.

33. Orvidas LJ, Lewis JE, Weaver AL, Bagniewski SM, Olsen KD. Adenocarcinoma of the nose and paranasal sinuses: a retrospective study of diagnosis, histologic characteristics, and outcomes in 24 patients. *Head Neck*. 2005;27:370-375.
34. Skalova A, Cardesa A, Leivo I, et al. Sinonasal tubulopapillary low-grade adenocarcinoma. Histopathological, immunohistochemical and ultrastructural features of poorly recognised entity. *Virchows Arch*. 2003;443:152-158.
35. Neto AG, Pineda-Daboin K, Luna MA. Sinonasal tract seromucous adenocarcinomas: a report of 12 cases. *Ann Diagn Pathol*. 2003;7:154-159.
36. Wenig BM, Heffner DK. Respiratory epithelial adenomatoid hamartomas of the sinonasal tract and nasopharynx: a clinicopathologic study of 31 cases. *Ann Otol Rhinol Laryngol*. 1995;104:639-645.
37. Weinreb I, Gnepp DR, Laver NM, et al. Seromucinous hamartomas: a clinicopathological study of a sinonasal glandular lesion lacking myoepithelial cells. *Histopathology*. 2009;54:205-213.
38. Andreasen S, Kiss K, Melchior LC, Laco J. The ETV6-RET gene fusion is found in ETV6-rearranged low-grade sinonasal adenocarcinoma without NTRK3 involvement. *Am J Surg Pathol*. 2018;42:985-988.
39. Andreasen S, Skalova A, Agaimy A, et al. ETV6 gene rearrangements characterize a morphologically distinct subset of sinonasal low-grade non-intestinal-type adenocarcinoma: a novel translocation-associated carcinoma restricted to the sinonasal tract. *Am J Surg Pathol*. 2017;41:1552-1560.
40. Villatoro TM, Mardekian SK. Two cases of sinonasal non-intestinal-type adenocarcinoma with squamoid morules expressing nuclear beta-catenin and CDX2: a curious morphologic finding supported by molecular analysis. *Case Rep Pathol*. 2018;2018:8741017.
41. Zur KB, Brandwein M, Wang B, Som P, Gordon R, Urken ML. Primary description of a new entity, renal cell-like carcinoma of the nasal cavity: van Meegeren in the house of Vermeer. *Arch Otolaryngol Head Neck Surg*. 2002;128:441-447.
42. Stelow EB, Jo VY, Mills SE, Carlson DL. A histologic and immunohistochemical study of high-grade non-intestinal sinonasal adenocarcinomas. *Am J Surg Pathol* 2011;35(7):971-980.
43. Bishop JA. Newly described tumor entities in sinonasal tract pathology. *Head Neck Pathol*. 2016;10:23-31.
44. Stelow EB, Mills SE, Jo VY, Carlson DL. Adenocarcinoma of the upper aerodigestive tract. *Adv Anat Pathol*. 2010;17:262-269.
45. Barnes L, Bedetti C. Oncocytic Schneiderian papilloma: a reappraisal of cylindrical cell papilloma of the sinonasal tract. *Hum Pathol*. 1984;15:344-351.
46. Kapadia SB, Barnes L, Pelzman K, Mirani N, Heffner DK, Bedetti C. Carcinoma ex oncocytic schneiderian (cylindrical cell) papilloma. *Am J Otolaryngol*. 1993;14:332-338.
47. Maitra A, Baskin LB, Lee EL. Malignancies arising in oncocytic schneiderian papillomas: a report of 2 cases and review of the literature. *Arch Pathol Lab Med*. 2001;125:1365-1367.
48. Shah AA, Jain D, Ababneh E, et al. SMARCB1 (INI-1)-deficient adenocarcinoma of the sinonasal tract: a potentially under-recognized form of sinonasal adenocarcinoma with occasional yolk sac tumor-like features. *Head Neck Pathol*. 2019.
49. Bell D, Kupferman ME, Williams MD, Rashid A, El-Naggar AK. Primary colonic-type adenocarcinoma of the base of the tongue: a previously unreported phenotype. *Hum Pathol*. 2009;40:1798-1802.
50. Volchok J, Jaffer A, Cooper T, Al-Sabbagh A, Cavalli G. Adenocarcinoma arising in a lingual foregut duplication cyst. *Arch Otolaryngol Head Neck Surg*. 2007;133:717-719.
51. Masand RP, El-Mofty SK, Ma XJ, Luo Y, Flanagan JJ, Lewis JS Jr. Adenosquamous carcinoma of the head and neck: relationship to human papillomavirus and review of the literature. *Head Neck Pathol*. 2011;5:108-116.

8

NEURAL, NEUROECTODERMAL, AND NEUROENDOCRINE NEOPLASMS

A variety of neural, neuroectodermal, and neuroendocrine neoplasms can occur throughout the region of the upper aerodigestive tract. These lesions may show overlapping histologic features and be difficult to distinguish from one another by small biopsy. Nonetheless distinction from one another and from other neoplasms is important as these tumors have widely different prognoses and require markedly different treatments. This chapter discusses the clinicopathologic features of these neoplasms and methods for accurately diagnosing them.

NEURAL LESIONS

Most neural lesions found throughout the peripheral nervous system can occur in the upper aerodigestive tract (Table 8.1).[1] These include neurofibromas, schwannomas, granular cell tumors, neuromas, neurothekeomas, paragangliomas, and malignant peripheral nerve sheath tumors. Most may occur throughout the upper aerodigestive tract; however, many occur more frequently at particular sites in well-defined clinicopathologic circumstances. With small biopsies, it is not always possible to distinguish the lesions from one another, especially as knowing the overall architecture of the neoplasms is sometimes necessary for the diagnosis. In such cases, differential diagnoses can be supplied or more general diagnoses such as *benign nerve sheath tumor* or *benign neural tumor* can be used.

Traumatic neuromas can occur throughout the tract but most frequently arise in the lip, tongue, or mental nerve area.[1,2] They present as small nodules which are often painful to palpation. Like their counterparts throughout the body, they are composed of tangles of neural tissue composed of axons and schwann cells, often accompanied with dense sclerotic tissue (Fig. 8.1, eFig. 8.1). Ganglion cells have been reported in some lesions. An S100 immunostain can be used to highlight the neural nature of these lesions.

TABLE 8.1 Neural Lesions of the Upper Aerodigestive Tract

Traumatic neuroma
Mucosal neuroma
Neurofibroma
Schwannoma
Granular cell tumor
Neurothekeoma
Nerve sheath myxoma
Palisaded, encapsulated neuroma (solitary, circumscribed neuroma)
Malignant peripheral nerve sheath tumor
Paraganglioma
Olfactory neuroblastoma

The *mucosal neuromas* of multiple endocrine neoplasia (MEN) type 2b resemble traumatic neuromas and are composed of convoluted neural tissue with numerous axons surrounded by a thickened perineurium.[1,3] These lesions mostly involve the lips and tongue, but can also involve other oral and nasal sites. The syndrome is associated with familial mutations of the *RET* protooncogene and the development of medullary thyroid carcinoma and pheochromocytomas.[3,4] It is important to distinguish these lesions from neurofibromas as the lesions occur in vastly different syndromes and have different risks for subsequent diseases.

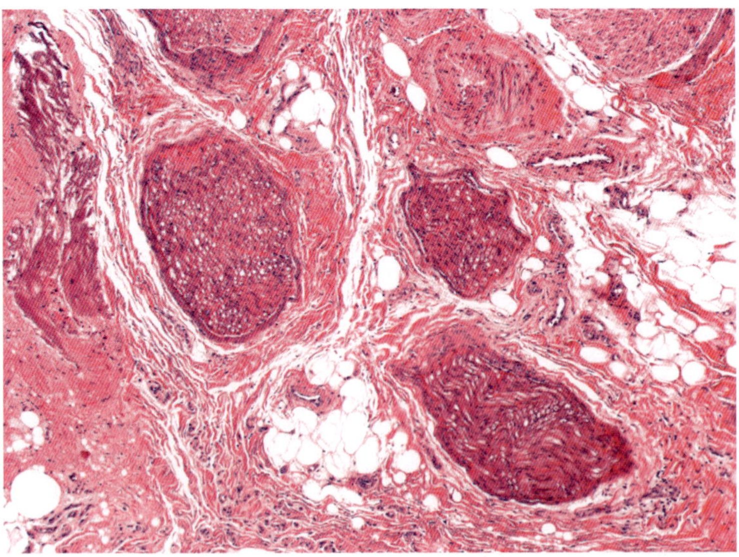

FIGURE 8.1 Traumatic neuroma with complex well-formed nerve.

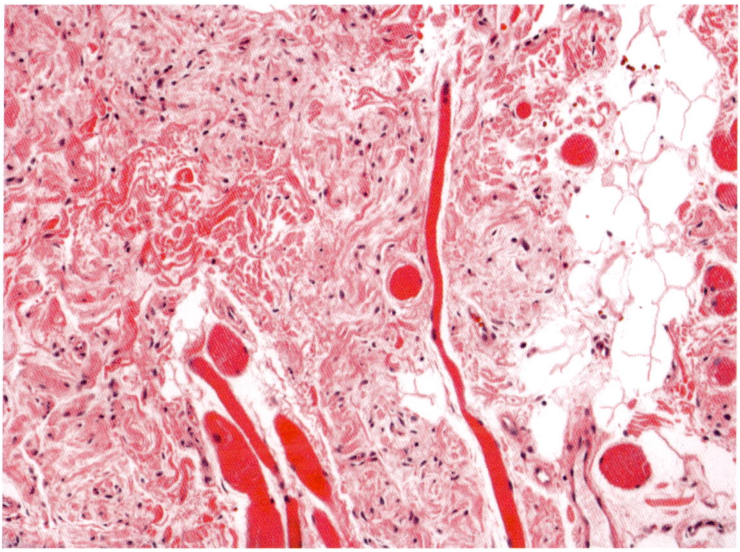

FIGURE 8.2 A plexiform neurofibroma infiltrating surrounding skeletal muscle.

Solitary and multiple neurofibromas can also occur throughout the upper aerodigestive tract and may be associated with neurofibromatosis type 1.[1,5–7] The distinction of these lesions from other neural tumors is thus important, as the diagnosis can allow for the identification of the other stigmata of the disease. Neurofibromas appear either somewhat circumscribed or plexiform (Fig. 8.2); however, even when they appear circumscribed, the interface of the lesion with the surrounding soft tissue is usually not discrete. The lesions are composed of intermixed spindled cells with serpentine or wavy nuclei, collagenous fibers, and myxoid matrix (eFig. 8.2). A mixture of S100 protein and CD34 immunoreactive cells can be identified by immunohistochemistry. Neurofibromas can usually be distinguished from other neural tumors because of their classic, rather uniform histology.

Schwannomas or neurilemomas also occur throughout the upper aerodigestive tract.[1,5,8,9] Aside from those which involve the ear, they appear to be most frequent in the sinonasal area. The tumors occur in older adults and usually present as polypoid masses with symptoms secondary to mass effect. Although benign, schwannomas may be associated with the destruction of surrounding bony tissues.[8] When not resected in a piecemeal fashion, the lesions will sometimes appear circumscribed and encapsulated although this feature seems to be less common than with peripheral schwannomas, and infiltration adjacent to mucosal epithelium may be seen.[8] Histologically, the tumors are similar to those seen at other sites of the body and are composed of variably cellular areas (cellular Antoni A and looser, less cellular Antoni B areas) (Fig. 8.3, eFig. 8.3). Cellular palisading or Verocay bodies can be identified in some cases,

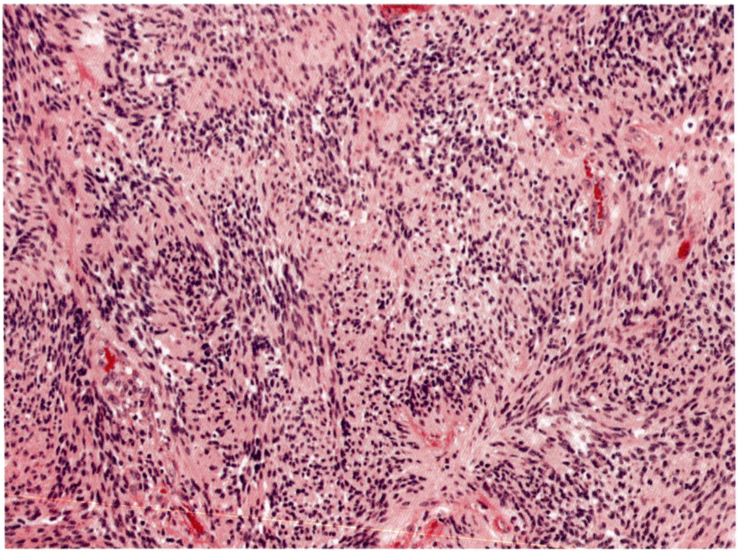

FIGURE 8.3 Schwannomas can be very cellular.

and hyalinized blood vessels can be found in most examples (eFigs. 8.4 and 8.5).[8,9] The tumors show strong and diffuse immunoreactivity with antibodies to S100. Although occasional cells may be immunoreactive with antibodies to CD34, such cells are much fewer in number than in neurofibromas.[8,9]

Granular cell tumors occur throughout the body, but the tongue is the most commonly involved anatomic site.[10,11] The lesions usually present as painless submucosal nodules. Frequently, the overlying squamous epithelium will show a significant amount of pseudoepitheliomatous hyperplasia, a well-described pitfall that has led some cases to be erroneously diagnosed as squamous cell carcinomas.[10,11] Granular cell tumors are circumscribed, but not encapsulated and neoplastic cells frequently infiltrate the surrounding soft tissues. The constituent cells are large and polygonal with abundant granular, eosinophilic cytoplasm (Fig. 8.4). Ultrastructurally, the granularity is due to numerous lysosomes filling the cytoplasm.[10] Nuclei are small and centrally located and rare cells may be multinucleated. Mitotic figures are uncommon, but occasional typical forms can be identified. By immunohistochemistry, the neoplastic cells react strongly and diffusely with antibodies to S100 protein (eFig. 8.6) and other markers of antigens associated with peripheral nerves.[12,13] Not surprisingly, the neoplastic cells react with antibodies to lysozyme and CD68.[14] Rare granular cell tumors are malignant, and as such are characterized by a larger size, necrosis, increased mitotic activity, and cellular atypia. Distinction of malignant tumors and multifocal granular cell tumors may be difficult.

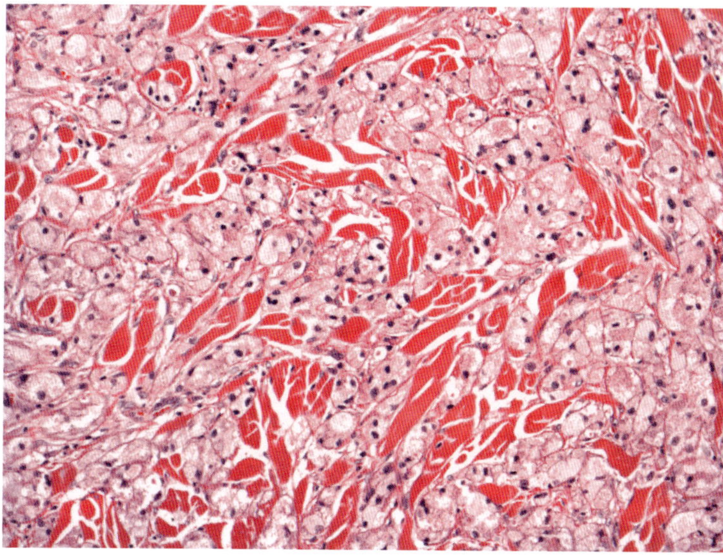

FIGURE 8.4 The large and polygonal cells of a granular cell tumor.

It is unclear how *congenital epulis* or *congenital granular cell tumor* relates to the typical adult granular cell tumor. These tumors present as large polypoid masses attached to the gingiva of newborns, almost always in girls.[15] By conventional H&E histology, they are identical to adult granular cell tumors (eFig. 8.7). The neoplastic cells do not react with antibodies to S100 protein, however.[16] Unlike nonneural granular cell tumors of the skin, congenital epulis does not appear to have *ALK* translocations.[17]

Nerve sheath myxomas and *neurothekeomas* are uncommon, benign tumors.[18–20] Both may involve the head and neck and when reported in the upper aerodigestive tract, they have almost exclusively involved the mouth. Histologically, nerve sheath myxomas are lobular and well-circumscribed although they do not have a capsule.[1,19] The lobules are composed of abundant myxoid stroma with intermixed spindled cells and are separated from one another by fibrous connective tissue that resembles perineurium (eFig. 8.8). These lesions show immunoreactivity with antibodies to S100 protein. Neurothekeomas are also typically well-circumscribed and grow as lobules of neoplastic cells separated by bands of collagen (Fig. 8.5). Frequently, some degree of myxoid matrix is present. The growth pattern is typically whirled although some fascicular growth may be present. Tumor cells are spindled and epithelioid with abundant eosinophilic cytoplasm. Only minimal to mild atypia is present in most cases and mitotic figures are usually infrequent. Osteoclastlike giant cells are sometimes present. Unlike nerve sheath myxomas, these lesions are not immunoreactive with antibodies to S100 protein. They are typically immunoreactive with antibodies

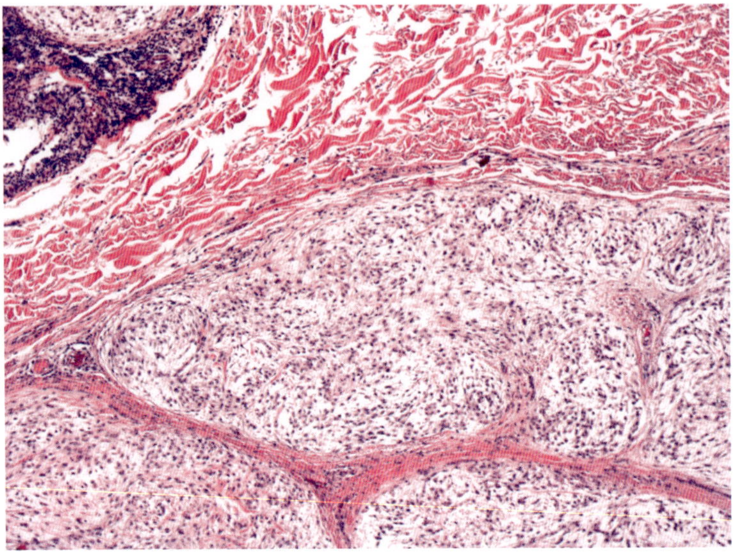

FIGURE 8.5 Neurothekeomas have a lobular and circumscribed growth pattern.

to NKI/C3, vimentin, and NSE. Frequently, they are immunoreactive with antibodies to MSA and SMA. Recently, some have suggested that these tumors may be related to fibrous histiocytomas.[21]

Palisaded, encapsulated neuroma or solitary circumscribed neuroma is a benign tumor of the peripheral nerve sheath that mostly occurs subcutaneously but may involve the mouth, especially in the region of the lips, gingiva, and palate.[22-24] The lesions are described as slow growing and painless and are mostly identified in adults. Histologically, they are well-circumscribed and partially encapsulated (Fig. 8.6). Tumors are composed of broad fascicles of spindled cells with little intervening eosinophilic stroma. Although the nuclei can focally appear vaguely parallel, palisading Verocay bodies akin to those seen with schwannomas are not usually seen with this tumor, in spite of its name.[22,24] Furthermore, hypocellular areas are also not seen. Small vessels are often noted, and hemorrhage and necrosis are not seen. Most tumor cells react with antibodies to S100 protein. Immunostaining for EMA will highlight the perineurium that surrounds the lesions.[22,23]

Malignant peripheral nerve sheath tumors (MPNSTs) also occur throughout the upper aerodigestive tract and have been frequently noted in the sinonasal area.[25-27] These tumors develop in older individuals and most often occur in patients who do not have neurofibromatosis. Unlike schwannomas, MPNSTs are infiltrative and destructive and after resection, tend to recur and eventually metastasize.[26,27] MPNSTs are usually highly cellular and generally have a histologic pattern reminiscent of a fibrosarcoma, although a prominent herringbone pattern is usually not seen and the nuclei tend to appear more irregular and wavy (Fig. 8.7).[26,27]

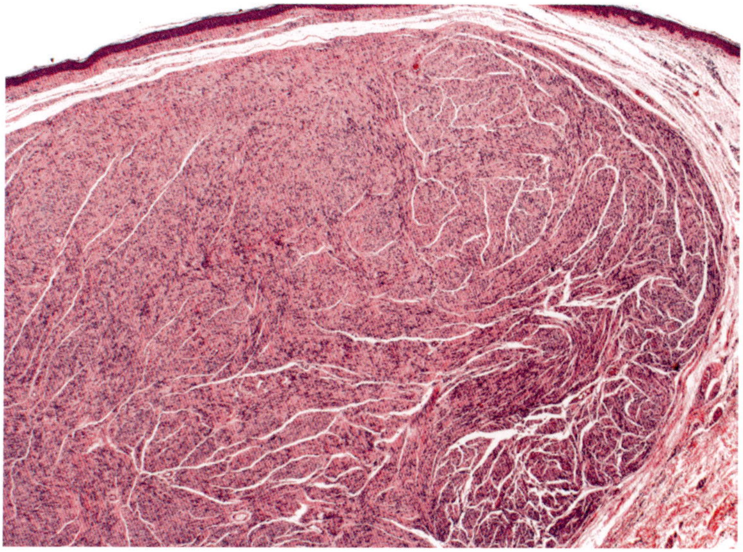

FIGURE 8.6 A solitary circumscribed neuroma of the lip.

MPNSTs also have been noted to have alternating less cellular (eFig. 8.9) areas and rare nuclear palisading. Compared to benign neurogenic tumors, mitotic figures in MPNSTs are usually increased in number and geographic necrosis can sometimes be found (Fig. 8.8). To assist in the diagnosis, immunohistochemistry can be helpful, especially if the tumor

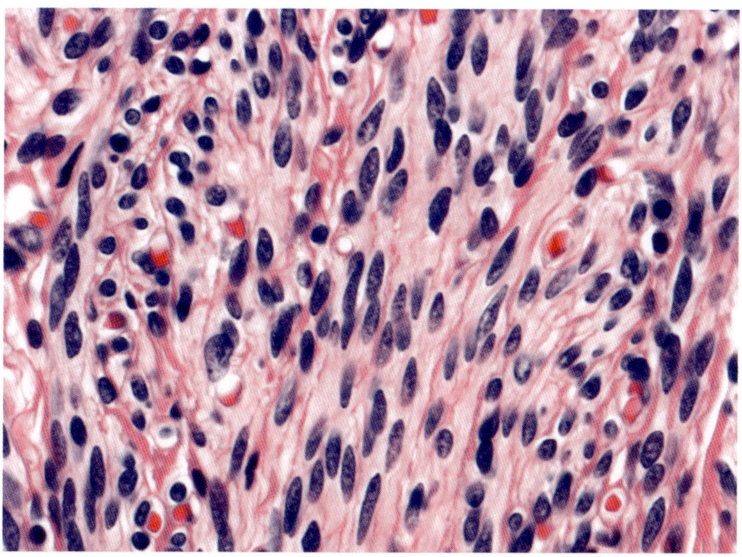

FIGURE 8.7 A cellular area within a malignant peripheral nerve sheath tumor with somewhat wavy nuclei.

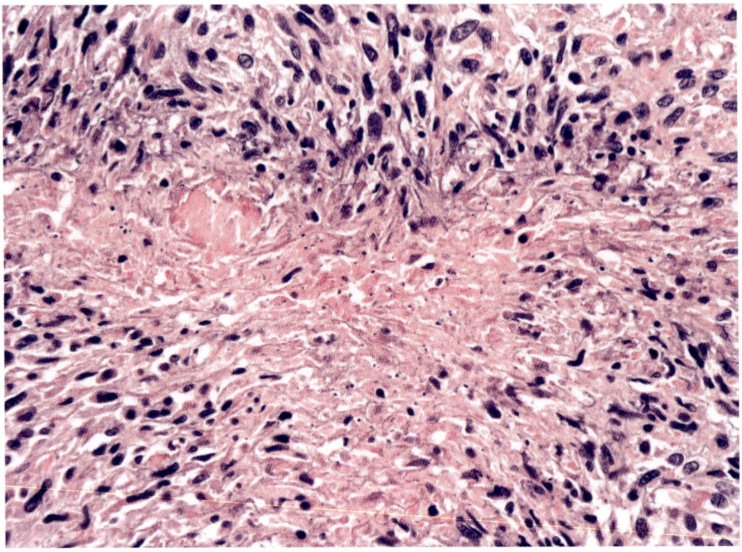

FIGURE 8.8 Geographic necrosis seen in a malignant peripheral nerve sheath tumor.

is immunoreactive with antibodies to S100 protein.[26,27] Staining for CD56 is more sensitive but less specific (eFig. 8.10). Importantly, with small biopsies, positive staining with antibodies to S100 protein does not clinch a diagnosis of MPNST and malignant melanoma must be excluded.[26] Also of note, up to 15% of MPNSTs are immunoreactive with antibodies to TLE1, an antibody generally used to diagnose synovial sarcoma.[28] A significant portion of tumors originally classified as MPNSTs of the sinonasal tract likely represent biphenotypic sinonasal sarcoma and will thus express S100 and SMA and have *PAX3* translocations (see Chapter 11).[29–31]

Most *paragangliomas* of the head and neck arise at the carotid body, the vagal body, or the middle ear. Those that arise in the upper aerodigestive tract usually arise within the nasal cavity and larynx.[32–34] Occasional tumors, likely arising in the vagal body, will present as nasopharyngeal masses. Paragangliomas develop in both sexes, usually in adults. Those that arise in the head and neck present almost exclusively with mass-related symptoms, or other nonspecific symptoms related to their site of presentation (e.g., epistaxis when in the nasal cavity).[32,34] Head and neck paragangliomas almost never produce symptoms secondary to hormone production, especially catecholamine production. Some pheochromocytomas and extra-adrenal paragangliomas are familial and can be seen with mutations of the *VHL* gene, *RET* proto-oncogene, and the genes encoding for subunits of succinate dehydrogenase (e.g., *SDHB*).[35]

The tumors have a typical histology, akin to that seen with pheochromocytomas of the adrenal gland.[33,34] They tend to be well-circumscribed and partially encapsulated. The tumors are composed of nests of epithelioid

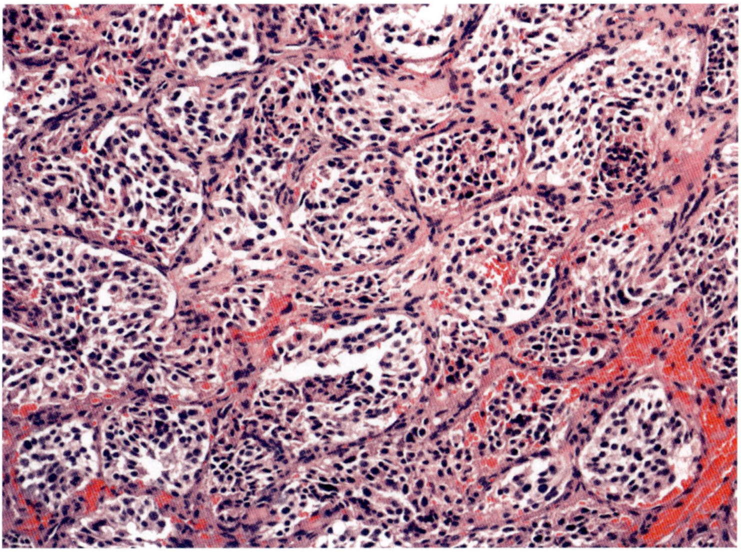

FIGURE 8.9 A laryngeal paraganglioma showing an obvious nested pattern.

cells with finely granular, eosinophilic cytoplasm and round to oval nuclei (Fig. 8.9, eFig. 8.11). The nuclei may have granular chromatin, and occasional prominent nucleoli may be seen (Fig. 8.10). Atypia may be present and should not be considered a feature suggestive of malignancy. Mitotic figures are rare. Surrounding the nests are slender sustentacular cells and a rich network of capillaries. By immunohistochemistry,

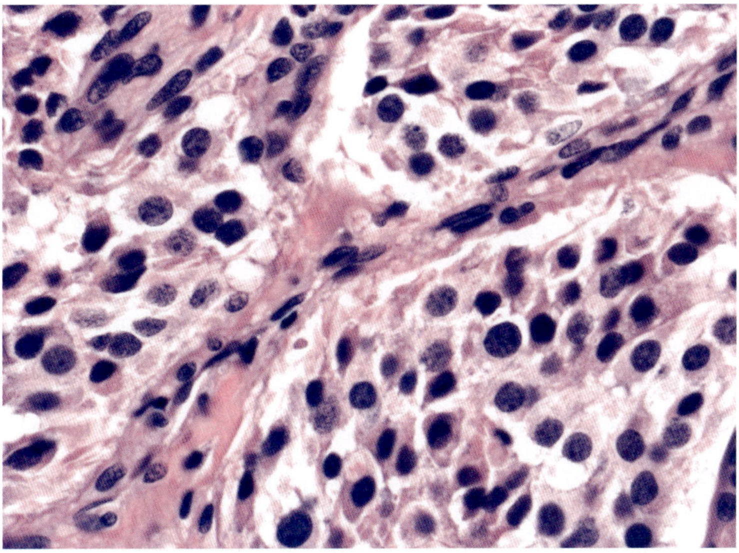

FIGURE 8.10 Most of the nuclei of paragangliomas have granular chromatin.

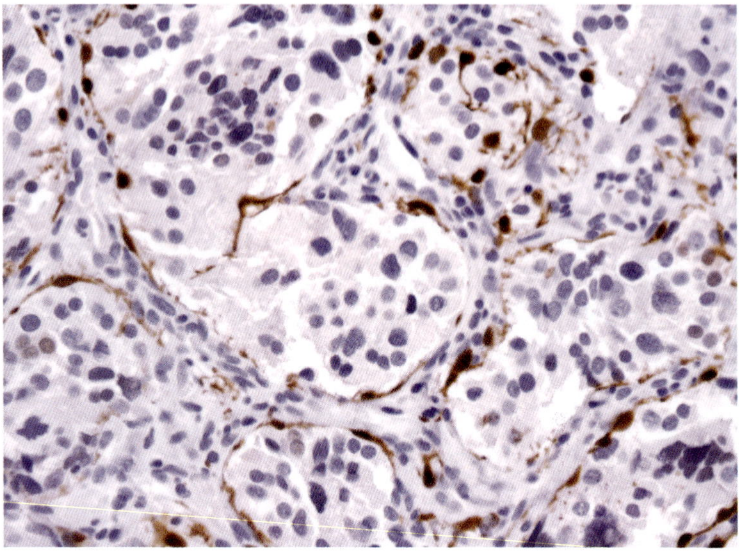

FIGURE 8.11 S100 immunostaining of a laryngeal paraganglioma highlights the sustentacular cells.

neoplastic cells will react with antibodies to chromogranin, synaptophysin, and NSE.[36,37] They do not react with antibodies to cytokeratins. Supporting sustentacular cells will react with antibodies to S100 protein (Fig. 8.11). Although some tumors will behave in a malignant fashion, histology provides little clues to distinguish benign and malignant tumors. Some have suggested that a lack of sustentacular cells, identified by an absence of S100 protein staining, may help to identify malignant tumors.[38]

Olfactory neuroblastomas (ONBs) are rare tumors that develop in the upper nasal cavity in the area of the olfactory epithelium.[39-41] The tumors show a bimodal age incidence and occur most frequently in adolescents and older adults. The tumors do not show a predilection for either sex or race. Patients with these malignancies present with nonspecific symptoms including nasal stuffiness, epistaxis, nasal discharge, headache, and anosmia. Occasionally, visual changes can be present.

The tumors are usually polypoid and occur high in the nasal cavity in the region of the cribriform plate, superior turbinate, and ethmoid sinuses.[39,41] The location of the tumor and its phenotypic characteristics have led most to consider it to be a malignancy of the olfactory epithelium. As biopsy specimens are received piecemeal and as patients are usually treated prior to surgical resection, staging is usually performed clinically and radiographically, based on the extent of the tumor according to the method originally described by Kadish (Table 8.2).[41] Molecular changes are complex, similar to most epithelial malignancies.[42] ONB is not a member of the Ewing sarcoma group of tumors and the typical t(11;22) seen in

TABLE 8.2 Kadish Staging System for Olfactory Neuroblastoma

Stage A	Limited to the nasal cavity
Stage B	Limited to the nasal cavity and paranasal sinuses
Stage C	Local or distant spread beyond the nasal cavity and paranasal sinuses

those tumors is not seen with ONBs, despite an early paper claiming the contrary.[43–45] With current multimodality treatments, patients with ONB do quite well and some have reported survival rates at 10 years to be greater than 80%.[46,47]

Microscopically, tumor cells grow either diffusely or in discrete, circumscribed nests that are separated by fibrous or edematous stroma (Figs. 8.12 and 8.13).[39,41] About 25% of cases have definitive Homer Wright rosettes with annular arrays of neoplastic cells surrounding central, eosinophilic fibrils (Fig. 8.14, eFig. 8.12). Many more will show more equivocal rosette formations surrounding fibrillary material and the remainder lack even rudimentary rosettes. An eosinophilic fibrillary background can be found in most cases (Fig. 8.15, eFig. 8.13) and calcification will be seen with some cases (eFig. 8.14). Vascular invasion and necrosis, either as single-cell apoptosis or as large zones, are often seen. Mature ganglion cells are also identified in some cases (eFig. 8.15). The neoplastic cells are small and usually have minimal eosinophilic cytoplasm.

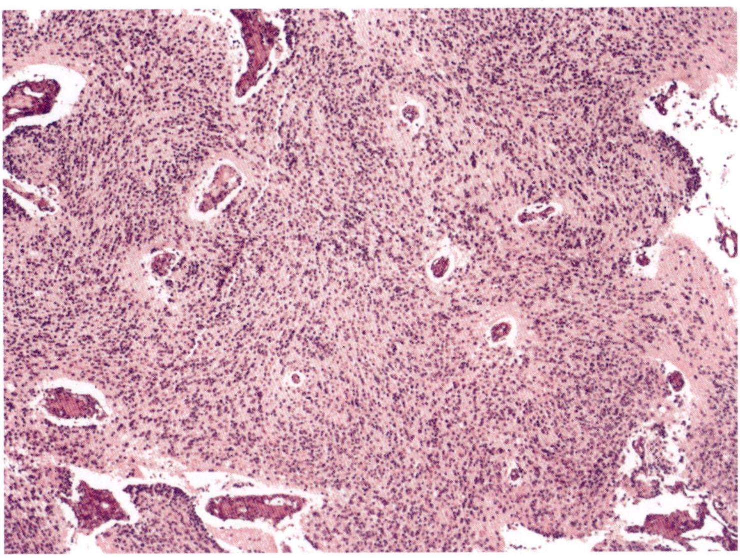

FIGURE 8.12 Olfactory neuroblastoma with a diffuse growth pattern.

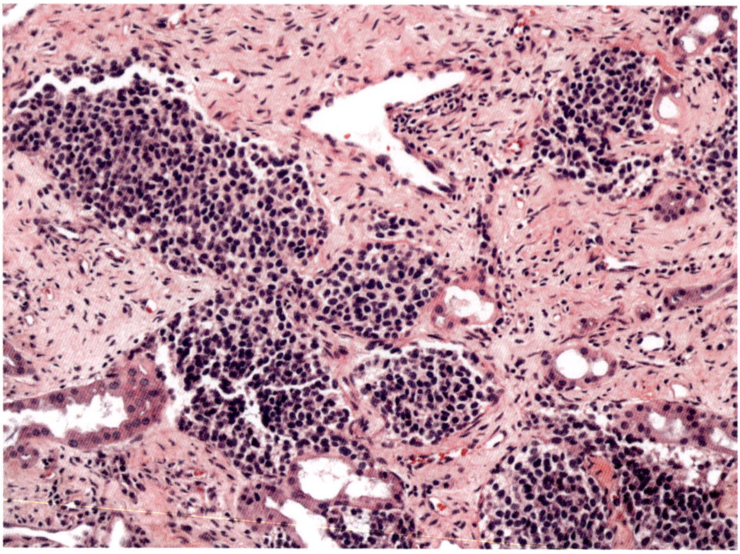

FIGURE 8.13 Olfactory neuroblastoma with a nested growth pattern.

The nuclei often appear monomorphic and round with delicate granular chromatin. Prominent nucleoli and mitotic figures are usually absent. The tumor can, however, display a wide range of atypia and some cases may show marked variation in nuclear size and shape. Mitotic activity can also vary greatly and some cases have been noted to have more than 10

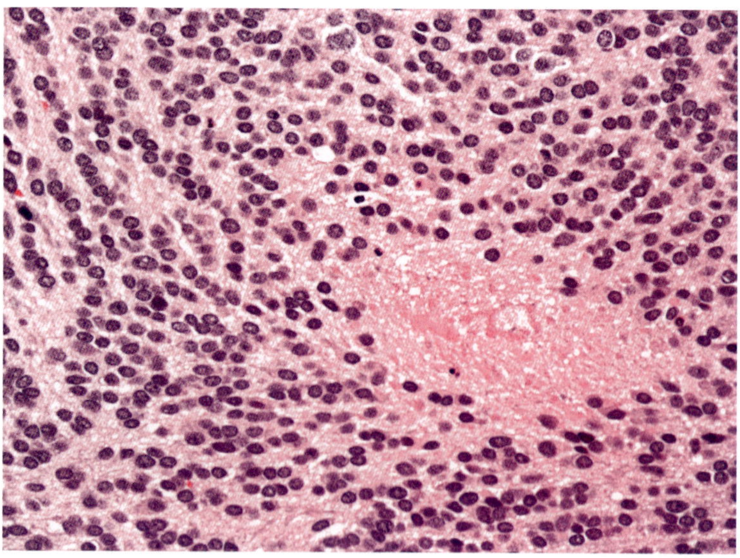

FIGURE 8.14 Homer Wright rosettes can be found in many olfactory neuroblastomas.

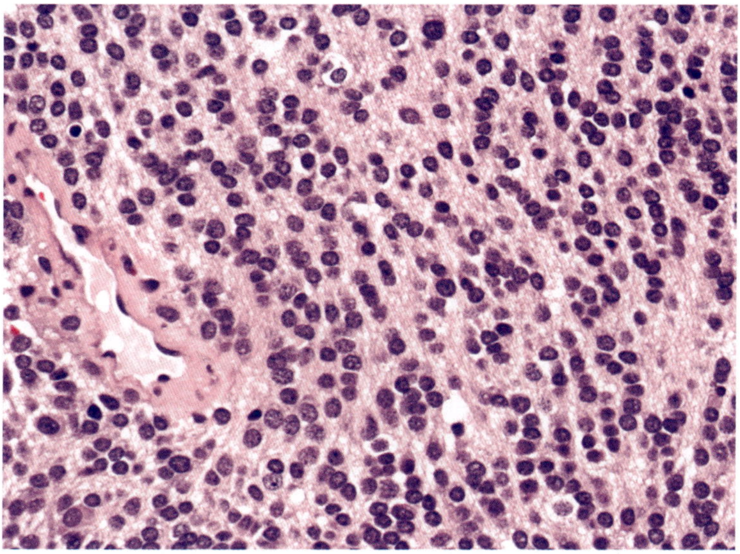

FIGURE 8.15 A neurofibrillary background can be seen with most cases of olfactory neuroblastoma.

mitotic figures per high-powered field. ONBs have been graded according to the Hyams grading system (Table 8.3) which takes into account tumor architecture, nuclear atypia, mitotic activity, necrosis, and the presence or absence of background fibrillary material.[48] There have been mixed reports regarding the utility of this grading system, and it should be noted that it was developed prior to the distinction of other high-grade neuroendocrine

TABLE 8.3 **Hyams Grading Scheme for Olfactory Neuroblastoma**

Histology	Grade 1	Grade 2	Grade 3	Grade 4
Lobular architecture	Predominant	Predominant	Occasional	Infrequent
Nuclear Pleomorphism	Minimal	Mild	Moderate	Marked
Mitotic figures	Rare	Occasional	Abundant	Abundant
Calcification	Sometimes present	Sometimes present	None	None
Necrosis	None	None	Some	Abundant
Fibrillary background	Abundant	Abundant	Less frequent	Not seen
H-W rosettes	Often seen	Often seen	Not seen	Not seen

H-W, Homer Wright.

tumors of the sinonasal tract, including sinonasal undifferentiated carcinoma (which may have originally been reported as grade 4 ONBs). As a result, most ONBs that we now see would be considered to be grade 1 or 2 neoplasms.

Although many ONBs can be diagnosed based on histology alone, immunohistochemistry is often prudently used for a number of reasons (Table 8.5).[40,49] The distinction of these lesions from other sinonasal tumors such as sinonasal undifferentiated carcinomas has significant prognostic value. Furthermore, biopsy specimens are often limited in both tumor quantity and quality, frequently exhibiting marked crush artifact. Most ONBs will show immunoreactivity with antibodies to synaptophysin or chromogranin, as well as with antibodies to less specific markers of neural or neuroendocrine differentiation such as NSE and CD56 (Fig. 8.16). Although most ONBs do not react with antibodies to cytokeratins, occasional tumors will display focal positivity and thus cytokeratin reactivity should not dissuade one from making the diagnosis. In our experience, strong reactivity with antibodies to cytokeratin is very rare with ONBs. S100 immunoreactivity, when present, is usually limited to the supporting or sustentacular cells that surround the neoplastic nests (Fig. 8.17). Occasional tumor cells may show limited reactivity with antibodies to S100; however, staining for other markers of melanoma, such as HMB45, should not be seen. Finally, membranous reactivity with antibodies to CD99 should not be seen nor should nuclear staining with antibodies to FLI1.

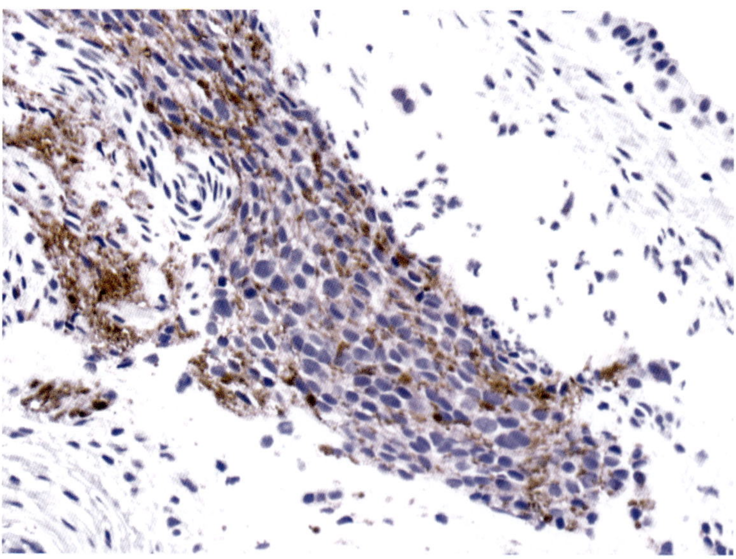

FIGURE 8.16 Olfactory neuroblastomas are generally immunoreactive with antibodies to synaptophysin.

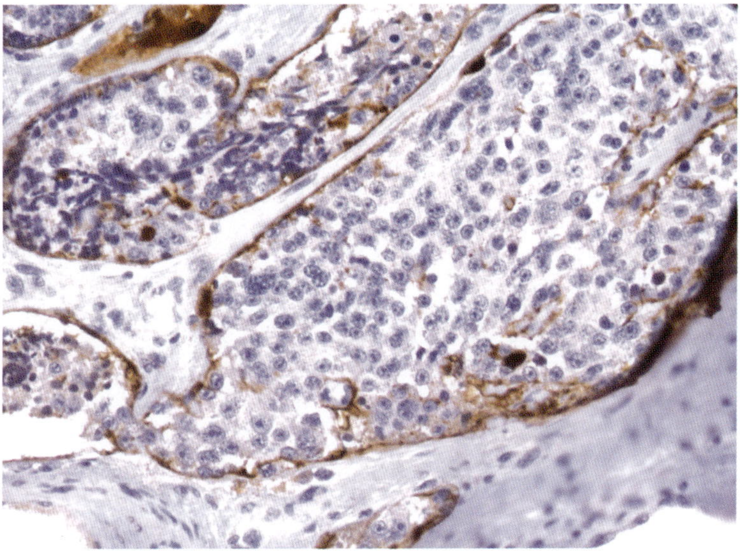

FIGURE 8.17 Sustentacular cells of olfactory neuroblastomas can be highlighted with an S100 immunostain.

NEUROECTODERMAL LESIONS

Melanotic Neuroectodermal Tumor of Infancy

This rare tumor can occur throughout the head and neck but usually involves maxilla or, less commonly, the mandible.[50-54] Patients are more often males and are usually younger than 1, although melanotic neuroectodermal tumors of infancy (MNTIs) sometimes present in older children. The prognosis for MNTI is good, and although tumors can recur, they only rarely metastasize.[52] The lesions usually are less than 5 cm in greatest dimension and appear grossly lobulated and circumscribed although capsules are not present. On cut surface the tumors may appear gray-white to darkly pigmented.[52]

Histologically, two cell populations are present. Larger, epithelioid cells with vesicular nuclei and prominent nucleoli and abundant eosinophilic cytoplasm that contains dark brown granular melanin pigment arrange themselves together in loose alveolar or tubular structures while small, round to oval cells with hyperchromatic nuclei and scant cytoplasm form small nests, cords, or sheets usually surrounded by the larger, epithelioid cells (Figs. 8.18 and 8.19, eFigs. 8.16–8.18).[51,52] Dense collagenous stroma separates the alveoli, pseudoglandular spaces, tubular structures, and small nests of neoplastic cells from one another. Occasionally, a more fibrillary stroma is identified within the islands of smaller cells. Neoplastic cells infiltrate into adjacent bone and soft tissue. Histologic features of a high-grade malignancy such as abundant mitotic figures or necrosis are not noted.

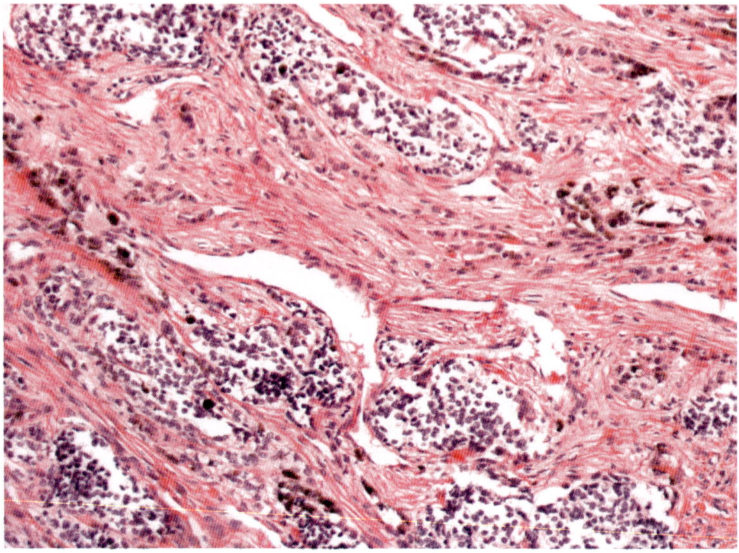

FIGURE 8.18 Melanotic neuroectodermal tumor of infancy showing a mixture of larger, pigmented epithelioid cells and smaller cells.

Reports regarding immunohistochemistry have been somewhat varied.[50–53] Both the larger and smaller cells are usually noted to show immunoreactivity with antibodies to NSE, synaptophysin, and HMB-45 along with other melanocytic antigens, while the larger cells will typically show

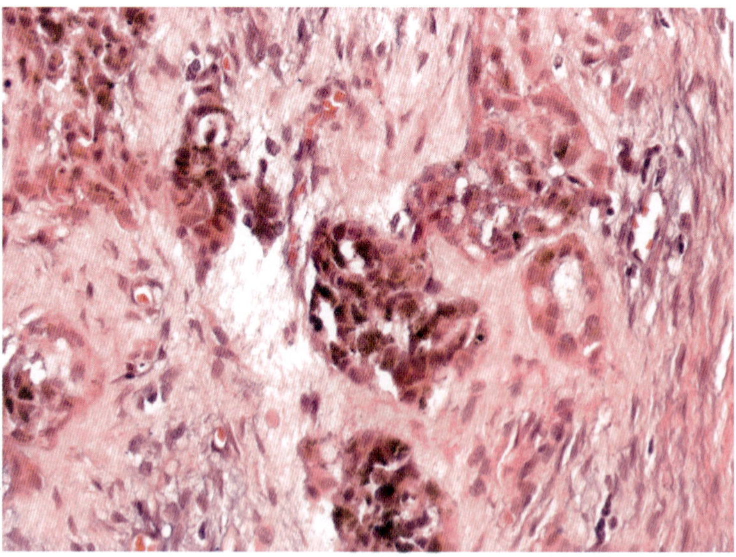

FIGURE 8.19 The larger, epithelioid cells of melanotic neuroectodermal tumor of infancy show abundant melanin pigment.

immunoreactivity with antibodies to epithelial antigens such as cytokeratins and EMA. It is interesting to note that neither cell will typically show immunoreactivity with antibodies to S-100 protein. Neoplastic cells are typically not reactive with antibodies to CD99.

Primitive Neuroectodermal Tumor/Ewing Family Tumors

Primitive neuroectodermal tumors (PNETs) can occur throughout the body and seldom involve the head and neck region.[55–58] When they do develop here, they often involve the sinonasal area.[59] PNETs may develop at any age but usually occur in the first three decades of life. Symptoms are nonspecific and related to either the primary mass or metastases. Although originally having a very poor prognosis, PNETs now have decent 5-year survival rates with multimodality treatment, especially when they are of lower stage.[60]

The tumors are grossly tan-white and have somewhat circumscribed borders. Histologically, these lesions are composed of small blue cells and thus must be differentiated from other small blue cell tumors.[61] The neoplastic cells are arranged in sheets and nests of cells, sometimes with intervening fibrous bands (Fig. 8.20). Homer Wright–like rosettes with centrally located fibrillary material are sometimes seen (eFigs. 8.19 and 8.20). The individual cells have high nuclear to cytoplasmic ratios with hyperchromatic nuclei. Mitotic figures are frequent.

To distinguish these tumors from other small blue cell tumors, ancillary studies such as immunohistochemistry are generally required (Table 8.5). If tissue is received fresh, it should be submitted for cytogenetic

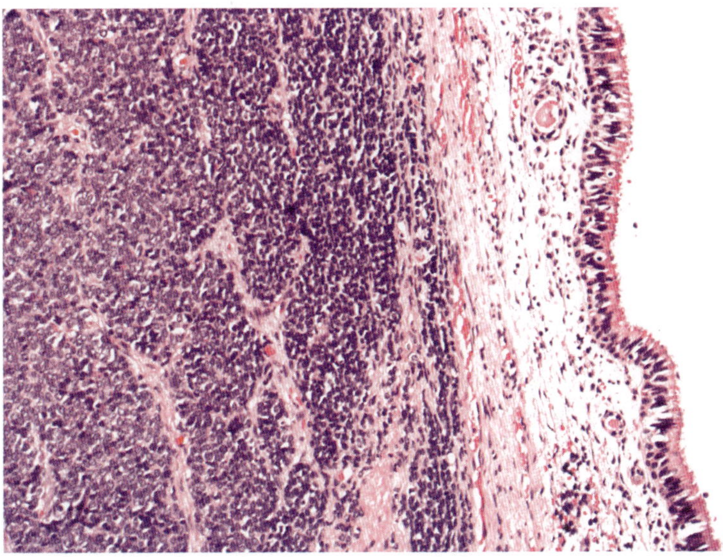

FIGURE 8.20 Sheets of small blue cells seen with a nasal primitive neuroectodermal tumor.

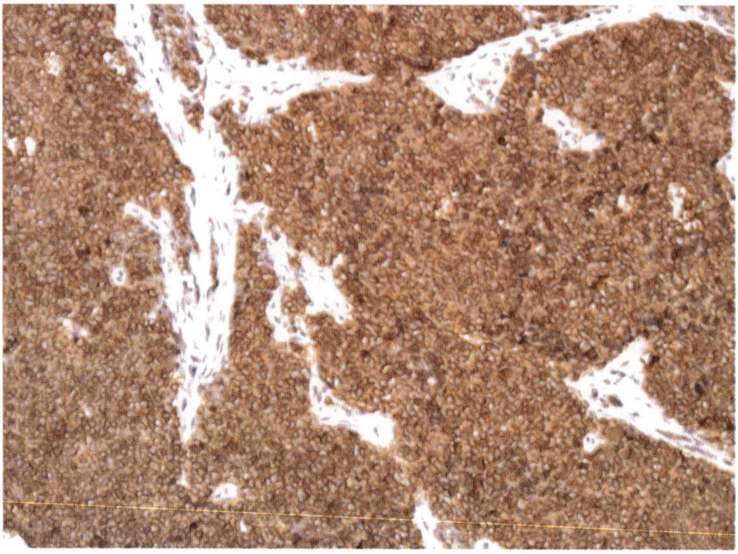

FIGURE 8.21 Strong membranous staining with antibodies to CD99 should be seen with primitive neuroectodermal tumors.

analysis and touch imprints should be made. Identification of the t(11;22)(q24;q12) is characteristic for PNET; it can be shown by conventional cytogenetic analysis, RT-PCR, or FISH.[62] Intracytoplasmic glycogen can often be demonstrated by PAS stain. By immunohistochemistry, most cases show immunoreactivity with antibodies to synaptophysin, NSE, S100, and CD99 (Fig. 8.21, eFig. 8.21).[61] Only rarely, will immunoreactivity with antibodies to muscle antigens be seen. Antibodies to FLI1 may also prove helpful since these tumors express this antigen secondary to their classic translocation that unites the *EWS* gene on chromosome 22 with the *FLI1* gene on chromosome 11 (eFig. 8.22).[63]

While PNETs frequently express keratins focally, an epithelial-appearing PNET has been described in the head and neck (so-called adamantinoma-like Ewing tumor).[64] The sinonasal tract and salivary glands have been the sites most commonly reported to be involved. The tumors resemble basaloid or nonkeratinizing squamous cell carcinomas and may even show keratin pearl formation. They are diffusely immunoreactive with antibodies to keratins and p40/p63. Like conventional PNETs, they also are immunoreactive with antibodies to CD99. Demonstrating *EWSR1* rearrangement, typically by FISH, is necessary for diagnosis.

Mucosal Melanocytic Lesions

Melanocytic neoplasms can occur throughout the upper aerodigestive tract and are most commonly identified in the sinonasal area and within the mouth. Benign lesions are almost always identified in the mouth,

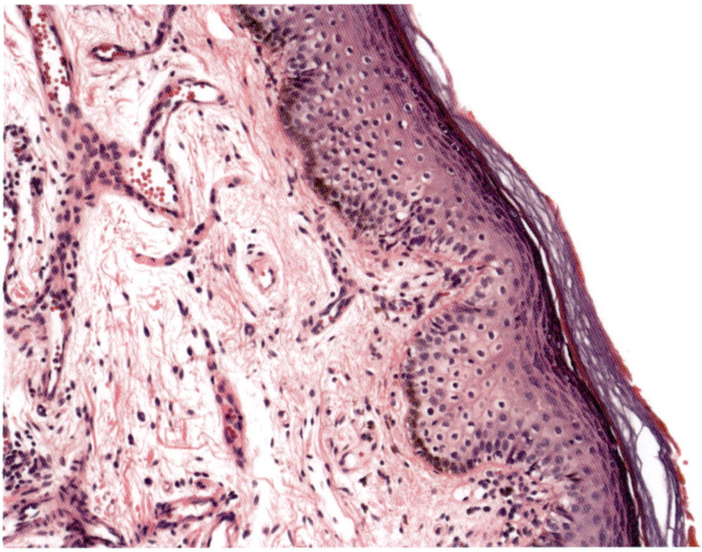

FIGURE 8.22 Melanotic macule of the lip showing increased basal pigmentation without increased numbers of melanocytes.

as they generally present as asymptomatic macules. Melanomas most often present as masses and are usually identified in the sinonasal area or mouth.

Benign pigmented lesions include melanotic macules, melanocytic "hyperplasia" (lentigo simplex), and nevi.[65] *Melanotic macules* are usually less than a centimeter in size, occur more frequently in women, and most commonly involve the lower lip, palate, gingiva, and buccal mucosa, in descending order of frequency.[52] Histologically, they are characterized by the deposition of melanin pigment in the basal cell layer of the squamous epithelium and within the lamina propria (Fig. 8.22, eFig. 8.23). Increased numbers of melanocytes should not be present.

Melanocytic "hyperplasia" or *lentigo simplex* is very uncommon in the mouth.[66] The few cases reported have been predominately in women and less than a centimeter in size. Histologically, the lesion is characterized by an increased number of benign, basal melanocytes, not meeting the criteria for a diagnosis of junctional nevus. The lesions are pigmented, obviously, as they would otherwise not be biopsied.

Melanoacanthomas are interesting and rare lesions that occur most frequently in black women.[65] The lesions are somewhat larger than typical melanotic macules and may raise clinical suspicion for melanoma. They are characterized by parakeratosis and acanthosis and numerous pigmented dendritic melanocytes are located throughout the squamous epithelium. The lesions are not believed to have malignant potential and are likely reactive in nature.

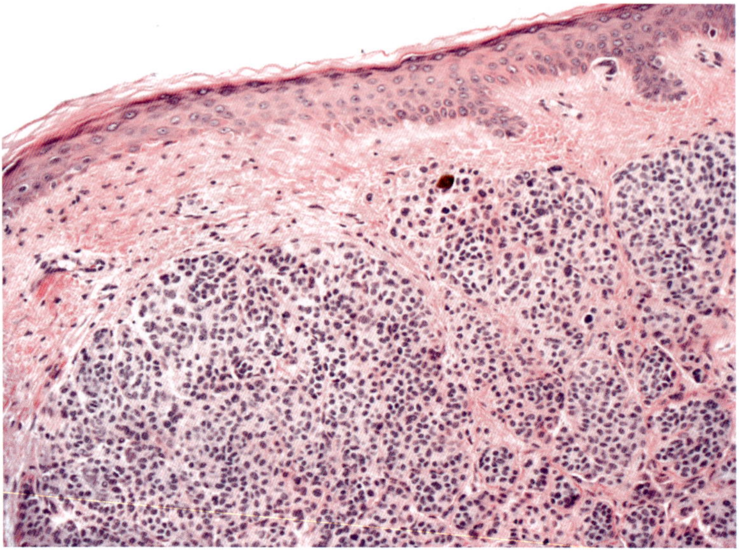

FIGURE 8.23 Intramucosal nevus of the lip.

The benign nevi of the mouth are similar histologically to cutaneous nevi and include *intramucosal, junctional, compound*, and *blue nevi*.[67,68] In larger series, most of the nevi are located in the hard palate, buccal mucosa, lip, and gingiva, in descending order of frequency, and the vast majority are either intramucosal or blue nevi (Fig. 8.23). As with other melanocytic lesions, they occur more frequently in women. The majority present in patients between 20 and 40 years of age and are less than a centimeter in size.

Most intramucosal or compound nevi will show some degree of pigmentation. The overlying epithelium may be normal; however, hyperplasia is usually present. The melanocytes mature toward the base of the lesion, becoming less epithelioid and more spindled (eFig. 8.24). Multinucleated "giant cells" are usually present. Blue nevi are universally pigmented and have normal surface epithelium. A zone of collagen of varying thickness separates the nevus cells from the surface epithelium. The spindled melanocytes of the blue nevus can extend into the deep lamina propria.

Occasional melanocytic lesions of the mouth have been termed *dysplastic nevi* when the interpreting pathologists believed that some histologic features were worrisome for melanoma.[69] We do not advise the use of such a term and instead prefer to call such lesions *atypical melanocytic lesions* and recommend conservative surgical management. The use of these terms for any pigmented oral lesion should be very rare.

Malignant melanomas may occur throughout the upper aerodigestive tract, although almost all the cases develop in the nasal cavity, paranasal sinuses, and mouth.[70–75] Rare primary malignant melanomas of the larynx have, however, also been reported.[76] Unlike cutaneous lesions, the majority of melanocytic lesions of the upper aerodigestive tract are malignant. This may be because the lesions present as masses rather than easily observable changes in pigmentation. As such, the lesions are often large and of advanced stage at the time of diagnosis. Furthermore, it is rarely difficult to distinguish these lesions from their benign counterparts. It is interesting to note that most mucosal melanomas lack *BRAF* mutations and that comparative genomic hybridization has identified chromosomal abnormalities such as 1q and 6p gains not usually seen with cutaneous melanomas.[77,78] Activating *KIT* mutations have been identified in a minority of oral melanomas and in up to 22% of sinonasal melanoma, similar to *NRAS* mutations.[79,80] Translocations involving *EWSR1*, typical of clear cell sarcomas, are not seen with mucosal melanomas of the head and neck.[81]

Malignant melanomas of the sinonasal area typically present in older patients with many of the cases identified in patients older than 70 years.[70,74,75] Oral lesions are more likely to present as intraepithelial malignancies; however, overall survival rates are similar.[82] Overall, the 5-year survival for patients diagnosed with mucosal melanoma of the head and neck is only about 30% and less than 20% for patients with nodal metastases.[75] Studies have found varying rates of sex and race predilection.

The surface epithelium may be ulcerated, especially with sinonasal melanomas; however, when epithelium is present, intraepithelial disease can often be identified with clusters of atypical melanocytes and single melanocytes spreading through all levels of the epithelium.[70,74] The invasive component can show a number of histologic patterns, often within the same tumor. The neoplastic cells may have a spindled, epithelioid, plasmacytoid, rhabdoid, or undifferentiated phenotype and usually show significant cytologic atypia with prominent nucleoli, intranuclear pseudoinclusions, and many mitotic figures (Figs. 8.24–8.26, eFigs. 8.25–8.27).[70,74] Intracellular melanin pigment is most often seen; however, up to a quarter of cases may be amelanotic. A background chronic inflammatory infiltrate may be present. Both perineural and vascular invasion are common. A desmoplastic variant with prominent sclerosis has been described in the mouth.[82]

More than half of sinonasal cases and many oral lesions can show an undifferentiated phenotype and be difficult to distinguish histologically from other undifferentiated lesions (Table 8.5).[70,74] Furthermore, spindled cell variants, including desmoplastic types, may be difficult to distinguish from other neoplastic and nonneoplastic conditions. For this reason, immunohistochemistry is often necessary for diagnosing these lesions. A number of studies have been performed specifically investigating

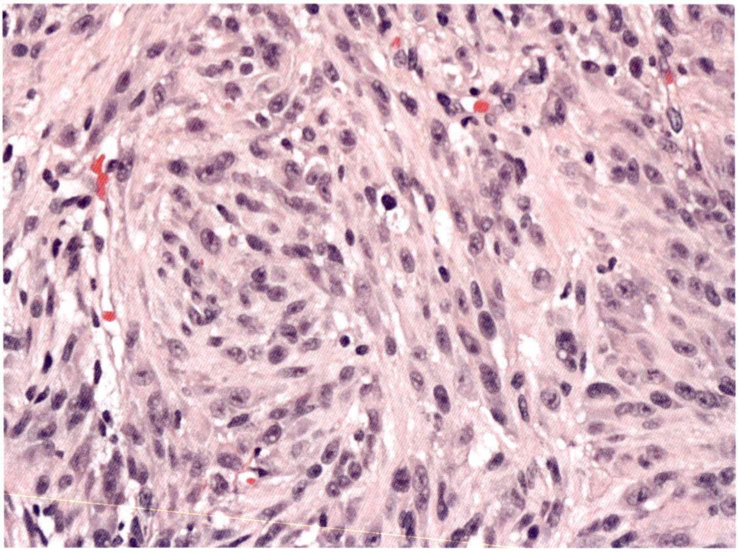

FIGURE 8.24 A sinonasal melanoma composed of spindled cells.

the immunophenotype of mucosal melanomas.[70,74,83–85] Nearly all tumors express S100 protein and most are found to be immunoreactive with other more specific melanocytic antigens such as HMB45, tyrosinase, Melan A, and microphthalmia transcription factor (Fig. 8.27, eFig. 8.28). Endocrine antigens, such as NSE, have been noted to be expressed in some cases. While most have found no expression of cytokeratins or EMA, focal immunoreactivity has been noted by some.[86]

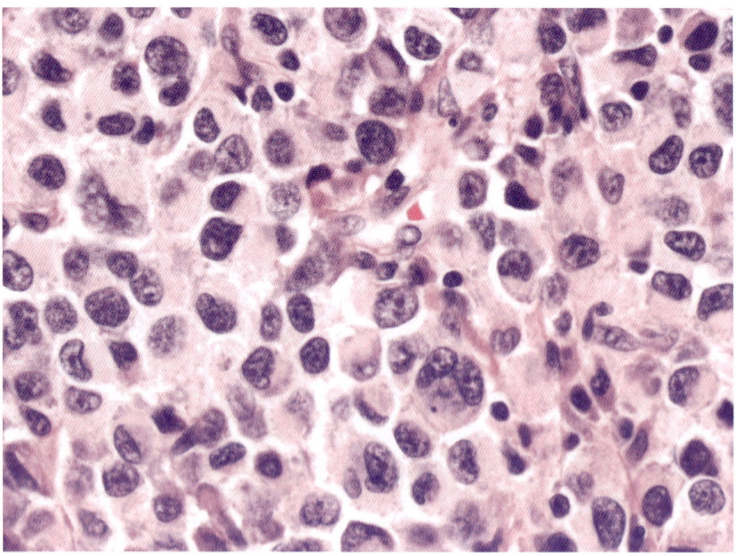

FIGURE 8.25 A sinonasal melanoma composed of more epithelioid cells.

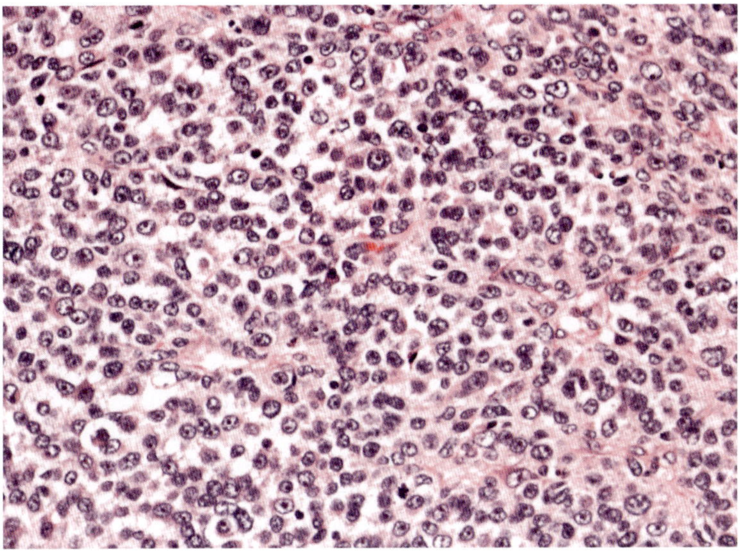

FIGURE 8.26 An undifferentiated area in a sinonasal melanoma.

NEUROENDOCRINE CARCINOMAS

Sinonasal Undifferentiated Carcinoma

Sinonasal undifferentiated carcinoma (SNUC) is a rare, aggressive malignancy of the sinonasal area.[87–91] The tumor was originally described by Frierson et al. in 1986 and is still considered a distinct entity by the

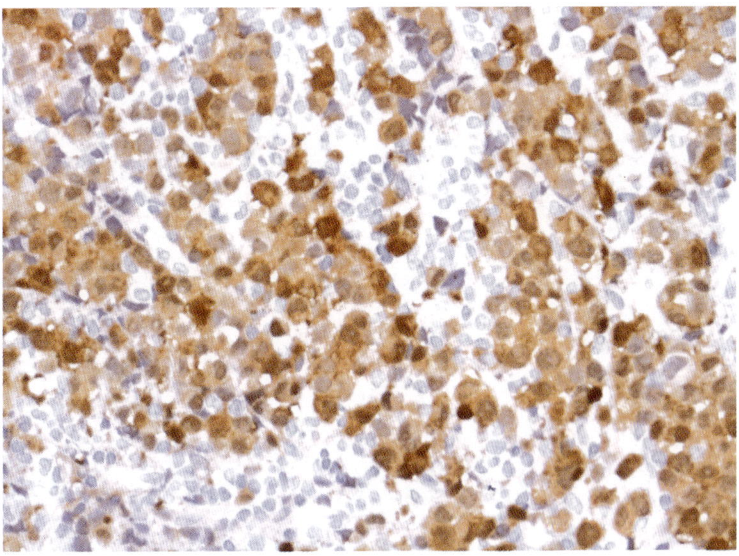

FIGURE 8.27 A sinonasal melanoma showing strong immunoreactivity with antibodies to S100 protein.

WHO. The mean age of diagnosis is in the sixth decade of life, but SNUCs have been reported in patients as young as 14 years of age. These tumors grow quickly and involve the nasal cavity and sinuses with frequent extension into surrounding tissues, including extension into the cranial cavity. Patients usually present with nasal obstruction and epistaxis or symptoms secondary to local invasion (e.g., proptosis, diplopia). The tumors behave poorly and result in the death of most patients in spite of aggressive multimodality therapy.[90,91] Tumors have been shown frequently to have *IDH2* mutations (and less commonly *IDH1* mutations).[92,93]

Histologically, the tumors are undifferentiated and consist of medium-sized cells that grow in nests, wide trabeculae, ribbons, and sheets (Fig. 8.28, eFigs. 8.29–8.31).[87] Nuclei are round to oval, pleomorphic, and hyperchromatic and usually display prominent nucleoli. Many cells have a small amount of eosinophilic cytoplasm. Mitotic figures and apoptotic bodies are numerous. Larger areas of necrosis are also sometimes noted along with prominent vascular invasion. Dysplasia of the overlying schneiderian mucosa has been identified by some authors who have suggested that the tumors originate there. Although the tumors are technically undifferentiated, some authors have allowed for focal squamous differentiation.[89]

Because of the numerous tumors throughout the sinonasal area that can histologically appear similar, the diagnosis of SNUC tends to be a diagnosis of exclusion usually after immunohistochemical staining (Table 8.5). The tumors should show strong immunoreactivity with antibodies to cytokeratin (pankeratins or simple keratins) (Fig. 8.29).[94] This feature alone helps to differentiate the tumors from olfactory neuroblastomas and

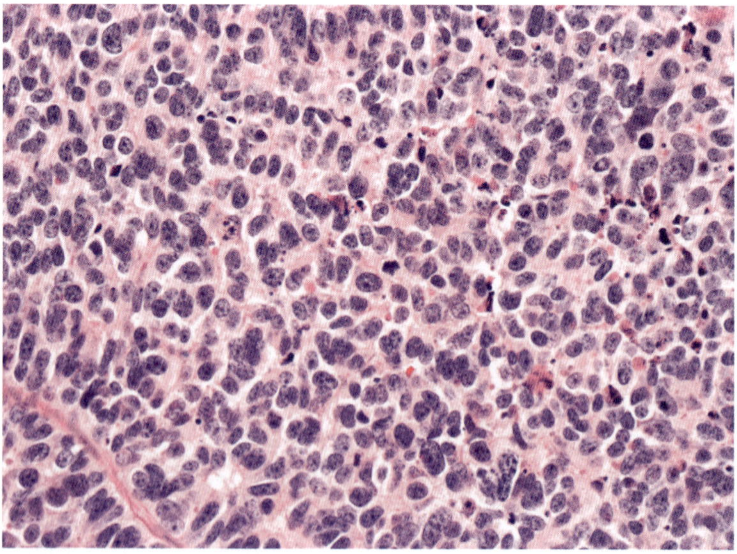

FIGURE 8.28 Sinonasal undifferentiated carcinomas are high-grade undifferentiated malignancies.

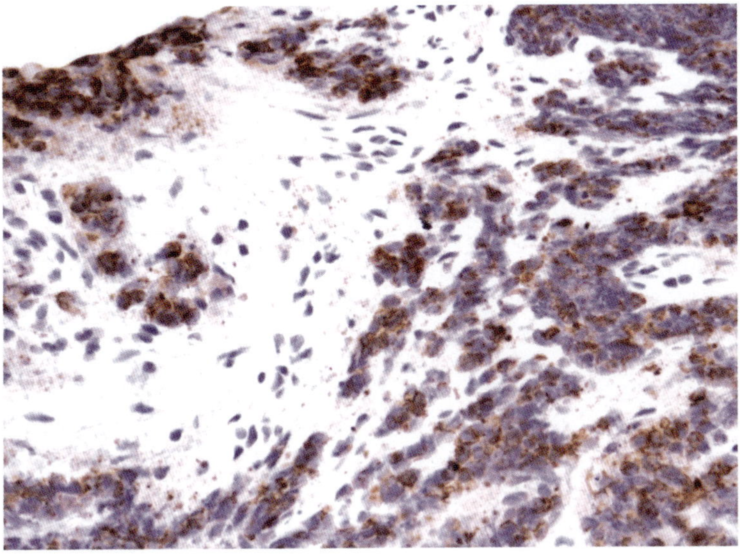

FIGURE 8.29 Immunoreactivity with antibodies to cytokeratins is seen with sinonasal undifferentiated carcinoma.

lymphomas, among other tumors. The tumors may show some reactivity with antibodies to neuroendocrine antigens such as NSE or synaptophysin but should not stain as intensely as ONBs (Fig. 8.30, eFig. 8.32). Focal S-100 immunoreactivity may be seen but not with the typical

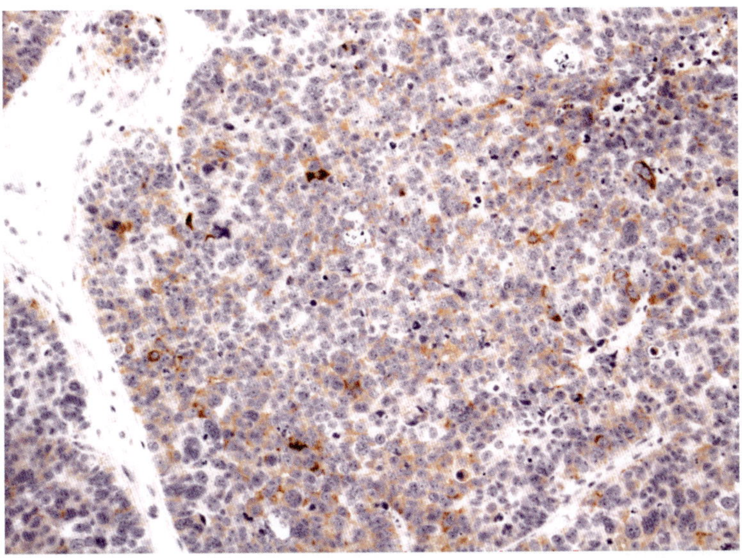

FIGURE 8.30 Weak immunoreactivity with antibodies to synaptophysin is often seen with sinonasal undifferentiated carcinomas.

nest-rimming pattern observed with ONBs. The tumors do not contain EBV particles and are negative both immunohistochemically and by in situ hybridization for the virus, unlike nasopharyngeal undifferentiated carcinoma (lymphoepithelioma).[95] Lymphoid, myogenous, and melanocytic antigens are also not expressed. In our hands, these tumors do not usually express p63, although that may be because we do not allow for squamous differentiation with this diagnosis.[96] IDH1/2 protein expression loss may assist in the diagnosis.[93] Before we make a diagnosis of SNUC, we exclude HR-HPV and EBV-related undifferentiated carcinomas, NUT carcinomas, SMARCB1 (or SMARCA4)-deficient sinonasal carcinomas, and so-called adamantinoma-like Ewing tumor.

Carcinoids, Atypical Carcinoids, and High-Grade Neuroendocrine Carcinomas

All grades of neuroendocrine carcinomas have been identified throughout the upper aerodigestive tract, most commonly in the larynx.[97-104] Distinguishing these tumors from one another and from other neoplasms on biopsy is very important as the tumors have vastly different prognoses and require different types of therapy (Tables 8.4 and 8.5).

Carcinoid tumors or *well-differentiated neuroendocrine carcinomas* are by far the rarest of these malignancies.[98-100] As with the other neuroendocrine carcinomas, these tumors are found most frequently in the supraglottic larynx. These tumors most often arise in the sixth to seventh decade of life and have been identified almost exclusively in men. These cases were not found to have regional lymph node metastases at the time of surgery; however, up to a third of the patients eventually developed distant metastases.[100] Mortality has been reported to be less than 10%.

The tumors are located in the submucosa and resemble carcinoid tumors from other sites.[98-100] The architecture is organoid with nests, ribbons, and trabeculae of small and uniform epithelioid cells (Fig. 8.31, eFig. 8.33). These cells may have a variable amount of cytoplasm that can sometimes appear granular or oncocytic. The nuclei are usually also uniform in size and are round to ovoid. The chromatin is most often described as granular although the nuclei may appear more vesicular and prominent nucleoli can be seen. Mitotic figures are usually not seen and necrosis is absent. A fibrous stroma can be present and may appear hyalinized. Amyloid may even be noted.

Histochemical stains, such as argyrophil and argentaffin stains, can be helpful, as can electron microscopy, but such methods are largely historical. Immunohistochemistry is instead used to definitively diagnose these tumors and they are usually immunoreactive for antibodies to keratins, NSE, chromogranin, synaptophysin, and specific endocrine antigens, such as serotonin.[99] It is important to differentiate these tumors from paragangliomas, which can have a remarkably similar nested and low grade appearance and also occur in the larynx but metastasize far less frequently.

TABLE 8.4 Clinical and Pathologic Features of Neuroendocrine Carcinomas of the Upper Aerodigestive Tract

	Carcinoid Tumor	Atypical Carcinoid Tumor	Small Cell Carcinoma	Poorly Differentiated, Large Cell Neuroendocrine Carcinoma (including SNUC)
Age	50–60	50–60	50–60	50–60
Sex	M ≫ F	M > F	M > F	M > F
Site	Supraglottic larynx	Supraglottic larynx	Supraglottic larynx and other sites including oropharynx and sinonasal tract	All sites, especially larynx and sinonasal tract
Survival, 5 y	>90%	Approx. 50%	<10%	<10%[a]
Atypia	None	Mild-moderate	Marked	Marked
Mitoses	None	Few scattered	Numerous	Numerous
Necrosis	None	None-little	Abundant	Abundant

F, females; M, males; SNUC, sinonasal undifferentiated carcinoma.

[a]Some studies report very high rates of survival for SNUCs possibly secondary to the inclusion of some nasopharyngeal carcinomas.

Paragangliomas should not be immunoreactive with antibodies to keratins and should show the typical sustentacular staining pattern when stained with antibodies to S100 protein.

Upper aerodigestive tract *atypical carcinoid tumors* or *moderately differentiated neuroendocrine carcinomas* are more than 10 times as common as typical carcinoid tumors. These tumors also present most frequently submucosally in the supraglottic larynx.[98–100] They are also more commonly found in men and present most frequently in the fifth to sixth decades of life. The tumors behave worse than the typical carcinoid tumors. Nearly half of these tumors present with regional lymph node metastases and less than one half of patients survive 5 years.[100]

The tumors have much the same histologic appearance as typical carcinoid tumors; however, they show more variable architecture

TABLE 8.5 Differential Diagnosis of Un-/Poorly Differentiated Neoplasia of the Sinonasal Tract With Immunophenotype

Tumor	CK	NSE	SYN	CHR	S100	HMB45[a]	LCA	Desmin	MYO	FLI	CD99	EBV[b]	HPV[c]	NUT[d]	INI1
SNUC	+	+[e]	+[e]	+[e]	–	–	–	–	–	–	–	–	–	–	+
HGNEC	+	+	+[f]	+[f]	–	–	–	–	–	–	–	–	–/+	–	+
EBVUC[g]	+	–	–	–	–	–	–	–	–	–	–	+	–	–	+
HPVUC	+	–	–	–	–	–	–	–	–	–	–	–	+	–	+
NC	+	–	–	–	–	–	–	–	–	–	–	–	–	+	+
SBDSC	+	–	–	–	–	–	–	–	–	–	–	–	–	–	–
ONB	–[h]	+	+	+	+[i]	–	–	–	–	–	–	–	–	–	+
Melanoma	–	–	-	–	+	+	–	–	–	–	–	–	–	–	+
Lymphoma[j]	–	–	–	–	–	–	+	–	–	–[k]	–[k]	–[l]	–	–	+
RMS	–[m]	–	–	–	–	–	–	+	+	–	–	–	–	–	+
PNET	+/–[n]	+	+/–	–	+/–	–	–	–	–	+	+	–	–	–	+
PA	+	+	+	+	–	–	–	–	–	–	–	–	–	–	+
MC	–	+	–	–	+	–	–	+/–	–	–	+	–	–	–	+

CHR, chromogranin; CK, cytokeratin; EBV, Epstein-Barr virus; EBVUC, undifferentiated carcinoma associated with EBV (nasopharyngeal carcinoma, etc.); HGNEC, high-grade neuroendocrine carcinoma (most are small cell carcinoma); HPV, human papillomavirus; HPVUC, undifferentiated carcinoma associated with HR-HPV; LCA, leukocyte common antigen; MC, mesenchymal chondrosarcoma; MYO, myogenin; NC, NUT carcinoma; NSE, neuron-specific enolase; NUT, nuclear protein in testis; ONB, olfactory neuroblastoma, RMS, rhabdomyosarcoma (embryonal and alveolar); PA, pituitary adenoma; PNET, peripheral neuroectodermal tumor; SBDSC, SMARCB1-deficient sinonasal carcinoma; SNUC, sinonasal undifferentiated carcinoma; SYN, synaptophysin.

[a]Or other specific melanocytic markers.

[b]EBV status may be assessed by a variety of means including in situ hybridization.

[c]High-risk HPV status is usually assessed with in situ hybridization outside the oropharynx.

[d]The status of nuclear protein of the testis may be assessed by immunohistochemistry or break-apart fluorescent in situ hybridization.

[e]Markers for neuroendocrine differentiation tend to stain SNUCs focally.

[f]Small cell carcinomas frequently lack staining for more specific endocrine markers.

[g]Also known as nasopharyngeal nonkeratinizing squamous cell carcinoma.

[h]ONBs may show focal immunoreactivity with antibodies to cytokeratins.

[i]S100 immunoreactivity in ONBs is limited primarily to peripheral staining of the sustentacular cells.

[j]Including most of the hematologic malignancies that may be found throughout this area (e.g., extranodal NK/T-cell lymphoma, nasal type, plasmacytoma).

[k]Lymphoblastic lymphomas often react with antibodies to CD99 and FLI1.

[l]Most lymphomas will not show diffuse, strong in situ hybridization for EBV-related nucleic acids or immunoreactivity with antibodies to EBV-related proteins. The notable exceptions include posttransplant lymphoproliferative disorders and extranodal NK/T-cell lymphoma, nasal type. In such patients, other markers may be needed.

[m]Keratin immunoreactivity seen in a small blue cell tumor of the upper aerodigestive tract that also expresses skeletal muscle markers should raise suspicion of a desmoplastic small round cell tumor.

[n]Conventional PNETs can sometimes show limited immunoreactivity with antibodies to low-molecular-weight keratins. So-called adamantinoma-like Ewing tumor will show diffuse keratin immunoreactivity and p63 immunoreactivity.

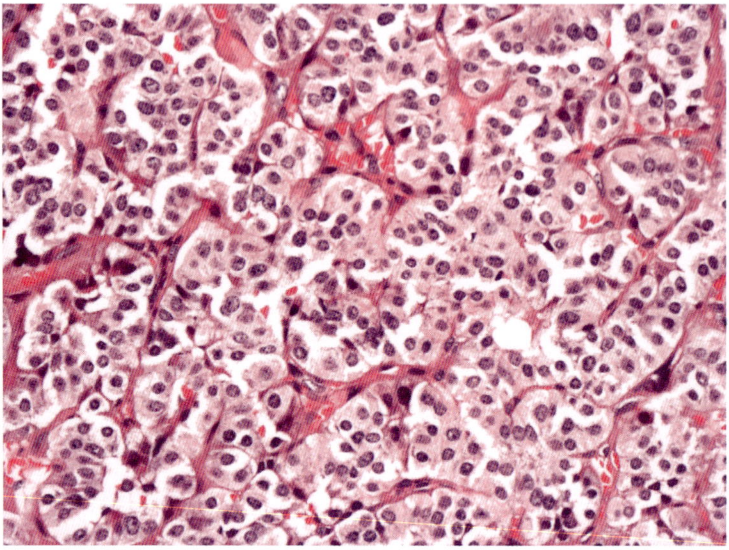

FIGURE 8.31 A laryngeal carcinoid tumor showing a prominent nesting pattern.

and can focally display sheetlike growth (Fig. 8.32).[98–100] Atypical carcinoid tumors also have abundant nuclear and cellular pleomorphism, can have occasional mitotic figures, and can have necrosis (eFig. 8.34). Oncocytic and mucinous changes have been noted and amyloid can also be found.

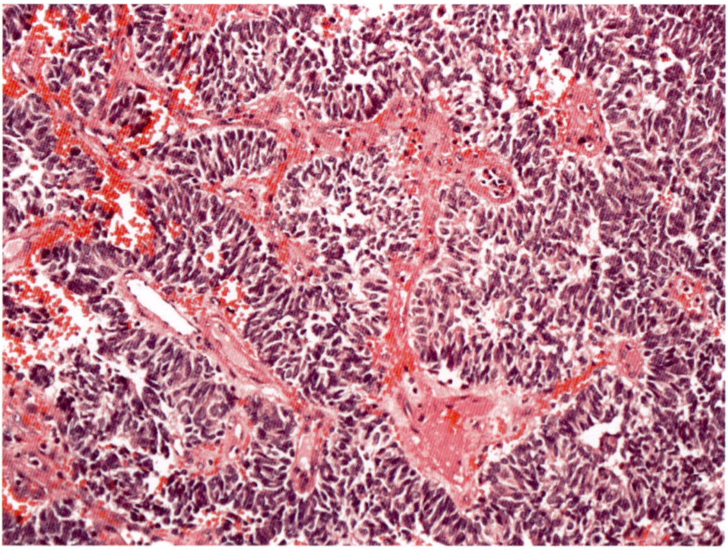

FIGURE 8.32 An atypical carcinoid tumor of the larynx with high cellularity and a trabecular architecture.

The tumors show a similar immunohistochemical staining pattern to typical carcinoid tumors and will react with antibodies to keratins and neuroendocrine antigens. Interestingly, up to 75% of these tumors react with antibodies to calcitonin.[105] That, combined with the occasional presence of amyloid, has led some authors to state that these tumors more closely resemble medullary thyroid cancers than pulmonary carcinoid tumors.

Small cell carcinomas or *poorly differentiated neuroendocrine carcinomas* are nearly as common as atypical carcinoid tumors in the upper aerodigestive tract.[98–102] Although they also most often involve the supraglottic larynx, the tumors occur more frequently than the other neuroendocrine carcinomas at other sites throughout the tract, especially in the sinonasal and oropharyngeal regions.[103,106] Laryngeal tumors occur more frequently in men, usually in the sixth to seventh decades of life and have a dismal prognosis, with less than 5% of patients diagnosed with these lesions alive at 5 years. The epidemiology and prognosis of sinonasal lesions is much harder to sort out as there is likely diagnostic confusion in some cases with both olfactory neuroblastomas and sinonasal undifferentiated carcinomas. These lesions occur more frequently in men and develop most often in the sixth decade of life. Patients usually die of disease within 5 years of diagnosis.[100] Oropharyngeal tumors have only begun to be reported.[106] These tumors are associated with high-risk human papillomavirus (HPV) infection and the patient demographics may be found to be different when compared to other small cell carcinomas of the upper aerodigestive tract. The prognosis appears to be worse for these tumors when compared to other HPV-related malignancies of the oropharynx.

Histologically, small cell carcinomas are characterized by variably sized sheets, cords, nests, and ribbons of small cells with little identifiable cytoplasm (Fig. 8.33, eFig. 8.35).[98–103] Fibrous cords often separate tumor cells. Large areas of confluent necrosis are often seen. Nuclear molding and focal crush artifact are often also seen with abundant mitotic figures and single cell apoptotic figures (Fig. 8.34). Tumor cell nuclei are hyperchromatic and have granular chromatin without prominent nucleoli. The Azzopardi effect is often noted as is true vascular invasion. The tumors may contain areas diagnostic of non–small cell carcinoma and varying differentiation has been noted throughout the upper aerodigestive tract.[99,106]

Immunohistochemically, small cell carcinomas will generally react with antikeratin antibodies with a characteristic "dotlike" staining pattern (Fig. 8.35).[98,99] The cells will show variable reactivity with antibodies to endocrine antigens, with the less specific markers such as NSE and CD56 having the greatest sensitivity. Chromogranin and/or synaptophysin immunoreactivity is preserved at least focally in most cases (eFig. 8.36); however, many cases will lack staining with these antibodies. P16 immunoreactivity has been noted with oropharyngeal small cell carcinomas as

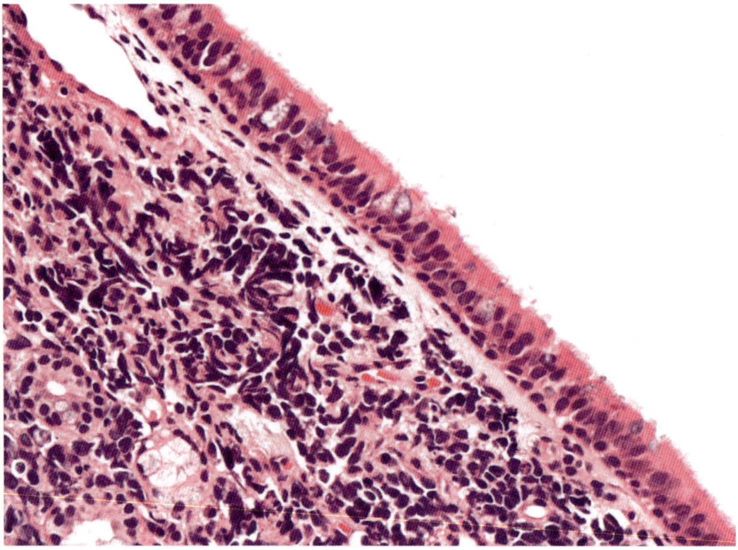

FIGURE 8.33 A sinonasal small cell carcinoma located beneath the normal appearing columnar, ciliated epithelium.

has positive testing for high-risk HPV by in situ hybridization. We are not sure, however, how well p16 immunohistochemistry will work as a surrogate test for HPV with these tumors, as small cell carcinomas not related to HPV at other sites often overexpress p16.

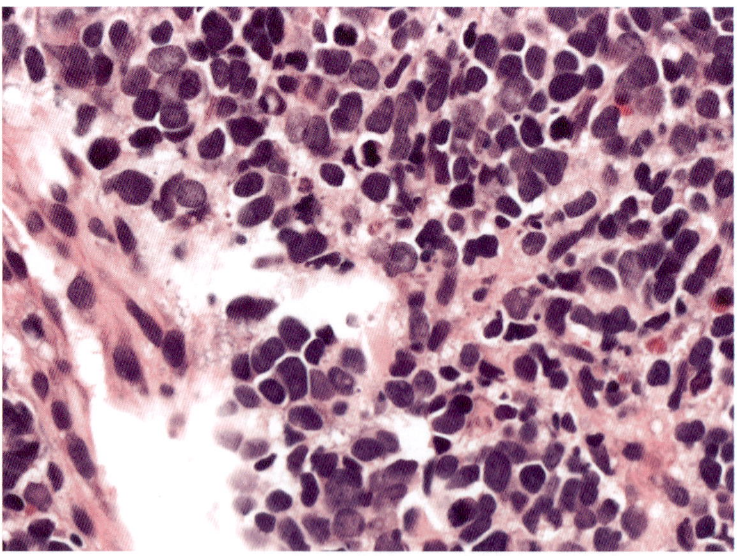

FIGURE 8.34 Small cell carcinomas of the upper aerodigestive tract have similar cytologic features to pulmonary small cell carcinomas with nuclear molding, granular chromatin, and frequent mitotic figures and apoptotic bodies.

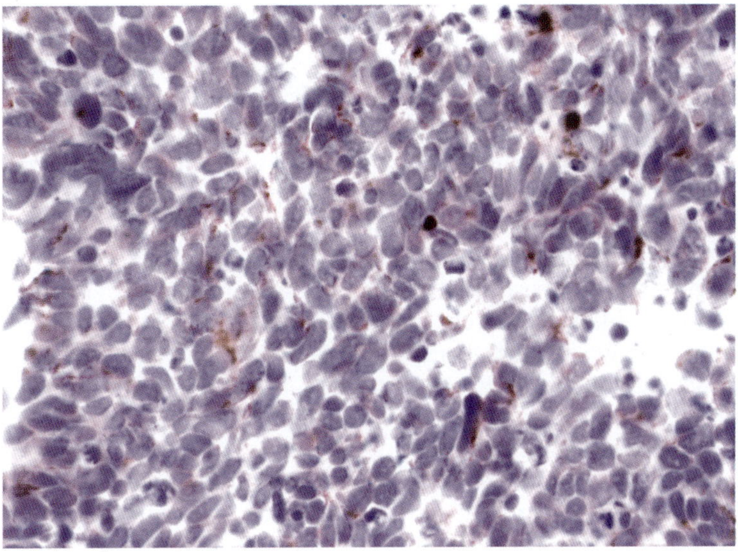

FIGURE 8.35 A sinonasal small cell carcinoma showing dotlike immunoreactivity with antibodies to cytokeratin.

The diagnosis of most laryngeal small cell carcinomas is straightforward; however, the diagnosis of these lesions at other sites, especially in the sinonasal area, can be difficult due to the vast differential diagnosis for such lesions at that site (Table 8.5). Larger cell carcinomas such as sinonasal undifferentiated carcinomas, other undifferentiated carcinomas, and basaloid squamous cell carcinomas need to be separated primarily by phenotype although basaloid squamous cell carcinomas should show p63 immunoreactivity and nasopharyngeal undifferentiated carcinomas often show evidence of EBV infection by in situ hybridization.[95,107] Small cell carcinomas and sinonasal undifferentiated carcinomas show considerable immunophenotypic overlap and should be differentiated using the criteria that one uses to distinguish pulmonary poorly differentiated large cell neuroendocrine carcinomas from small cell carcinomas.[108]

High-grade large cell neuroendocrine carcinomas of the upper aerodigestive tract have been variably reported. Part of the variability is due to how they are diagnosed and to be distinguished from poorly differentiated or undifferentiated carcinomas with neuroendocrine features and small cell carcinomas. Recently, some have suggested that to be diagnosed as a large cell neuroendocrine carcinoma, a tumor must have cells with moderate to abundant cytoplasm, features of neuroendocrine differentiation such as organoid, trabecular, or nesting growth, rosette formation and peripheral palisading of nuclei, a high mitotic rate (>10 per 10 high powered fields), and confirmation of neuroendocrine differentiation by immunohistochemistry.[109] Of the 10 laryngeal cases reviewed, 9 were from the supraglottis. Only one patient with significant follow-up was alive without disease.

USUAL CNS NEOPLASMS

Tumors usually restricted to the central nervous system (CNS) can present in the upper aerodigestive tract, particularly in the sinonasal and nasopharyngeal areas, either secondary to direct extension or through neoplastic transformation of heterotopic tissues. The most commonly noted neoplasms that occur in these areas include those seen in the area of the sella turcica, including pituitary adenomas, craniopharyngiomas, and meningiomas.

Sinonasal meningiomas occur with equal frequency in men and women over a wide age range.[110] Most patients present with symptoms of a mass lesion or epistaxis. Rarely, patients may present with visual changes. Most cases involve the nasal cavity alone or the nasal cavity and paranasal sinuses although some tumors only involve the paranasal sinuses. The tumors have histologic features identical to typical meningiomas and most are classified as meningotheliomatous and are composed of whorled nodules of plump spindled cells (Fig. 8.36, eFig. 8.37). The individual cells have bland, oval nuclei with occasional intranuclear pseudoinclusions. Mitotic figures and cellular atypia should be rare and when present raise the question of an *atypical meningioma*. Occasional cases will have more spindled cells and some will have metaplastic change usually with lipidized cells. Psammoma bodies can be found in about one-third of the cases. Most cases will show infiltration of the surrounding normal tissues.

Because of the rarity of these tumors, immunohistochemistry is often helpful and reassuring. Neoplastic cells will react with antibodies to EMA and vimentin.[110] About 50% of cases will show immunoreactivity with

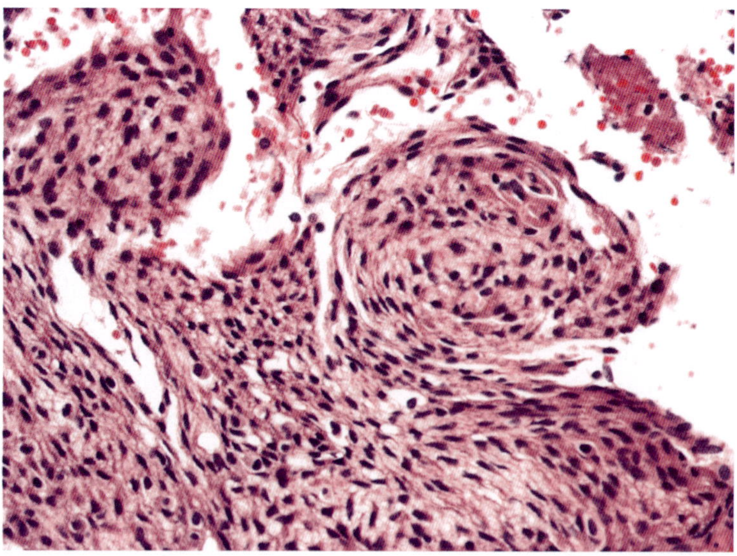

FIGURE 8.36 A meningioma involving the sinus with a whorled meningotheliomatous appearance.

antibodies to progesterone receptor and a limited number will show reactivity with antibodies to cytokeratins and estrogen receptor.

Pituitary adenomas can also present as sinonasal lesions or nasopharyngeal masses, usually through the direct extension of tumor from the sella turcica or, rarely, through the development of tumor from presumed ectopic pituitary tissue.[111] The tumors typically present as mass lesions; however, endocrine disturbances such as Cushing syndrome or acromegaly also may be present. The tumors typically have features of lower grade neuroendocrine carcinomas with nests, rosettes, ribbons, and pseudoglandular structures composed of monomorphic epithelioid or plasmacytoid cells (Fig. 8.37, eFig. 8.38). Mitotic figures are usually infrequent and the chromatin pattern is typically granular. Nuclear atypia and nucleoli may sometimes be seen and tumors may even resemble poorly differentiated carcinomas (eFig. 8.39). Immunohistochemistry can be helpful and most tumors (but not all) will react with antibodies to cytokeratins and endocrine antigens such as synaptophysin and chromogranin. Staining for specific peptide hormones such as prolactin, ACTH, human growth hormone can also be helpful.

Rarely, *craniopharyngiomas* will present in the nasopharynx.[112] Patients are usually younger than 30 year and will present with nonspecific findings, occasionally with visual problems. The tumors are composed of nests and cords of maturing squamous cells that keratinize and have a reticular appearance akin to that of ameloblastoma. Indeed, without a known site of biopsy, the tumors are impossible to distinguish from ameloblastomas and odontogenic cysts.

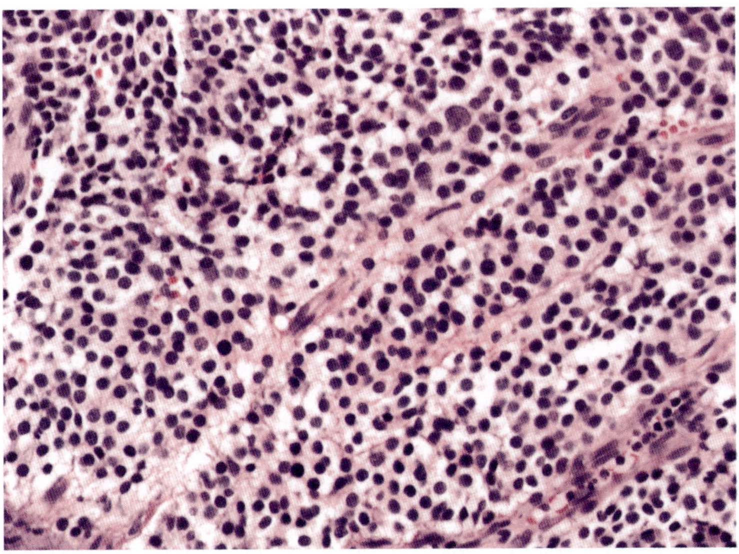

FIGURE 8.37 A pituitary adenoma involving the nasal cavity with a somewhat organoid appearance and monomorphic epithelioid cells.

REFERENCES

1. Wright BA, Jackson D. Neural tumors of the oral cavity. A review of the spectrum of benign and malignant oral tumors of the oral cavity and jaws. *Oral Surg Oral Med Oral Pathol.* 1980;49:509-522.
2. Daneshvar A. Pharyngeal traumatic neuromas and traumatic neuromas with mature ganglion cells (pseudoganglioneuromas). *Am J Surg Pathol.* 1990;14:565-570.
3. Gorlin RJ, Sedano HO, Vickers RA, Cervenka J. Multiple mucosal neuromas, pheochromocytoma and medullary carcinoma of the thyroid–a syndrome. *Cancer.* 1968;22:293-299.
4. Hofstra RM, Landsvater RM, Ceccherini I, et al. A mutation in the RET proto-oncogene associated with multiple endocrine neoplasia type 2B and sporadic medullary thyroid carcinoma. *Nature.* 1994;367:375-376.
5. Perzin KH, Panyu H, Wechter S. Nonepithelial tumors of the nasal cavity, paranasal sinuses and nasopharynx. A clinicopathologic study. XII: Schwann cell tumors (neurilemoma, neurofibroma, malignant schwannoma). *Cancer.* 1982;50:2193-2202.
6. Geist JR, Gander DL, Stefanac SJ. Oral manifestations of neurofibromatosis types I and II. *Oral Surg Oral Med Oral Pathol.* 1992;73:376-382.
7. Cangiarella J, Jagirdar J, Adelman H, Budzilovich G, Greco MA. Mucosal neuromas and plexiform neurofibromas: an immunocytochemical study. *Pediatr Pathol.* 1993;13:281-288.
8. Hasegawa SL, Mentzel T, Fletcher CD. Schwannomas of the sinonasal tract and nasopharynx. *Mod Pathol.* 1997;10:777-784.
9. Buob D, Wacrenier A, Chevalier D, et al. Schwannoma of the sinonasal tract: a clinicopathologic and immunohistochemical study of 5 cases. *Arch Pathol Lab Med.* 2003;127:1196-1199.
10. Lack EE, Worsham GF, Callihan MD, et al. Granular cell tumor: a clinicopathologic study of 110 patients. *J Surg Oncol.* 1980;13:301-316.
11. Regezi JA, Batsakis JG, Courtney RM. Granular cell tumors of the head and neck. *J Oral Surg.* 1979;37:402-406.
12. Nathrath WB, Remberger K. Immunohistochemical study of granular cell tumours. Demonstration of neurone specific enolase, S 100 protein, laminin and alpha-1-antichymotrypsin. *Virchows Arch A Pathol Anat Histopathol.* 1986;408:421-434.
13. Mazur MT, Shultz JJ, Myers JL. Granular cell tumor. Immunohistochemical analysis of 21 benign tumors and one malignant tumor. *Arch Pathol Lab Med.* 1990;114:692-696.
14. Filie AC, Lage JM, Azumi N. Immunoreactivity of S100 protein, alpha-1-antitrypsin, and CD68 in adult and congenital granular cell tumors. *Mod Pathol.* 1996;9:888-892.
15. Lack EE, Worsham GF, Callihan MD, Crawford BE, Vawter GF. Gingival granula cell tumors of the newborn (congenital "epulis"): a clinical and pathologic study of 21 patients. *Am J Surg Pathol.* 1981;5:37-46.
16. Lifshitz MS, Flotte TJ, Greco MA. Congenital granular cell epulis. Immunohistochemical and ultrastructural observations. *Cancer.* 1984;53:1845-1848.
17. Cohen JN, Yeh I, Jordan RC, et al. Cutaneous non-neural granular cell tumors harbor recurrent ALK gene fusions. *Am J Surg Pathol.* 2018;42:1133-1142.
18. Fetsch JF, Laskin WB, Hallman JR, Lupton GP, Miettinen M. Neurothekeoma: an analysis of 178 tumors with detailed immunohistochemical data and long-term patient follow-up information. *Am J Surg Pathol.* 2007;31:1103-1114.
19. Fetsch JF, Laskin WB, Miettinen M. Nerve sheath myxoma: a clinicopathologic and immunohistochemical analysis of 57 morphologically distinctive, S-100 protein- and GFAP-positive, myxoid peripheral nerve sheath tumors with a predilection for the extremities and a high local recurrence rate. *Am J Surg Pathol.* 2005;29:1615-1624.

20. Hornick JL, Fletcher CD. Cellular neurothekeoma: detailed characterization in a series of 133 cases. *Am J Surg Pathol.* 2007;31:329-340.
21. Sheth S, Li X, Binder S, Dry SM. Differential gene expression profiles of neurothekeomas and nerve sheath myxomas by microarray analysis. *Mod Pathol.* 2011;24:343-354.
22. Fletcher CD. Solitary circumscribed neuroma of the skin (so-called palisaded, encapsulated neuroma). A clinicopathologic and immunohistochemical study. *Am J Surg Pathol.* 1989;13:574-580.
23. Magnusson B. Palisaded encapsulated neuroma (solitary circumscribed neuroma) of the oral mucosa. *Oral Surg Oral Med Oral Pathol Oral Radiol Endod.* 1996;82:302-304.
24. Koutlas IG, Scheithauer BW. Palisaded encapsulated ("solitary circumscribed" neuroma of the oral cavity: a review of 55 cases. *Head Neck Pathol.* 2010;4:15-26.
25. Hillstrom RP, Zarbo RJ, Jacobs JR. Nerve sheath tumors of the paranasal sinuses: electron microscopy and histopathologic diagnosis. *Otolaryngol Head Neck Surg.* 1990;102:257-263.
26. Hellquist HB, Lundgren J. Neurogenic sarcoma of the sinonasal tract. *J Laryngol Otol.* 1991;105:186-190.
27. Heffner DK, Gnepp DR. Sinonasal fibrosarcomas, malignant schwannomas, and "Triton" tumors. A clinicopathologic study of 67 cases. *Cancer.* 1992;70:1089-1101.
28. Foo WC, Cruise MW, Wick MR, Hornick JL. Immunohistochemical staining for TLE1 distinguishes synovial sarcoma from histologic mimics. *Am J Clin Pathol.* 2011;135:839-844.
29. Fritchie KJ, Jin L, Wang X, et al. Fusion gene profile of biphenotypic sinonasal sarcoma: an analysis of 44 cases. *Histopathology.* 2016;69:930-936.
30. Huang SC, Ghossein RA, Bishop JA, et al. Novel PAX3-NCOA1 fusions in biphenotypic sinonasal sarcoma with focal rhabdomyoblastic differentiation. *Am J Surg Pathol.* 2016;40:51-59.
31. Stelow EB, Bishop JA. Update from the 4th edition of the World Health Organization classification of head and neck tumours: tumors of the nasal cavity, paranasal sinuses and skull base. *Head Neck Pathol.* 2017;11:3-15.
32. Lack EE, Cubilla AL, Woodruff JM, Farr HW. Paragangliomas of the head and neck region: a clinical study of 69 patients. *Cancer.* 1977;39:397-409.
33. Lack EE, Cubilla AL, Woodruff JM. Paragangliomas of the head and neck region. A pathologic study of tumors from 71 patients. *Hum Pathol.* 1979;10:191-218.
34. Barnes L. Paraganglioma of the larynx. A critical review of the literature. *ORL J Otorhinolaryngol Relat Spec.* 1991;53:220-234.
35. Neumann HP, Bausch B, McWhinney SR, et al. Germ-line mutations in nonsyndromic pheochromocytoma. *N Engl J Med.* 2002;346:1459-1466.
36. Kliewer KE, Wen DR, Cancilla PA, Cochran AJ. Paragangliomas: assessment of prognosis by histologic, immunohistochemical, and ultrastructural techniques. *Hum Pathol.* 1989;20:29-39.
37. Johnson TL, Zarbo RJ, Lloyd RV, Crissman JD. Paragangliomas of the head and neck: immunohistochemical neuroendocrine and intermediate filament typing. *Mod Pathol.* 1988;1:216-223.
38. Achilles E, Padberg BC, Holl K, Kloppel G, Schroder S. Immunocytochemistry of paragangliomas–value of staining for S-100 protein and glial fibrillary acid protein in diagnosis and prognosis. *Histopathology.* 1991;18:453-458.
39. Mills SE, Frierson HF Jr. Olfactory neuroblastoma. A clinicopathologic study of 21 cases. *Am J Surg Pathol.* 1985;9:317-327.
40. Frierson HF Jr, Ross GW, Mills SE, Frankfurter A. Olfactory neuroblastoma. Additional immunohistochemical characterization. *Am J Clin Pathol.* 1990;94:547-553.

41. Kadish S, Goodman M, Wang CC. Olfactory neuroblastoma. A clinical analysis of 17 cases. *Cancer*. 1976;37:1571-1576.
42. Guled M, Myllykangas S, Frierson HF Jr, Mills SE, Knuutila S, Stelow EB. Array comparative genomic hybridization analysis of olfactory neuroblastoma. *Mod Pathol*. 2008;21:770-778.
43. Sorensen PH, Wu JK, Berean KW, et al. Olfactory neuroblastoma is a peripheral primitive neuroectodermal tumor related to Ewing sarcoma. *Proc Natl Acad Sci U S A*. 1996;93:1038-1043.
44. Kumar S, Perlman E, Pack S, et al. Absence of EWS/FLI1 fusion in olfactory neuroblastomas indicates these tumors do not belong to the Ewing's sarcoma family. *Hum Pathol*. 1999;30:1356-1360.
45. Argani P, Perez-Ordonez B, Xiao H, Caruana SM, Huvos AG, Ladanyi M. Olfactory neuroblastoma is not related to the Ewing family of tumors: absence of EWS/FLI1 gene fusion and MIC2 expression. *Am J Surg Pathol*. 1998;22:391-398.
46. Loy AH, Reibel JF, Read PW, et al. Esthesioneuroblastoma: continued follow-up of a single institution's experience. *Arch Otolaryngol Head Neck Surg*. 2006;132:134-138.
47. Diaz EM Jr, Johnigan RH III, Pero C, et al. Olfactory neuroblastoma: the 22-year experience at one comprehensive cancer center. *Head Neck*. 2005;27:138-149.
48. Mills SE, Gaffey MJ, Frierson HF: *Neural, neuroendocrine, and neuroectodermal neoplasia*. In: *Tumors of the Upper Aerodigestive Tract and Ear*. 3rd ed. Washington, DC: AFIP; 2000:159.
49. Hirose T, Scheithauer BW, Lopes MB, et al. Olfactory neuroblastoma. An immunohistochemical, ultrastructural, and flow cytometric study. *Cancer*. 1995;76:4-19.
50. Stirling RW, Powell G, Fletcher CD. Pigmented neuroectodermal tumour of infancy: an immunohistochemical study. *Histopathology*. 1988;12:425-435.
51. Pettinato G, Manivel JC, d'Amore ES, Jaszcz W, Gorlin RJ. Melanotic neuroectodermal tumor of infancy. A reexamination of a histogenetic problem based on immunohistochemical, flow cytometric, and ultrastructural study of 10 cases. *Am J Surg Pathol*. 1991;15:233-245.
52. Kapadia SB, Frisman DM, Hitchcock CL, Ellis GL, Popek EJ. Melanotic neuroectodermal tumor of infancy. Clinicopathological, immunohistochemical, and flow cytometric study. *Am J Surg Pathol*. 1993;17:566-573.
53. Barrett AW, Morgan M, Ramsay AD, Farthing PM, Newman L, Speight PM. A clinicopathologic and immunohistochemical analysis of melanotic neuroectodermal tumor of infancy. *Oral Surg Oral Med Oral Pathol Oral Radiol Endod*. 2002;93:688-698.
54. Kruse-Losler B, Gaertner C, Burger H, Seper L, Joos U, Kleinheinz J. Melanotic neuroectodermal tumor of infancy: systematic review of the literature and presentation of a case. *Oral Surg Oral Med Oral Pathol Oral Radiol Endod*. 2006;102:204-216.
55. Jones JE, McGill T. Peripheral primitive neuroectodermal tumors of the head and neck. *Arch Otolaryngol Head Neck Surg*. 1995;121:1392-1395.
56. Jurgens H, Bier V, Harms D, et al. Malignant peripheral neuroectodermal tumors. A retrospective analysis of 42 patients. *Cancer*. 1988;61:349-357.
57. Nikitakis NG, Salama AR, O'Malley BW Jr, Ord RA, Papadimitriou JC. Malignant peripheral primitive neuroectodermal tumor-peripheral neuroepithelioma of the head and neck: a clinicopathologic study of five cases and review of the literature. *Head Neck*. 2003;25:488-498.
58. Windfuhr JP. Primitive neuroectodermal tumor of the head and neck: incidence, diagnosis, and management. *Ann Otol Rhinol Laryngol*. 2004;113:533-543.
59. Hafezi S, Seethala RR, Stelow EB, et al. Ewing's family of tumors of the sinonasal tract and maxillary bone. *Head Neck Pathol*. 2011;5:8-16.

60. Ahmad R, Mayol BR, Davis M, Rougraff BT. Extraskeletal Ewing's sarcoma. *Cancer.* 1999;85:725-731.
61. Folpe AL, Goldblum JR, Rubin BP, et al. Morphologic and immunophenotypic diversity in Ewing family tumors: a study of 66 genetically confirmed cases. *Am J Surg Pathol.* 2005;29:1025-1033.
62. Turc-Carel C, Aurias A, Mugneret F, et al. Chromosomes in Ewing's sarcoma. I. An evaluation of 85 cases of remarkable consistency of t(11;22)(q24;q12). *Cancer Genet Cytogenet.* 1988;32:229-238.
63. Folpe AL, Hill CE, Parham DM, O'Shea PA, Weiss SW. Immunohistochemical detection of FLI-1 protein expression: a study of 132 round cell tumors with emphasis on CD99-positive mimics of Ewing's sarcoma/primitive neuroectodermal tumor. *Am J Surg Pathol.* 2000;24:1657-1662.
64. Bishop JA, Alaggio R, Zhang L, Seethala RR, Antonescu CR. Adamantinoma-like Ewing family tumors of the head and neck: a pitfall in the differential diagnosis of basaloid and myoepithelial carcinomas. *Am J Surg Pathol.* 2015;39:1267-1274.
65. Eisen D, Voorhees JJ. Oral melanoma and other pigmented lesions of the oral cavity. *J Am Acad Dermatol.* 1991;24:527-537.
66. Buchner A, Merrell PW, Hansen LS, Leider AS. Melanocytic hyperplasia of the oral mucosa. *Oral Surg Oral Med Oral Pathol.* 1991;71:58-62.
67. Buchner A, Hansen LS. Pigmented nevi of the oral mucosa: a clinicopathologic study of 32 new cases and review of 75 cases from the literature. Part I: a clinicopathologic study of 32 new cases. *Oral Surg Oral Med Oral Pathol.* 1979;48:131-142.
68. Buchner A, Hansen LS. Pigmented nevi of the oral mucosa: a clinicopathologic study of 36 new cases and review of 155 cases from the literature. Part I: a clinicopathologic study of 36 new cases. *Oral Surg Oral Med Oral Pathol.* 1987;63:566-572.
69. Umeda M, Komatsubara H, Shibuya Y, Yokoo S, Komori T. Premalignant melanocytic dysplasia and malignant melanoma of the oral mucosa. *Oral Oncol.* 2002;38:714-722.
70. Franquemont DW, Mills SE. Sinonasal malignant melanoma. A clinicopathologic and immunohistochemical study of 14 cases. *Am J Clin Pathol.* 1991;96:689-697.
71. Hicks MJ, Flaitz CM. Oral mucosal melanoma: epidemiology and pathobiology. *Oral Oncol.* 2000;36:152-169.
72. Barker BF, Carpenter WM, Daniels TE, et al. Oral mucosal melanomas: the WESTOP Banff workshop proceedings. Western Society of Teachers of Oral Pathology. *Oral Surg Oral Med Oral Pathol Oral Radiol Endod.* 1997;83:672-679.
73. Rapini RP, Golitz LE, Greer RO Jr, Krekorian EA, Poulson T. Primary malignant melanoma of the oral cavity. A review of 177 cases. *Cancer.* 1985;55:1543-1551.
74. Thompson LD, Wieneke JA, Miettinen M. Sinonasal tract and nasopharyngeal melanomas: a clinicopathologic study of 115 cases with a proposed staging system. *Am J Surg Pathol.* 2003;27:594-611.
75. Chang AE, Karnell LH, Menck HR. The National Cancer Data Base report on cutaneous and noncutaneous melanoma: a summary of 84,836 cases from the past decade. The American College of Surgeons Commission on Cancer and the American Cancer Society. *Cancer.* 1998;83:1664-1678.
76. Wenig BM. Laryngeal mucosal malignant melanoma. A clinicopathologic, immunohistochemical, and ultrastructural study of four patients and a review of the literature. *Cancer.* 1995;75:1568-1577.
77. Cohen Y, Rosenbaum E, Begum S, et al. Exon 15 BRAF mutations are uncommon in melanomas arising in nonsun-exposed sites. *Clin Cancer Res.* 2004;10:3444-3447.
78. van Dijk M, Sprenger S, Rombout P, et al. Distinct chromosomal aberrations in sinonasal mucosal melanoma as detected by comparative genomic hybridization. *Genes Chromosomes Cancer.* 2003;36:151-158.

79. Rivera RS, Nagatsuka H, Gunduz M, et al. C-kit protein expression correlated with activating mutations in KIT gene in oral mucosal melanoma. *Virchows Arch*. 2008;452:27-32.
80. Wroblewska JP, Mull J, Wu CL, et al. SF3B1, NRAS, KIT, and BRAF mutation; CD117 and cMYC expression; and tumoral pigmentation in sinonasal melanomas: an analysis with newly found molecular alterations and some population-based molecular differences. *Am J Surg Pathol*. 2019;43:168-177.
81. Lyle PL, Amato CM, Fitzpatrick JE, Robinson WA. Sinonasal tract melanoma or clear cell sarcoma? Molecular evaluation of 4 cases diagnosed as malignant melanoma. *Mod Pathol*. 2008;21:238A.
82. Prasad ML, Busam KJ, Patel SG, Hoshaw-Woodard S, Shah JP, Huvos AG. Clinicopathologic differences in malignant melanoma arising in oral squamous and sinonasal respiratory mucosa of the upper aerodigestive tract. *Arch Pathol Lab Med*. 2003;127:997-1002.
83. Wick MR, Stanley SJ, Swanson PE. Immunohistochemical diagnosis of sinonasal melanoma, carcinoma, and neuroblastoma with monoclonal antibodies HMB-45 and anti-synaptophysin. *Arch Pathol Lab Med*. 1988;112:616-620.
84. Prasad ML, Jungbluth AA, Iversen K, Huvos AG, Busam KJ. Expression of melanocytic differentiation markers in malignant melanomas of the oral and sinonasal mucosa. *Am J Surg Pathol*. 2001;25:782-787.
85. Snyder ML, Paulino AF. Melan-A as a useful diagnostic immunohistochemical stain for the diagnosis of primary sinonasal melanomas. *Head Neck*. 2002;24:52-55.
86. Feeley C, Theaker J. Epithelial markers in primary sinonasal mucosal melanoma. *Histopathology*. 2004;45:96-98.
87. Frierson HF Jr, Mills SE, Fechner RE, Taxy JB, Levine PA. Sinonasal undifferentiated carcinoma. An aggressive neoplasm derived from schneiderian epithelium and distinct from olfactory neuroblastoma. *Am J Surg Pathol*. 1986;10:771-779.
88. Jeng YM, Sung MT, Fang CL, et al. Sinonasal undifferentiated carcinoma and nasopharyngeal-type undifferentiated carcinoma: two clinically, biologically, and histopathologically distinct entities. *Am J Surg Pathol*. 2002;26:371-376.
89. Ejaz A, Wenig BM. Sinonasal undifferentiated carcinoma: clinical and pathologic features and a discussion on classification, cellular differentiation, and differential diagnosis. *Adv Anat Pathol*. 2005;12:134-143.
90. Enepekides DJ. Sinonasal undifferentiated carcinoma: an update. *Curr Opin Otolaryngol Head Neck Surg*. 2005;13:222-225.
91. Musy PY, Reibel JF, Levine PA. Sinonasal undifferentiated carcinoma: the search for a better outcome. *Laryngoscope*. 2002;112:1450-1455.
92. Dogan S, Chute DJ, Xu B, et al. Frequent IDH2 R172 mutations in undifferentiated and poorly-differentiated sinonasal carcinomas. *J Pathol*. 2017;242:400-408.
93. Mito JK, Bishop JA, Sadow PM, et al. Immunohistochemical detection and molecular characterization of IDH-mutant sinonasal undifferentiated carcinomas. *Am J Surg Pathol*. 2018;42:1067-1075.
94. Iezzoni JC, Mills SE. "Undifferentiated" small round cell tumors of the sinonasal tract: differential diagnosis update. *Am J Clin Pathol*. 2005;124 suppl:S110-S121.
95. Cerilli LA, Holst VA, Brandwein MS, Stoler MH, Mills SE. Sinonasal undifferentiated carcinoma: immunohistochemical profile and lack of EBV association. *Am J Surg Pathol*. 2001;25:156-163.
96. Bourne TD, Bellizzi AM, Stelow EB, et al. p63 Expression in olfactory neuroblastoma and other small cell tumors of the sinonasal tract. *Am J Clin Pathol*. 2008;130:213-218.
97. Logue JP, Banerjee SS, Slevin NJ, Vasanthan S. Neuroendocrine carcinomas of the larynx. *J Laryngol Otol*. 1991;105:1031-1035.

98. Ferlito A, Barnes L, Rinaldo A, Gnepp DR, Milroy CM. A review of neuroendocrine neoplasms of the larynx: update on diagnosis and treatment. *J Laryngol Otol.* 1998;112:827-834.

99. Ferlito A, Friedmann I. Review of neuroendocrine carcinomas of the larynx. *Ann Otol Rhinol Laryngol.* 1989;98:780-790.

100. Batsakis JG, el-Naggar AK, Luna MA. Neuroendocrine tumors of larynx. *Ann Otol Rhinol Laryngol.* 1992;101:710-714.

101. Mills SE, Cooper PH, Garland TA, Johns ME. Small cell undifferentiated carcinoma of the larynx. Report of two patients and review of 13 additional cases. *Cancer.* 1983;51:116-120.

102. Gnepp DR, Ferlito A, Hyams V. Primary anaplastic small cell (oat cell) carcinoma of the larynx. Review of the literature and report of 18 cases. *Cancer.* 1983;51:1731-1745.

103. Perez-Ordonez B, Caruana SM, Huvos AG, Shah JP. Small cell neuroendocrine carcinoma of the nasal cavity and paranasal sinuses. *Hum Pathol.* 1998;29:826-832.

104. Lewis JS Jr, Ferlito A, Gnepp DR, et al. Terminology and classification of neuroendocrine neoplasms of the larynx. *Laryngoscope.* 2011;121:1187-1193.

105. Woodruff JM, Huvos AG, Erlandson RA, Shah JP, Gerold FP. Neuroendocrine carcinomas of the larynx. A study of two types, one of which mimics thyroid medullary carcinoma. *Am J Surg Pathol.* 1985;9:771-790.

106. Bishop JA, Westra WH. Human papillomavirus-related small cell carcinoma of the oropharynx. *Am J Surg Pathol.* 2011;35:1679-1684.

107. Zhang H, Liu J, Cagle PT, Allen TC, Laga AC, Zander DS. Distinction of pulmonary small cell carcinoma from poorly differentiated squamous cell carcinoma: an immunohistochemical approach. *Mod Pathol.* 2005;18:111-118.

108. Mills SE. Neuroectodermal neoplasms of the head and neck with emphasis on neuroendocrine carcinomas. *Mod Pathol.* 2002;15:264-278.

109. Lewis JS Jr, Spence DC, Chiosea S, Barnes EL Jr, Brandwein-Gensler M, El-Mofty SK. Large cell neuroendocrine carcinoma of the larynx: definition of an entity. *Head Neck Pathol.* 2010;4:198-207.

110. Thompson LD, Gyure KA. Extracranial sinonasal tract meningiomas: a clinicopathologic study of 30 cases with a review of the literature. *Am J Surg Pathol.* 2000;24:640-650.

111. Luk IS, Chan JK, Chow SM, Leung S. Pituitary adenoma presenting as sinonasal tumor: pitfalls in diagnosis. *Hum Pathol.* 1996;27:605-609.

112. Byrne MN, Sessions DG. Nasopharyngeal craniopharyngioma. Case report and literature review. *Ann Otol Rhinol Laryngol.* 1990;99:633-639.

9

HEMATOPOIETIC AND LYMPHOID DISORDERS

Abundant mucosa-associated lymphoid tissue is present within the upper aerodigestive tract that can be involved by both nonneoplastic proliferations and malignancies.[1–25] The remaining tract may be involved by hematopoietic and lymphoid lesions more specific to certain sites (e.g., the sinonasal tract and extranodal natural killer [NK]/T-cell lymphomas), while the entire tract can be involved by other processes (e.g., extramedullary plasmacytomas or diffuse, large B-cell lymphoma). This chapter will methodically discuss hematopoietic and lymphoid disorders of this area, first discussing the benign proliferations and then discussing the malignant entities. Those tumors that occur most frequently throughout these sites will be discussed in the most detail.

Ancillary studies, including immunohistochemistry, flow cytometry, cytogenetics, and molecular studies that test for immunoglobulin or T-cell receptor rearrangements or various fusion transcripts, are now extremely important for the correct diagnosis of these lesions. Thus, the better one is prepared at the time of biopsy, the better the tissue will be triaged and the more likely one will be able to make a concise and correct diagnosis. Unfortunately, because these diagnoses are often unsuspected, many must be rendered using formalin-fixed tissue and immunohistochemistry.

NONNEOPLASTIC AND BENIGN PROLIFERATIONS

Most benign lymphoid proliferations of the upper aerodigestive tract occur within Waldeyer ring, most often in children. Because of obstructive symptoms or recurrent infections, the lymphoid tissue from this area is sometimes removed via tonsillectomy and adenoidectomy. Most specimens from these procedures will show a combination of follicular and interfollicular hyperplasia (Fig. 9.1, eFigs. 9.1 and 9.2).[26] The follicles will be enlarged and somewhat variable in size with well-formed germinal centers and mantle zones that typically are "zonated." The reactive germinal centers will contain abundant mitotic figures and tingible body macrophages. Some degree of interfollicular expansion is also usually present and can show variable changes. Generally, the paracortex and sinuses will have

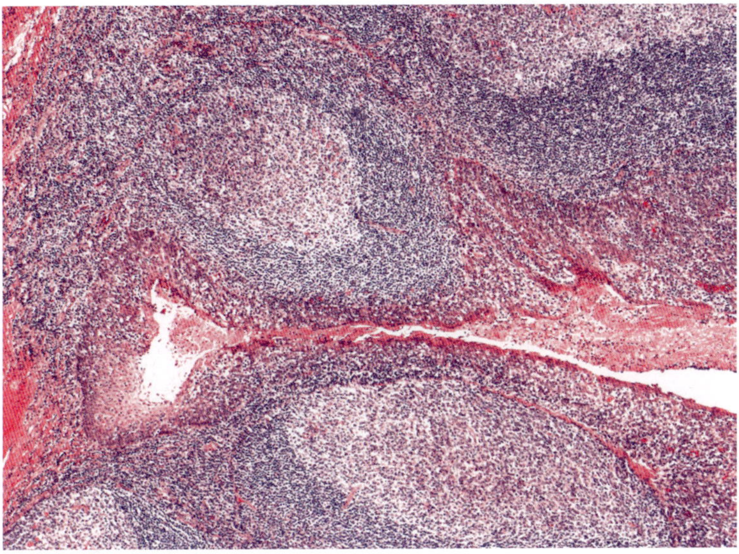

FIGURE 9.1 Follicular and interfollicular hyperplasia.

mixed smaller and larger lymphocytes with macrophages, immunoblasts, plasma cells, and acute inflammatory cells. Sometimes the overall growth pattern and particular cell types present allow for the identification of the cause of the hyperplasia. Certain reactive conditions can clinically and histologically be worrisome for malignancy.

Infectious mononucleosis secondary to Epstein-Barr virus (EBV) infection can be associated with massive tonsillar enlargement.[5,18,27] Indeed, the portal of entry for this virus is generally believed to be Waldeyer ring. Histologically, some degree of follicular hyperplasia is usually seen, together with marked interfollicular expansion by numerous immunoblasts, lymphocytes, and plasma cells (Fig. 9.2). The immunoblasts can be particularly prominent and may surround focal areas of necrosis (Fig. 9.3, eFigs. 9.3 and 9.4). Some immunoblasts may have multiple nuclei and mimic Reed-Sternberg cells, forcing one to consider a diagnosis of interfollicular involvement by Hodgkin lymphoma.[5,18,27] Immunohistochemistry can be helpful here, as immunoblasts should typically react with antibodies to CD20 and not with antibodies to CD15. Confusing the matter, however, is the fact that immunoblasts frequently react with antibodies to CD30 and background granulocytes may react with antibodies to CD15.[28] In situ hybridization or immunohistochemistry demonstrating infection by EBV is not necessarily helpful, as lymphomas also frequently show infection.[18,29]

Although infection with human immunodeficiency virus (HIV) puts patients at a much increased risk for lymphoma, benign *HIV-induced hyperplasias* are also common. While these lesions may occur in lymph nodes at any site, they can also develop in Waldeyer ring.[23] Here, they may even represent the initial manifestation of the patient's HIV infection.

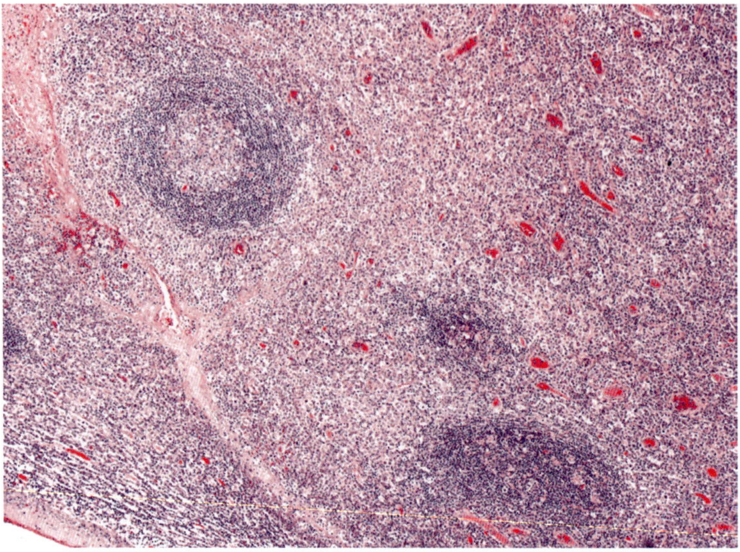

FIGURE 9.2 Marked interfollicular expansion seen in a case of infectious mononucleosis.

These lesions are histologically characterized by florid follicular hyperplasia with markedly enlarged germinal centers that are irregular in shape or "serpentine" (Fig. 9.4). Follicular fragmentation or lysis may be noted, as smaller lymphocytes extend into the germinal centers and give them

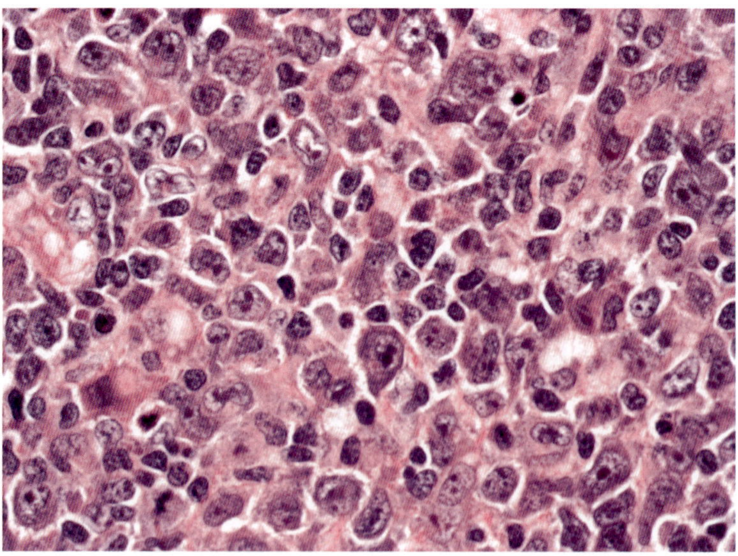

FIGURE 9.3 A proliferation of immunoblasts seen in a case of infectious mononucleosis.

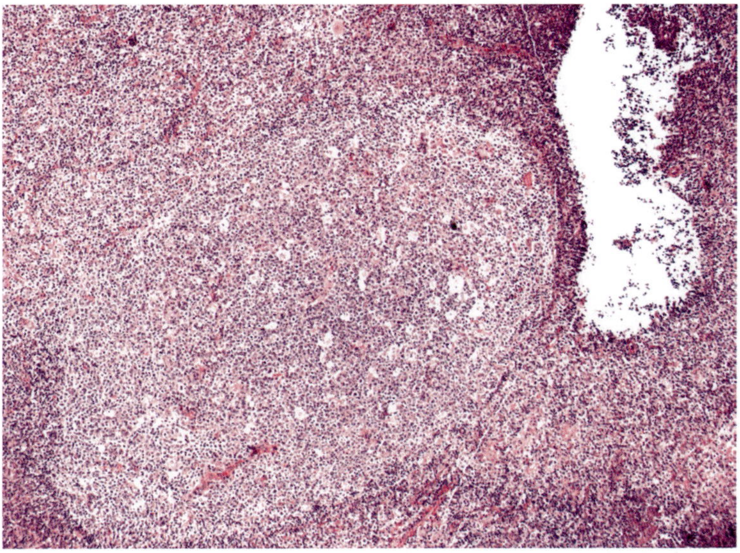

FIGURE 9.4 Marked follicular hyperplasia seen in a patient infected with human immunodeficiency virus.

a somewhat "moth-eaten" appearance. Interfollicular expansion can be present due to numerous monocytoid lymphocytes, immunoblasts, and plasma cells. Interfollicular hemorrhage is also often noted, as are multinucleated giant cells (Fig. 9.5). The giant cells can be located anywhere

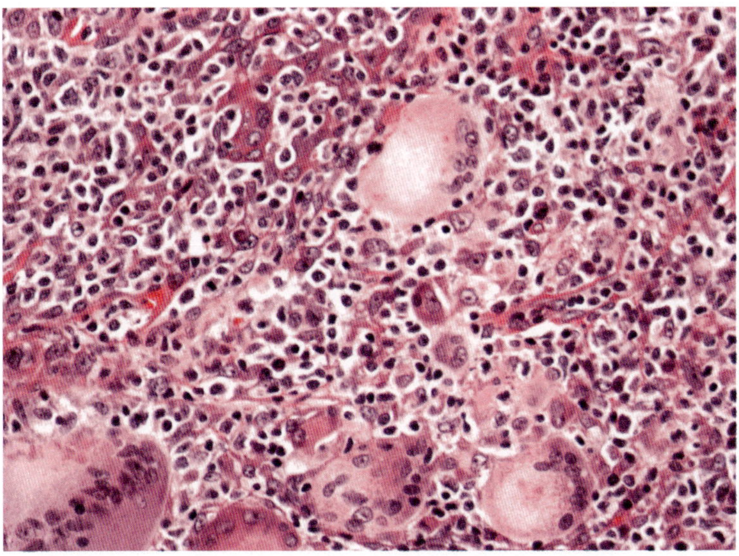

FIGURE 9.5 Multinucleated giant cells can be found in the reactive lymph nodes of patients infected with human immunodeficiency virus.

throughout the tissue but are frequently noted just adjacent to the surface epithelium. These cells have multiple medium-sized nuclei that are usually located at the periphery of the cell. It has been noted that these giant cells are less commonly seen in advanced disease.

Sinus histiocytosis with massive lymphadenopathy is believed to be a reactive condition that may involve lymph nodes or extranodal sites.[30,31] The disease may affect individuals at any age; however, it frequently develops in young patients and the mean reported age is around 20 years. Although it affects all races, it is more common in black individuals. Sinus histiocytosis with massive lymphadenopathy most commonly presents with cervical lymphadenopathy; however, extranodal sites in the head and neck can be involved either with or without concomitant adenopathy.[7,22] In the upper aerodigestive tract, the disease often involves Waldeyer ring, but it also can involve other sites, especially the sinonasal area.[32] Symptoms are nonspecific and include fever, obstruction, epistaxis, and changes secondary to mass effect. Although the disease is benign and nonneoplastic, it frequently recurs after excision either locally or at other sites. Patients rarely die from the disease or from its treatment.

Histologically, sinus histiocytosis with massive lymphadenopathy has a biphasic appearance with darker areas composed mostly of lymphocytes and more pale areas composed of histiocytes intermixed with lymphocytes and plasma cells (Fig. 9.6, eFig. 9.5).[7,22,30] The process diffusely involves subepithelial tissues while the overlying epithelia and underlying seromucinous glands remain intact. Fibrotic bands can by be prominent. The lymphoid areas are composed of small, mature lymphocytes with occasional histiocytes. Germinal center formation is not observed

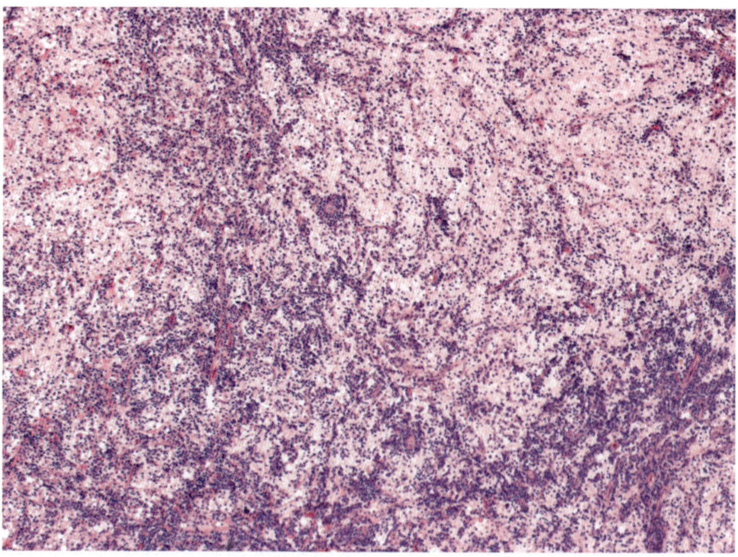

FIGURE 9.6 Sinus histiocytosis with massive lymphadenopathy.

within these areas. The histiocytes, generally better viewed in the less cellular areas, have round to oval nuclei with vesicular chromatin and abundant amphiphilic to eosinophilic, granular to foamy cytoplasm. Prominent emperipolesis characterizes this process, and the phagocytized cells can be lymphocytes, plasma cells, erythrocytes, or neutrophils (Fig. 9.7, eFig. 9.6). The process can extend into surrounding soft tissue and bone. If special stains are performed, organisms should not be identified.

A process termed *atypical marginal zone hyperplasia of mucosa-associated lymphoid tissue* has been described, primarily affecting Waldeyer ring in children.[1] The affected children presented with unilateral or bilateral tonsillar enlargement. Histologically, these cases were characterized by follicular hyperplasia with expansion of the marginal zones that can extend into the germinal centers. The expanded marginal zones showed light-chain restriction by immunohistochemistry; however, clonality was not found by molecular methods. The few cases reported received no additional therapy to the initial resection, and all patients remained free of lymphoma during the follow-up period.

MYELOID MALIGNANCIES

Myeloid sarcomas (extramedulary myeloid tumors, chloromas, etc.) can present anywhere throughout the body and have been noted to involve the upper aerodigestive tract.[33-40] When they do involve this location, they most commonly affect the oral tissue or mucosal lymphoid tissue of Waldeyer ring and are associated with cervical lymphadenopathy. These

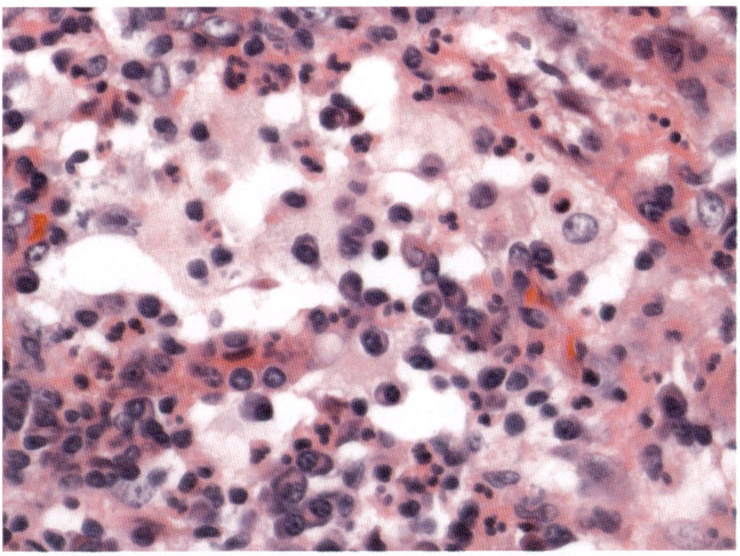

FIGURE 9.7 Marked emperipolesis seen in a case of sinus histiocytosis with massive lymphadenopathy.

lesions may be associated with acute myeloid leukemias, myeloproliferative disorders, or myelodysplastic syndromes. Rarely, myeloid sarcomas can occur as isolated lesions. Patients with myeloid sarcomas fare poorly, and in some cases, the lesions may signify a blast transformation of a preexistent myeloproliferative disorder and myelodysplastic syndrome. When the lesions are isolated, however, they can be associated with good outcomes.[33]

Myeloid sarcomas are infiltrative lesions that histologically display a sheetlike growth pattern (Figs. 9.8 and 9.9).[33,35,37] Neoplastic cells show varying degrees of differentiation and phenotype. Some tumors will be immature and show predominately myeloblasts, large, atypical cells with scanty cytoplasm, round to slightly convoluted nuclei, delicate chromatin, and prominent nuclei (eFig. 9.7). Other cases show more granulocytic or monocytic differentiation. Auer rods are seen in some cases.

Outside of a setting of known hematopoietic neoplasia, the diagnosis of a myeloid sarcoma can be difficult, mostly because it is not considered. Immunohistochemistry is generally needed to confirm a diagnosis and neoplastic cells will react with antibodies to myeloperoxidase (eFig. 9.8).[14,36,37] Other antigens expressed by the immature myelocytes and blasts can be identified by flow cytometry or immunohistochemistry and include CD13, CD33, and CD117.[39] Immunoreactivity with antibodies to CD34 can be seen in the blasts. Frequently, neoplasms will show immunoreactivity with antibodies to lysozyme and CD68. Cytogenetic abnormalities typical of myeloid neoplasia can be identified in many cases.[38]

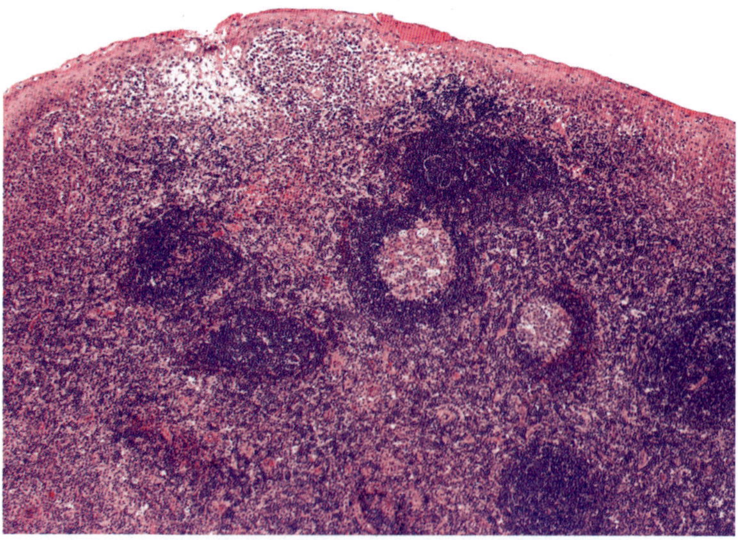

FIGURE 9.8 Partial tonsillar effacement by a myeloid sarcoma.

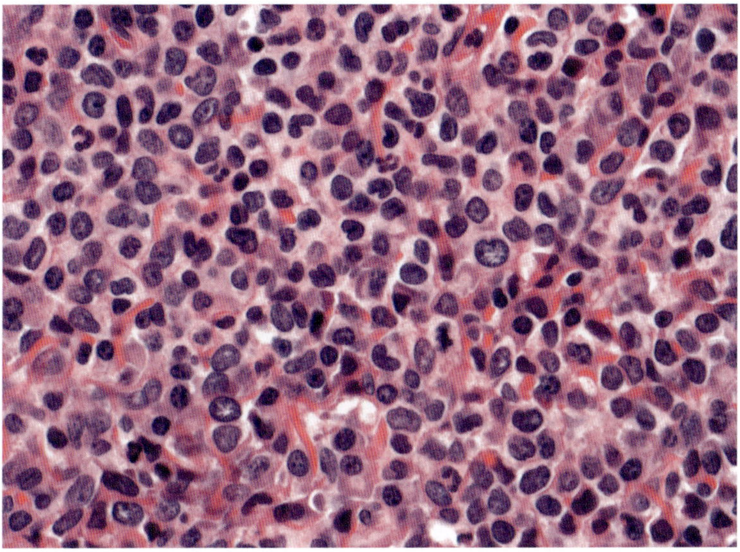

FIGURE 9.9 Sheets of myeloblasts found with a myeloid sarcoma.

Precursor B- and T-cell Malignancies

The most common hematolymphoid malignancies to involve Waldeyer ring in children are precursor B- and T-lymphoblastic lymphomas and Burkitt lymphomas.[41] As most precursor B-cell neoplasms also involve the bone marrow and blood, they are usually diagnosed as acute leukemias. Also, although these lesions are most common in children, adults can be affected by both precursor B- and T-cell malignancies.

Patients with leukemia generally present with systemic symptoms secondary to bone marrow replacement. These include symptoms secondary to anemia, leukopenia, and thrombocytopenia. Patients with involvement of Waldeyer ring often have involvement of other lymph nodes and more widespread adenopathy. Symptoms secondary to a pharyngeal mass can also be noted, and patients can have speech, eating, or breathing difficulties. Although patients without bone marrow and blood involvement usually present secondary to more widespread adenopathy, occasional patients will present with symptoms secondary to unilateral tonsillar enlargement. Indeed, although the vast majority of tonsils removed in children are removed because of reactive hyperplasia, most of us have encountered the rare tonsillectomy specimen found "incidentally" to contain lymphoblastic lymphoma. We have seen cases submitted for "gross examination only" that were later found to have lymphoblastic lymphoma when the patient presented with more widespread adenopathy.

The tonsillar tissue is effaced by sheets of lymphoblasts, although some cases may show only partial nodal involvement (Fig. 9.10).[42] The blasts are characteristically small to medium sized and have only a small

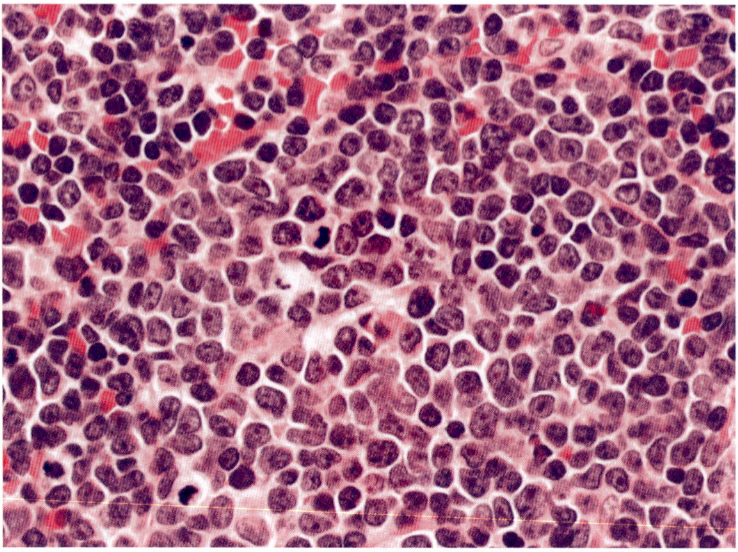

FIGURE 9.10 Sheets of lymphoblasts seen in a case of tonsillar lymphoblastic lymphoma.

amount of amphiphilic cytoplasm (eFig. 9.9). The nuclear contours can vary from smooth to convoluted, and the chromatin usually appears fine. Prominent nucleoli may be noted with many mitotic figures. Some degree of maturation is sometimes seen, and some of the lymphocytes can appear smaller, with more condensed chromatin and less prominent nucleoli. Numerous tingible body macrophages can be present, reminiscent of a Burkitt lymphoma.

Antigen expression in precursor B- and T-cell leukemias/lymphomas depends on the lineage and maturity of the neoplastic cells. Lesions not involving the marrow and blood are more likely to have a precursor T-cell phenotype and express CD3 (cytoplasmic) with variable expression of other T-cell antigens such as CD2, CD4, CD5, CD7, and CD8.[42,43] The cells should also express terminal deoxynucleotidyl transferase (TdT) and, often, CD10 (eFig. 9.10 and 9.11). Markers of myeloid or B-cell differentiation can also be present and do not necessarily exclude a diagnosis of precursor T-cell lymphoma/leukemia. Lesions that also have bone marrow and blood involvement are more likely to have a precursor B-cell phenotype and will express B-cell antigens such as CD19 and CD79a and others such as CD20 and CD22. The neoplastic blasts should also express TdT and will frequently express CD10. Although these tumors can be diagnosed with immunohistochemistry, flow cytometry is generally the method of choice for assessing antigen expression.

Cytogenetic analysis is very important with these tumors and provides prognostic information that may influence therapy.[42] This is especially true with precursor B-cell malignancies and certain translocations such as t(9;22)(q34; q11.2), t(4;11)(q21;q23), and t(1;19)(q23;p13.3) are considered "unfavorable" whereas others, such as t(12;21)(p12;q22) are considered "favorable." Cases with a hyperdiploid karyotype are also considered "favorable," whereas those that are hypodiploid are considered "unfavorable."

Mature B-cell Malignancies

Most types of mature B-cell neoplasia have been noted to involve the upper aerodigestive tract (Table 9.1).[3,4,14–17,19,21,24,41,44–56] These tumors, especially the lower grade lesions, primarily affect Waldeyer ring. Some, such as diffuse, large B-cell lymphomas, can involve both mucosa-associated lymphoid tissue and other sites, while others, such as extramedullary plasmacytomas, often occur outside of Waldeyer ring. Of the lesions involving Waldeyer ring, diffuse large B-cell lymphomas are the most common, followed by mantle cell lymphomas and follicular lymphomas. Nearly all mature B-cell lymphomas have been noted to involve Waldeyer ring, however. Of the mature B-cell malignancies involving other sites, diffuse, large B-cell lymphomas are again the most common malignancies. When involving Waldeyer ring, many of these lymphomas efface the normal lymphoid tissue; however, each may only partially involve the tissue. As with other hematolymphoid malignancies, ancillary studies are often necessary for diagnosis. Many of these malignancies can be properly diagnosed with immunohistochemistry; however, flow cytometry is very helpful. Molecular diagnostic studies and cytogenetic analysis can be useful as many of these tumors show recurrent cytogenetic abnormalities. Finally, immunoglobulin and T-cell receptor gene rearrangement studies can be helpful with very small specimens when a definitive diagnosis of lymphoma cannot be made for one reason or another.

Diffuse large B-cell lymphoma is the most common type of non-Hodgkin lymphoma of adults in Western countries.[57,58] While the lymphoma most frequently occurs in older individuals, it can develop in patients of any age. This lymphoma generally presents as a rapidly growing mass and is usually considered to be primary, that is to say there is no clinical knowledge of previous lower grade lymphomas. Sometimes, though, the tumor evolves from lower grade malignancy such as chronic lymphocytic leukemia/small lymphocytic lymphoma (CLL/SLL), follicular lymphoma, or extranodal marginal zone lymphoma.

Histologically, diffuse large B-cell lymphomas have "large" neoplastic cells intermixed with smaller, more mature, normal-appearing lymphocytes (Fig. 9.11, eFig. 9.12).[58] In general, the larger, neoplastic cells predominate; however, in some cases, they may be few in number and can even be hard to identify, as they are obscured by numerous, small T-cells (T-cell–rich variant of diffuse large B-cell lymphoma). The tumor nuclei are at least two times the size of a resting mature lymphocyte. They can have scant to moderate amounts of basophilic cytoplasm and

TABLE 9.1 The More Common Hematopoietic and Lymphoid Malignancies of the Upper Aerodigestive Tract[4,14,16,21,44,48,49,51,53–56]

Waldeyer ring (approximately 70% of UADT lymphomas)
Diffuse large B-cell lymphoma
Mantle cell lymphoma
Follicular lymphoma
Extranodal marginal zone lymphoma
Burkitt lymphoma
T-cell lymphoma (various)[a]
Other (lymphoblastic lymphoma, plasmacytoma, Hodgkin lymphoma, posttransplant lymphoproliferative disorder, etc.)
Oral cavity (approximately 13% of UADT lymphomas)
Diffuse large B-cell lymphoma
Plasmablastic lymphoma
Follicular lymphoma
Mantle cell lymphoma
Extranodal marginal zone lymphoma
Plasmacytoma
Lymphoblastic lymphoma
Other (Burkitt lymphoma, Hodgkin lymphoma, myeloid sarcoma, etc.)
Sinonasal tract (approximately 13% of UADT lymphomas)
Diffuse large B-cell lymphoma
T-cell lymphoma (predominately NK/T-cell lymphomas, nasal type)[a]
Follicular lymphoma
Small lymphocytic lymphoma
Lymphoblastic lymphoma
Burkitt lymphoma
Other (extranodal marginal aone lymphoma, Hodgkin lymphoma, etc.)
Larynx (approximately 4% of UADT lymphomas)
Diffuse large B-cell lymphoma
Plasmacytoma
Other (lymphoblastic lymphoma, Burkitt lymphoma, etc.)

UADT, upper aerodigestive tract.

[a]The proportion of lymphomas at each site that are T-cell lymphomas varies according to the geographic location of the study population. Eastern populations are more frequently affected by T-cell lymphomas secondary to human T-cell leukemia virus infection. Natural killer (NK)/T-cell lymphomas of the nasal-type, driven by Epstein-Barr virus (EBV) infection, also vary in their frequencies across different populations.

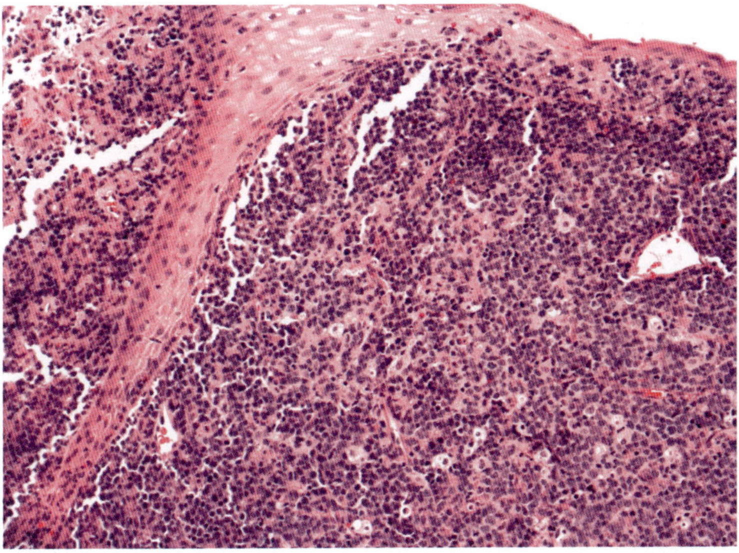

FIGURE 9.11 A diffuse large B-cell lymphoma involving the tonsil.

have pleomorphic nuclei with irregular contours and vesicular chromatin (Fig. 9.12, eFig. 9.13). Some cases have cells that appear more centroblastic, with more scanty cytoplasm and two to four nucleoli that are often associated with the nuclear membrane. Other cases have cells that appear more immunoblastic with moderate amounts of cytoplasm and single,

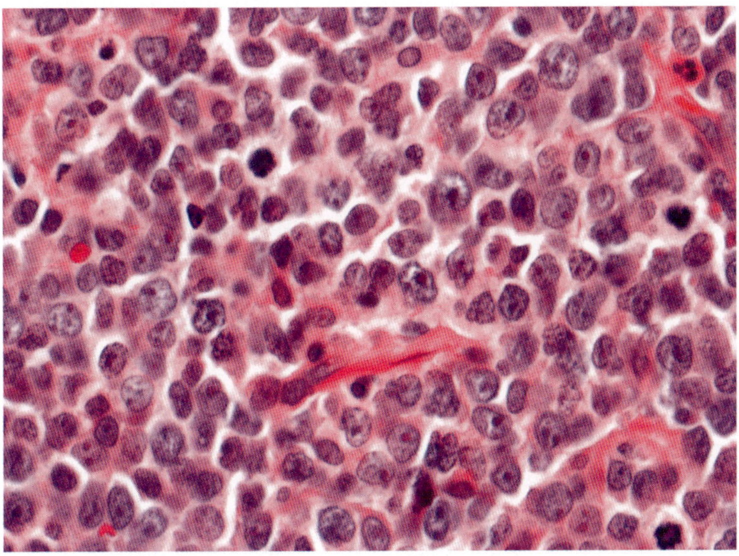

FIGURE 9.12 This diffuse large B-cell lymphoma is composed of cells resembling immunoblasts.

centrally located nucleoli. Regardless of the appearance, mitotic figures are usually easy to identify. Prominent background sclerosis can sometimes be present. Rarely, background necrosis may be noted.

Immunophenotypically, the neoplastic cells should show evidence of B-cell differentiation and usually express CD19, CD20, CD22, and CD79a (eFig. 9.14).[58] Occasional cases will express CD5 or CD10. These tumors do not express cyclin D1 (BCL1), which allows them to be distinguished from mantle cell lymphomas. Because patients who have tumors with a "germinal center" immunophenotype fare better than those with tumors that have an "activated" immunophenotype, additional immunohistochemistry is performed on most of these cases.[59,60] Expression of BCL6 and CD10 correlates with a "germinal center" phenotype, whereas expression of mum1 is consistent with an "activated" phenotype. EBV infection can be noted with some cases by immunohistochemistry or in situ hybridization; however, infection is more common in those lymphomas developing in patients who are immunocompromised.

Diffuse large B-cell lymphomas can show a variety of cytogenetic and molecular abnormalities. Some cases show the t(14;18), typical of follicular lymphomas.[59] This can occur both in cases believed to represent true progression and in cases believed to be primary. Also, chromosomal rearrangements of 3q27 are sometimes noted, leading to activation of BCL6.[61]

Plasmablastic lymphoma is an aggressive lymphoma that occurs most frequently in patients infected with HIV.[46,47,50,62,63] While these malignancies can develop at any site, they frequently involve the oral cavity. Histologically, the tumors resemble diffuse large B-cell lymphomas that have a more immunoblastic phenotype with medium to large cells with a moderate amount of cytoplasm and a single prominent nucleolus (Fig. 9.13, eFig. 9.15). Mitotic figures and single cell necrosis are frequent, and binucleated or multinucleated tumor cells are often seen (eFig. 9.16). The neoplastic cells react with antibodies to CD45 but do not generally react with antibodies to CD20, PAX5, and BCL6 and show variable reactivity with antibodies to CD79a.[47,50,63] Instead reactivity for plasma cell antigens such as CD38 and CD138 is usually seen. While most cases will show evidence of EBV infection by in situ hybridization for EBV-encoded RNA and evidence of human herpes virus 8 (HHV8) infection by polymerase chain reaction (PCR), neither marker is typically identified by immunohistochemistry (EBV-LMP or HHV8).[46,47,50,63] Cytoplasmic light-chain restriction can usually be identified by immunohistochemistry (eFig. 9.17).

Mantle cell lymphoma is the second most common mature B-cell lymphoma of Waldeyer ring which appears to be involved in at least 20% of cases of mantle cell lymphoma at time of diagnosis.[14,64,65] These lymphomas occur in older patients and are more common in men.[57,58,66] The disease usually presents at high stage, often with bone marrow involvement. It is a relentless disease, and the majority of patients die within 5 years of their diagnosis.

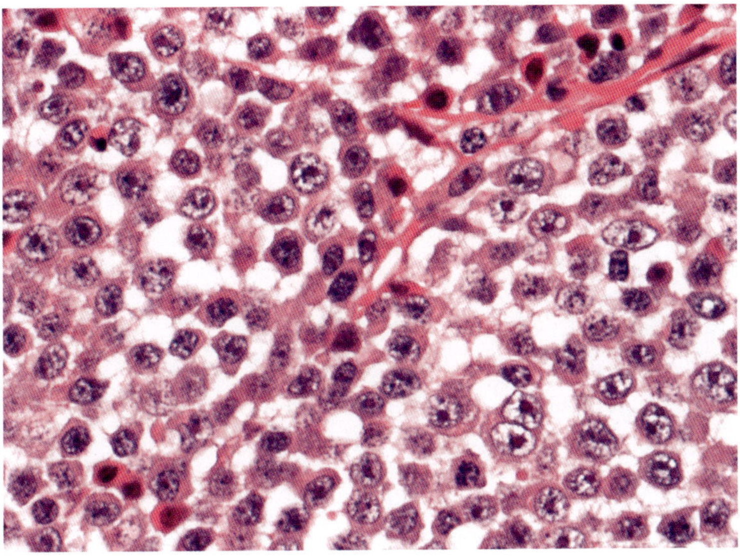

FIGURE 9.13 The neoplastic cells of a plasmablastic lymphoma are similar to immunoblasts.

Mantle cell lymphoma is histologically characterized by effacement of the lymphoid tissue by a diffuse or vaguely nodular lymphoid infiltrate (Fig. 9.14).[58,66] The neoplastic lymphocytes are small to medium sized and show irregular nuclear membranes (Fig. 9.15). The chromatin

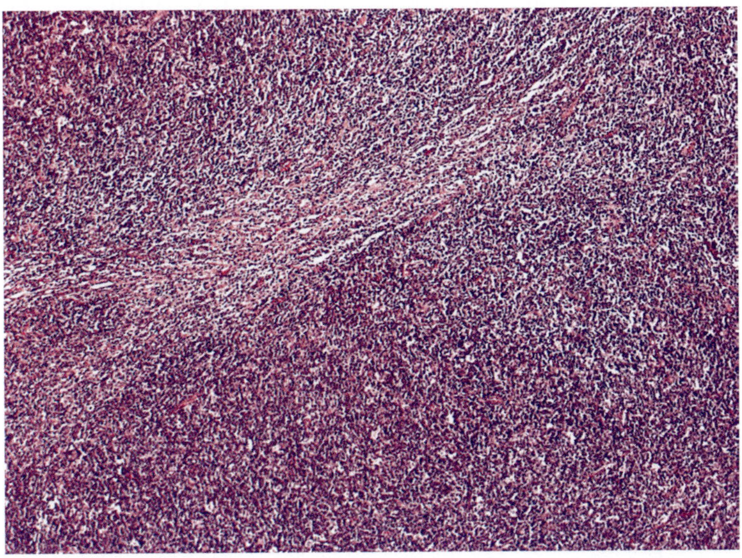

FIGURE 9.14 Mantle cell lymphomas have a somewhat nodular appearance under low power.

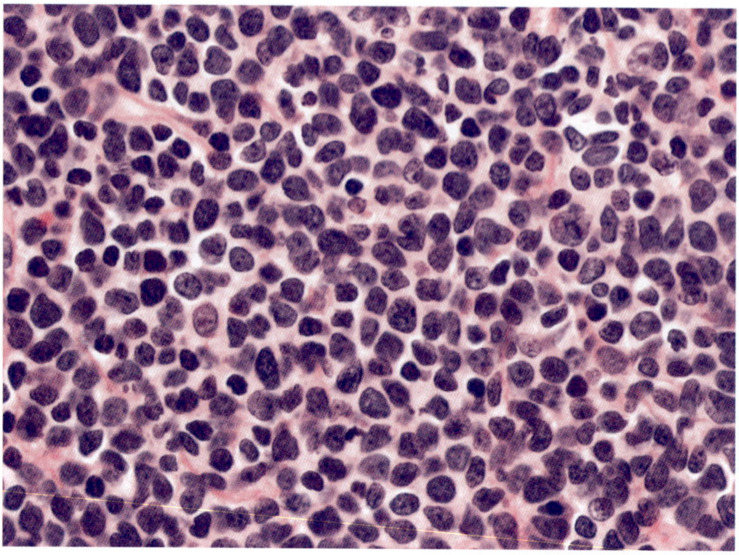

FIGURE 9.15 The neoplastic cells of a mantle cell lymphoma have irregular nuclear contours.

appears somewhat granular, and nucleoli are usually not seen. Mitotic figures are variable in number but can be frequent. Intermixed "clean" macrophages are usually seen as are small, hyalinized vessels (eFigs. 9.18 and 9.19). Occasional cases will progressively develop a more blastic appearance (blastoid variant). With these cases, the neoplastic cells may appear slightly larger and have fine or dispersed chromatin. These cases also have more frequent mitotic figures (>10/10 hpfs) (eFig. 9.20).

Mantle cell lymphomas express B-cell antigens such as CD19, CD20, and CD79a.[58,66] The neoplastic cells are also immunoreactive with antibodies to CD5, CD43, BCL2, and cyclin D1 (eFig. 9.21). Most mantle cell lymphomas do not express CD10 or CD23. Cytogenetically, the tumors characteristically have the t(11;14)(q13;q32) which juxtaposes the immunoglobulin heavy chain gene and the cyclin D1 gene. All tumors suspected of being mantle cell lymphomas should be confirmed as such either by demonstrating cyclin D1 expression or the t(11;14)(q13;q32).

Follicular lymphoma is a common non-Hodgkin lymphoma in the Western world, and it does not infrequently involve Waldeyer ring. Patients typically present with widespread adenopathy, and follicular lymphomas are usually high stage at the time of the diagnosis.[57,58] As with other low-grade B-cell lymphomas, this is a malignancy usually diagnosed in older patients. That said, some follicular lymphomas are seen in children and these appear to have a greater predilection for involvement of Waldeyer ring. Lower grade follicular lymphomas are typically not curable; however, many patients live more than 10 years after they are diagnosed with this malignancy. Although higher grade follicular lymphomas are more aggressive, they tend to be treated with more aggressive chemotherapeutic regimens and some patients can actually be cured of their disease.

Lower grade follicular lymphomas typically show effacement of the normal lymphoid tissue by neoplastic follicles (Fig. 9.16, eFig. 9.22).[57,67] The follicles are relatively uniform in size, are poorly defined, lack mantle zones, lack tingible body macrophages, and frequently merge together. Some lower grade lesions and, more frequently, higher grade lesions will show a more diffuse pattern of growth. The follicular and diffuse patterns are often noted together in the same case and some advocate the reporting of the proportions of these patterns. The neoplastic cells resemble centrocytes and centroblasts, and the relative proportion of these two cell types (or, more accurately, the number of centroblasts present) is used for the grading of these tumors (Fig. 9.17). Centrocytes are smaller cells with scanty cytoplasm and folded or clefted nuclei that typically do not have nucleoli. Centroblasts are larger cells that have slightly more cytoplasm and larger nuclei. These cells have more vesicular chromatin than centrocytes and typically have multiple small, peripheral nucleoli. The current WHO scheme for the diagnosis of lymphoid tumors suggests grading these tumors based the absolute number of centroblasts present in neoplastic follicles.[68] Grade 1 follicular lymphomas have 0 to 5 centroblasts/hpf; grade 2 follicular lymphomas have 6 to 15 centroblasts/hpf; and grade 3 have more than 15 centroblasts/hpf.

Follicular lymphomas are mature B-cell lymphomas and as such express CD19, CD20, and CD79a.[58] Most express CD10 and BCL2 and do not express CD5 or CD23 (eFig. 9.23). Exceptions have been noted, however. The expression of the bcl-2 protein can be used to distinguish these

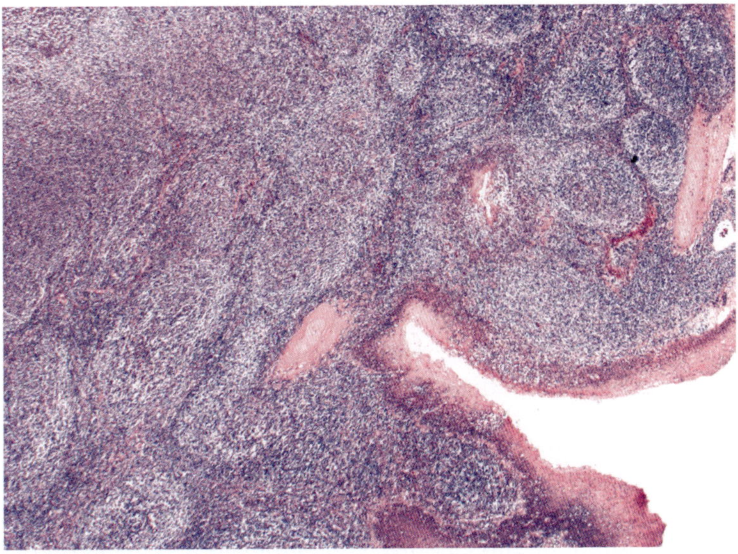

FIGURE 9.16 Tonsillar involvement in a follicular lymphoma.

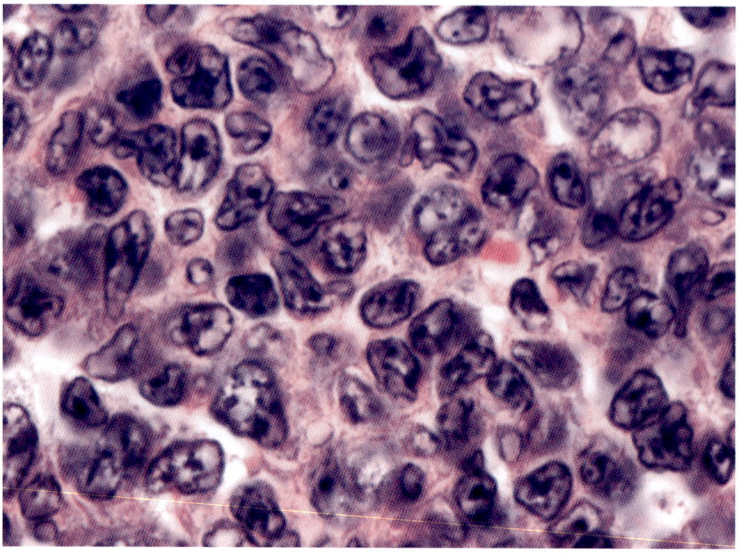

FIGURE 9.17 Small-sized and medium-sized cleaved nuclei are seen with follicular lymphomas.

lesions from nonneoplastic follicular hyperplasia as the B-lymphocytes within the germinal centers of nonneoplastic, reactive conditions do not express the protein. Follicular lymphoma is characterized by the t(14;18)(q23;q21) that juxtaposes the immunoglobulin heavy chain with the *BCL2* gene. Other translocations involving *BCL2* have also been noted, however.

As was stated, follicular lymphomas are uncommon in children; however, when they develop in this population, they frequently involve Waldeyer ring and are more common in boys (*pediatric-type follicular lymphoma*).[13,15,19,24] Unlike adult follicular lymphomas, these tumors are often localized and of lower stage. Furthermore, they are also more likely to be higher grade and appear to be curable in the majority of patients. The histology is nearly identical to that of adult follicular lymphomas except that the follicles appear larger and may even appear "floral." The neoplastic cells express B-cell antigens and typically express CD10 and BCL6. They do not usually express BCL2, however, and the typical t(14;18) seen in adult cases is infrequently identified in these cases.[13,19]

Extranodal marginal zone lymphomas of mucosa-associated lymphoid tissue (MALTomas) can involve Waldeyer ring or any mucosal site throughout the upper aerodigestive tract.[57,58,69,70] Outside of Waldeyer ring, the lesions often involve the seromucinous glands and can arise is patients with a history of Sjogren syndrome. These tumors occur most frequently in older patients (older than 50 years) and are slightly more common in women, perhaps because of their association with autoimmune disease. The tumors are indolent and can often be managed with local therapy only. Some cases will transform into diffuse large B-cell lymphomas.

Extranodal marginal zone lymphomas often appear to occur in the setting of chronically inflamed tissue.[58,69,70] Generally, one sees residual reactive lymphoid follicles, sometimes partially obliterated by expanded marginal zones (Fig. 9.18). The neoplastic cells then efface the surrounding tissues. The tumor cells appear centrocytic with smaller and folded nuclei or have a moderate amount of pale to clear cytoplasm and resemble the monocytoid B-cells seen between the follicles in some reactive conditions (eFig. 9.24). Some degree of differentiation is usually seen throughout these tumors with some cells that appear more immunoblastic and others that appear plasmacytoid. In some cases, these more differentiated cells predominate. The more plasmacytoid cells can have eosinophilic intranuclear pseudoinclusions or Dutcher bodies. In areas with abundant seromucinous glands, numerous lymphoepithelial lesions can be found. Involvement of the overlying squamous epithelium does not qualify as a lymphoepithelial lesion; however, especially in Waldeyer ring, as such lesions are frequently seen in benign, nonneoplastic situations.[71]

Extranodal marginal zone lymphomas show a mature B-cell immunophenotype and express CD19, CD20, and CD79a.[58] Tumors cells should not react with antibodies to CD5, CD10, or CD23 and will generally not show immunoreactivity with antibodies to plasma cell antigens such as CD38 or CD138. A number of translocations have been seen with these malignancies including t(11;18)(q21;q21), t(14;18)(q32;q21), t(3;14)(p14.1;q32), and t(1;14)(p22;q32).[72] Each translocation occurs more frequently at a specific site, and tumors involving the salivary glands infrequently have these translocations.

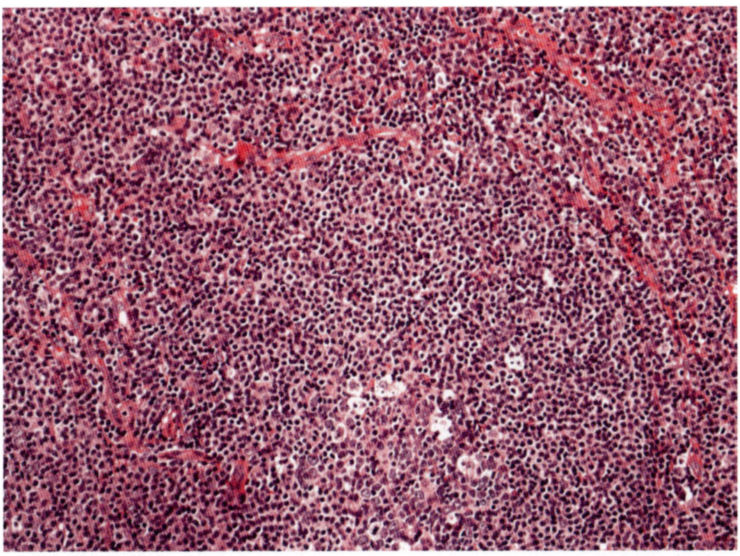

FIGURE 9.18 Germinal center "colonization" by an extranodal marginal zone lymphoma.

Extraosseous plasmacytomas are defined as monoclonal proliferations of plasma cells that occur at extraosseus sites in patients without concomitant bone marrow involvement by the disease.[73] Up to 20% of patients, however, have a monoclonal gammopathy. While these are relatively uncommon tumors, they have a predilection for the head and neck and frequently involve the mucosa of the upper aerodigestive tract.[2,3,17,45,52] They can involve any site throughout this area and most frequently affect the sinonasal area and Waldeyer ring. These lesions arise in older patients with a median age of presentation in the sixth decade of life. The prognosis for these patients is good, and the disease is usually cured with local therapy. Up to a quarter recur, however, and approximately 15% of patients are later found to have myeloma.[45]

Histologically, extraosseous plasmacytomas characteristically have sheets of plasma cells with abundant amphiphilic cytoplasm and eccentrically placed round to oval nuclei with granular (clock-faced) chromatin (Fig. 9.19, eFig. 9.25).[2,3,17,52] Occasional cases will have cells that show more cytologic atypia or have a more "plasmablastic" phenotype with larger nuclei, finer chromatin, and more prominent nucleoli. Mott cells and Russell bodies are frequently encountered. Neoplastic cells often fail to express some of the typical B-cell antigens such as CD19 and CD20.[74] They typically express CD79a, CD38, and CD138 and will show light-chain restriction by immunohistochemistry or in situ hybridization (eFigs. 9.26 and 9.27).[74,75] Some cases may be difficult to distinguish from extranodal marginal zone lymphomas that show plasma cell differentiation.[3] Nonneoplastic, plasma cell–rich inflammatory lesions should be excluded by their lack of light-chain restriction.[76]

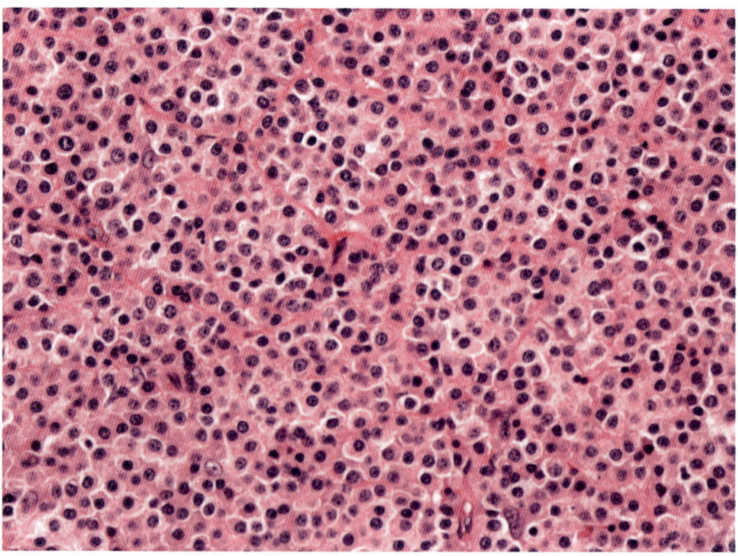

FIGURE 9.19 Sheets of plasma cells are seen in plasmacytomas.

A number of other mature B-cell lymphomas can involve the upper aerodigestive tract, especially Waldeyer ring.[4,14,16,21,44,48,49,51,53,56] These include *chronic lymphocytic leukemia/small lymphocytic lymphoma, Burkitt lymphoma, lymphoplasmacytic lymphoma*, and *lymphomatoid granulomatosis*. Most cases of chronic lymphocytic leukemia/small lymphoblastic lymphoma that involve the upper aerodigestive tract present with widespread adenopathy and often have bone marrow and blood involvement. Immunohistochemistry is generally sufficient for the diagnosis of this disease and the small, neoplastic lymphocytes, aside from expressing B-cell antigens, typically express CD5 and CD23.[58] Lymphoplasmacytic lymphoma can also usually be diagnosed with histology and immunohistochemistry and should histologically lack features of other low-grade B-cell lymphomas that can have a plasmacytoid phenotype.[58] Immunophenotypically, these lymphomas express B-cell antigens and often CD38 and CD23, do not express CD10, and usually lack CD5.[58,77] Burkitt lymphoma can present in younger patients or immunocompromised patients and will show the well-known "starry-sky" histologic appearance (Fig. 9.20, eFig. 9.28).[58] These tumors also express B-cell antigens, CD10, and BCL6 and show a high ki-67 index (virtually 100% of tumor nuclei stain), but do not express TdT.[58,78] Whether one can accurately distinguish Burkitt lymphoma from diffuse large B-cell lymphomas without showing evidence of *MYC* rearrangement remains to be seen, and lymphomas with combined features are sometimes seen.

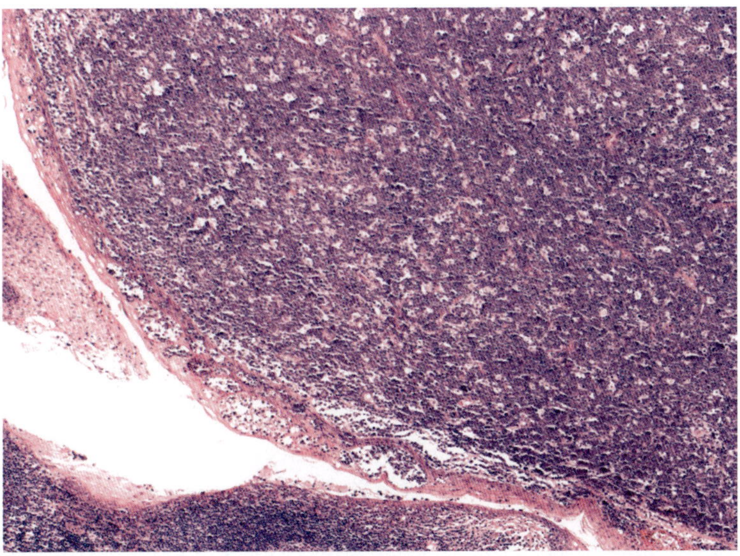

FIGURE 9.20 A tonsil involved in Burkitt lymphoma.

Mature T-cell/NK-cell Malignancies

In the Western world, T-cell or NK-cell malignancies of the upper aerodigestive tract are uncommon and most often are extranodal NK/T-cell lymphomas of the nasal type.[79] In other parts of the world, however, other T-cell malignancies are more common and, as such, represent a greater number of the lymphomas found throughout the upper aerodigestive tract.

Extranodal NK/T-cell lymphoma, nasal type is a disease of older adults with a mean age at presentation of 50 years.[79–82] The malignancies usually present as midline nasal septal destruction and represent many cases of what was once called "lethal midline granuloma" or "idiopathic midline destructive lesion." Larger tumors can be associated with more clinical abnormalities including those secondary to involvement of the palate and eye. The tumors are very aggressive, often in spite of multimodality therapy. These lymphomas are associated with infection with EBV, and common cytogenetic abnormalities include deletions of 6q and 1p with gains of 2q.[81–84]

Histologically, extranodal NK/T-cell lymphomas, nasal type can be quite varied.[79–82] Some cases will be composed of small neoplastic cells that are similar to normal mature lymphocytes, while others will have very large, markedly atypical cells with irregular nuclear contours and prominent nucleoli. Many cases have a mixture of small- to medium-sized cells that have a moderate amount of cytologic atypia, with abundant apoptotic cells and mitotic figures (Figs. 9.21 and 9.22, eFigs. 9.29 and 9.30).

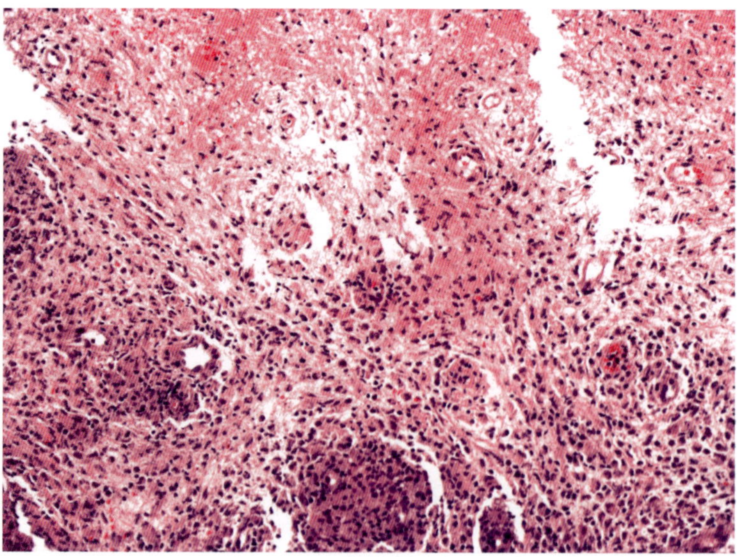

FIGURE 9.21 Necrosis and atypical cellular infiltrate seen in a case of extranodal natural killer (NK)/T-cell lymphoma, nasal type.

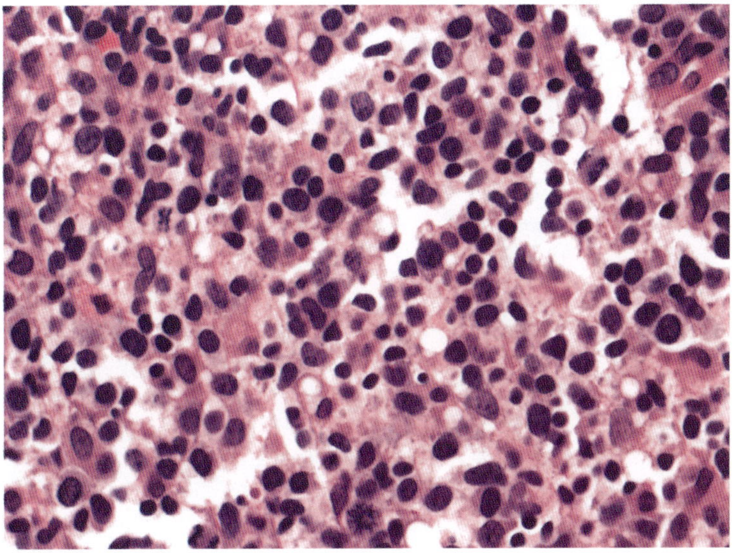

FIGURE 9.22 Large, markedly atypical cells are seen in this extranodal natural killer (NK)/T-cell lymphoma, nasal type.

Angiocentricity and angioinvasion are frequently also seen with large areas of necrosis. A mixture of other inflammatory cells is also usually present and may be so marked as to actually obscure the neoplastic cells.

Ancillary studies are necessary for the diagnosis of extranodal NK/T-cell lymphomas. Tumor cells should be immunoreactive with antibodies to CD45 (leukocyte common antigen). In situ hybridization for EBV can be very helpful, and almost all cases should be positive (Fig. 9.23).[82,85] The neoplastic cells may express some T-cell antigens including CD2 and CD3 (cytoplasmic, not surface); however, clonal T-cell receptor arrangements are not seen with these tumors.[79] Most cases will be immunoreactive with antibodies to CD56 but not with antibodies to CD57 (eFig. 9.31).[79,86,87]

Other mature T-cell malignancies occur throughout the upper aerodigestive tract, although the incidences of these tumors are hard to determine as larger studies investigating these tumors at these sites predate our current classification system. It appears, nonetheless, that extranodal NK/T-cell lymphoma predominates, even in other parts of the world; however, anaplastic large cell lymphomas and adult T-cell lymphomas/leukemias can certainly involve the area (eFigs. 9.32 and 9.33).[4,14,16,56] Furthermore, both mucosal and cutaneous T-cell malignancies have been noted to involve the upper aerodigestive tract, including intestinal T-cell lymphomas and mycosis fungoides/Sezary syndrome.[88,89] The diagnosis of these T-cell lymphomas must be based on the same criteria used to diagnosis them at other sites and requires immunophenotyping, either with flow cytometry of immunohistochemistry. Molecular studies used to identify T-cell receptor gene rearrangements may also be

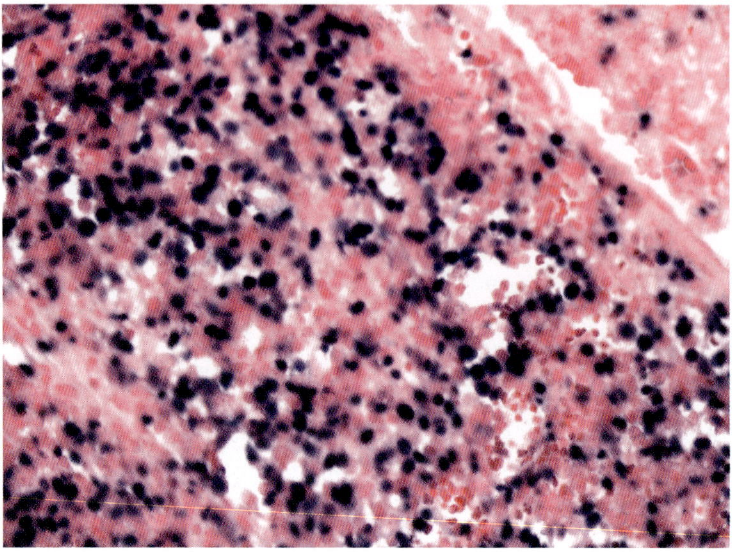

FIGURE 9.23 Positive in situ hybridization for Epstein-Barr virus–encoded RNA is seen with this extranodal natural killer (NK)/T-cell lymphoma, nasal type.

needed, especially with small biopsies of lower grade lesions. It should here be noted that traumatic ulcerative granuloma of the tongue (discussed in Chapter 14) frequently has atypical CD30-positive cells and may have clonal T-cell receptor rearrangements.[90] It is debated whether this lesion is truly a lymphoproliferative disorder and how it overlaps with cutaneous CD30-positive tumors.[91]

Hodgkin Lymphoma

Classic Hodgkin lymphoma has been described involving the upper aerodigestive tract; most often it affects Waldeyer ring.[6,10,20] It is much less common then non-Hodgkin lymphoma throughout the tract (Fig. 9.24). When it presents here, it is frequently low stage. Approximately half the cases reported to involve Waldeyer ring have been classified as mixed cellularity. The second most frequent pattern noted is nodular sclerosis. A broad age range has been reported, and patients fare similar to those patients diagnosed with nodal disease of similar stage. As with classic Hodgkin lymphomas at other sites, the diagnosis rests with the identification of Reed-Sternberg cells or Reed-Sternberg cell variants, large, atypical single cells with single or multiple atypical nuclei that typically have convoluted membranes, vesicular chromatin, and prominent nucleoli (Fig. 9.25, eFigs. 9.34 and 9.35). These cells should be immunoreactive with antibodies to CD15 and CD30 and usually not with antibodies to CD45 (eFigs. 9.36 and 9.37).[10]

Also, it should be noted that rare cases of nodular lymphocyte–predominant Hodgkin lymphoma have been reported to involve Waldeyer

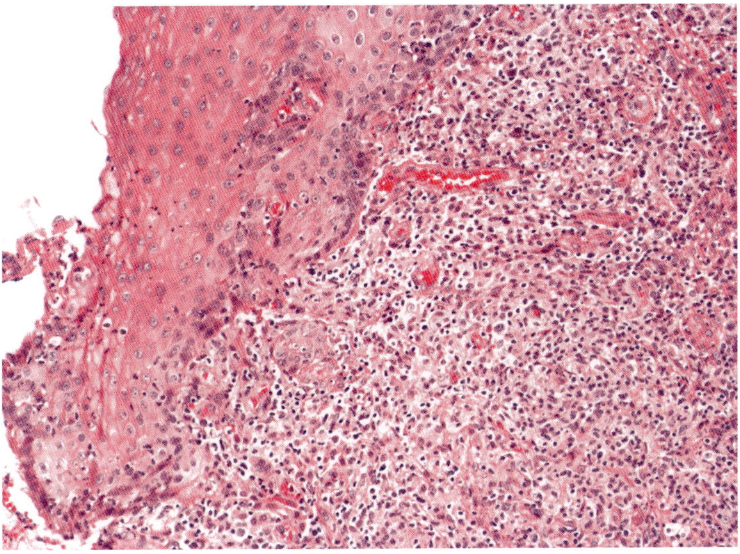

FIGURE 9.24 Tongue involvement in a classical Hodgkin lymphoma.

ring.[92] The immunophenotype for these neoplasms is different from classic Hodgkin lymphoma, and the neoplastic cells will typically cxpress CD45 and CD20 and will not express CD15 or CD30. Some authors have noted that Hodgkin lymphomas of Waldeyer ring are more likely to show evidence of EBV infection by in situ hybridization.[10]

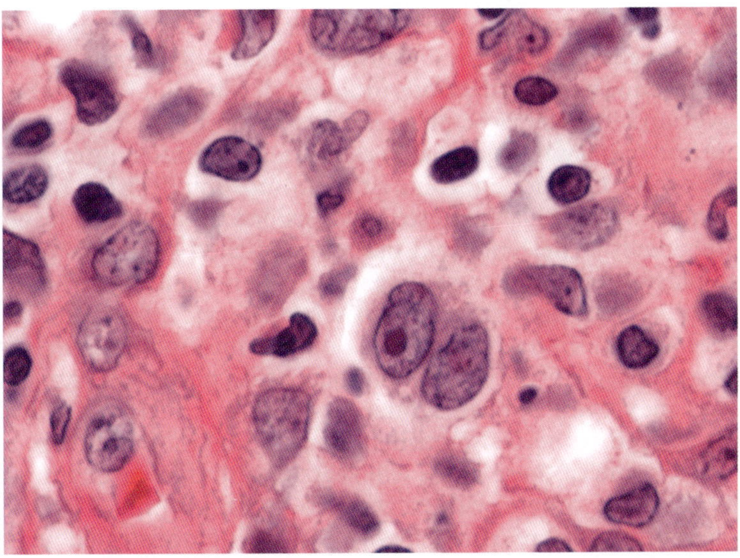

FIGURE 9.25 Reed-Sternberg cells typify classical Hodgkin lymphoma.

Immunodeficiency-Associated Lymphoproliferative Disorders

Patients infected with HIV are at up to a 100-fold increased risk for the development of a lymphoma.[93] Thus, any tonsillar tissue removed from a patient infected with HIV should be worked up for lymphoma. In general, these lymphomas should be classified using the criteria applied to lesions from patients who are immunocompetent. The most common lymphomas affecting these patients include Burkitt lymphoma, diffuse large B-cell lymphoma, and plasmablastic lymphoma (see above). Other lymphomas can also be seen including Hodgkin lymphoma, extranodal marginal zone lymphoma, etc. Some lymphomas more specifically affecting patients with HIV have also been described, such as primary effusion lymphoma. This disease can rarely present as a mass lesion involving the upper aerodigestive tract.[94]

Patients who are recipients of solid organ or bone marrow transplants are at increased risk for the development of lymphoproliferative disease because of their immunocompromised states. As such, these diseases are widely classified as *posttransplant lymphoproliferative disorders* (PTLDs).[8,11,25] Because most cases of PTLDs appear to be related to infection with EBV and as the tonsils are the portal of entry for this virus, it should not be surprising that Waldeyer ring is frequently involved by these proliferations.[12,95] Also, EBV can be demonstrated by immunohistochemistry or in situ hybridization in most of these processes. Finally, the diseases occur on a continuum and distinguishing one lesion from another can be difficult as the processes progress.

PTLDs are categorized as early lesions, polymorphic PTLDs, monomorphic PTLDs, and Hodgkin lymphoma PTLD (Table 9.2).[8,11,25] Early lesions show some degree of residual typical follicular hyperplasia with partial effacement of the tissue by either plasma cells (plasmacytic hyperplasia) or immunoblasts (infectious mononucleosis–like PTLD). Some histologic overlap between these processes is often present. These lesions are not clonal and many will regress with decreased immunosuppression. Some cases may evolve into polymorphic or monomorphic PTLDs, however.[8]

Polymorphic PTLDs are destructive lesions that often show complete tissue effacement.[8] The lymphoid tissue is replaced by sheets of lymphocytes and plasma cells that show, in general, a complete spectrum of differentiation with small- and medium-sized lymphocytes, immunoblasts, and plasma cells (Fig. 9.26, eFig. 9.38). Some immunoblasts are enlarged and appear cytologically atypical, and focal areas of necrosis are common. These cells may even appear similar to Reed-Sternberg cells and occasional cases need to be distinguished from Hodgkin lymphoma. As with early lesions, some of these cases will regress with decreased immunosuppression; however, others will progress to monomorphic PTLDs. Clonal immunoglobulin gene rearrangements can be demonstrated in most of these cases.[11]

TABLE 9.2 Posttransplant Lymphoproliferative Disorders

Disorder	Histology	Clonality	EBV	Behavior
Early lesion (nondestructive)	Some architectural preservation with plasmacytic or immunoblastic proliferation	Polyclonal	+	Most regress with reduction in immunosuppression
Plasmacytic hyperplasia				
Infectious (mononucleosis-like)				
Polymorphic	Effaced architecture with plasma cells, lymphocytes and immunoblasts	Monoclonal	+	Some regress with reduction in immunosupression
Monomorphic	Effaced architecture with monomorphic lymphoid population (appearance will vary, most often cells resemble immunoblasts)	Monoclonal	+	Rarely regress with reduction in immunosuppression
Hodgkin Lymphoma	Effaced architecture with Hodgkin lymphoma	Monoclonal	+	Not known

EBV, Epstein-Barr virus.

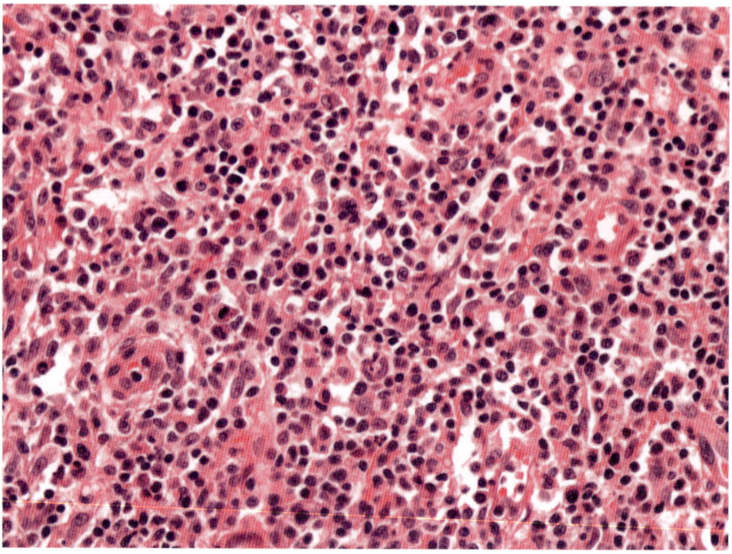

FIGURE 9.26 A polymorphic posttransplant lymphoproliferative disorder involving the tonsil.

Monomorphic PTLDs can either show a B-cell or a T-/NK-cell phenotype.[8] These lymphomas should be classified as they would in patients who have not undergone transplantation; however, the term "PTLD" should appear in the diagnosis. Most of the B-cell lymphomas will be diffuse large B-cell lymphomas; however, Burkitt lymphoma, plasmacytoma, and others have also been reported (Fig. 9.27, eFigs. 9.39 and 9.40). Monoclonality is demonstrated by immunohistochemistry or molecular studies. As stated above, infection by EBV can be demonstrated with in situ hybridization or other methods (Fig. 9.28).

Finally, occasional cases of classic Hodgkin lymphoma PTLD occur.[8,25] Hodgkin lymphoma should be diagnosed when the histologic and immunohistochemical features are identical to those seen in Hodgkin lymphomas developing in patients who have not had transplants (eFig. 9.41). The neoplastic cells of these lesions can be shown to harbor EBV in the majority of cases (Fig. 9.29).

An EBV-associated ulcerative disease developing in immunocompromised patients has been described (*EBV-positive mucocutaneous ulcer*).[96] The lesions developed in older patients, usually immunocompromised only through their age (immunosenescence), and more than 60% of the cases involved the oral or oropharyngeal mucosa. Histologically, the lesions were shallow and well circumscribed. The inflammatory infiltrate was polymorphous with mostly lymphocytes and immunoblasts; intermixed plasma cells, histiocytes, and eosinophils were also present. Occasional larger cells were present, reminiscent of Reed-Sternberg cells. Larger cells are frequently immunoreactive with antibodies to CD45, CD20, CD30,

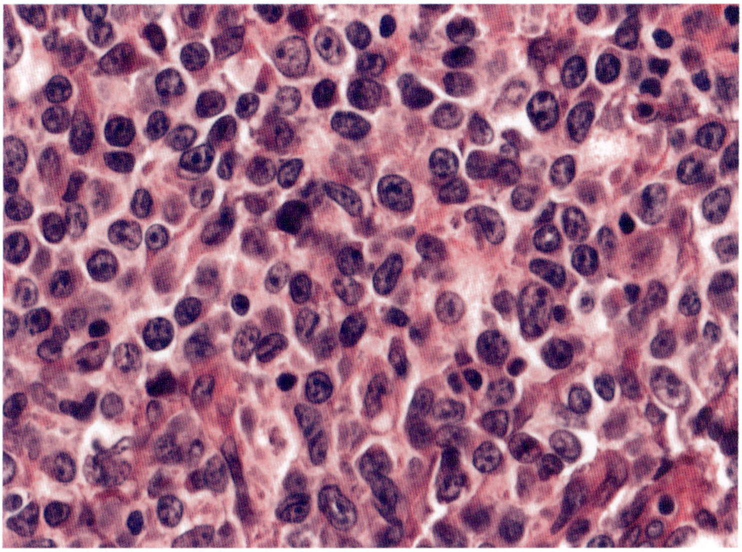

FIGURE 9.27 A diffuse large B-cell lymphoma involving the tonsil in a patient having undergone solid organ transplantation.

and sometimes CD15. EBV can be demonstrated by in situ hybridization in many cells, including the larger, atypical cells. Monoclonal immunoglobulin or T-cell receptor rearrangements can be identified in most cases. These lesions typically regress, with or without treatment.

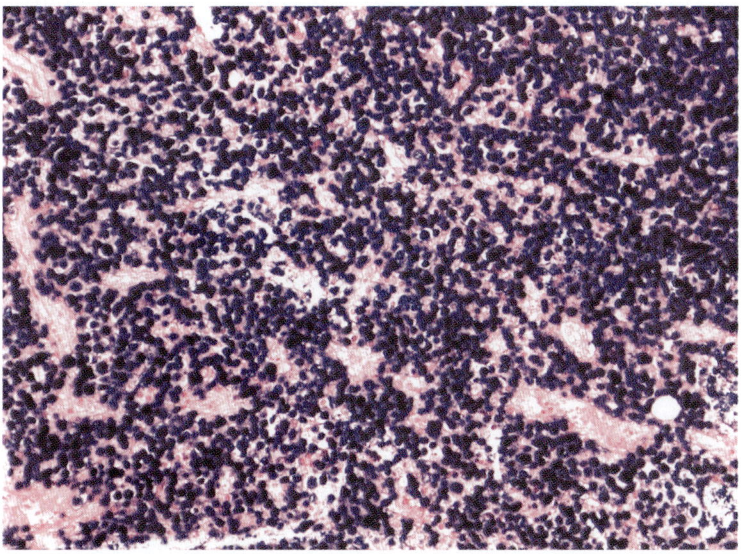

FIGURE 9.28 Strong and diffuse positivity for Epstein-Barr virus–encoded RNA by in situ hybridization is seen with this case of monomorphic posttransplant lymphoproliferative disorder.

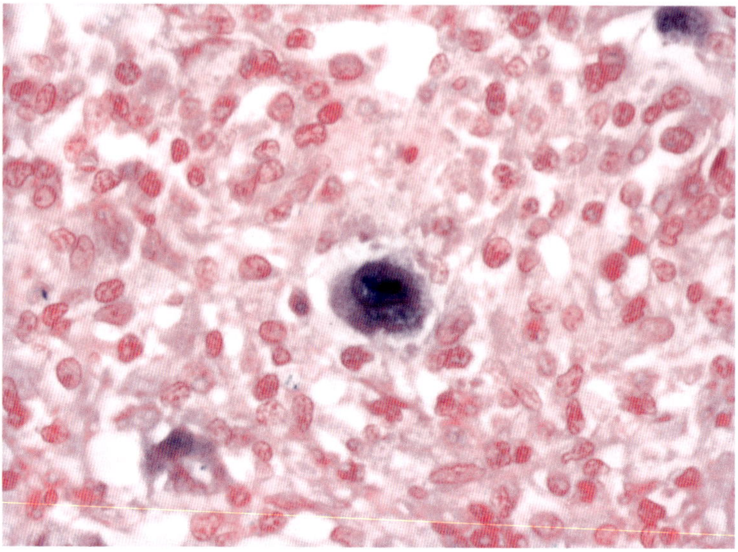

FIGURE 9.29 Reed-Sternberg cells in posttransplant Hodgkin lymphoma are more likely to be associated with Epstein-Barr virus.

Histiocytic and Dendritic Cell Malignancies

Neoplasms composed of cells resembling macrophages or antigen-presenting dendritic cells are uncommon. Most of these diseases, such as histiocytic sarcoma, Langerhans cell histiocytosis, and Langerhans cell sarcoma, rarely involve the upper aerodigestive tract.[97] When Langerhans cell histiocytosis does involve the upper aerodigestive tract, it usually is an extension of a primary bone tumor.[98] The dendritic cell tumors, especially follicular dendritic cell sarcomas have been reported throughout this area, however, and they should be considered in the differential diagnosis for spindle cell tumors in the head and neck.[97,99-101]

Follicular dendritic cell sarcoma often occurs at extranodal sites and frequently involves the upper aerodigestive tract, especially the mouth and Waldeyer ring.[99,101,102] These tumors of antigen-presenting cells occur slightly more frequently in women and over a broad age range, with a mean age of approximately 44 years. These neoplasms have been noted to behave more akin to low-grade sarcomas than other hematopoietic neoplasms. Nearly half of the cases recur or metastasize, and the most frequent site of metastasis is the lung. A little more than 5% of patients have expired secondary to their disease.

Grossly, follicular dendritic cell sarcomas appear circumscribed and have fleshy cut surfaces.[99,101,102] Histologically, the lesions appear hypercellular and are composed of plump spindled and epithelioid cells. Tumor cells frequently have a syncytial growth pattern and are noted to have a moderate amount of fibrillary cytoplasm with indistinct cell borders (Fig. 9.30, eFig. 9.42). The nuclei are round to oval and have

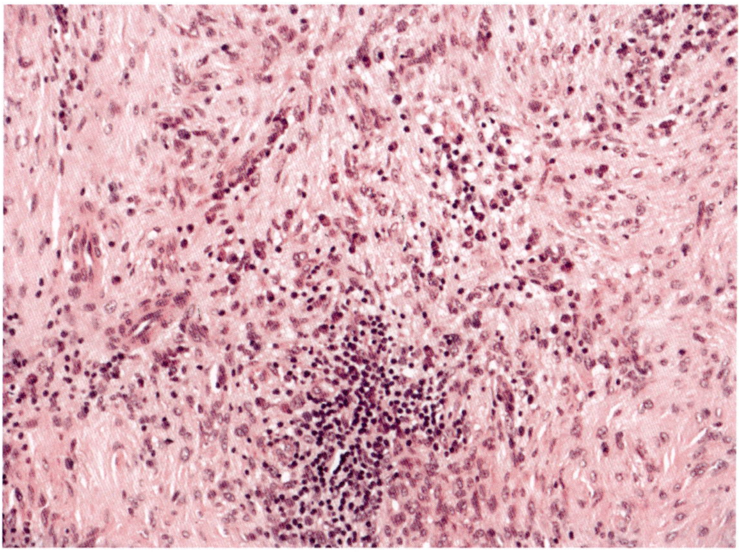

FIGURE 9.30 Syncytia of spindled cells with admixed lymphocytes in a case of follicular dendritic cell sarcoma.

wrinkled nuclear membranes, typically with vesicular appearing chromatin and without prominent nucleoli (Fig. 9.31). Mitotic activity can vary greatly but is usually low with a mean of approximately 3/10 hpfs (eFig. 9.43). Tumors cells are intermixed with numerous small lymphocytes, and

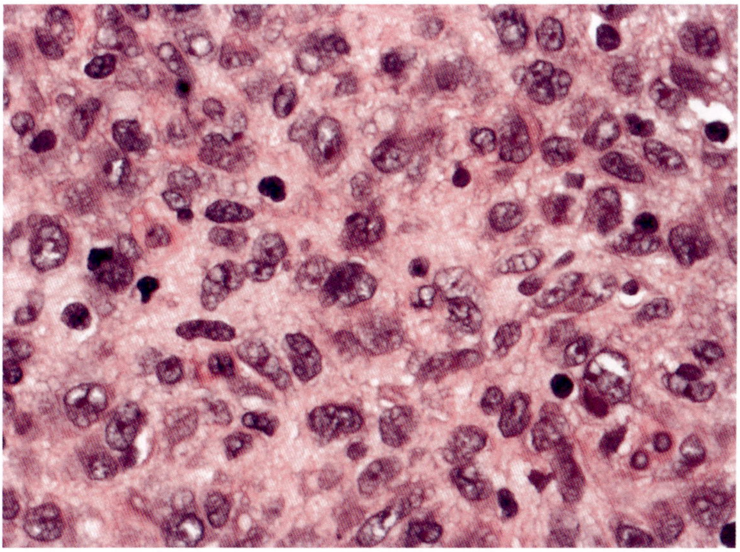

FIGURE 9.31 Atypical nuclei with vesicular chromatin are seen in this follicular dendritic cell sarcoma.

coagulative necrosis has been seen in 30% of cases. Occasional cells may be multinucleated or have intranuclear inclusions.

The differential diagnosis for follicular dendritic cell sarcomas includes other spindled cells neoplasms and thus must include spindle cell carcinoma, melanoma, and many different mesenchymal neoplasms. Immunohistochemistry typically proves itself very helpful with these cases (see Chapter 11). The neoplastic cells of follicular dendritic cell sarcomas are reactive with antibodies to CD21, CD35, clusterin, and fascin in most cases and will react with antibodies to S100 and CD68 in approximately one-third of cases.[97,101] While most cases will react with antibodies to epithelial membrane antigen (EMA), cytokeratin immunoreactivity is rare. Recently, it has been shown that D2-40 is a good marker for these tumors.[103] Follicular dendritic cell sarcomas have been shown to have clonal immunoglobulin receptor gene rearrangements.[104]

As was mentioned, other histiocytic or dendritic cell tumors can also involve the upper aerodigestive tract. *Interdigitating dendritic cell sarcomas* should be distinguished from follicular dendritic cell sarcomas as the two have different prognoses.[100] Interdigitating dendritic cell sarcomas have a variable prognosis and sometimes present with disseminated disease. Histologically, the tumors may resemble follicular dendritic cell tumors; however, the neoplastic cells may sometimes appear more epithelioid (Fig. 9.32). Neoplastic cells are reactive with antibodies to S100 protein and weakly with antibodies to CD68 and not with antibodies to CD21 (eFig. 9.44).[97,100]

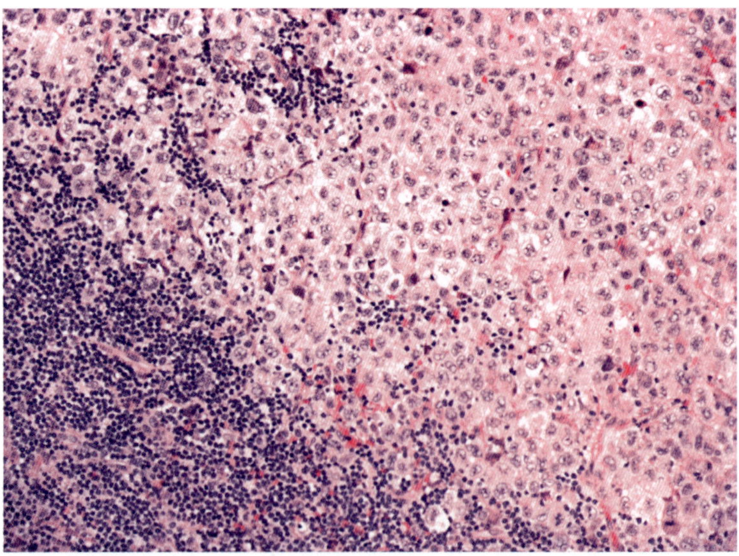

FIGURE 9.32 An interdigitating dendritic cell sarcoma of the nasopharynx.

REFERENCES

1. Attygalle AD, Liu H, Shirali S, et al. Atypical marginal zone hyperplasia of mucosa-associated lymphoid tissue: a reactive condition of childhood showing immunoglobulin lambda light-chain restriction. *Blood.* 2004;104(10):3343-3348.
2. Batsakis JG, Fries GT, Goldman RT, Karlsberg RC. Upper respiratory tract plasmacytoma. *Arch Otolaryngol.* 1964;79:613-618.
3. Batsakis JG, Medeiros JL, Luna MA, El-Naggar AK. Plasma cell dyscrasias and the head and neck. *Ann Diagn Pathol.* 2002;6(2):129-140.
4. Chan JK, Ng CS, Lo ST. Immunohistological characterization of malignant lymphomas of the Waldeyer's ring other than the nasopharynx. *Histopathology.* 1987;11(9):885-899.
5. Childs CC, Parham DM, Berard CW. Infectious mononucleosis. The spectrum of morphologic changes simulating lymphoma in lymph nodes and tonsils. *Am J Surg Pathol.* 1987;11(2):122-132.
6. Colby TV, Hoppe RT, Warnke RA. Hodgkin's disease: a clinicopathologic study of 659 cases. *Cancer.* 1982;49(9):1848-1858.
7. Foucar E, Rosai J, Dorfman RF. Sinus histiocytosis with massive lymphadenopathy. *Arch Otolaryngol.* 1978;104(12):687-693.
8. Harris NL, Ferry JA, Swerdlow SH. Posttransplant lymphoproliferative disorders: summary of Society for Hematopathology Workshop. *Semin Diagn Pathol.* 1997;14(1):8-14.
9. Joshi VV, Gagnon GA, Chadwick EG, et al. The spectrum of mucosa-associated lymphoid tissue lesions in pediatric patients infected with HIV: a clinicopathologic study of six cases. *Am J Clin Pathol.* 1997;107(5):592-600.
10. Kapadia SB, Roman LN, Kingma DW, Jaffe ES, Frizzera G. Hodgkin's disease of Waldeyer's ring. Clinical and histoimmunophenotypic findings and association with Epstein-Barr virus in 16 cases. *Am J Surg Pathol.* 1995;19(12):1431-1439.
11. Knowles DM, Cesarman E, Chadburn A, et al. Correlative morphologic and molecular genetic analysis demonstrates three distinct categories of posttransplantation lymphoproliferative disorders. *Blood.* 1995;85(2):552-565.
12. Lones MA, Mishalani S, Shintaku IP, Weiss LM, Nichols WS, Said JW. Changes in tonsils and adenoids in children with posttransplant lymphoproliferative disorder: report of three cases with early involvement of Waldeyer's ring. *Hum Pathol.* 1995;26(5):525-530.
13. Lorsbach RB, Shay-Seymore D, Moore J, et al. Clinicopathologic analysis of follicular lymphoma occurring in children. *Blood.* 2002;99(6):1959-1964.
14. Menarguez J, Mollejo M, Carrion R, et al. Waldeyer ring lymphomas. A clinicopathological study of 79 cases. *Histopathology.* 1994;24(1):13-22.
15. Pinto A, Hutchison RE, Grant LH, Trevenen CL, Berard CW. Follicular lymphomas in pediatric patients. *Mod Pathol.* 1990;3(3):308-313.
16. Shima N, Kobashi Y, Tsutsui K, et al. Extranodal non-Hodgkin's lymphoma of the head and neck. A clinicopathologic study in the Kyoto-Nara area of Japan. *Cancer.* 1990;66(6):1190-1197.
17. Stout AP, Kenney FR. Primary plasma-cell tumors of the upper air passages and oral cavity. *Cancer.* 1949;2:261-278.
18. Strickler JG, Fedeli F, Horwitz CA, Copenhaver CM, Frizzera G. Infectious mononucleosis in lymphoid tissue. Histopathology, in situ hybridization, and differential diagnosis. *Arch Pathol Lab Med.* 1993;117(3):269-278.
19. Swerdlow SH. Pediatric follicular lymphomas, marginal zone lymphomas, and marginal zone hyperplasia. *Am J Clin Pathol.* 2004;122(Suppl):S98-S109.
20. Todd GB, Michaels L. Hodgkin's disease involving Waldeyer's lymphoid ring. *Cancer.* 1974;34(5):1769-1778.
21. Vega F, Lin P, Medeiros LJ. Extranodal lymphomas of the head and neck. *Ann Diagn Pathol.* 2005;9(6):340-350.

22. Wenig BM, Abbondanzo SL, Childers EL, Kapadia SB, Heffner DR. Extranodal sinus histiocytosis with massive lymphadenopathy (Rosai-Dorfman disease) of the head and neck. *Hum Pathol.* 1993;24(5):483-492.
23. Wenig BM, Thompson LD, Frankel SS, et al. Lymphoid changes of the nasopharyngeal and palatine tonsils that are indicative of human immunodeficiency virus infection. A clinicopathologic study of 12 cases. *Am J Surg Pathol.* 1996;20(5):572-587.
24. Winberg CD, Nathwani BN, Bearman RM, Rappaport H. Follicular (nodular) lymphoma during the first two decades of life: a clinicopathologic study of 12 patients. *Cancer.* 1981;48(10):2223-2235.
25. Swerdlow JB, Webber SA, Chadburn A, Ferry JA. Post-transplant lymphoproliferative disorders. In: Swerdlow JB, Campo E, Harris NL, et al, eds. *WHO Classification of Tumours of Haematopoietic and Lymphoid Tissues.* Lyon: IARC Press; 2017:453-464.
26. van der Valk P, Meijer CJLM. Lymph nodes. In: Mills SE, ed. *Histology for Pathologists.* Philadelphia: Lippincott Williams and Wilkins; 2007:763-781.
27. Salvador AH, Harrison EG Jr, Kyle RA. Lymphadenopathy due to infectious mononucleosis: its confusion with malignant lymphoma. *Cancer.* 1971;27(5):1029-1040.
28. Segal GH, Kjeldsberg CR, Smith GP, Perkins SL. CD30 antigen expression in florid immunoblastic proliferations. A clinicopathologic study of 14 cases. *Am J Clin Pathol.* 1994;102(3):292-298.
29. Niedobitek G, Hamilton-Dutoit S, Herbst H, et al. Identification of Epstein-Barr virus-infected cells in tonsils of acute infectious mononucleosis by in situ hybridization. *Hum Pathol.* 1989;20(8):796-799.
30. Rosai J, Dorfman RF. Sinus histiocytosis with massive lymphadenopathy: a pseudolymphomatous benign disorder. Analysis of 34 cases. *Cancer.* 1972;30(5):1174-1188.
31. Rosai J, Dorfman RF. Sinus histiocytosis with massive lymphadenopathy. A newly recognized benign clinicopathological entity. *Arch Pathol.* 1969;87(1):63-70.
32. Ojha J, Rawal YB, Hornick JL, et al. Extra nodal Rosai-Dorfman disease originating in the nasal and paranasal complex and gnathic bones: a systematic analysis of seven cases and review of literature. *Head Neck Pathol.* 2019.
33. Meis JM, Butler JJ, Osborne BM, Manning JT. Granulocytic sarcoma in nonleukemic patients. *Cancer.* 1986;58(12):2697-2709.
34. Menasce LP, Banerjee SS, Beckett E, Harris M. Extra-medullary myeloid tumour (granulocytic sarcoma) is often misdiagnosed: a study of 26 cases. *Histopathology.* 1999;34(5):391-398.
35. Neiman RS, Barcos M, Berard C, et al. Granulocytic sarcoma: a clinicopathologic study of 61 biopsied cases. *Cancer.* 1981;48(6):1426-1437.
36. Quintanilla-Martinez L, Zukerberg LR, Ferry JA, Harris NL. Extramedullary tumors of lymphoid or myeloid blasts. The role of immunohistology in diagnosis and classification. *Am J Clin Pathol.* 1995;104(4):431-443.
37. Traweek ST, Arber DA, Rappaport H, Brynes RK. Extramedullary myeloid cell tumors. An immunohistochemical and morphologic study of 28 cases. *Am J Surg Pathol.* 1993;17(10):1011-1019.
38. Pileri SA, Ascani S, Cox MC, et al. Myeloid sarcoma: clinico-pathologic, phenotypic and cytogenetic analysis of 92 adult patients. *Leukemia.* 2007;21(2):340-350.
39. Pileri SA, Orazi A, Falini B. Myeloid sarcoma. In: Swerdlow JB, Campo E, Harris NL, et al, eds. *WHO Classification of Tumours of Haematopoietic and Lymphoid Tumors.* Lyon: IARC Press; 2017:167-168.
40. Campidelli C, Agostinelli C, Stitson R, Pileri SA. Myeloid sarcoma: extramedullary manifestation of myeloid disorders. *Am J Clin Pathol.* 2009;132(3):426-437.
41. Sayed K, Van Savell H Jr, Hutchison RE, et al. Review of tonsillar lymphoma in pediatric patients from the pediatric oncology group: what can be learned about some indications for microscopic examination?. *Pediatr Dev Pathol.* 2005;8(5):533-540.

42. Reddy KS, Perkins SL. Advances in the diagnostic approach to childhood lymphoblastic malignant neoplasms. *Am J Clin Pathol.* 2004;122(suppl):S3-S18.
43. Cairo MS, Raetz E, Lim MS, Davenport V, Perkins SL. Childhood and adolescent non-Hodgkin lymphoma: new insights in biology and critical challenges for the future. *Pediatr Blood Cancer.* 2005;45(6):753-769.
44. Abbondanzo SL, Wenig BM. Non-Hodgkin's lymphoma of the sinonasal tract. A clinicopathologic and immunophenotypic study of 120 cases. *Cancer.* 1995;75(6):1281-1291.
45. Alexiou C, Kau RJ, Dietzfelbinger H, et al. Extramedullary plasmacytoma: tumor occurrence and therapeutic concepts. *Cancer.* 1999;85(11):2305-2314.
46. Cioc AM, Allen C, Kalmar JR, Suster S, Baiocchi R, Nuovo GJ. Oral plasmablastic lymphomas in AIDS patients are associated with human herpesvirus 8. *Am J Surg Pathol.* 2004;28(1):41-46.
47. Colomo L, Loong F, Rives S, et al. Diffuse large B-cell lymphomas with plasmablastic differentiation represent a heterogeneous group of disease entities. *Am J Surg Pathol.* 2004;28(6):736-747.
48. Cuadra-Garcia I, Proulx GM, Wu CL, et al. Sinonasal lymphoma: a clinicopathologic analysis of 58 cases from the Massachusetts General Hospital. *Am J Surg Pathol.* 1999;23(11):1356-1369.
49. Fellbaum C, Hansmann ML, Lennert K. Malignant lymphomas of the nasal cavity and paranasal sinuses. *Virchows Arch A Pathol Anat Histopathol.* 1989;414(5):399-405.
50. Folk GS, Abbondanzo SL, Childers EL, Foss RD. Plasmablastic lymphoma: a clinicopathologic correlation. *Ann Diagn Pathol.* 2006;10(1):8-12.
51. Frierson HF Jr, Innes DJ Jr, Mills SE, Wick MR. Immunophenotypic analysis of sinonasal non-Hodgkin's lymphomas. *Hum Pathol.* 1989;20(7):636-642.
52. Fu YS, Perzin KH. Nonepithelial tumors of the nasal cavity, paranasal sinuses and nasopharynx. A clinicopathologic study. IX. Plasmacytomas. *Cancer.* 1978;42(5):2399-2406.
53. Handlers JP, Howell RE, Abrams AM, Melrose RJ. Extranodal oral lymphoma. Part I. A morphologic and immunoperoxidase study of 34 cases. *Oral Surg Oral Med Oral Pathol.* 1986;61(4):362-367.
54. Morgan K, MacLennan KA, Narula A, Bradley PJ, Morgan DA. Non-Hodgkin's lymphoma of the larynx (stage IE). *Cancer.* 1989;64(5):1123-1127.
55. Swerdlow JB, Merl SA, Davey FR, Gacek RR, Gottlieb AJ. Non-Hodgkin's lymphoma limited to the larynx. *Cancer.* 1984;53(11):2546-2549.
56. van der Waal RI, Huijgens PC, van der Valk P, van der Waal I. Characteristics of 40 primary extranodal non-Hodgkin lymphomas of the oral cavity in perspective of the new WHO classification and the International Prognostic Index. *Int J Oral Maxillofac Surg.* 2005;34(4):391-395.
57. Armitage JO, Weisenburger DD. New approach to classifying non-Hodgkin's lymphomas: clinical features of the major histologic subtypes. Non-Hodgkin's Lymphoma Classification Project. *J Clin Oncol.* 1998;16(8):2780-2795.
58. Harris NL, Jaffe ES, Stein H, et al. A revised European-American classification of lymphoid neoplasms: a proposal from the International Lymphoma Study Group. *Blood.* 1994;84(5):1361-1392.
59. De Paepe P, De Wolf-Peeters C. Diffuse large B-cell lymphoma: a heterogeneous group of non-Hodgkin lymphomas comprising several distinct clinicopathological entities. *Leukemia.* 2007;21(1):37-43.
60. Muris JJ, Meijer CJ, Vos W, et al. Immunohistochemical profiling based on Bcl-2, CD10 and MUM1 expression improves risk stratification in patients with primary nodal diffuse large B cell lymphoma. *J Pathol.* 2006;208(5):714-723.
61. Kawasaki C, Ohshim K, Suzumiya J, et al. Rearrangements of bcl-1, bcl-2, bcl-6, and c-myc in diffuse large B-cell lymphomas. *Leuk Lymphoma.* 2001;42(5):1099-1106.

62. Delecluse HJ, Anagnostopoulos I, Dallenbach F, et al. Plasmablastic lymphomas of the oral cavity: a new entity associated with the human immunodeficiency virus infection. *Blood.* 1997;89(4):1413-1420.
63. Dong HY, Scadden DT, de Leval L, Tang Z, Isaacson PG, Harris NL. Plasmablastic lymphoma in HIV-positive patients: an aggressive Epstein-Barr virus-associated extramedullary plasmacytic neoplasm. *Am J Surg Pathol.* 2005;29(12):1633-1641.
64. Jaffe ES. Lymphoid lesions of the head and neck: a model of lymphocyte homing and lymphomagenesis. *Mod Pathol.* 2002;15(3):255-263.
65. Zucca E, Fontana S, Roggero E, Pedrinis E, Pampallona S, Cavalli F. Treatment and prognosis of centrocytic (mantle cell) lymphoma: a retrospective analysis of twenty-six patients treated in one institution. *Leuk Lymphoma.* 1994;13(1-2):105-110.
66. Argatoff LH, Connors JM, Klasa RJ, Horsman DE, Gascoyne RD. Mantle cell lymphoma: a clinicopathologic study of 80 cases. *Blood.* 1997;89(6):2067-2078.
67. Jaffe ES, Harris NL, Swerdlow JB, et al. Follicular lymphoma. In: Swerdlow JB, Campo E, Harris NL, et al, eds. *WHO CLassification of Tumours of Haematopoietic and Lymphoid Tissues.* Lyon: IARC Press; 2017:266-277.
68. Swerdlow SH, Campo E, Harris NL, et al. *WHO Classification of Tumours of the Haematopoietic and Lymphoid Tissues.* Lyon: IARC Press; 2017.
69. Nathwani BN, Anderson JR, Armitage JO, et al. Marginal zone B-cell lymphoma: a clinical comparison of nodal and mucosa-associated lymphoid tissue types. Non-Hodgkin's Lymphoma Classification Project. *J Clin Oncol.* 1999;17(8):2486-2492.
70. Paulsen J, Lennert K. Low-grade B-cell lymphoma of mucosa-associated lymphoid tissue type in Waldeyer's ring. *Histopathology.* 1994;24(1):1-11.
71. Winther B, Innes DJ. The human adenoid. A morphologic study. *Arch Otolaryngol Head Neck Surg.* 1994;120(2):144-149.
72. Remstein ED, Dogan A, Einerson RR, et al. The incidence and anatomic site specificity of chromosomal translocations in primary extranodal marginal zone B-cell lymphoma of mucosa-associated lymphoid tissue (MALT lymphoma) in North America. *Am J Surg Pathol.* 2006;30(12):1546-1553.
73. McKenna RW, Kyle RA, Kuehl WM, Harris NL, Coupland RW, Fend F. Plasma cell neoplasms. In: Swerdlow JB, Campo E, Harris NL, et al, eds. *WHO Classification of Tumours of Haematopoietic and Lymphoid Tissues.* Lyon: IARC Press; 2017:241-258.
74. Strickler JG, Audeh MW, Copenhaver CM, Warnke RA. Immunophenotypic differences between plasmacytoma/multiple myeloma and immunoblastic lymphoma. *Cancer.* 1988;61(9):1782-1786.
75. Grogan TM, Van Camp B, Kyle RA, Muller-Hermelink HK, Harris NL. Plasma cell neoplasms. In: Jaffe ES, Stein H, Vardiman JW, eds. *Pathology and Genetics of Tumours of Heamatopoietic and Lymphoid Tissues.* Lyon: IARC Press; 2001:142-156.
76. Brix WK, Nassau SR, Patterson JW, Cousar JB, Wick MR. Idiopathic lymphoplasmacellular mucositis-dermatitis. *J Cutan Pathol.* 2010;37(4):426-431.
77. Konoplev S, Medeiros LJ, Bueso-Ramos CE, Jorgensen JL, Lin P. Immunophenotypic profile of lymphoplasmacytic lymphoma/Waldenstrom macroglobulinemia. *Am J Clin Pathol.* 2005;124(3):414-420.
78. Haralambieva E, Boerma EJ, van Imhoff GW, et al. Clinical, immunophenotypic, and genetic analysis of adult lymphomas with morphologic features of Burkitt lymphoma. *Am J Surg Pathol.* 2005;29(8):1086-1094.
79. Jaffe ES, Chan JK, Su IJ, et al. Report of the workshop on nasal and related extranodal angiocentric T/natural killer cell lymphomas. Definitions, differential diagnosis, and epidemiology. *Am J Surg Pathol.* 1996;20(1):103-111.
80. Jaffe ES, Krenacs L, Kumar S, Kingma DW, Raffeld M. Extranodal peripheral T-cell and NK-cell neoplasms. *Am J Clin Pathol.* 1999;111(1 suppl 1):S46-S55.

81. Nava VE, Jaffe ES. The pathology of NK-cell lymphomas and leukemias. *Adv Anat Pathol.* 2005;12(1):27-34.
82. Strickler JG, Meneses MF, Habermann TM, et al. Polymorphic reticulosis: a reappraisal. *Hum Pathol.* 1994;25(7):659-665.
83. Kanavaros P, Lescs MC, Briere J, et al. Nasal T-cell lymphoma: a clinicopathologic entity associated with peculiar phenotype and with Epstein-Barr virus. *Blood.* 1993;81(10):2688-2695.
84. Iqbal J, Kucuk C, Deleeuw RJ, et al. Genomic analyses reveal global functional alterations that promote tumor growth and novel tumor suppressor genes in natural killer-cell malignancies. *Leukemia.* 2009;23(6):1139-1151.
85. Harabuchi Y, Imai S, Wakashima J, et al. Nasal T-cell lymphoma causally associated with Epstein-Barr virus: clinicopathologic, phenotypic, and genotypic studies. *Cancer.* 1996;77(10):2137-2149.
86. Emile JF, Boulland ML, Haioun C, et al. CD5-CD56+ T-cell receptor silent peripheral T-cell lymphomas are natural killer cell lymphomas. *Blood.* 1996;87(4):1466-1473.
87. Schwartz EJ, Molina-Kirsch H, Zhao S, Marinelli RJ, Warnke RA, Natkunam Y. Immunohistochemical characterization of nasal-type extranodal NK/T-cell lymphoma using a tissue microarray: an analysis of 84 cases. *Am J Clin Pathol.* 2008;130(3):343-351.
88. Shiboski CH, Greenspan D, Dodd CL, Daniels TE. Oral T-cell lymphoma associated with celiac sprue. A case report. *Oral Surg Oral Med Oral Pathol.* 1993;76(1):54-58.
89. Sirois DA, Miller AS, Harwick RD, Vonderheid EC. Oral manifestations of cutaneous T-cell lymphoma. A report of eight cases. *Oral Surg Oral Med Oral Pathol.* 1993;75(6):700-705.
90. Salisbury CL, Budnick SD, Li S. T-cell receptor gene rearrangement and CD30 immunoreactivity in traumatic ulcerative granuloma with stromal eosinophilia of the oral cavity. *Am J Clin Pathol.* 2009;132(5):722-727.
91. Agarwal M, Shenjere P, Blewitt RW, et al. CD30-positive T-cell lymphoproliferative disorder of the oral mucosa–an indolent lesion: report of 4 cases. *Int J Surg Pathol.* 2008;16(3):286-290.
92. Chang KL, Kamel OW, Arber DA, Horyd ID, Weiss LM. Pathologic features of nodular lymphocyte predominance Hodgkin's disease in extranodal sites. *Am J Surg Pathol.* 1995;19(11):1313-1324.
93. Carbone A, Gloghini A. AIDS-related lymphomas: from pathogenesis to pathology. *Br J Haematol.* 2005;130(5):662-670.
94. Mate JL, Navarro JT, Ariza A, et al. Oral solid form of primary effusion lymphoma mimicking plasmablastic lymphoma. *Hum Pathol.* 2004;35(5):632-635.
95. Montone KT, Hodinka RL, Salhany KE, Lavi E, Rostami A, Tomaszewski JE. Identification of Epstein-Barr virus lytic activity in post-transplantation lymphoproliferative disease. *Mod Pathol.* 1996;9(6):621-630.
96. Dojcinov SD, Venkataraman G, Raffeld M, Pittaluga S, Jaffe ES. EBV positive mucocutaneous ulcer–a study of 26 cases associated with various sources of immunosuppression. *Am J Surg Pathol.* 2010;34(3):405-417.
97. Pileri SA, Grogan TM, Harris NL, et al. Tumours of histiocytes and accessory dendritic cells: an immunohistochemical approach to classification from the International Lymphoma Study Group based on 61 cases. *Histopathology.* 2002;41(1):1-29.
98. Madrigal-Martinez-Pereda C, Guerrero-Rodriguez V, Guisado-Moya B, Meniz-Garcia C. Langerhans cell histiocytosis: literature review and descriptive analysis of oral manifestations. *Med Oral Patol Oral Cir Bucal.* 2009;14(5):E222-E228.
99. Chan JK, Tsang WY, Ng CS, Tang SK, Yu HC, Lee AW. Follicular dendritic cell tumors of the oral cavity. *Am J Surg Pathol.* 1994;18(2):148-157.

100. Gaertner EM, Tsokos M, Derringer GA, Neuhauser TS, Arciero C, Andriko JA. Interdigitating dendritic cell sarcoma. A report of four cases and review of the literature. *Am J Clin Pathol.* 2001;115(4):589-597.

101. Shia J, Chen W, Tang LH, et al. Extranodal follicular dendritic cell sarcoma: clinical, pathologic, and histogenetic characteristics of an underrecognized disease entity. *Virchows Arch.* 2006;449(2):148-158.

102. Duan GJ, Wu F, Zhu J, et al. Extranodal follicular dendritic cell sarcoma of the pharyngeal region: a potential diagnostic pitfall, with literature review. *Am J Clin Pathol.* 2010;133(1):49-58.

103. Yu H, Gibson JA, Pinkus GS, Hornick JL. Podoplanin (D2-40) is a novel marker for follicular dendritic cell tumors. *Am J Clin Pathol.* 2007;128(5):776-782.

104. Chen W, Lau SK, Fong D, et al. High frequency of clonal immunoglobulin receptor gene rearrangements in sporadic histiocytic/dendritic cell sarcomas. *Am J Surg Pathol.* 2009;33(6):863-873.

10

GERM CELL TUMORS

It is extremely uncommon for extragonadal germ cell tumors to involve the head and neck and even more uncommon for them to actually arise from the upper aerodigestive tract. Tumors reported to involve this area include teratomas (and dermoids), yolk sac tumors (endodermal sinus tumors), choriocarcinomas, and teratocarcinosarcomas. Mixed tumors with teratomatous and yolk sac components also have been described. Definitive, concise diagnosis requires assessment of the entire tumor and thus one should be careful diagnosing small biopsies too specifically.

TERATOMA

Teratomas are germ cell neoplasms that recapitulate normal immature and mature tissues that represent the three germinal layers of endoderm, mesoderm, and ectoderm. In the head and neck, these tumors occur in both sexes and are almost always identified in infants or young children.[1-5] They have been described within the nasal cavity, nasopharynx, oropharynx, and mouth. When they are very large, they may be associated with stillbirth. If a malignant component is not identified (somatic malignancy or yolk sac tumor) and the tumor is resectable, both immature and mature teratomas tend to behave well and most patients survive, free of recurrences.[3,5]

Histologically, the tumors may show mature or immature differentiation or a mixture of the two. When immature differentiation is present, a prominent neuroepitheliomatous component may be noted, and it is important to distinguish these tumors from neural or neuroectodermal malignancies that can be found in the upper aerodigestive tract.[2] Careful attention should be paid in order to identify other germ cell components, especially elements of yolk sac tumor or somatic malignancy.

The diagnosis of a mature teratoma is usually straightforward; however, nonneoplastic lesions such as glial heterotopia and hairy polyps need to be excluded; this can be done be identifying endodermally, mesodermally, and ectodermally derived tissues.[2] Abundant maturing, stratified squamous epithelium is usually present with juxtaposed dermal appendages. Neural, adipose tissue, muscle, cartilage, and bone all may also be seen (Fig. 10.1, eFig. 10.1), as may epithelium that shows respiratory or gastrointestinal differentiation.

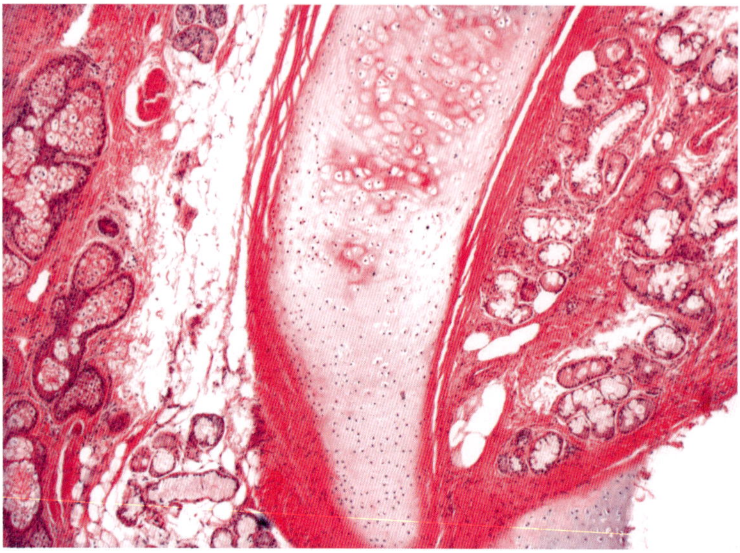

FIGURE 10.1 A mature teratoma with prominent cartilage formation.

DERMOID CYSTS

Unlike teratomas, dermoid cysts are probably not neoplasms, but instead represent developmental abnormalities.[2,5] In the upper aerodigestive tract, the lesions are usually located in the nasal cavity or in the floor of the mouth. Most patients are newborns or young adults. The tumors are composed of only ectodermally and mesodermally derived tissues and, as such, usually form large cystic structures lined by a maturing, stratified squamous epithelium replete with appendages (Fig. 10.2). A small amount of surrounding fibrous tissue and adipose tissue is also usually present. Immature elements and malignancy should not be seen. With resection, the lesions infrequently recur.[5]

YOLK SAC TUMOR

Yolk sac tumors or endodermal sinus tumors can occur throughout the head and neck region and infrequently involve the upper aerodigestive tract where they have been reported in the nose, paranasal sinuses, nasopharynx, oropharynx, and mouth.[3,6] They occur mostly in childhood but have been noted in middle-aged adults. The tumors show no obvious male or female predilection. Many reported patients have died secondary to local or disseminated disease; however, it is unclear how these tumors would behave given today's more effective multimodality treatments. Patients present with symptoms secondary to mass effect or with nonspecific symptoms such as epistaxis. Serum concentrations of α-fetoprotein

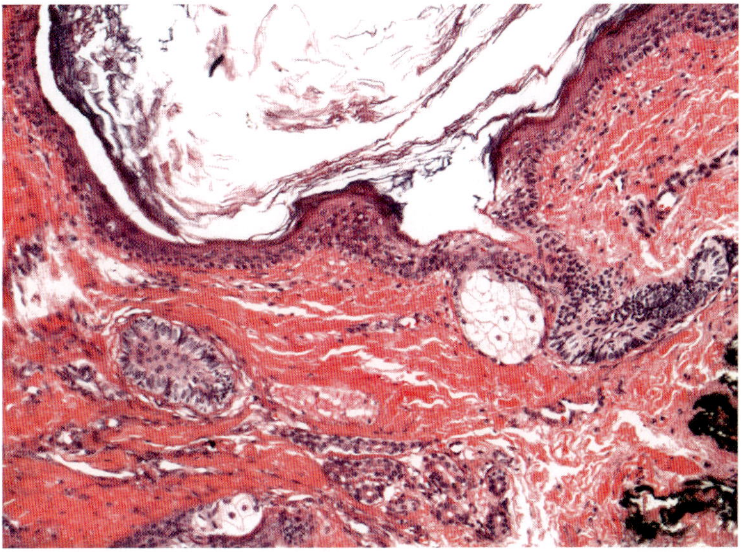

FIGURE 10.2 A squamous-lined dermoid cyst with appendages.

(AFP) are frequently high.[6] It should be noted that yolk sac differentiation is sometimes seen focally with some carcinomas, especially adenocarcinomas with SMARCB-1 loss.[7] Such tumors should be classified first as carcinomas, and the yolk sac differentiation should be considered a secondary change.

Like their counterparts throughout the body, yolk sac tumors of the head and neck can show a variety of architectural patterns.[6] Microcystic, macrocystic, solid, alveolar, glandular, polyvesicular, vesicular vitelline, myxomatous, papillary, hepatoid, and intestinal patterns have all been noted (Fig. 10.3, eFig. 10.2). Many tumors, at least, focally show a perivascular arrangement of tumor cells with well-formed Schiller-Duval bodies (Fig. 10.4). The tumor cells are usually large and can range from a polygonal to a more flattened appearance. A moderate amount of clear to eosinophilic cytoplasm is present with at least moderate cellular and nuclear pleomorphism. The nuclei appear vesicular and usually have distinct nucleoli. Occasional mitotic figures are often seen. Eosinophilic, PAS-positive, and diastase-resistant globules are also often noted (eFig. 10.3). The tumors frequently have an associated teratomatous component.[3,6]

Immunohistochemically, the neoplastic cells will show reactivity with antibodies to AFP and cytokeratins (Fig. 10.5, eFig. 10.4).[8] Tumor cells usually do not react with antibodies to EMA and CD30. Reports regarding the immunoreactivity with antibodies to PLAP have been variable.

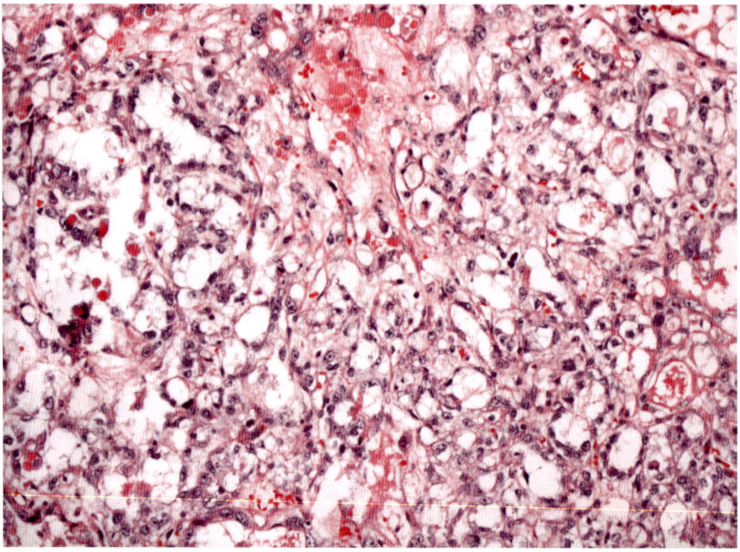

FIGURE 10.3 A yolk sac tumor with a prominent cystic architecture.

CHORIOCARCINOMA

Choriocarcinomas have been very rarely reported to primarily involve the upper aerodigestive tract.[9] It is imperative to first exclude metastatic choriocarcinoma.[10,11] The cases reported have involved the sinonasal tract. They are hemorrhagic and composed of a dual population of cells. Smaller,

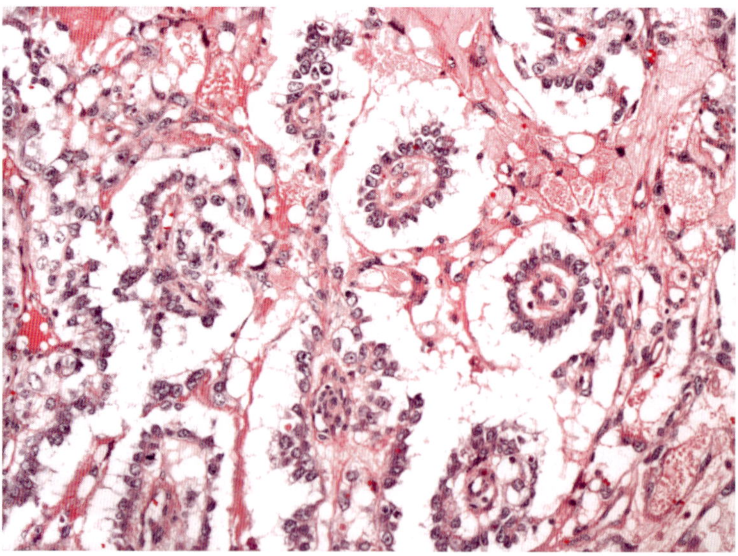

FIGURE 10.4 Numerous Schiller-Duval bodies in a yolk sac tumor.

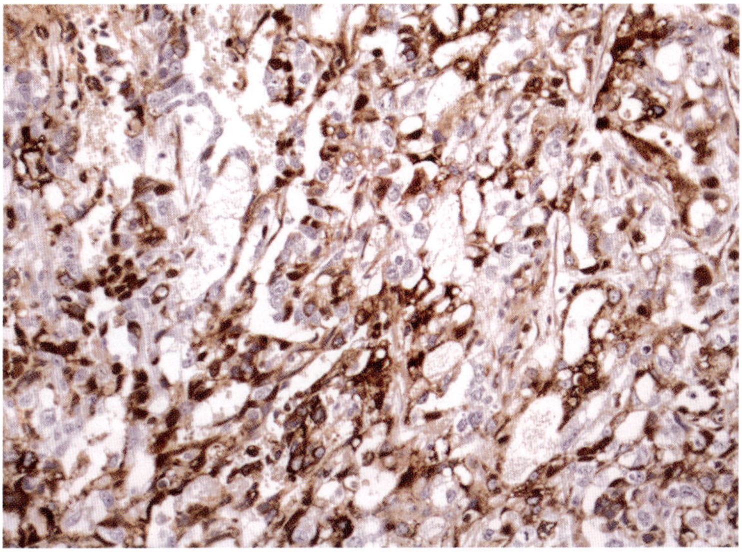

FIGURE 10.5 Strong immunoreactivity with antibodies to α-fetoprotein can be seen with most yolk sac tumors.

mononuclear, round to polygonal cells resemble cytotrophoblasts; and large, multinucleated giant cells resemble syncytiotrophoblasts. The cells should have large nuclei with prominent nucleoli. The multinucleated cells are immunoreactive with antibodies to β-HCG. All cells are immunoreactive with antibodies to pankeratin.

TERATOCARCINOSARCOMA

Teratocarcinosarcomas are rare malignancies that develop more commonly in older adult men (more than half of patients are older than 60 years).[12,13] The tumors almost always arise in the nasal cavity and sinuses and present with nonspecific symptoms such as nasal obstruction, epistaxis, and head ache. In the original studies, the tumors behaved poorly and about half of the patients died secondary to their malignancies in spite of resection or other therapy.[12] Larger studies using today's treatment modalities have not been published. How these lesions relate to other true germ cell tumors such as teratomas is not understood and it is striking that most conventional teratomas occur in childhood while teratocarcinosarcomas occur almost exclusively in adults. This suggests that there may be fundamental differences in the origin and biology of these tumors.

The lesions are usually received piecemeal and have been described as friable and purple-red.[12,13] Histologically, the tumors show an extremely variegated appearance, which can lead to much difficulty with diagnosis when only a small biopsy is received. Both epithelial and mesenchymal components are present and these range in appearance

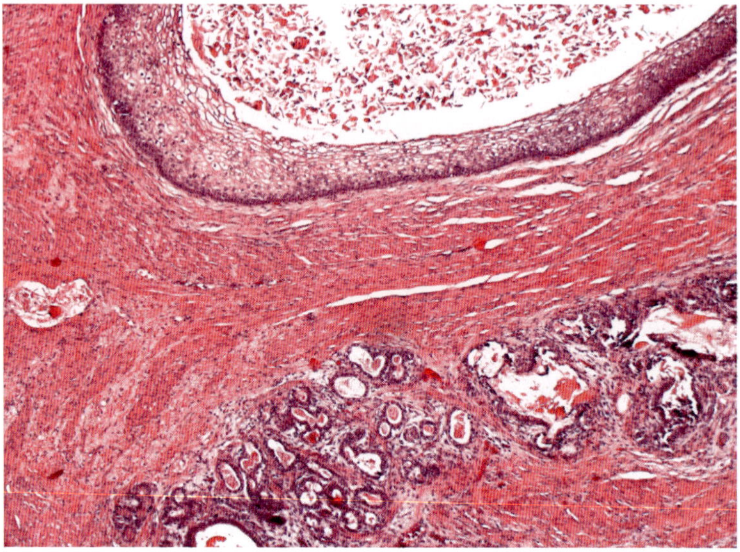

FIGURE 10.6 More mature-appearing epithelial and mesenchymal tissue in a teratocarcinosarcoma.

from mature to immature to malignant (Fig. 10.6). The mesenchymal component usually shows smooth muscle, fibroblastic, and neural differentiation and can sometimes show chondroid or osseous differentiation (eFigs. 10.5 and 10.6). Abundant, mature smooth muscle is usually seen adjacent to epithelial structures and can give rise to an organoid appearance; however, more malignant-appearing muscle (rhabdomyosarcomatous) tissue is often also seen with cellular atypia, mitotic figures, and necrosis. A varying degree of differentiation is also seen with the fibromatous component, which can be myxoid or densely sclerotic. The neural component may be relatively mature appearing with occasional ganglion cells and abundant neuropil, but often appears immature and reminiscent of neuroblastoma (Fig. 10.7). Indeed, the malignant neural component can sometimes predominate and such tumors may be mistaken for olfactory neuroblastomas, especially when only small biopsies are obtained.[14]

The epithelial component usually consists of well-differentiated squamous epithelium that has prominent clear cell change and haphazardly arranged glandular structures that may merge abruptly with the squamous epithelium (eFig. 10.7).[12,13] Along with the more mature-appearing epithelial structures, malignant-appearing epithelium is also seen. This is usually poorly differentiated but obviously epithelial and often has gland formation. Other components of germ cell neoplasia are not seen. Immunoreactivity will recapitulate the apparent phenotype. Of note, blastomatous elements have shown immunoreactivity with antibodies to neuroendocrine antigens, CD 99 and S100 protein.[13]

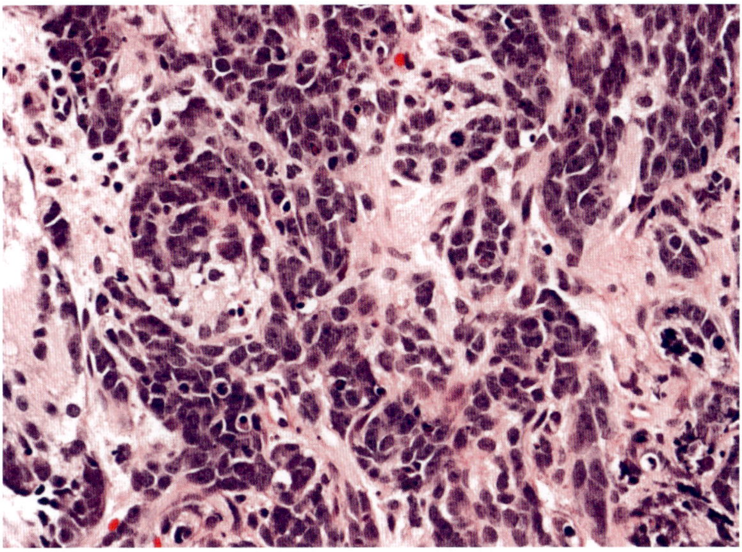

FIGURE 10.7 **Malignant blastic-appearing component of a teratocarcinosarcoma.**

REFERENCES

1. Dehner LP. Gonadal and extragonadal germ cell neoplasia of childhood. *Hum Pathol.* 1983;14:493-511.
2. Heffner DK. Problems in pediatric otorhinolaryngic pathology, III. Teratoid and neural tumors of the nose, sinonasal tract, and nasopharynx. *Int J Pediatr Otorhinolaryngol.* 1983;6:1-21.
3. Lack EE. Extragonadal germ cell tumors of the head and neck region: review of 16 cases. *Hum Pathol.* 1985;16:56-64.
4. Stephenson JA, Mayland DM, Kun LE, Etcubanas E, Thompson EI, Gross CW. Malignant germ cell tumors of the head and neck in childhood. *Laryngoscope.* 1989;99:732-735.
5. Coppit GL III, Perkins JA, Manning SC. Nasopharyngeal teratomas and dermoids: a review of the literature and case series. *Int J Pediatr Otorhinolaryngol.* 2000;52:219-227.
6. Devaney KO, Ferlito A. Yolk sac tumors (endodermal sinus tumors) of the extracranial head and neck regions. *Ann Otol Rhinol Laryngol.* 1997;106:254-260.
7. Shah AA, Jain D, Ababneh E, et al. SMARCB1 (INI-1)-Deficient adenocarcinoma of the sinonasal tract: a potentially under-recognized form of sinonasal adenocarcinoma with occasional yolk sac tumor-like features. *Head Neck Pathol.* 2019. doi:10.1007/s12105-019-01065-7.
8. Ulbright TM. Germ cell tumors of the gonads: a selective review emphasizing problems in differential diagnosis, newly appreciated, and controversial issues. *Mod Pathol.* 2005;18(suppl 2):S61-S79.
9. Bell DM, Porras G, Tortoledo ME, Luna MA. Primary sinonasal choriocarcinoma. *Ann Diagn Pathol.* 2009;13:96-100.
10. Salimi R. Metastatic choriocarcinoma of the nasal mucosa. *J Surg Oncol.* 1977;9:301-305.
11. Alici S, Bavbek SE, Eralp Y, et al. An atypical presentation of metastatic gestational choriocarcinoma with maxillary sinus and subcutaneous involvement; report of a case with literature review. *J Balk Union Oncol.* 2002;7:373-376.

12. Heffner DK, Hyams VJ. Teratocarcinosarcoma (malignant teratoma?) of the nasal cavity and paranasal sinuses A clinicopathologic study of 20 cases. *Cancer*. 1984;53:2140-2154.
13. Carrizo F, Pineda-Daboin K, Neto AG, Luna MA. Pharyngeal teratocarcinosarcoma: review of the literature and report of two cases. *Ann Diagn Pathol*. 2006;10:339-342.
14. Naresh KN, Pai SA. Foci resembling olfactory neuroblastoma and craniopharyngioma are seen in sinonasal teratocarcinosarcomas. *Histopathology*. 1998;32:84.

11

SOFT TISSUE TUMORS

All categories of soft tissue tumors have been reported to involve the upper aerodigestive tract. These include neoplasms that show fibroblastic, myofibroblastic, vascular, myogenous, and neural differentiation. Some neoplasms appear more unique to the area, e.g., angiofibroma, while most can occur throughout the soft tissues of the entire body. This chapter will discuss the more common soft tissue tumors that involve this area (neural tumors have been discussed in Chapter 8; bone and cartilagenous tumors will be discussed in Chapter 12).

It should be noted that the vast majority of neoplasms of the upper aerodigestive tract are epithelial and that some of these can show a spindle cell phenotype, e.g., spindle cell or sarcomatoid carcinoma and myoepitheliomas. Also, melanomas frequently show a spindled cell phenotype when they involve this area. These tumors have markedly different prognoses and require different treatments than those for soft tissue tumors. Because of this, one should be comfortable using immunohistochemistry or other methods with the diagnosis of these lesions, and to help exclude epithelial or melanocytic neoplasms (Table 11.1).[1]

FIBROBLASTIC/MYOFIBROBLASTIC TUMORS

Fibroblastic or myofibroblastic tumors make up the majority of soft tissue tumors of the aerodigestive tract and range from nonneoplastic or benign proliferations (fibromas) to high-grade malignancies (undifferentiated high-grade pleomorphic sarcomas). Distinguishing between these tumors is important because they have vastly different prognoses (Table 11.2). Such distinctions cannot always be made with small biopsy specimens, however, although high-grade malignancies can usually be distinguished from lower grade neoplasia and reactive conditions.

"Fibroma"

A variety of benign fibrous lesions that may or may not be neoplastic can be found within the upper aerodigestive tract and have been termed "fibromas." These include nasal and oral fibromas (traumatic/irritation fibromas, peripheral ossifying fibromas, cementifying fibromas, etc.). One should be cautious regarding the use of the term fibroma within the upper aerodigestive tract outside of these lesions.

TABLE 11.1 Immunohistochemical Profiles of Spindled Cell Neoplasms of the Upper Aerodigestive Tract

	CK	EMA	S100	HMB	SMA	DES	Myo	β-Cat[a]	Bcl-2	CD31	CD34	HHV	CD21	ALK	PAX3
SC	+	+	–[b]	–	–	–		+/–		–	–		–		
Melanoma	–	–	+	+[c]	–	–		–	+/–	–	–		–		
Nodular fasciitis	–		–		+	–	–	–	–		–		–	–	
Fibromatosis	–	–	–		+	–/+	–/+	+	–	–	–		–	–	
Myofibroma	–		–		+	–	–/+							–	
SFT	–		–	–	–	–		+/–	+	–	+				–
IMT	–/+	–	–		+	+/–	–	–	–					–/+	
LGMFS	–	–	–		+	+/–[d]	–				–/+		–		
Fibrosarcoma	–	–	–	–	–/+	–		–/+	+	–	+/–		–		
UHGPS	–	–	–	–	+/–	–	–	–	–/+	–	–		–		
LM/LMS	–	–	–	–	+	+	–	–	–	–	–		–	–	
Rhabdomyoma	–	–	+/–		+/–	+	+	–		–			–		
ERMS	–	–	–	–	+/–	+	+	–/+		–	–		–	–/+	–/+
Angiofibroma[e]	–		–		–	–		+		–					
Glomangiopericytoma	–	–	–		+	–		+	–	–	–				–
Angiosarcoma	–	–	–	–	–	–		–/+	+	+	+	+[f]	–		
Spindle cell lipoma	–	–	–	–	–	–		–	+	–	+		–		
Synovial sarcoma[g]	+	+	–/+	–	–	–	–	+/–	+	–	–		–	–	–
BSS	–	–	+	–	+	+/–	–/+	–/+			–/+				+

Neurofibroma	–	–	+	–	–	–		–	–	–	+	–		
Schwannoma	–	–	+	–	–	–		–	+/–	–	+/–	–		–
Neurothekoma	–	–	+	–	–	–				–		–		
MPNST	–	–	+/–	–	–	–	–	–	–/+	–	–	–	+/–	–
Meningioma	–/+	+	–	–	–	–				–		–		
FDCT	–	–	+/–		–	–						+		

β-cat, β-catenin; ALK, anaplastic lymphoma kinase; BSS, biphenotypic sinonasal sarcoma; CK, cytokeratin; Des, desmin; EMA, epithelial membrane antigen; ERMS, embryonal rhabdomyosarcoma; FDCT, follicular dendritic cell tumor; HHV, human herpes virus 8; HMB, HMB45; IMT, inflammatory myofibroblastic tumor; LGMFS, low-grade myofibroblastic sarcoma; MPNST, malignant peripheral nerve sheath tumor; Myo, myogenin; SC, sarcomatoid carcinoma; SFT, solitary fibrous tumor; SMA, smooth muscle actin; UHGPS, undifferentiated high-grade pleomorphic sarcoma.

[a]Nuclear localization.

[b]Sarcomatoid carcinomas can show variable reactivity with antibodies to traditionally mesenchymal antigens (e.g., S100, SMA).

[c]Other more specific markers for melanoma (e.g., Melan A) can also be used.

[d]Some LGMFSs are immunoreactive with antibodies to desmin and not with antibodies to SMA.

[e]The pattern listed is for the spindled cell component of the tumor.

[f]Kaposi sarcoma.

[g]The pattern listed is for the spindled component of the tumor.

TABLE 11.2 Fibroblastic/Myofibroblastic Lesions of the Upper Aerodigestive Trace

Tumor	Site	Helpful Clinical	Helpful Histology	Helpful IHC, etc.
"Fibroma"	Nasal (nasal fibroma) Oral (traumatic, etc.)	Small (<1 cm), often incidental	Low cellular and collagenized	None
Nodular fasciitis	Mouth	Recent, rapidly growing lesion	Loose with chronic inflammation and extravasated red cells	*USP6* translocation
Fibromatosis	Throughout the UADT	More common in women	Dense collagen Little atypia or mitotic activity	Nuclear staining with antibodies to β-catenin more likely than with other F/MFLUADT
Myofibroma	Most common in the mouth	Often in children May be multiple	Characteristic hypocellular and hypercellular areas	None
Solitary fibrous tumor	Throughout the UADT	Rarely associated with hypoglycemia	Variable cellularity with hemangiopericytoma-like vasculature	Strong and diffuse immunoreactivity with antibodies to CD34 and STAT6
Inflammatory myofibroblastic tumor	Throughout the UADT	Can be associated with fever, anemia, and thrombocytosis	Different growth patterns with looser, NF-like areas with mixed inflammation, more compact, storiform areas with plasma cells, and more sclerotic areas	Immunoreactivity with antibodies to ALK more likely than with other F/MFLUADT
Low-grade myofibroblastic sarcoma	Most common in the mouth, esp., the tongue	Seen in adults More often in men	Usually hypercellular with low-grade spindled cells arranges in short fascicles	Immunoreactivity with desmin more likely than with other F/MFLUADT

Fibrosarcoma	Throughout the UADT, more common in the sinonasal area	Most often occur in older adults	Very cellular with "herringbone" growth pattern Only mild cellular atypia	None; diagnosis of exclusion
Undifferentiated high-grade pleomorphic sarcoma	Throughout UADT	Most often occurs in older adults	Marked atypia and abundant mitotic activity Often has storiform architecture May have multinucleated giant cells or marked inflammation	Giant cells may be reactive with antibodies to CD68

F/MFLUADT, fibroblastic/myofibroblastic lesions of the upper aerodigestive tract; UADT, upper aerodigestive tract.

Nasal fibromas or fibrous polyps are small, smooth polypoid lesions that develop in or near the nasal vestibule.[2] They are usually less than 1 cm in size and frequently present incidentally. Histologically, mature fibroblasts are arranged haphazardly within dense collagen (Fig. 11.1, eFigs. 11.1 and 11.2). More than mild cytologic atypia is not seen and mitotic figures are usually not present. The lesions are benign and do not recur after resection.

A number of different lesions occur in the mouth, which have been termed *fibroma*.[3,4] These lesions all appear to be reactive, yet have a few differences between them. *Traumatic* or *irritation fibromas* are the most common. These are polypoid lesions that are composed of subepithelial, haphazardly arranged, bland fibroblasts within a collagenous stroma. The overlying squamous epithelium can be normal or can show changes consistent with continued trauma such as parakeratosis or acanthosis. The lesions can be ulcerated and chronically inflamed (*epulis fissuratum*), may have large, stellate fibroblasts (*giant cell fibroma*), and may contain odontogenic epithelium (*retrocuspid papule*).[4] Some mesenchymal cells of the gingiva may have a pluripotent nature and be able to differentiate into either osteoblasts or cementoblasts; thus some apparently reactive fibromas within the mouth can form osteoid or cementum (*peripheral ossifying fibroma* or *peripheral cementifying fibroma*, respectively) (Figs. 11.2 and 11.3, eFig. 11.3).[4] (Ossifying fibroma of the bone will be discussed in Chapter 12.)

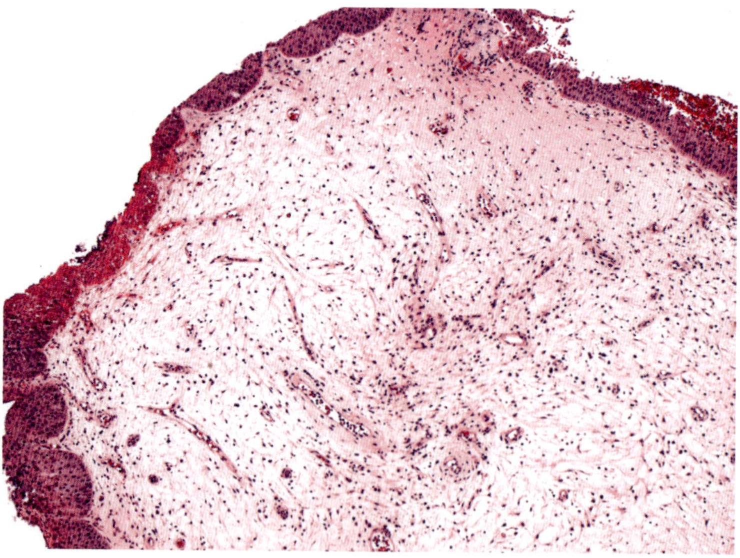

FIGURE 11.1 Nasal fibroma with low cellular, somewhat edematous stroma.

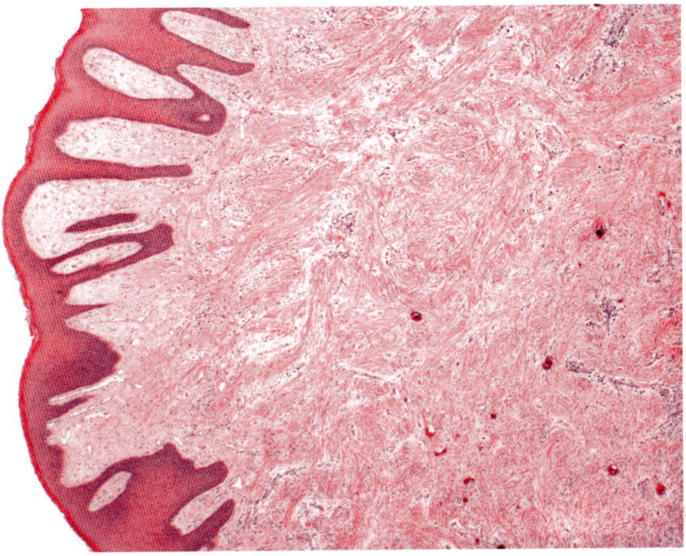

FIGURE 11.2 Oral peripheral cementifying fibroma with overlying pseudoepitheliomatous hyperplasia.

Nodular Fasciitis

Nodular fasciitis and its related lesions usually affect the subcutaneous soft tissue.[5–8] These lesions have rarely been reported in the mouth and very rarely in the nasal cavity, and one should be wary of diagnosing them elsewhere in the upper aerodigestive tract.[9,10] They characteristically affect

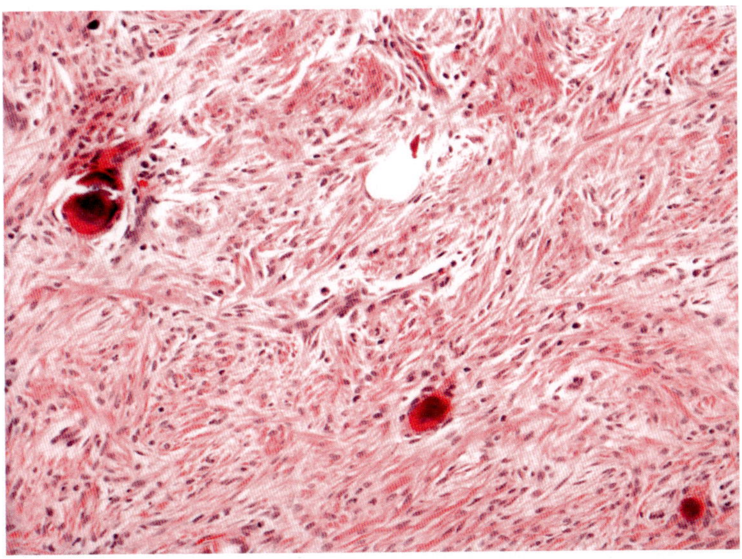

FIGURE 11.3 Cement formation in an oral peripheral cementifying fibroma.

young adults. Clinically, they present as rapidly enlarging, solitary, and often tender masses and are usually less than 2 cm in size. The lesions do not recur if they are completely resected. They are now considered neoplastic and characteristically have *MYH9-USP6* translocations.[11]

Nodular fasciitis is well-circumscribed; however some minor degree of infiltration into surrounding skeletal muscle can be present.[5] The tumors are composed of proliferating fibroblasts and myofibroblasts arranged in a haphazard or somewhat storiform appearance in a background loose, somewhat myxoid stroma (Fig. 11.4, eFig. 11.4).[5-7,10] Zonation, a characteristic feature consisting of alternating degrees of cellularity within single intermediate-power fields, is usually present. The fibroblasts may be plump but usually show only minimal cytologic or nuclear atypia (Fig. 11.5). Older lesions may have a more collagenized stroma (eFig. 11.5). The number of mitotic figures varies greatly from case to case, but can be high. Background mixed inflammatory cells and extravasated red cells are usually seen (eFig. 11.6). As with other myofibroblastic lesions, the spindled cells are typically immunoreactive with antibodies to SMA (Fig. 11.6).

As nodular fasciitis is neither aggressive nor malignant, it is important to distinguish it from other fibroblastic or myofibroblastic lesions of the area such as fibromatosis and inflammatory myofibroblastic tumor (Table 11.2). Fibromatosis usually does not present as a rapidly growing mass and is not well-circumscribed. Furthermore, while some areas of fibromatosis may be more proliferative, the tumors are generally much more collagenized. Immunostaining with antibodies to β-catenin may also be helpful (see below). Distinguishing nodular fasciitis from inflammatory myofibroblastic

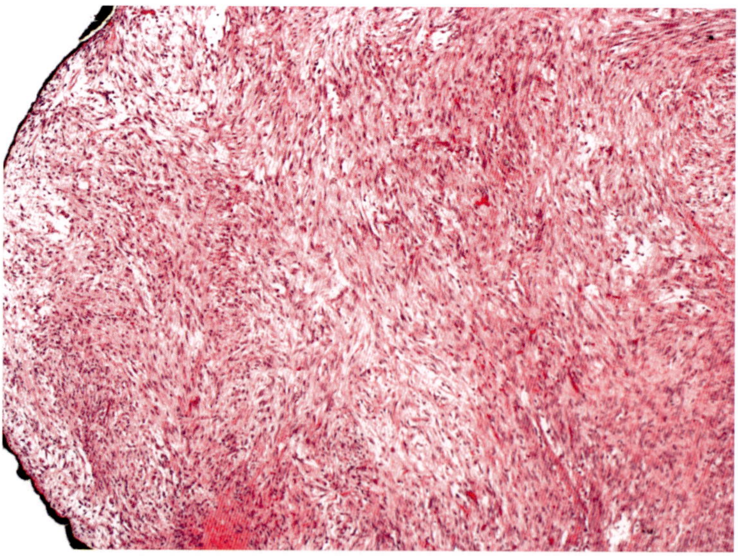

FIGURE 11.4 Nodular fasciitis of the floor of the mouth with a storiform architecture.

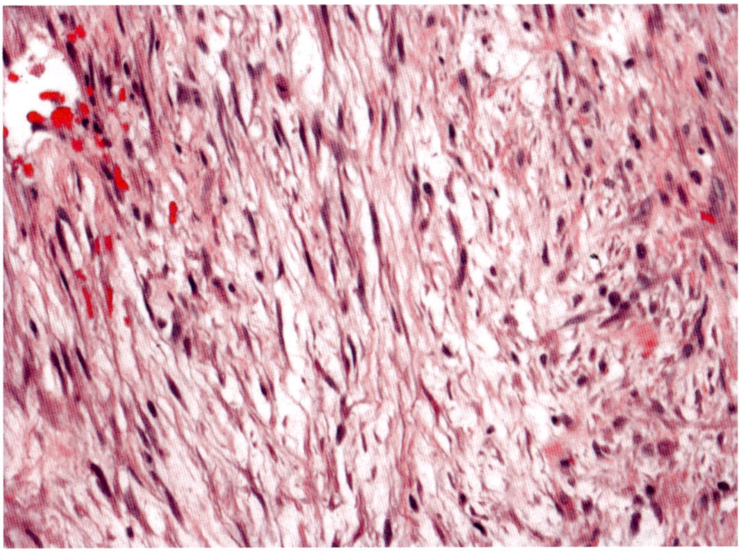

FIGURE 11.5 Loose stroma and bland spindled cells in a case of nodular fasciitis.

tumors in small biopsy specimens may be impossible. Inflammatory myofibroblastic tumors can appear more inflamed and have more sclerotic areas; however, they often have areas very reminiscent of nodular fasciitis. Clinical history and immunostaining with antibodies to ALK1 (see below) may be helpful. Identifying a *USP6* translocation, usually with break-apart FISH, can clinch a diagnosis.[11]

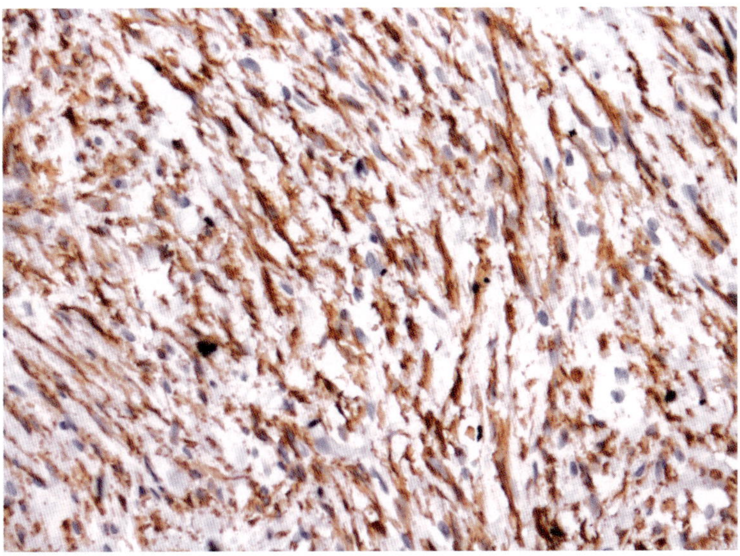

FIGURE 11.6 Strong SMA immunoreactivity seen with nodular fasciitis.

Fibromatosis

Aggressive or desmoid-type fibromatosis can involve the head and neck and may occasionally be sampled in biopsies from the upper aerodigestive tract.[2,12,13] In one study, involvement of the neck was noted in roughly 20% of the extra-abdominal desmoid tumors studied.[12] The tumors can occur at any age and are somewhat evenly distributed throughout the first five decades of life. Extra-abdominal desmoids occur slightly more often in women, although they are not usually associated with pregnancy. The tumors frequently recur, especially when wide excision is not an option (some have noted that sinonasal tract fibromatoses recur less commonly than other extra-abdominal fibromatosis).[13] Although the tumors do not, by definition, metastasize, they can cause death due to the local destruction and entanglement of vital structures. This is especially true in the head and neck. Fibromatoses are neoplastic, and cytogenetic abnormalities can frequently be identified, especially involving the long arm of chromosome 5.[14] This is interesting as abdominal fibromatoses have long been recognized to occur with familial adenomatous polyposis syndrome (Gardner syndrome), a hereditary disorder characterized by mutations of the *adenomatous polyposis coli* (*APC*) gene, which is located on the long arm of chromosome 5.[15,16]

Grossly, the tumors are white-tan and rubbery and appear whorled and infiltrative.[2,12,13] Histologically, they are composed of interlacing bundles and fascicles of spindled to plump myofibroblasts (Figs. 11.7 and 11.8, eFigs. 11.7 and 11.8). Collagen deposition is usually seen and can vary in amount within a tumor, thus rendering some areas hypocellular in appearance while other areas appear moderately cellular. The margins of

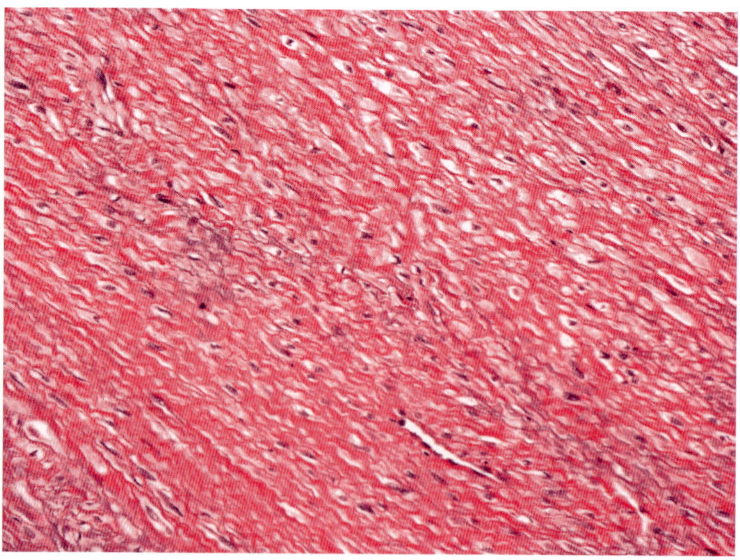

FIGURE 11.7 A low cellular area in a case of extra-abdominal fibromatosis.

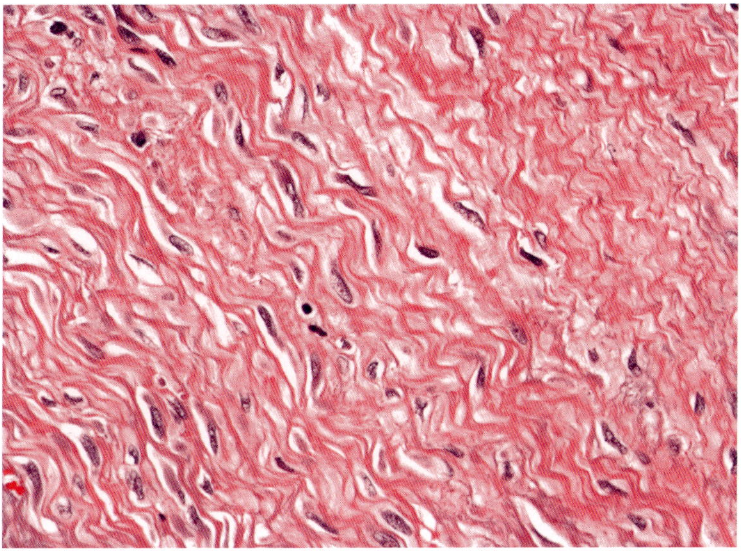

FIGURE 11.8 Bland spindled cells and abundant collagen seen in a case of extra-abdominal fibromatosis.

fibromatoses are infiltrative and fascicles of spindled myofibroblasts can be seen dissecting through adjacent soft tissues. Frequently, entrapped skeletal muscle can be seen with degenerating changes, and it is important not to confuse these changes with epithelial or multinucleated giant cells (Fig. 11.9, eFig. 11.9). Occasional mitotic figures may be present; however, more than mild cellular or nuclear atypia should exclude the diagnosis.

The neoplastic cells of fibromatoses have an immunophenotype similar to other myofibroblastic tumors and are immunoreactive with antibodies to vimentin and SMA. Focal desmin immunoreactivity can be observed. It has recently been noted that most of these tumors, regardless of whether they actually have *β-catenin* or *APC* mutations, will show nuclear localization of β-catenin by immunohistochemistry, and that this can be helpful for distinguishing these tumors from other fibroblastic or myofibroblastic tumors.[17]

Myofibroma/Myofibromatosis

Myofibromas are uncommon tumors that have a marked predilection for the head and neck and are somewhat more common in boys and men.[18–22] The tumors can be solitary or multifocal (myofibromatosis). Most solitary myofibromas and cases of myofibromatosis occur in children, although both can be diagnosed at any age. These tumors are most often identified in the mouth when they involve the upper aerodigestive tract. They are generally benign and have even been noted to regress. Multifocal tumors that involve vital structures can sometimes lead to the death of the patient.

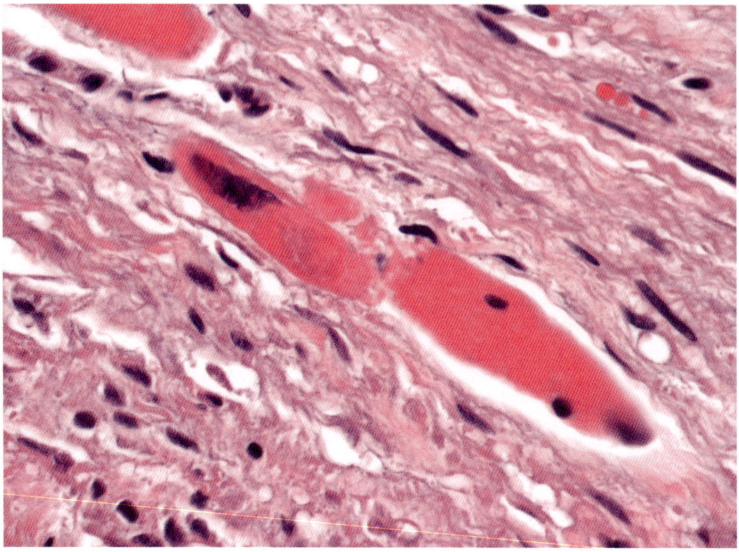

FIGURE 11.9 Entrapped, degenerating skeletal muscle cells in a case of extra-abdominal fibromatosis.

Myofibromas can vary in size and are circumscribed but not encapsulated with a whorled or lobulated cut surface.[18] Microscopically, the tumors are composed of haphazardly arranged, interweaving bundles and short fascicles of plump spindled cells (Fig. 11.10).[18–21] The cytoplasm is pale and eosinophilic and can rarely have small vacuoles. The spindled cells

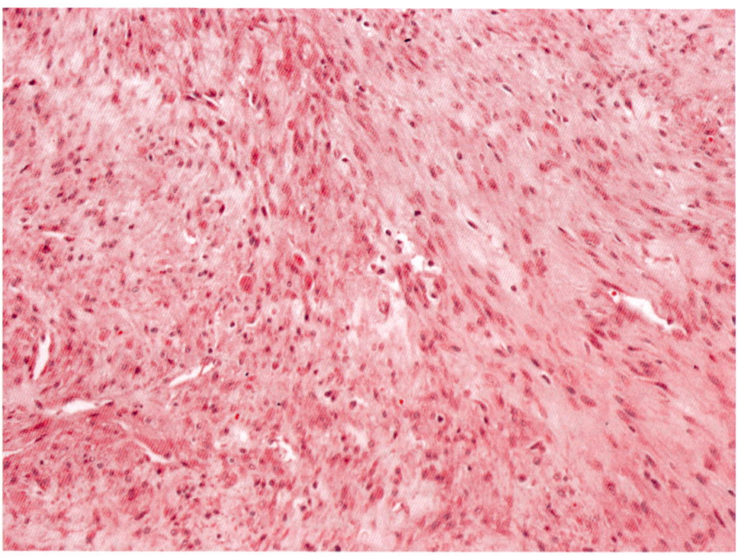

FIGURE 11.10 Haphazardly arranged myofibroblasts seen in a myofibroma.

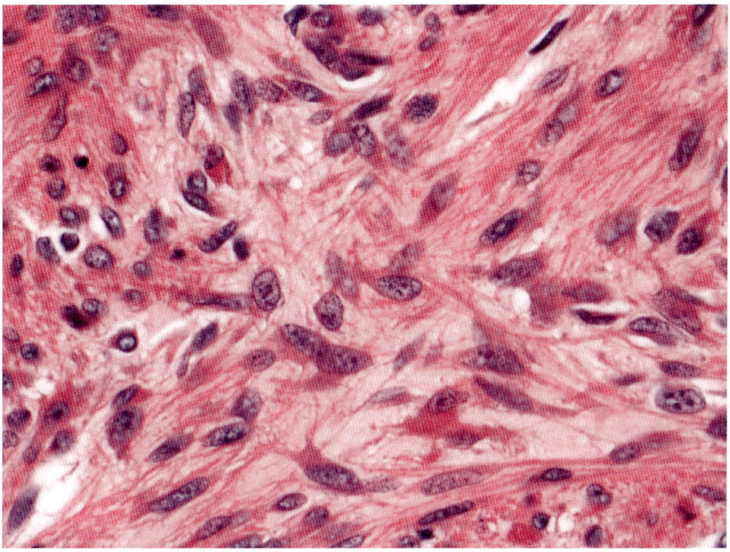

FIGURE 11.11 **Bland spindled and somewhat stellate cells are seen in this myofibroma.**

have oval, rounded, or tapered nuclei with vesicular chromatin and small, indistinct nucleoli (Fig. 11.11). The tumors often have hypocellular and hypercellular areas with many small slitlike vessels. In the more cellular areas, the vessels may display a hemangiopericytoid appearance often with the intravascular polypoid projection of tumor (eFig. 11.10). Occasional mitotic figures may be noted (up to 5 per 10 high-powered fields). Despite their gross appearance of circumscription, infiltration of surrounding tissue is usually present with entrapped soft tissue elements (e.g., peripheral nerved or skeletal muscle) (eFig. 11.11). Multinucleated giant cells can be present, as can degenerative myxoid changes and necrosis (eFigs. 11.12 and 11.13). Some cases have abundant stromal collagen.

Immunohistochemically, the tumor cells express SMA and MSA (eFig. 11.14).[18–21] Antibodies to desmin are usually nonreactive. Focal reactivity with antibodies to S100 protein has been described but most tumors are nonreactive. These tumors need to be distinguished from other myofibroblastic lesions that can be seen with biopsy (Table 11.2). They lack the inflammatory background of inflammatory myofibroblastic tumors and of nodular fasciitis, and the less cellular areas of myofibromas do not have the loose appearance of either of those tumors. The alternating hypocellular and hypercellular areas seen with these tumors are not present in low-grade myofibroblastic sarcomas or fibromatoses, at least not to the same degree.

Extrapleural Solitary Fibrous Tumor

Many sinonasal tract tumors originally described as "hemangiopericytomas" appear to be more closely related to glomus tumors (see below).[23] In fact, once such tumors are reclassified, true solitary fibrous tumors of the upper aerodigestive tract are found to be much less common than they were once believed to be. Nonetheless, small series have been published of these tumors within the sinonasal area and the mouth, while a few scattered case reports have described these tumors in the larynx.[24-29] The tumors arise submucosally in adults of either sex and may either appear as lumps or as polypoid masses. Solitary fibrous tumors are mostly benign, but some (10%–15%) will behave aggressively and may recur or even metastasize.[30] Most tumors have a *NAB2-STAT6* translocation.[31]

These tumors are characteristically well-circumscribed rubbery lesions, although circumscription would obviously be difficult to assess with the piecemeal specimens removed for the sinonasal tract.[24-27,30] They usually have admixed hypercellular and hypocellular areas and may have focal myxoid change. The neoplastic cells are bland, spindled to ovoid, haphazardly arranged, and have oval to polygonal nuclei with fine chromatin and inconspicuous nucleoli. These cells are intertwined between collagen fibers of varying thicknesses (Fig. 11.12, eFig. 11.15). Mitotic activity can be present but is usually low (less than 2 mitotic figures per 10 high powered fields), and necrosis should not be seen. In fact, when increased mitotic activity (>3 mitotic figures per 10 high-powered fields), necrosis, marked cytologic atypia, or infiltrative margins are seen, the tumors are more likely to behave malignantly.[30,32,33] Many thin-walled, small to medium-sized vessels are present that often have a prominent “staghorn” appearance and can focally have a thickened, collagenous cuff (eFig. 11.16). Mast cells are usually present. While some entrapped normal tissue may be present, the lesions rarely infiltrate bony tissues (eFig. 11.17).

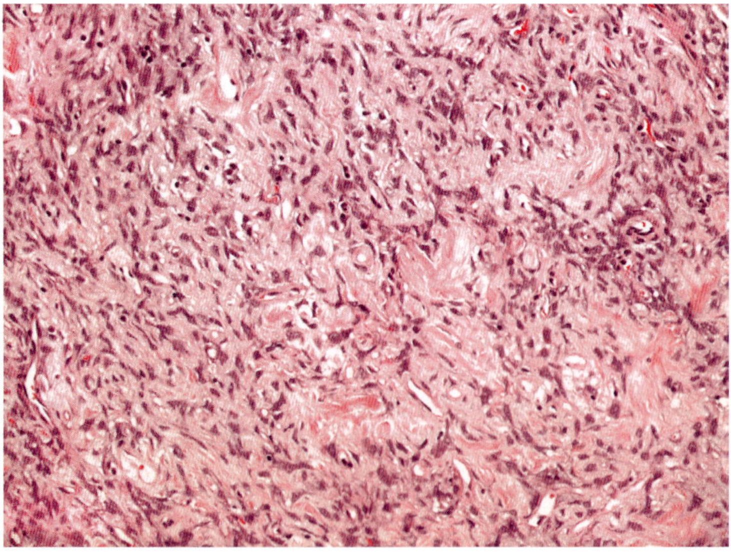

FIGURE 11.12 A solitary fibrous tumor of the nasal cavity with numerous spindled cells and entrapped collagen.

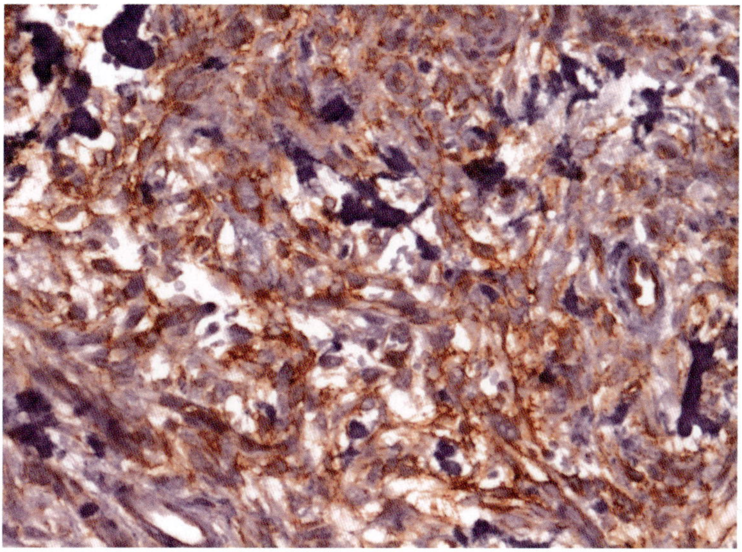

FIGURE 11.13 Strong immunoreactivity with antibodies to CD34 is seen with solitary fibrous tumors.

Immunohistochemically, solitary fibrous tumors react strongly with antibodies to STAT6, vimentin, CD34, and bcl-2 (Fig. 11.13).[24,34] Some staining, albeit weak, is often seen with antibodies to CD99. Antibodies to specific vascular and muscle markers are usually nonreactive (weak, focal reactivity with antibodies to SMA may rarely be seen). The differential diagnosis for solitary fibrous tumors is broad, and the diagnosis is often considered a diagnosis to be made after the exclusion of numerous other entities. In the sinonasal area, glomangiopericytomas must be excluded. This is easily accomplished by immunostaining the tumors with antibodies to STAT6, CD34, β-catenin, and SMA. At all sites, other tumors, such as synovial sarcomas, fibrosarcomas, myofibroblastic tumors, and various neural tumors, must be excluded (Table 11.1). Unlike synovial sarcomas, solitary fibrous tumors do not express TLE1.[35]

Inflammatory Myofibroblastic Tumor

Extrapulmonary inflammatory myofibroblastic tumors occur throughout the body. A little more than 10% of these involve the upper aerodigestive tract.[36–40] The tumors can be found in patients of all ages, but children are more frequently affected. Within the upper aerodigestive tract, they present with the nonspecific symptoms of a mass lesion; however, clinical features can include fever and anemia. Infrequently patients may be found to have thrombocytosis or hypergammaglobulinemia. Some inflammatory myofibroblastic tumors have rearrangements of *ALK* on the short arm of chromosome 2.[41] The tumors occasionally recur (approximately 20%); however, death from disease is rare.

Grossly, the tumors can range from fleshy to firm and may have hemorrhage, necrosis, or calcification.[36,37] The histologic features seen with these tumors can be quite variable and have been generally described as having three different patterns, all of which may be seen in any particular tumor. One pattern resembles granulation tissue or nodular fasciitis and is composed of loosely arrayed, stellate to plump spindled cells with abundant eosinophilic cytoplasm (Figs. 11.14 and 11.15, eFig. 11.18). The cells are embedded within a myxoid or edematous stroma with numerous small blood vessels, a mixed inflammatory infiltrate, and extravasated red cells. Mitotic figures are common but atypical forms are not present. Another pattern is more compact, with the myofibroblasts having a fascicular or storiform growth pattern. Plasma cells are abundant with this pattern and typical mitotic figures can frequently be found (eFigs. 11.19 and 11.20). The third pattern is characteristically less cellular with dense collagen (Fig. 11.16). Fewer mitotic figures are identified in these areas and the inflammatory infiltrate tends to be less prominent. Calcifications can sometimes be seen in these areas.

Immunohistochemically, the myofibroblasts show immunoreactivity with antibodies to vimentin, SMA, and MSA (eFig. 11.21).[36] Limited reactivity with antibodies to desmin can be seen; however, tumor cells have not been found to be immunoreactive with antibodies to myoglobin.[42] Immunoreactivity with antibodies to cytokeratin is seen in up to 36% of the cases. Consistent with the activation of *ALK*, approximately 30% can be found to overexpress ALK1 by immunohistochemistry.[43]

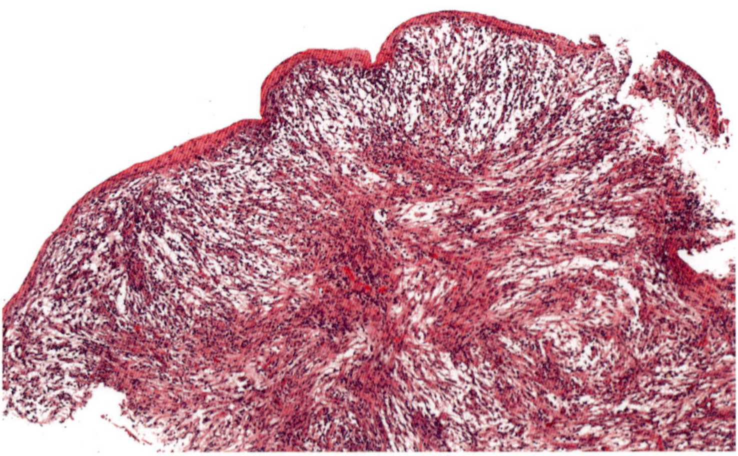

FIGURE 11.14 An inflammatory myofibroblastic tumor of the larynx with a cellular appearance somewhat akin to nodular fasciitis.

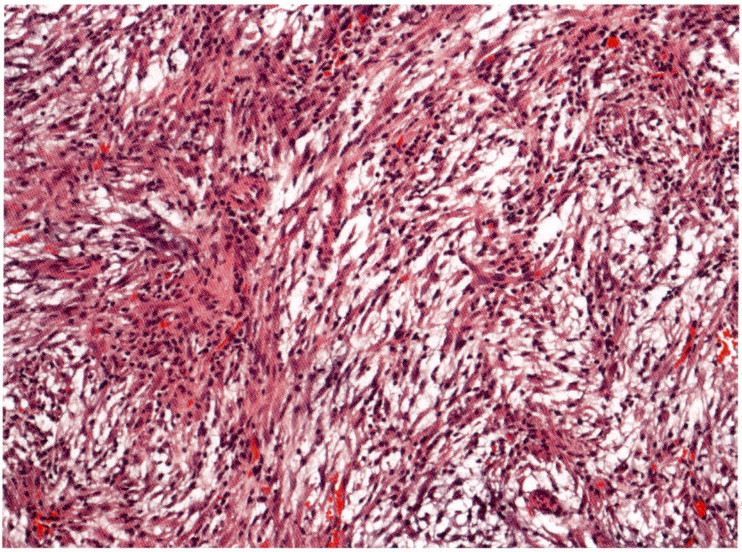

FIGURE 11.15 A nodular fasciitislike area within an inflammatory myofibroblastic tumor.

These tumors can be distinguished from other myofibroblastic tumors by their characteristic inflammatory infiltrate and variable growth patterns. Occasionally ALK1 immunostaining may be helpful, especially when the tumor expresses the protein; however, some have shown ALK1 staining not

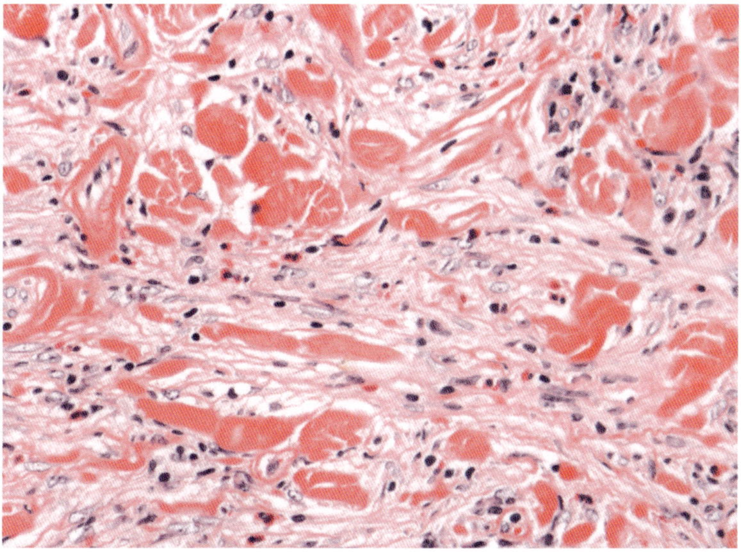

FIGURE 11.16 A more collagenized area within an inflammatory myofibroblastic tumor.

to be unique to inflammatory myofibroblastic tumors.[43] The large spindled cells with eosinophilic cytoplasm may occasionally appear reminiscent of the rhabdomyoblasts or strap cells seen with embryonal rhabdomyosarcomas. Cross striations and less differentiated areas should not be seen with inflammatory myofibroblastic tumors nor should immunoreactivity with antibodies to myogenin. The characteristic inflammatory cell infiltrate seen with inflammatory myofibroblastic tumors is not usually seen with embryonal rhabdomyosarcomas.

Low-Grade Myofibroblastic Sarcoma

Myofibroblastic differentiation is common in soft tissue neoplasms. The diagnosis of low-grade myofibroblastic sarcoma is used to connote what is believed to be a specific clinicopathologic entity.[44,45] In the two largest reports discussing these lesions, they have been noted to occur more frequently in men and have been limited to adults (although some case reports discuss younger patients). Approximately a quarter of these tumors have been found to develop in the mouth.[46] The tumors recur in approximately 40% of cases; however, less than 10% have been found to metastasize.

Low-grade myofibroblastic sarcomas are firm and fibrous and most have ill-defined margins; however, they can appear distinctly circumscribed.[44,45] Histologically, the tumors usually appear to infiltrate surrounding soft tissues. Neoplastic cells are arranged in fascicles of varying lengths; however, herringbone, hemangiopericytoid, and storiform growth patterns have been noted. Cellularity can vary, but areas of hypercellularity are always found (Figs. 11.17 and 11.18, eFigs. 11.22 and 11.23). Tumor cells

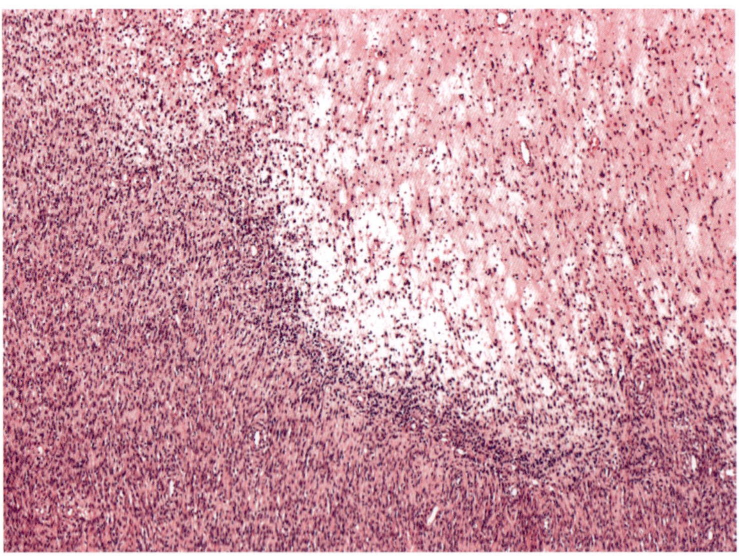

FIGURE 11.17 Most cases of low-grade myofibroblastic sarcoma have areas of high cellularity.

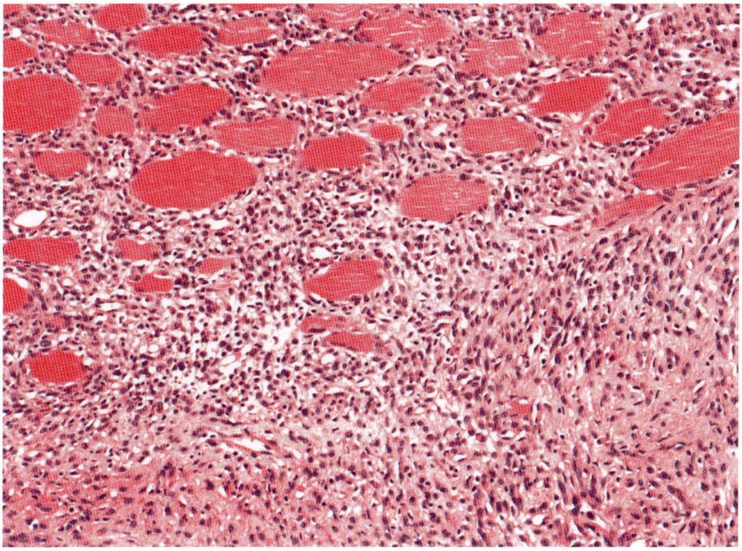

FIGURE 11.18 A low-grade myofibroblastic sarcoma with infiltration into surrounding skeletal muscle.

are spindled and have pale, eosinophilic cytoplasm with tapered nuclei (eFig. 11.24). The nuclei have fine or vesicular chromatin and inconspicuous nucleoli. Most cases have little atypia, although occasional examples display moderate atypia with enlarged, pleomorphic, hyperchromatic nuclei and prominent nucleoli. Occasional stellate cells with elongated cell processes may be seen. Mitotic activity is present and up to 10 mitotic figures per 10 high-powered fields have been found. Tumor necrosis may is noted focally in rare cases.

Immunohistochemically, these tumors react with antibodies to vimentin and SMA and frequently with antibodies to desmin (eFig. 11.25).[44,45] They do not react with antibodies to cytokeratins or S100 protein. Most do not react with antibodies to CD34, although occasional cases may have limited weak staining. This immunohistochemical staining pattern of these tumors should help to distinguish them from other spindle cell lesions, such as neural tumors, solitary fibrous tumor, sarcomatoid carcinoma, and malignant melanoma. It is obviously not very helpful for distinguishing the tumors from smooth muscle tumors or other myofibroblastic proliferations. Low-grade myofibroblastic sarcomas have more atypia than leiomyomas and they have infiltrating borders. Also, the fascicular cell arrangement of leiomyomas is much more pronounced, and the individual cells of those tumors are more eosinophilic with blunted rather than tapered nuclei. Leiomyosarcomas also have more eosinophilic cells and often have a more prominent fascicular appearance. They typically have more cytologic atypia than low-grade myofibroblastic sarcomas.

Distinguishing low-grade myofibroblastic sarcomas from the various other myofibroblastic lesions of the upper aerodigestive tract may be particularly challenging (Table 11.2). Low-grade myofibroblastic sarcomas should be more cellular and show more cytologic atypia than fibromatoses, and fibromatoses are much less frequently immunoreactive with antibodies to desmin. Myofibromas have more plump cells and typically show less cytologic atypia than low-grade myofibroblastic sarcomas. Although, the cellularity of low-grade myofibroblastic sarcomas can vary, the typical biphasic cellularity seen with myofibromas is not seen with these tumors. Like fibromatoses, myofibromas infrequently show immunoreactivity with antibodies to desmin. Finally, inflammatory myofibroblastic tumors typically have a more pronounced inflammatory cell infiltrate and have areas with looser stroma than in low-grade myofibroblastic sarcomas. They also frequently have *ALK* rearrangements and express ALK1 by immunohistochemistry.[47]

Fibrosarcoma

Fibrosarcomas have been reported to involve the upper aerodigestive tract, especially the sinonasal area.[2,48–50] Most patients are adults, although rare cases of infantile fibrosarcomas have been reported. Adult fibrosarcomas typically arise in middle-aged or older individuals. Patients present with nonspecific complaints such as pain, obstruction, or bleeding. Destruction of adjacent bone is often seen by imaging. The tumors often metastasize, especially to the lungs, and 5-year survival rate is approximately 50% for adult fibrosarcomas that are grade 2 or higher.[50]

Most adult fibrosarcomas are highly cellular and usually show only limited collagen production (although it is typically present, at least focally) (Fig. 11.19, eFig. 11.26).[2,51] Less cellular areas may, however, be seen within a tumor. The elongated spindled cells are arranged in bundles that often intersect to form the classic "herringbone" pattern (Fig. 11.20, eFig. 11.27). Most tumors have rather uniform cells with spindled to oval nuclei and little pleomorphism. Mitotic figures are usually abundant. Immunohistochemically, fibrosarcomas will react with antibodies to vimentin and may have limited reactivity with antibodies to SMA.[52]

Adult fibrosarcomas need to be distinguished from a number of lesions including the other fibroblastic and myofibroblastic tumors discussed in this chapter (Tables 11.1 and 11.2). In general, fibrosarcomas are typically more cellular and mitotically active than benign or the lower grade malignancies. Low-grade fibrosarcomas have been reported at this site that are difficult to distinguish from fibromatoses and may have a better prognosis than higher grade (grade 2 or above) fibrosarcomas (eFig. 11.28). Some have suggested using a mitotic count to distinguish these lesions, designating tumors with 6 to 10 mitotic figures per 10 high-powered fields as "borderline" and those with more than 10 as fibrosarcomas. β-Catenin immunostaining may also be helpful. Other spindle celled tumors,

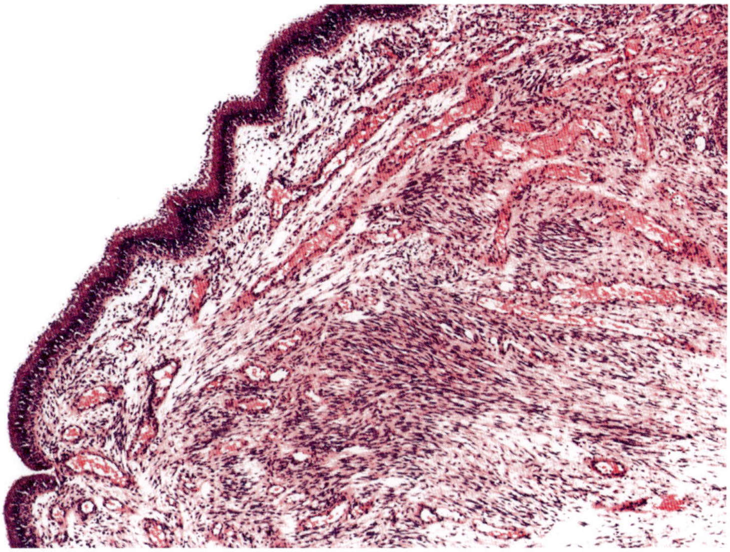

FIGURE 11.19 High cellularity is the norm for fibrosarcomas.

especially monophasic synovial sarcomas and malignant peripheral nerve sheath tumors, need to be distinguished from these malignancies. This can usually be accomplished with immunohistochemistry (Table 11.1). Adult fibrosarcomas typically have limited cellular atypia, and more pronounced

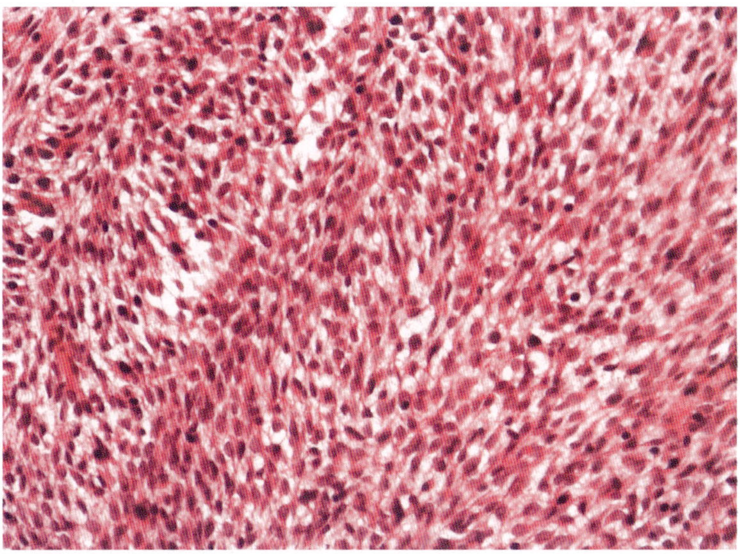

FIGURE 11.20 A "herringbone" growth pattern is seen with this fibrosarcoma of the maxillary sinus.

atypia should lead to a diagnosis of pleomorphic sarcoma. Finally, as with all spindle cell sarcomas of the upper aerodigestive tract, these tumors need to be distinguished from sarcomatoid carcinomas, especially after radiation therapy for squamous cell carcinoma. Intraepithelial neoplasia (squamous dysplasia) or focal squamous differentiation can often be identified with sarcomatoid carcinomas, and many sarcomatoid carcinomas show immunoreactivity with antibodies to cytokeratins.

Adult fibrosarcoma is a diagnosis now made only after other, better-defined entities have been excluded.[53] With this in mind, previous reports of fibrosarcoma of the upper aerodigestive tract should be interpreted with some caution, especially as there appears to be significant overlap between what some might call fibrosarcoma and others might call malignant peripheral nerve sheath tumors.[49] Recently, some have described a low-grade sarcoma of the sinonasal tract that can have limited myogenic and S100 immunoreactivity, that has both histologic and immunohistochemical features that overlap with these tumors (see below).[54]

Undifferentiated Sarcoma

Undifferentiated sarcomas usually involve the extremities, but have been noted within the upper aerodigestive tract.[48,55–58] The tumors occur in older adults, often in the sixth and seventh decades of life. Once other lesions such as sarcomatoid carcinomas or dedifferentiated liposarcomas are distinguished from these tumors, it appears that they have an overall poor prognosis with a 5-year survival rate of 50% to 60%.[48] Interestingly, some of these lesions involving the head and neck have been reported after radiotherapy, which has also been suggested as a risk factor for the transformation of conventional squamous cell carcinomas to a sarcomatoid carcinoma.[59]

Histologically, these tumors have a variable appearance and may appear spindled, epithelioid, round cell or pleomorphic. Pleomorphic tumors are characterized by marked cytologic and nuclear pleomorphism (Fig. 11.21, eFig. 11.29).[55–58] Many tumor cells will be spindled, but large round and polygonal tumors cells are often noted with atypical multinucleated tumor cells. Some cells will have abundant eosinophilic cytoplasm and some may appear finely vacuolated. Cellularity is usually high, although some tumors have a myxoid or fibrous background and appear less cellular. Mitotic figures are abundant and necrosis and hemorrhage are common. Osteoclastlike giant cells are often present and can be numerous (Fig. 11.22, eFigs. 11.30 and 11.31). Background inflammation may be present and can occasionally be prominent.

The diagnosis of undifferentiated sarcoma is one of exclusion. In the upper aerodigestive tract, a sarcomatoid or spindle cell carcinoma must first be ruled out. Immunostaining with antibodies to cytokeratin can be helpful, although a lack of staining does not exclude carcinoma. A careful search for a squamous component to the tumor or overlying squamous dysplasia should be made and the identification of either should lead one

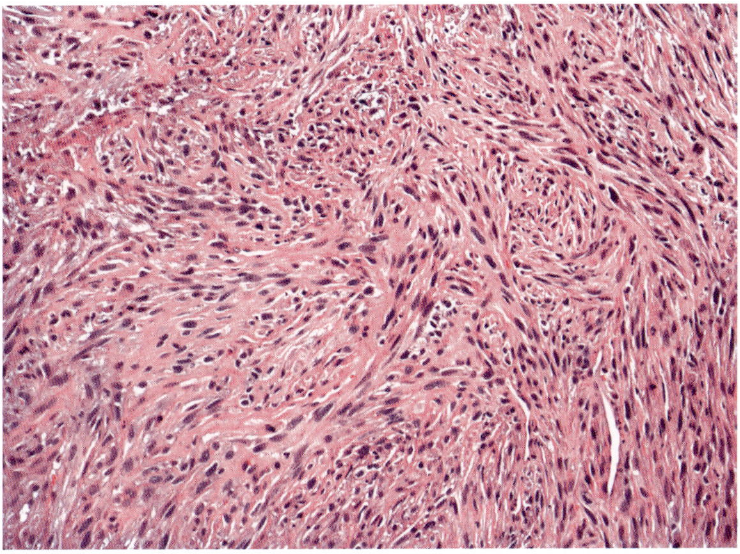

FIGURE 11.21 A storiform growth pattern and moderate cellular atypia is seen with this undifferentiated high-grade pleomorphic sarcoma of the tongue.

to diagnose the lesion as a sarcomatoid carcinoma. Dedifferentiated liposarcomas and chondrosarcomas as well as osteosarcomas should be distinguished from these lesions because of their different prognoses, and a careful search for well-differentiated liposarcoma or chondrosarcoma or

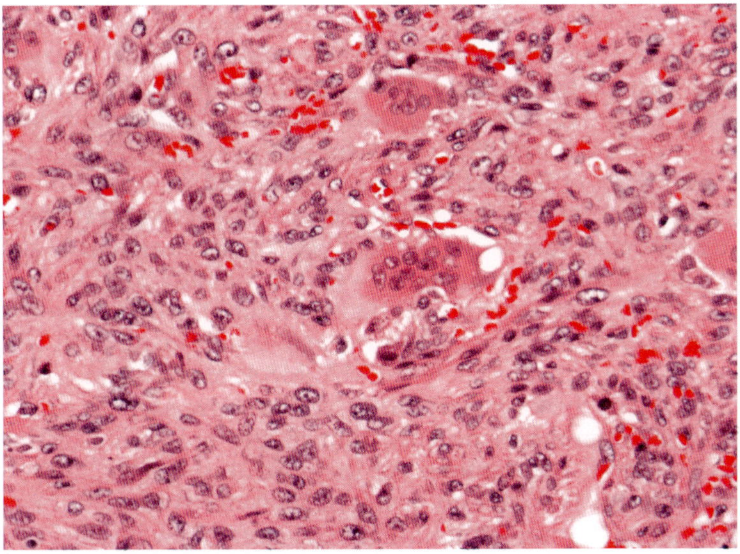

FIGURE 11.22 Numerous osteoclastlike giant cells can be seen with some undifferentiated high-grade pleomorphic sarcomas.

osteoid production should be made. Immunohistochemistry can be used when needed to distinguish leiomyosarcomas and angiosarcomas from these tumors.

Other Myofibroblastic Tumors

Other myofibroblastic tumors have rarely been reported to involve the upper aerodigestive tract, and these include *dermatofibromas* or *benign fibrous histiocytomas*, *dermatofibrosarcomas*, *giant cell angiofibroma*, *infantile fibrosarcomas*, low-grade fibromyxoid sarcoma, and *sclerosing epithelioid fibrosarcoma*, among others. One should keep in mind that most soft tissue tumors can develop in the head in neck and can, either primarily or through secondary extension, come to involve the upper aerodigestive tract.

MYOGENIC TUMORS

Neoplasms showing either smooth muscle or striated muscle differentiation have been identified in the upper aerodigestive tract. Other than rhabdomyosarcomas, most of these tumors occur in adults.

Leiomyomas

Leiomyomas have been described throughout the upper aerodigestive tract but have been most frequently identified in the mouth.[60–64] As with at other anatomic sites, they appear to be slightly more common in women. These tumors are usually described as small, often less than a centimeter in greatest dimension, and are noted to be circumscribed and rubbery (Fig. 11.23). A variety of histologic appearances have been documented and have been classified as solid or conventional, vascular (angioleiomyoma), and epithelioid. Conventional leiomyomas appear similar to leiomyomas from other sites in the body and are circumscribed, moderately cellular neoplasms with broad fascicles of oval to spindled cells that have a moderate amount of eosinophilic cytoplasm and oval, "cigar-shaped" nuclei (Fig. 11.24, eFig. 11.32). Mitotic figures should be rare and necrosis should not be present. Angioleiomyomas are similar except that they have numerous vascular spaces surrounded by thick, muscular walls (eFig. 11.33).[60] Epithelioid leiomyomas are very uncommon and are composed of large, epithelioid cells with abundant eosinophilic cytoplasm; spindled cells may be difficult to find.[63] Leiomyomas should react with antibodies to smooth muscle antigens such as SMA, MSA, and desmin (eFigs. 11.34 and 11.35).[63,64] For the most part, these tumors show a typical morphology, and with their immunophenotype, they should be readily distinguished from other spindle cell tumors. As their name indicates, these tumors behave in a benign fashion and have not been noted to recur or metastasize. If necessary, desmin immunoreactivity can usually be used to exclude tumors with pericytic differentiation (e.g., myopericytoma) that can appear similar to angioleiomyomas.[65]

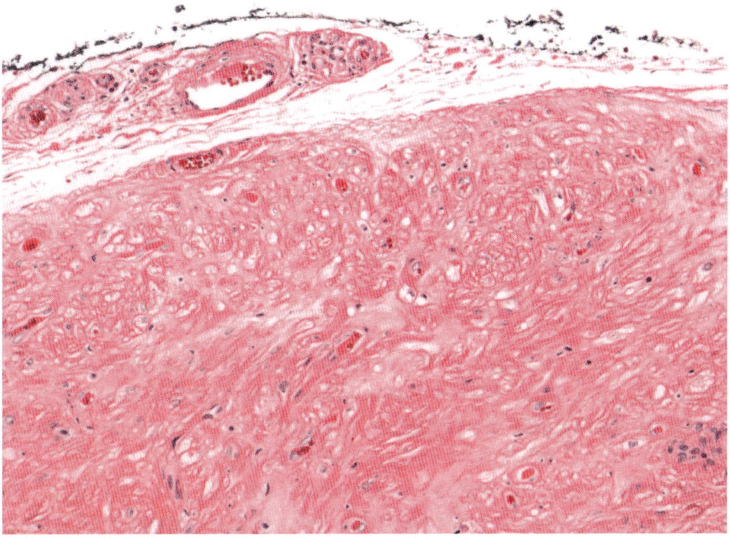

FIGURE 11.23 Leiomyomas are typically well-circumscribed.

Leiomyosarcomas

Leiomyosarcoma are very uncommon in the upper aerodigestive tract.[61,62,64,66–68] They have been noted in the mouth, sinonasal area, pharynx, and larynx. The tumors have mostly arisen in adults, and the small studies that exist have not shown a definitive sex predilection. The tumors

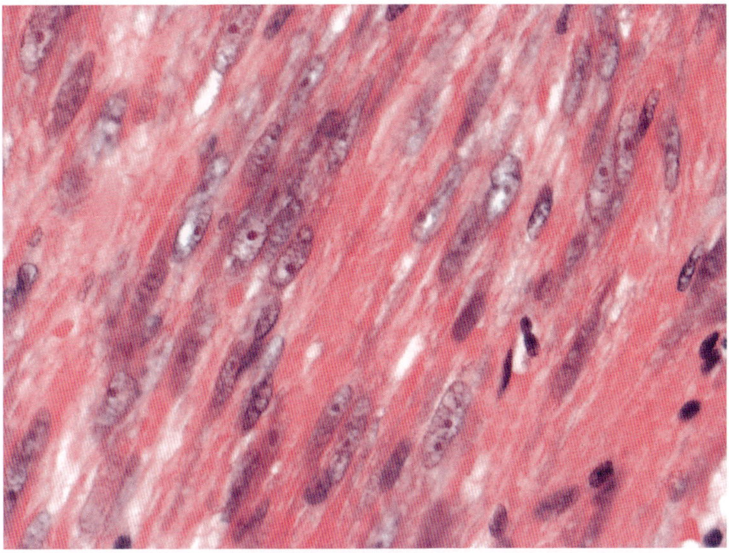

FIGURE 11.24 The typical cigar-shaped nuclei of a leiomyoma.

vary greatly in size, and a single tumor that was only 3 mm in greatest dimension has been reported.[66] Histologically, the tumors are infiltrative rather than circumscribed. They are composed of fascicles of spindled cells with eosinophilic cytoplasm; however, cytologic features of malignancy are also seen, with cellular and nuclear atypia, increased mitotic activity, and tumor necrosis (Fig. 11.25, eFig. 11.36). Smooth muscle differentiation should be identified by immunohistochemistry. Leiomyosarcomas metastasize in more than 50% of the patients affected, and nearly one-third of these patients may die of their disease.

Rhabdomyoma

Rhabdomyomas are benign tumors showing striated muscle differentiation. The adult and fetal forms have a marked predilection for involving the mucosa of the upper aerodigestive tract.[62,69–72] A single case has been reported in a patient with Birt-Hogg-Dube syndrome.[73]

Adult-type rhabdomyomas can occur at almost any age; however, they most often present in older adults, and the mean age of presentation is 60 years.[70,72] These tumors occur more frequently in men and typically involve the pharynx, oral cavity, and larynx. The tumors present as either single or multiple nodules and usually cause obstruction. Although nearly half recur after resection, none have metastasized or resulted in the death of the patient.

Grossly, adult-type rhabdomyomas are tan to red-brown, circumscribed, lobulated, and soft in consistency.[70,72] Histologically, the tumors are composed of closely packed round to polygonal cells with abundant,

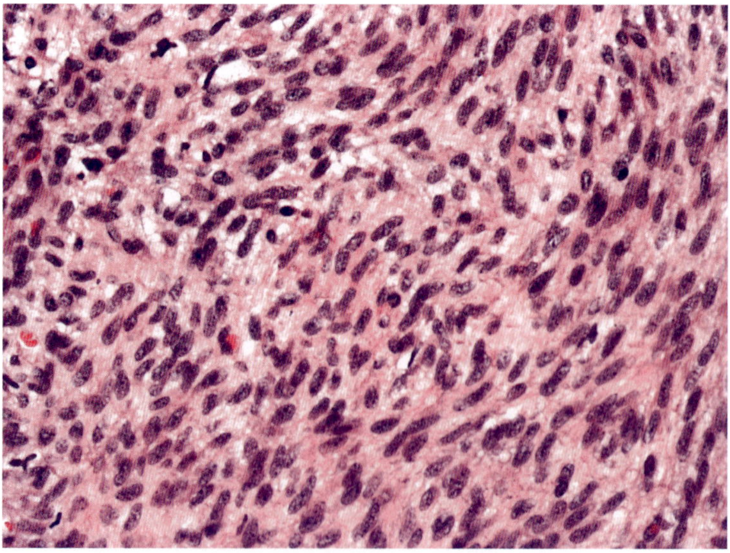

FIGURE 11.25 This leiomyosarcoma is highly cellular with easily identifiable mitotic figures.

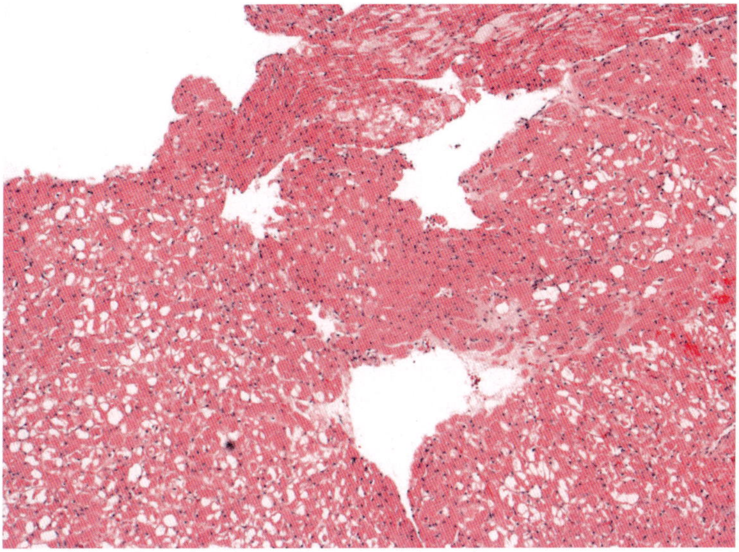

FIGURE 11.26 A biopsy of an adult-type rhabdomyoma of the larynx with large cells with abundant eosinophilic cytoplasm.

granular eosinophilic cytoplasm (Fig. 11.26). Striations may be seen but are often hard to identify. Many cells have clear or vacuolated cytoplasm that may be secondary to glycogen or lipid accumulation (Fig. 11.27, eFigs. 11.37 and 11.38). Strands of eosinophilic cytoplasm may remain in these cells and can give the impression of a spider web. Haphazardly

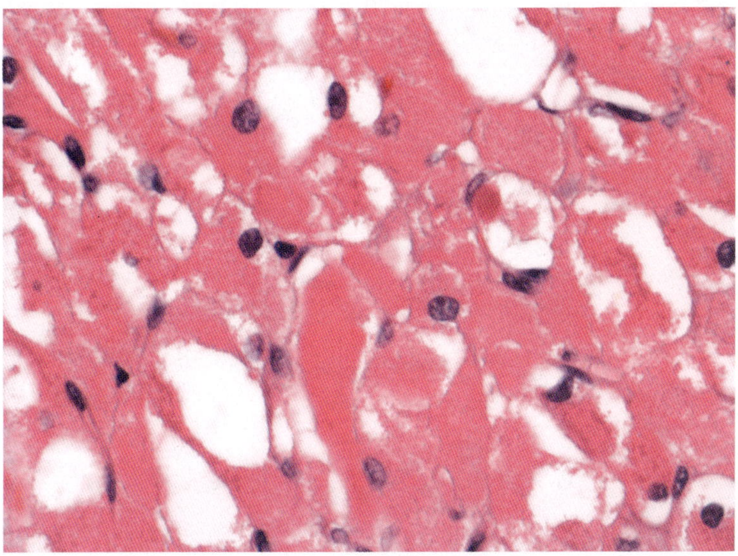

FIGURE 11.27 Some cells of a rhabdomyoma have clear cytoplasm.

arranged intracytoplasmic crystalloids can sometimes be seen. The nuclei are small and round, can be located centrally or peripherally, and have vesicular chromatin and prominent nucleoli. Mitotic figures and necrosis are not seen.

Fetal-type rhabdomyomas can also occur over a broad age range but, as the name suggests, usually occur in children, many of whom are younger than 1 year.[69,72] These tumors are also more common in boys and often present in the upper aerodigestive tract causing obstruction, most frequently in the nasopharynx and mouth. They only very rarely recur after resection.

Grossly, fetal-type rhabdomyomas are circumscribed, soft, gray-white to pink and somewhat mucoid on cut surface.[69,72] Histologically, the tumors remain circumscribed but are not encapsulated. These tumors have been noted to show varying degrees of differentiation. The classic type is composed of small, spindled cells with larger, slender, tapered, eosinophilic cells that display occasional cytoplasmic cross-striations (Fig. 11.28, eFig. 11.39). The cells are arranged haphazardly and the background stroma may appear myxoid or fibromyxoid. Cells showing skeletal muscle differentiation may be located separately or in small fascicles. The nuclei are small and oval with fine chromatin and indistinct nucleoli. The intermediate-form of feta-type rhabdomyoma usually has some component that appears classic, while other areas show more differentiation with prominent strap cells that have basophilic or eosinophilic cytoplasm, obvious cross striations, and larger nuclei with prominent nucleoli.[69] Focal areas with large, eosinophilic and vacuolated polygonal cells may also be seen, identical to those seen in adult rhabdomyomas.

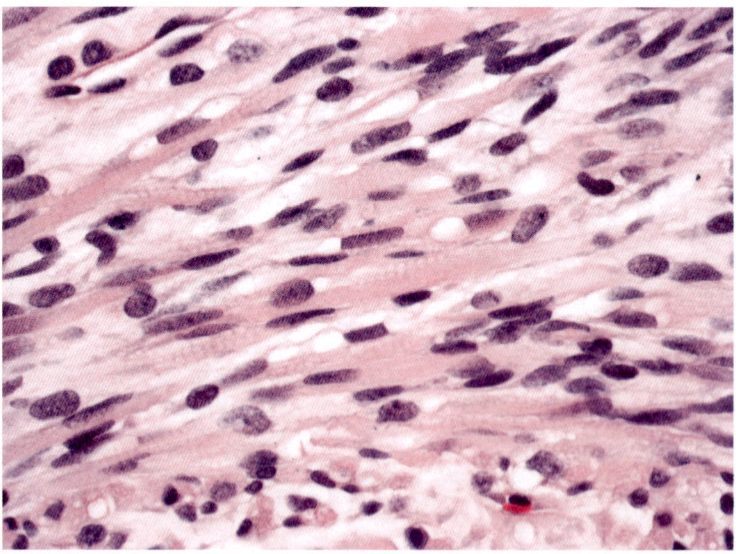

FIGURE 11.28 Fetal-type rhabdomyomas have spindled cells akin to fetal skeletal muscle.

By immunohistochemistry, desmin, MSA, and myoglobin are universally identified in both fetal-type and adult-type rhabdomyomas (eFig. 11.40).[69,70] Other muscle antigens such as SMA may also be identified by immunohistochemistry, especially with fetal rhabdomyomas, and immunoreactivity with antibodies to S100 protein is frequently identified. The differential diagnosis for adult rhabdomyomas is short and includes granular cell tumor and, less likely, hibernoma. The identification of myogenous differentiation helps to distinguish these tumors. Fetal-type rhabdomyomas must be distinguished from embryonal rhabdomyosarcomas which can be much more difficult (see below).

Rhabdomyosarcoma

It has long been recognized that malignancies can show skeletal muscle differentiation; however, the recognition of rhabdomyosarcomas in children did not gain favor until the early to middle of the 20th century. It is now known that rhabdomyosarcomas are the most prevalent soft tissue sarcomas of childhood.[74–78] Between one-third and one-half of rhabdomyosarcomas involve the head and neck, and, of these, between a quarter and a third involve the upper aerodigestive tract. These rhabdomyosarcomas are the pediatric variants, and the adult forms, e.g., pleomorphic rhabdomyosarcoma, generally involve the extremities and will not be discussed here.[79]

The majority of rhabdomyosarcomas occur in the first two decades of life.[74–78,80] The embryonal type occurs more often in younger patients, whereas the alveolar type develops in slightly older patients. Within the head and neck, nearly 70% of rhabdomyosarcomas are embryonal.[74] The overall prognosis for these tumors varies based upon the histologic classification and other factors, such as patient age, site of involvement, and stage.[75,77] All such factors are considered for the overall risk assignment and subsequent therapies. Considering histologic features alone, botryoid and spindle cell variants of embryonal rhabdomyosarcoma have the best prognoses with a 5-year survival of approximately 90%.[77] Other embryonal rhabdomyosarcomas behave in a more aggressive fashion and have an intermediate 5-year survival of 66%. Alveolar rhabdomyosarcomas and rhabdomyosarcomas with anaplasia have the worse prognoses. Five-year survivals for these tumors are around 50% to 60%.

The histologic classification system has varied somewhat over the years, but the major subtypes have remained unchanged. For the purpose of this review, we will discuss embryonal rhabdomyosarcoma, with attention to the conventional, botryoid and spindle cell–types, alveolar rhabdomyosarcoma, and anaplasia with the mention of a few caveats (Table 11.3).

Most embryonal rhabdomyosarcomas cannot be classified as botryoid or spindle cell and lack anaplasia.[74] They are thus classified as embryonal rhabdomyosarcomas, not otherwise specified. These tumors can vary greatly in their degree of differentiation and can range from

TABLE 11.3 Embryonal Versus Alveolar Rhabdomyosarcoma

	Embryonal	Alveolar
Clinical	Usually younger (<10 y/o) More likely to involve the head and neck	Slightly older population (10–30 y/o) Somewhat less likely to involve the head and neck
Variants	Spindle Botryoid Conventional	Solid Conventional
Histology	Spectrum of cellular differentiation ranging from small round cells to spindled rhabdomyoblasts (strap cells) More likely to be associated with anaplasia	Minimally differentiated round cells separated by fibrous septae into nests with central degeneration and discohesion May also grow in solid sheets Less likely to be associated with anaplasia
Helpful immunohisto-chemistry	More likely to show limited and weaker immunoreactivity with antibodies to myogenin and MyoD1	More likely to have strong and diffuse immunoreactivity with antibodies to myogenin and MyoD1
Cytogenetics	Frequent allelic loss at 11p15	t(1;13)(p36;q14) or t(2;13)(q35;q14)

very primitive-appearing tumors that are difficult to distinguish from other small, round cell tumors of childhood to tumors that appear similar to fetal skeletal muscle.[77,78,80] Most tumors show a spectrum of differentiation with both small round to ovoid undifferentiated cells and differentiated, larger round or spindled cells with eosinophilic cytoplasm and occasional identifiable cross-striations (strap cells) (Figs. 11.29 and 11.30, eFigs. 11.41–11.45). The number of strap cells differs significantly from case to case. The smaller, more primitive cells of these tumors are noted to have mildly pleomorphic, hyperchromatic nuclei with small nucleoli. Abundant mitotic figures are seen in areas composed of the more primitive-appearing cells. Larger rhabdomyoblasts have a granular or fibrillary eosinophilic cytoplasm and rarely undergo cellular division. The cellularity usually varies from field to field and the background matrix is myxoid. This low-power feature can be helpful for distinguishing embryonal rhabdomyosarcomas from alveolar rhabdomyosarcomas.

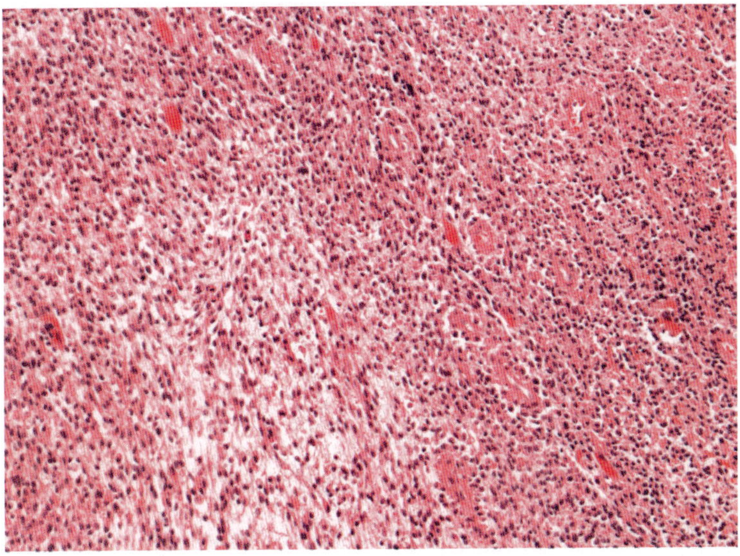

FIGURE 11.29 A highly cellular area in an embryonal rhabdomyosarcoma.

The botryoid-type of embryonal rhabdomyosarcoma is associated with mucosal surfaces and presents as a polypoid, edematous, grapelike mass.[77,80] It is characterized by a subepithelial condensation of tumor cells abutting the surface epithelium or separated from the surface epithelium

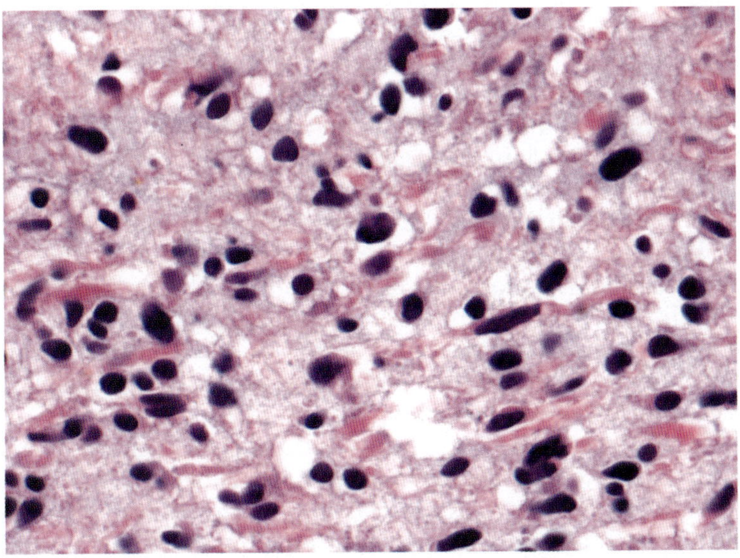

FIGURE 11.30 Occasional strap cells can be seen with most embryonal rhabdomyosarcomas.

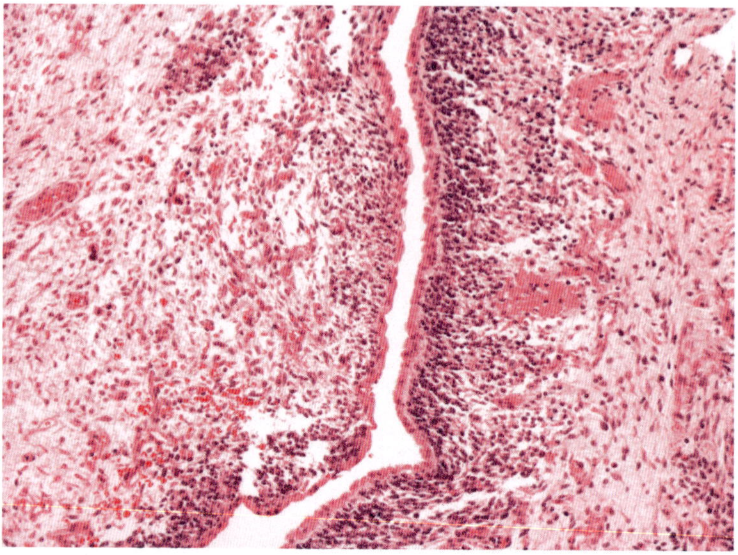

FIGURE 11.31 Condensation of tumor cells immediately below the epithelium was seen with this botryoid embryonal rhabdomyosarcoma.

by a narrow region of loose stroma (cambium layer) (Fig. 11.31). The thickness of the condensation can vary from tumor to tumor and may be only focally present. Histologically, the tumors are otherwise similar to conventional embryonal rhabdomyosarcomas.

The spindle cell–type of embryonal rhabdomyosarcoma is rare, accounting for less than 5% of rhabdomyosarcomas, and more commonly affects boys.[77,80,81] It is composed of elongated spindled cells with fibrillary, eosinophilic cytoplasm and oval-shaped nuclei with blunted ends. Cross striations may sometimes be seen. The tumor cells may make irregular fascicles and can appear reminiscent of leiomyosarcoma or fibrosarcoma. Some tumors may have abundant collagen (i.e., sclerosing rhabdomyosarcoma).

Alveolar rhabdomyosarcomas occur more frequently in the extremities but do occasionally involve the upper aerodigestive tract.[77,80] The tumors are described as either typical, i.e., alveolar, or solid. Typical alveolar rhabdomyosarcomas characteristically have fibrous bands that separate nests of minimally differentiated round cells (Fig. 11.32, eFig. 11.46). A layer of neoplastic cells clings to the fibrous tissue while the centrally located cells appear discohesive and aggregate within the centers of the alveolar spaces. The solid variant of alveolar rhabdomyosarcoma lacks the abundant fibrous bands (although some may be present) and the characteristic alveolar pattern, and is instead composed of larger nests and sheets of undifferentiated tumor cells (eFig. 11.47). The neoplastic cells are small with little cytoplasm and have round to oval hyperchromatic nuclei. Numerous mitotic figures are seen (eFig. 11.48). Often, larger multinucleated cells or cells with clear cytoplasm may be present (Fig. 11.33). Cross striations and

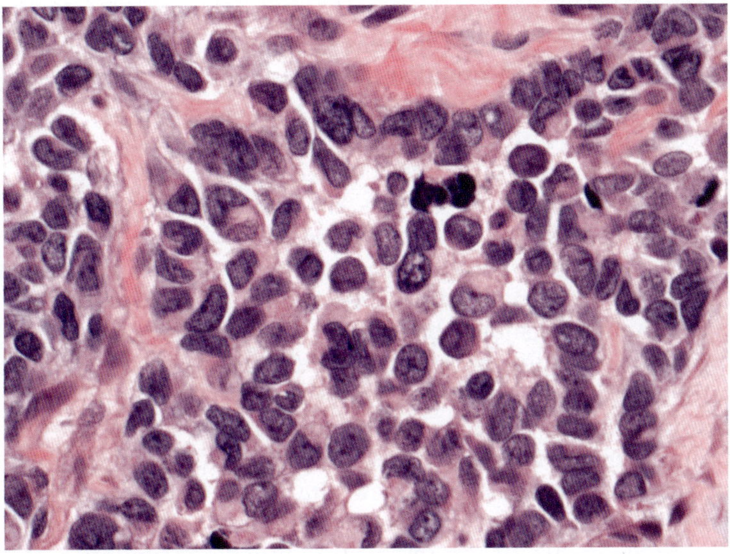

FIGURE 11.32 Primitive round cells with focal discohesion are seen in this alveolar rhabdomyosarcoma.

typical strap cells are not present in alveolar rhabdomyosarcoma; however, some tumors show a mixed phenotype with embryonal and alveolar areas (thus strap cells may be seen with some alveolar rhabdomyosarcomas). These tumors are considered alveolar, or at least treated as such.

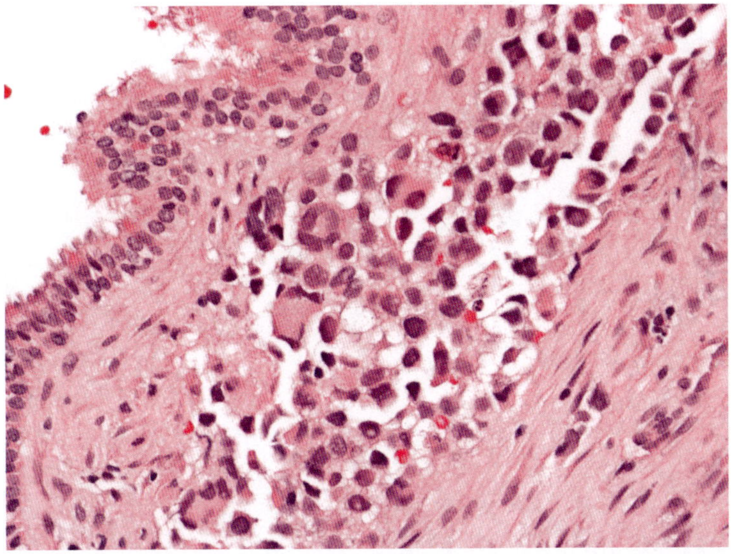

FIGURE 11.33 Larger, multinucleated cells are seen with this alveolar rhabdomyosarcoma.

Embryonal rhabdomyosarcomas (and, less commonly, alveolar rhabdomyosarcomas) can have focal areas of anaplasia characterized by cells with large, lobate hyperchromatic nuclei (three times the size of surrounding nuclei) and atypical mitotic figures (Fig. 11.34, eFig. 11.49).[77] This feature needs to be noted, as any amount of anaplasia carries a worse prognosis. Heterologous differentiation, usually neural, may also be seen (ectomesenchymoma). These tumors are best classified by their rhabdomyosarcoma component. Finally, posttreatment biopsies or resection specimen can show pronounced differentiation (eFig. 11.50). Inspection of these lesions for blastemal components should be performed and, if present, these components should be noted.

Ancillary techniques, such as molecular or cytogenetics, are extremely valuable for the classification of pediatric and young adult tumors. Furthermore, results may be necessary for the enrollment of patients into certain clinical trials. Unfortunately, by the time one is looking through a microscope at a rhabdomyosarcoma, many ancillary techniques are no longer possible. For this reason, the pathologist should be made aware of the impending biopsy of pediatric and young adult tumors. Tissue can then be collected for conventional cytogenetics and other studies, such as flow cytometry, and tissue can be frozen for other possible studies.

Alveolar rhabdomyosarcomas frequently have the t(1;13)(p36;q14) or t(2;13)(q35;q14) juxtaposing the *FKHR* gene with either the *PAX7* or *PAX3* genes, respectively.[74,75] These translocations can be identified by conventional cytogenetics, RT-PCR, or fluorescent in situ hybridization. Embryonal rhabdomyosarcomas do not have a characteristic translocation;

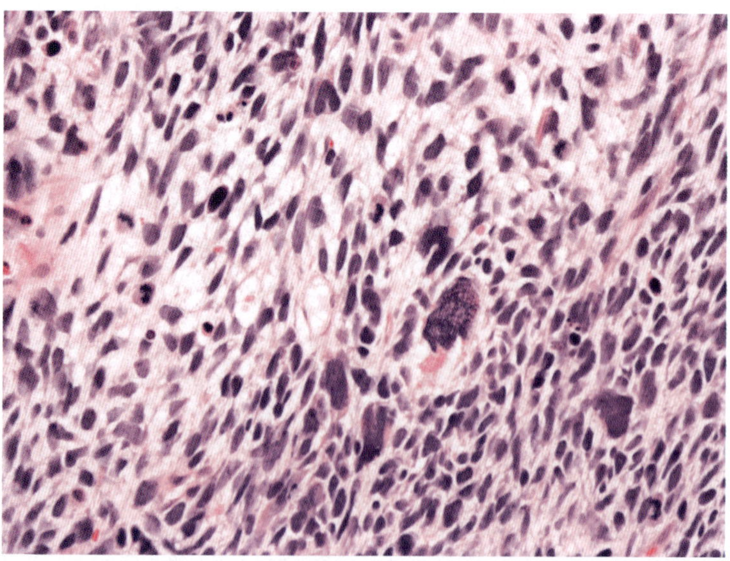

FIGURE 11.34 Anaplasia was identified in this embryonal rhabdomyosarcoma.

however, they frequently have been shown to have allelic loss at 11p15. Although, the diagnosis of these sarcomas is still based on histologic features, identification of the t(1;13) or t(2;13) should lead one to strongly favor a diagnosis of alveolar rhabdomyosarcoma.

Immunohistochemically, rhabdomyosarcomas express skeletal muscle antigens. Most tumors react with antibodies to desmin, MSA, myoglobin, myogenin, and MyoD1 (Figs. 11.35 and 11.36, eFigs. 11.51 and 11.52).[42,74,77,82] Most tumors do not show immunoreactivity with antibodies to S100 protein, cytokeratins, SMA, CD99, and lymphoid antigens; however, all have been noted in some cases.[77] Antibodies to FLI1 generally fail to react with these tumors.[83] Of note, some authors have found that alveolar rhabdomyosarcomas show more uniform and intense staining with antibodies to myogenin and MyoD1 than embryonal rhabdomyosarcomas.[84] PAX2, PAX5, and WT1 are more commonly expressed in alveolar rhabdomyosarcomas and may be helpful for distinguishing these tumors from embryonal rhabdomyosarcomas.[85–88] Cytoplasmic expression of p63 has also recently been shown to correlate with muscle differentiation.[89]

The differential diagnosis for rhabdomyosarcomas includes other small round cell tumors, especially the alveolar subtype. Histologically, the identification of differentiated rhabdomyoblasts is helpful; however, the diagnosis now rests to a great extent on the immunohistochemical findings. Embryonal rhabdomyosarcomas can be difficult to distinguish from rhabdomyomas and tumors with myofibroblastic differentiation, such as inflammatory myofibroblastic tumors (see above). Blastemal areas, increased mitotic activity, necrosis, and infiltrative borders all should lead

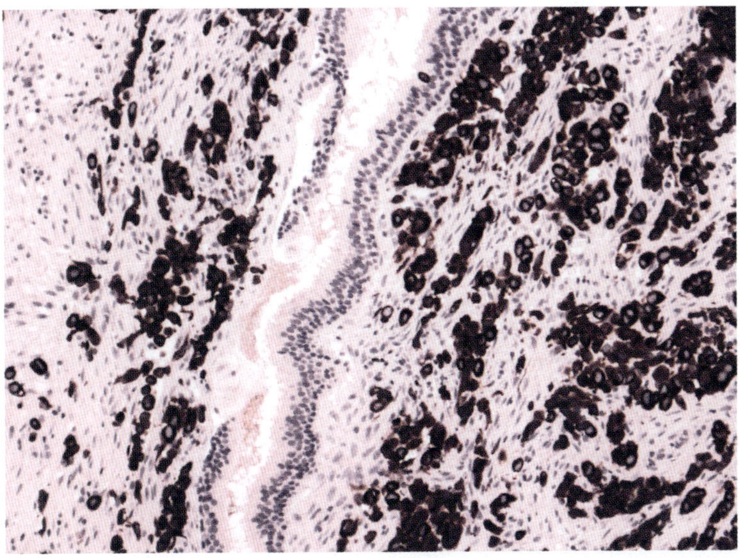

FIGURE 11.35 This rhabdomyosarcoma showed strong immunoreactivity with antibodies to desmin.

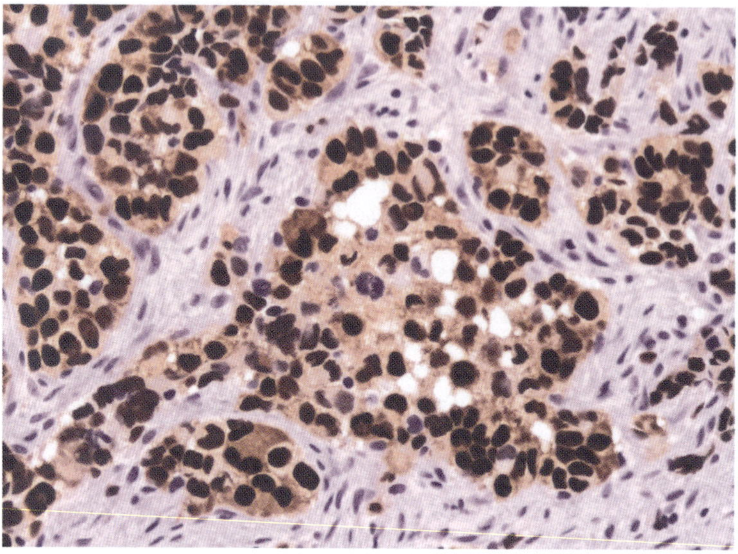

FIGURE 11.36 Strong and diffuse immunoreactivity is seen with antibodies to MyoD1 with this alveolar rhabdomyosarcoma.

one to favor a diagnosis of embryonal rhabdomyosarcoma. Also of note, DICER1-associated sarcomas can show abundant skeletal muscle differentiation similar to pleuropulmonary blastomas.[90]

VASCULAR TUMORS

Most vascular tumors can be identified within the upper aerodigestive tract; however, some seem especially prone to develop there, e.g., lobular capillary hemangioma and intravascular papillary endothelial hyperplasia (Table 11.4). Some tumors appear virtually unique to the area and do not show a definitive vascular phenotype, per se, but are nonetheless, classified as vascular neoplasms by convention (e.g., angiofibroma and glomangiopericytomas).

TABLE 11.4 Vascular Lesions of the Upper Aerodigestive Tract
Intravascular papillary endothelial hyperplasia
Hemangioma (lobular capillary, juvenile, cavernous)
Hemangioendothelioma (epithelioid)
Angiosarcoma (Kaposi, epithelioid, solid, not otherwise specified)
Angiofibroma
Glomangiopericytoma

Intravascular Papillary Endothelial Hyperplasia (Masson Tumor)

The endothelium of thrombosed vessels or other vascular lesions can undergo papillary hyperplasia and, as such, has been termed intravascular papillary endothelial hyperplasia.[91–93] These lesions can grow into masses and may occur in patients of any age, more often in women. They commonly involve the mouth, especially the lips and tongue. Intravascular papillary endothelial hyperplasia typically presents as a slow-growing mass that can measure up to 2 cm. Prior to biopsy, most are believed to be benign vascular proliferations. In the mouth, most involve single dilated vessels; however, lesions found elsewhere are often associated with lobular capillary or cavernous hemangiomas. Rarely, they develop outside of preexisting vascular structures in organizing hematomas. Tumors within vessels appear well-circumscribed, whereas those in hemangiomas retain the overall architecture of the preexisting lesion. The vascular spaces are filled with papillary fronds that fuse with one another and produce numerous slitlike spaces (Fig. 11.37). The stroma of the papillae may be either hyalinized or loose. The papillae are lined by a single layer of endothelial cells with large round to oval nuclei that project into the vascular spaces, producing in some cases a rather hobnail appearance (Fig. 11.38, eFig. 11.53). The nuclei can be atypical and hyperchromatic and mitotic figures can be identified.[92,93] Within the vascular spaces, fibrin thrombi and red cells are usually seen. By immunohistochemistry, the endothelial cells react with antibodies to CD31, CD34, and factor VIII–related antigen (eFig. 11.54).

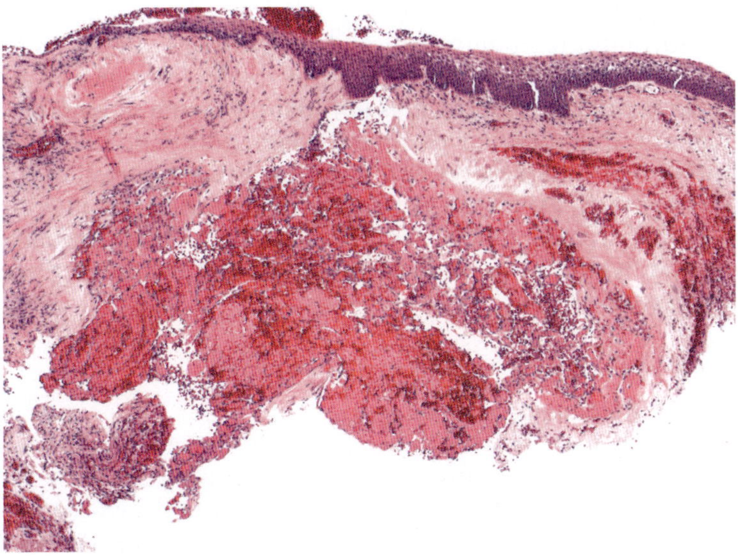

FIGURE 11.37 Intravascular papillary endothelial hyperplasia within a subepithelial clot.

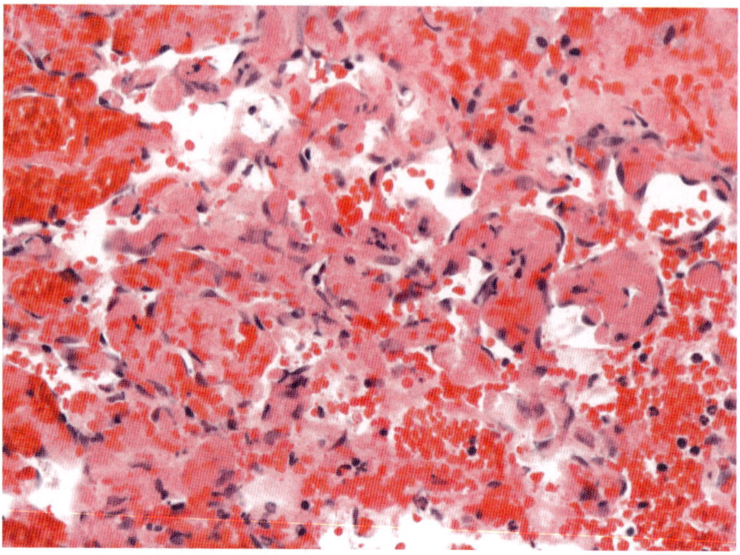

FIGURE 11.38 The endothelial cells of intravascular papillary endothelial hyperplasia show at most only mild atypia.

It is important to recognize intravascular papillary endothelial hyperplasia as it can be confused with angiosarcoma, and, less commonly, epithelioid hemangioendothelioma and papillary intralymphatic angioendothelioma (Dabska tumor). Intravascular papillary endothelial hyperplasia occurs in normal vessels or preexisting neoplastic vascular structures, unlike angiosarcomas. They also are associated with thrombotic material, show less cytologic atypia and mitotic activity than angiosarcomas, and do not exhibit tumor cell necrosis. Other intravascular tumors such as epithelioid hemangioendotheliomas and malignant endovascular papillary angioendotheliomas show more atypia and epithelioid features and have not been reported in the upper aerodigestive tract. Finally, a similar lesion to intravascular papillary endothelial hyperplasia called papillary intralymphatic angioendothelioma occurs in lymphatic vessels and has also not been described in the upper aerodigestive tract.[94]

Hemangioma

All forms of hemangioma occur throughout the upper aerodigestive tract.[95–99] The most common of these is the lobular capillary hemangioma, the so-called pyogenic granuloma or epulis of pregnancy.[98] These tumors most frequently involve the lip, nasal cavity, and oral mucosa and occur over a wide age range. It is interesting that most children affected are male, whereas affected young adults are more frequently female. Also of note, gingival lesions frequently are associated with pregnancy. Lobular capillary hemangiomas usually present with bleeding and are typically described as ulcerated and pedunculated red masses. These tumors are universally benign and only rarely recur.

Histologically, the tumors can appear pedunculated and may have a surrounding "collar" formed by the downward growth of squamous epithelium.[97,98] Most tumors extend to depths deeper than this epithelium, however. Lobules of closely packed, bland endothelial cells that show more obvious lumen formation toward the surface of the lesion are present in all lesions (Figs. 11.39 and 11.40, eFigs. 11.55–11.57). Deeper portions of these tumors have more dense-appearing stroma that surrounds the capillary lobules and contains scattered inflammatory cells (eFig. 11.58). The more superficial stroma has more edema and, when it is ulcerated, has many neutrophils. Fibrin and typical granulation tissue are usually seen in such cases (eFigs. 11.59 and 11.60). The number of mitotic figures can vary greatly, and abundant mitotic figures should not lead one to necessarily worry about malignancy (eFig. 11.61).

These tumors are easily distinguished from other vascular tumors that can be found throughout the upper aerodigestive tract. The lobular pattern of growth should distinguish them from granulation tissue, other types of hemangiomas, nasopharyngeal angiofibromas, or glomangiopericytomas. Furthermore, unlike nasopharyngeal angiofibromas, lobular capillary hemangiomas do not typically involve the nasopharynx. Small biopsies of mitotically active lobular capillary hemangiomas may lead one to consider a diagnosis of angiosarcoma. Lobular capillary hemangiomas should not be infiltrative nor do they have cytologic atypia. It should be noted that these tumors rarely occur in the larynx, and most lesions designated as

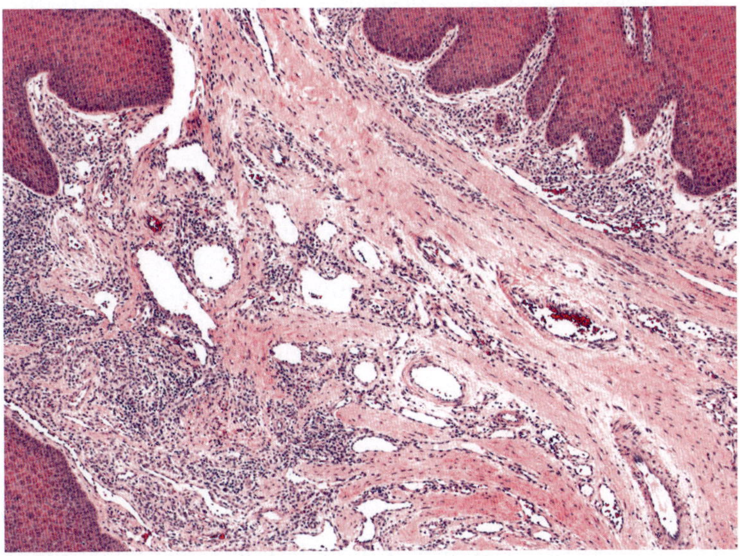

FIGURE 11.39 A lobular capillary hemangioma with intact overlying epithelium.

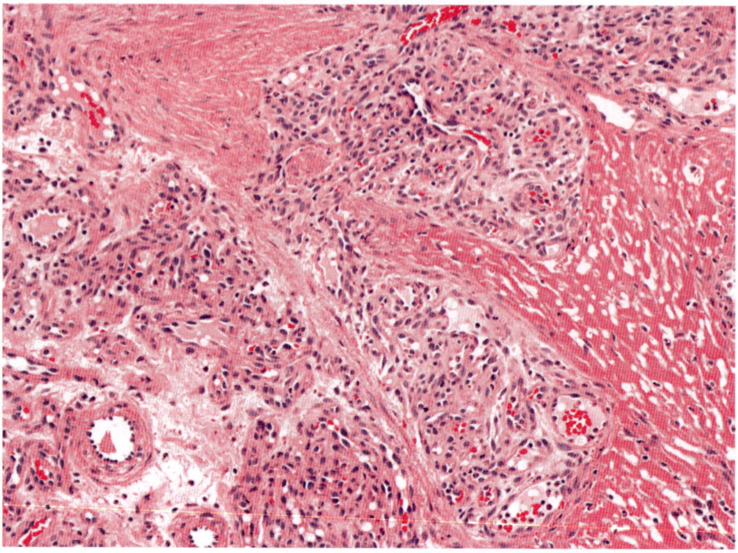

FIGURE 11.40 Lobules of capillaries are seen with lobular capillary hemangiomas.

such have been found to be granulation tissue, usually developing after trauma.[100] Immunohistochemically, the lesions react with antibodies to endothelial antigens such as CD31, CD34, ERG, and factor VIII–related antigen.[101,102] Despite their association with pregnancy, antibodies to estrogen and progesterone receptors are not reactive.

Cavernous hemangiomas also can occur within the upper aerodigestive tract and appear histologically similar to their counterparts throughout the body with large dilated vessels lined by a flattened and bland endothelium.[95,97] In the larynx, these lesions are glottic or supraglottic and are more common in men.

Juvenile or *infantile hemangiomas* are also seen throughout the upper aerodigestive tract and can be associated with cutaneous hemangiomas.[96,99] When these tumors present in the larynges of infants, they are usually subglottic and can cause obstructive airway symptoms. These tumors are characteristically hypercellular and nodular with plump endothelial cells that can show brisk mitotic activity. Early lesions have less obvious vascular spaces. This, however, changes as the lesions age and involute. First the vascular spaces dilate, the endothelial cells eventually flatten, and mitotic activity decreases. With more time, the lesions become fibrotic and the vascular channels disappear.

Cavernous Lymphangioma

Cavernous lymphangioma or cystic hygroma is generally identified in the head and neck region of newborns, although other sites can be involved.[96,103] Large tumors may extend into the floor of mouth, larynx, or pharynx and can lead to airway obstruction. The lesions are treated surgically and often require multiple resections because of recurrences. Although these tumors are rarely associated with mortality, their large size and extensive infiltration of normal tissues can lead to significant morbidity.

Grossly, cavernous lymphangiomas are lobulated and spongy.[96,103] They are histologically characterized by large, dilated lymphatics that contain lymph and lymphocytes. These are lined by a flattened, inconspicuous, layer of bland endothelial cells (Fig. 11.41, eFig. 11.62). Lymphoid tissue and smooth muscle may surround some of the larger lymphatic channels. The lesions can become acutely infected and will then contain an associated inflammatory infiltrate. Older lesions may show fibrosis.

Angiofibroma

Nasopharyngeal angiofibromas are tumors of male adolescents.[104–107] In fact, they almost universally arise during the second decade of life, consistent with the now widely accepted theory that they are androgen dependent. Some of the rare cases that have been reported in girls have been found to be other tumors when rereviewed.[107] The tumors extend from the posterior lateral nasal wall or the nasopharynx and often lead to nasal obstruction. Epistaxis and nasal drainage are also typically seen. Nasopharyngeal angiofibromas may sometimes be locally aggressive and can extend into surrounding tissues. Most, however, will behave in a benign fashion, and only 20% will recur. Even patients who have recurrent lesions can eventually be cured. Patients with familial adenomatous polyposis (FAP) have been found to be 25 times more likely to have nasopharyngeal angiofibromas

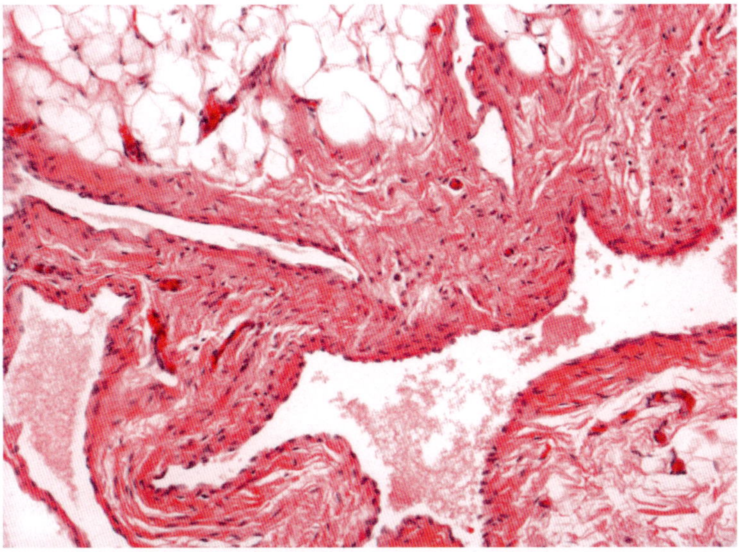

FIGURE 11.41 A cavernous lymphangioma has bland endothelium lining lymphatic spaces.

than the general public, implying that mutations of the adenomatous polyposis coli gene may be involved in the pathogenesis of these tumors.[108,109]

Nasopharyngeal angiofibromas are often not biopsied because their clinical features are considered diagnostic and biopsy can lead to severe bleeding. In controlled circumstances, however, our clinicians do feel comfortable biopsying these lesions when needed. Grossly, the tumors are polypoid and firm.[104–107] Histologically, they are composed of a rich network of variably sized, irregularly shaped vessels within a low to moderately cellular stroma (Fig. 11.42). The vessel wall thickness can vary from a single layer of endothelium to vessels with multiple layers of smooth muscle that can appear hyalinized or "padlike" (eFig. 11.63). The vessels can be thrombosed either naturally or, in the case of resected specimens, with preoperatively injected material (eFig. 11.64).

The stromal tissue is composed mostly of thick and thin fibrils of collagen and can appear variably cellular. Numerous oval to spindled to stellate stromal cells arrange themselves haphazardly throughout the lesions (Fig. 11.43, eFig. 11.65). These cells are bland and have a small to moderate amount of eosinophilic cytoplasm and bland oval nuclei with fine chromatin and small, indistinct nucleoli. Occasional atypical and multinucleated cells can be seen, but mitotic figures are rare. The overlying respiratory-type epithelium can be intact or eroded and, when intact, may undergo squamous metaplasia. Background mast cells are invariably present, often in large numbers. Rarely, these tumors undergo sarcomatous "transformation," almost invariably after the patients have received radiation therapy.[110,111]

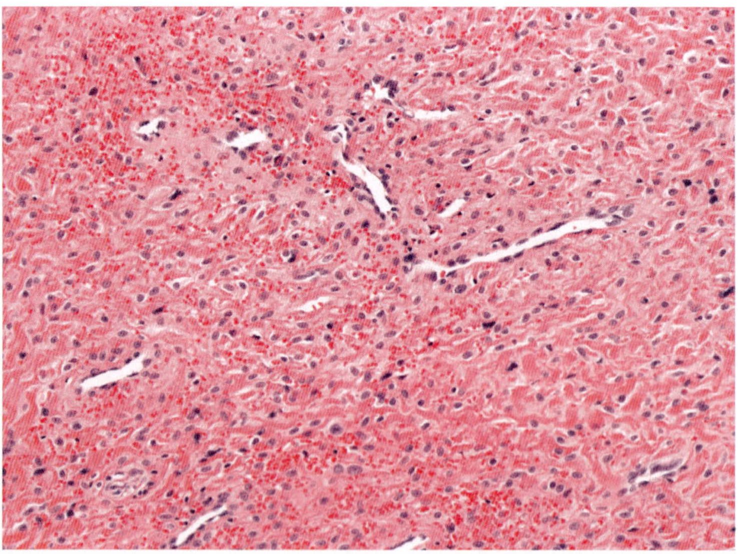

FIGURE 11.42 A moderately cellular stoma with numerous irregular shaped vessels is seen with this angiofibroma.

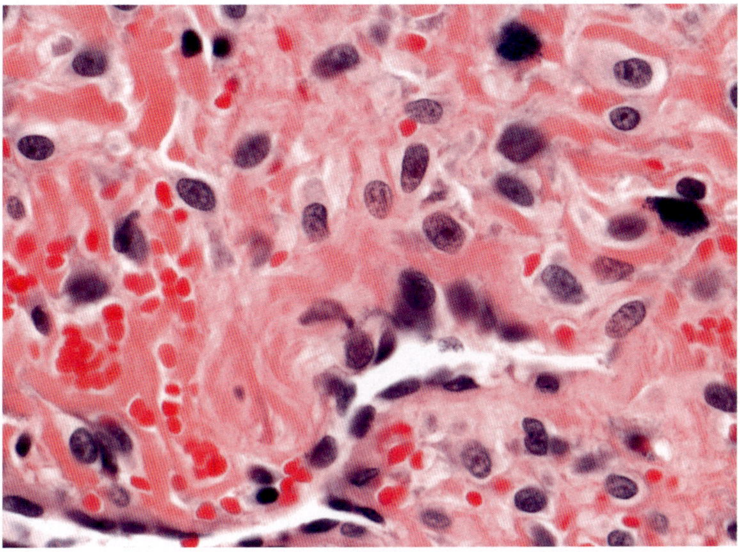

FIGURE 11.43 The stroma cells of an angiofibroma are bland and background mast cells can often be identified.

Immunohistochemically, the lesions show nonspecific but expected findings.[112] The endothelial cells react with antibodies to typical endothelial antigens such as CD31, CD34, or factor VIII–related antigen. The focal smooth muscle surrounding these vessels typically shows immunoreactivity with antibodies to SMA and can react with antibodies to desmin. The stromal cells are usually noted to show immunoreactivity only with antibodies to vimentin. Androgen receptors have been identified by immunohistochemistry in both the stromal and endothelial cells, whereas most cases will show no immunoreactivity with antibodies to estrogen or progesterone receptors.[113] Supporting a possible relationship to FAP, nuclear localization of β-catenin has also been reported.[114]

Glomangiopericytoma and Glomus Tumor

Most tumors previously classified as hemangiopericytomas of the sinonasal area are, in fact, more phenotypically and immunophenotypically similar to glomus tumors than to solitary fibrous tumors/hemangiopericytomas.[23,115,116] As such, the current WHO classification scheme for tumors of the nasal cavities and paranasal sinuses designates them as glomangiopericytomas.[117]

Glomangiopericytomas most frequently arise in the nasal cavities, or, less often, involve the paranasal sinuses.[23,115,118,119] The tumors are slightly more common in women and can arise at any age. The mean age of presentation is in the seventh decade. Patients present with nonspecific symptoms such as obstruction and epistaxis. The tumors behave very well and more than 95% of patients have no recurrence after initial surgical resection. Rare cases do behave more aggressively, however, and can eventually lead to the death of the patient.

Grossly, the lesions are typically described as polypoid and are noted to be free of surface ulceration.[23,115,118,119] Histologically, glomangiopericytomas are cellular neoplasms that usually have an intact overlying epithelium (Fig. 11.44, eFig. 11.66). The neoplastic cells efface most of the normal structures, but residual seromucinous glands can often be identified. The cells are spindle-shaped or oval and grow in fascicular, storiform, whorled, palisaded, and reticular patterns (Fig. 11.45, eFig. 11.67). The neoplastic cells have indistinct cell borders with a small amount of eosinophilic cytoplasm. Nuclei have blunt ends and rarely display more than mild atypia (Fig. 11.46, eFig. 11.68). Mitotic figures are infrequent. Numerous small, thin-walled vessels course through the tumors and typically have a "staghorn" appearance. Occasionally these vessels are surrounded by a small cuff of acellular fibrosis. Mast cells, eosinophils, and extravasated red cells are usually present.

Immunohistochemically, the neoplastic cells react with antibodies to SMA, MSA, and factor XIIIa (eFig. 11.69).[23] Of note, the neoplastic cells do not react with antibodies to cytokeratins, desmin, CD34, STAT6, S100 protein, bcl-2, factor VIII, and CD31.[34] The immunophenotype of these tumors is extremely helpful and allows for the ready distinction of these tumors from histologically similar tumors such as solitary fibrous tumors and the vast variety of vascular, smooth muscle, neural, and other mesenchymal tumors that may be considered (Table 11.1). Recently, these

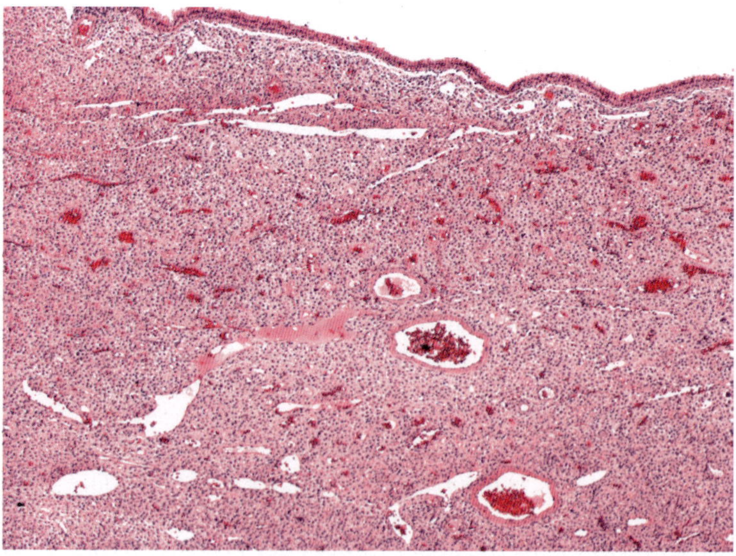

FIGURE 11.44 Glomangiopericytomas have a cellular stroma and numerous small vessels.

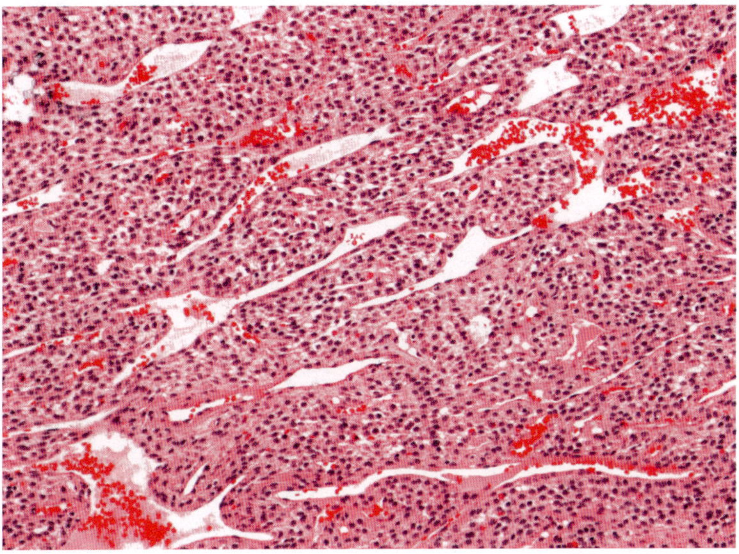

FIGURE 11.45 A hemangiopericytoid area in a glomangiopericytoma.

tumors have been shown to have gain-of-function mutations of *CTNNB1* and secondary strong nuclear expression of β-catenin (Fig. 11.47).[120]

More typical glomus tumors (not the misnamed paragangliomas) have rarely been noted to involve the upper aerodigestive tract and only few scattered reports of these tumors in the upper aerodigestive tract

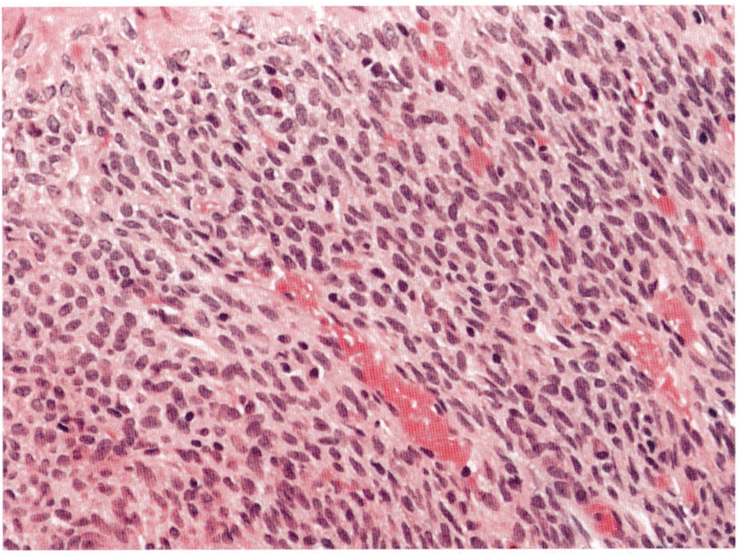

FIGURE 11.46 The stromal cells of this glomangiopericytoma are oval and bland with blunt-ended nuclei.

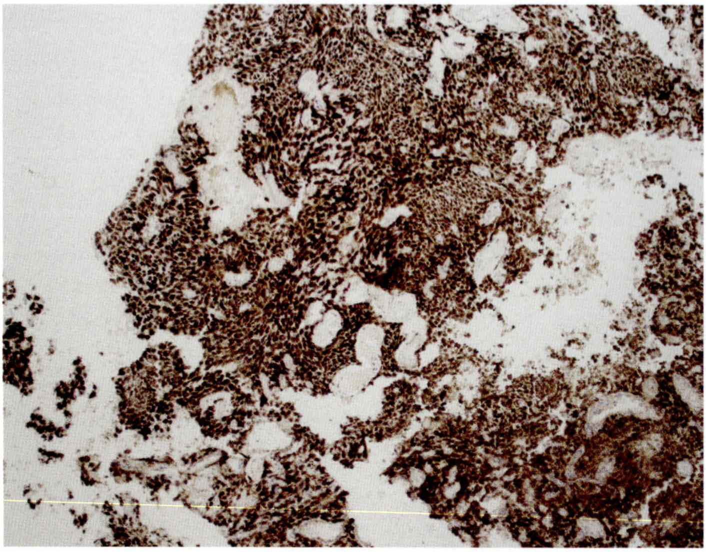

FIGURE 11.47 A glomangiopericytoma showing diffuse nuclear expression of β-catenin.

exist.[97,121] Here, they appear akin to those of the skin and are characterized by a cellular proliferation of small, round, monomorphic cells with centrally placed round nuclei. Numerous small vessels are usually noted which, in some cases, can be larger and more prominent. As with glomangiopericytomas, the neoplastic cells are immunoreactive with antibodies to SMA and not with antibodies to CD34.

Hemangioendothelioma

Hemangioendotheliomas are intermediate-grade vascular malignancies. They are subclassified based upon morphology into a few clinicopathologic entities (e.g., epithelioid hemangioendothelioma, retiform hemangioendothelioma, pseudomyogenic hemangioendothelioma). The most common variant to involve the mucosa of the upper aerodigestive tract is epithelioid hemangioendothelioma.

Epithelioid hemangioendothelioma is associated with a *WWTR1-CAMTA1* translocation.[122] The tumors occur slightly more often in women and can present in patients of any age.[123,124] They have been reported to involve most sites of the head and neck but appear to occur most commonly within the mouth.[125–128] Characteristically, tumors are composed of chains of epithelioid endothelial cells evenly dispersed within a myxohyaline stroma (Fig. 11.48). Intracytoplasmic vacuoles are present that deform the cells and give them a characteristic "blister cell" appearance. These sometimes contain red cells. Mild to moderate nuclear atypia may be seen along with occasional mitotic figures. The tumors should appear "less" malignant than epithelioid angiosarcomas. Neoplastic cells are

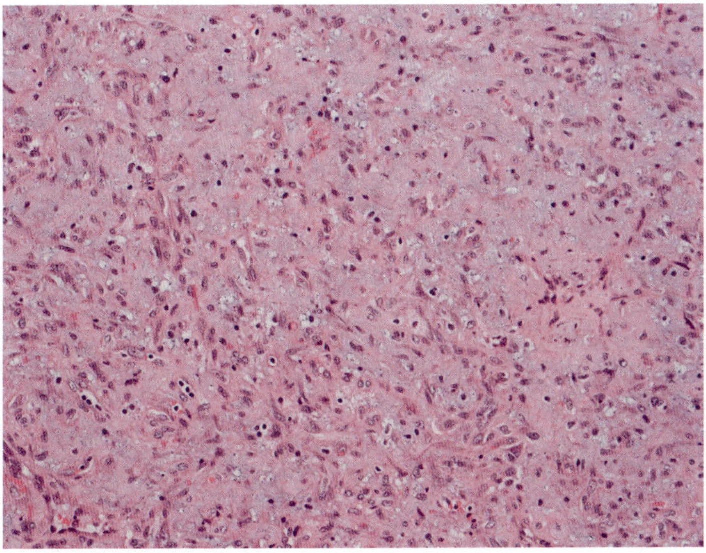

FIGURE 11.48 Epithelioid hemangioendothelioma with typical myxohyaline stroma.

immunoreactive with antibodies to vascular antigens such as CD31, CD34, and ERG.[102] Up to 40% of cases express keratins. The tumors are apt to recur; however, they metastasize infrequently.

Angiosarcoma

Variants of angiosarcoma have been described involving the upper aerodigestive tract.[97,129-135] By far, the most common is Kaposi sarcoma. In fact, Kaposi sarcoma represented approximately two-thirds of the oral spindle cell lesions seen at the University of San Francisco between 1982 and 2002.[132]

Kaposi sarcoma can develop in different scenarios and may be classic, endemic, iatrogenic, and AIDS-associated.[136] When it develops in the upper aerodigestive tract, it is almost always associated with AIDS; thus the lesions most commonly affect young to middle-aged men.[132] The tumors are now known to be secondary to HHV-8 infection. Kaposi sarcoma is considered an intermediate-grade vascular malignancy and is characterized by locally aggressive growth in HIV patients, typically with multisite involvement.

Kaposi sarcoma typically presents as a violaceous, nodular discoloration.[129,136] Histologically, the lesions differ somewhat throughout their natural history. Early lesions are characterized by nonspecific vascular proliferations. Eventually, the endothelial cells develop more atypia, become more infiltrative, and make less well-formed vessels. Once the tumors are fully developed and nodular, they are hypercellular and composed of spindled cells with mild cytologic atypia (Fig. 11.49, eFig. 11.70). Numerous slitlike vascular spaces are usually seen filled with red cells and hyaline droplets (eFig. 11.71).

Kaposi sarcoma must be distinguished from other spindle cell tumors. This can easily be done with immunohistochemistry, and the neoplastic cells of Kaposi sarcoma react diffusely and strongly with antibodies to endothelial antigens such as ERG, CD31, CD34, and factor VIII–related antigen.[102,132,136] Nuclear immunoreactivity with antibodies to HHV-8 will be seen and can help distinguish these tumors from other vascular lesions (Fig. 11.50, eFig. 11.72).[136] The main differential here is with Kaposiform hemangioendothelioma, a lesion that most commonly develops in children, rarely involves sites other than the retroperitoneum and distal extremities, and is not associated with HHV-8.[137]

More conventional types of angiosarcoma arise throughout the upper aerodigestive tract and the full spectrum of histologic appearances associated with this malignancy may be seen.[97,130,131,133–135] Angiosarcomas have been noted in the mouth, sinonasal area, and larynx and usually develop in adults, although the age range is large. Some patients reportedly received radiation treatment prior to the development of their tumors and some lesions that develop on the lips have been postulated to be secondary to sun exposure. The reported outcomes have been somewhat disparate, and, in one report, only two of eight patients with oral angiosarcoma with follow-up died of their disease.[130] A number of patients underwent wide excisions and were alive without disease more than 10 years after their original diagnoses. It should be emphasized that studies of these series have few patients and, we suspect, that some have included cases of intravascular papillary endothelial hyperplasia, lobular capillary hemangiomas, or reactive conditions.[138] If correctly diagnosed, these tumors should behave as dismally as other soft tissue angiosarcomas.

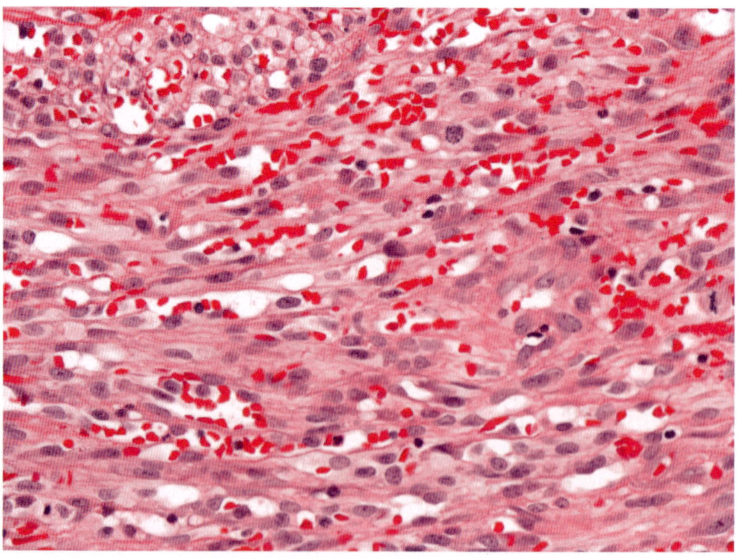

FIGURE 11.49 A Kaposi sarcoma with identifiable vascular channels.

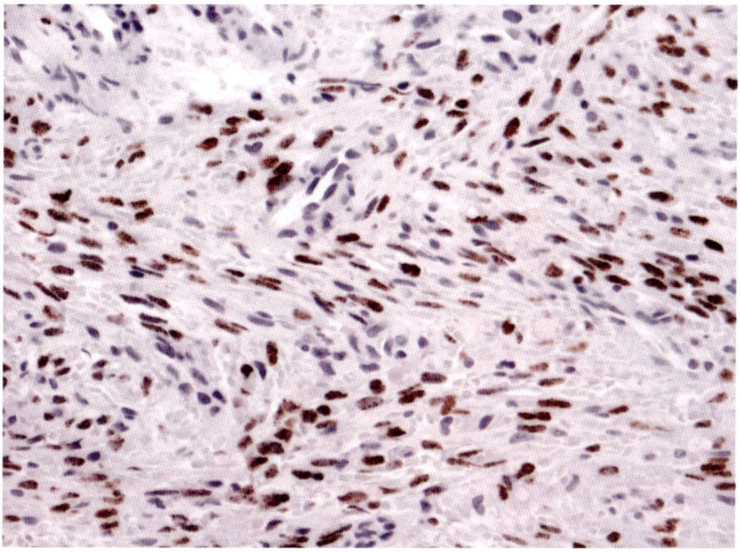

FIGURE 11.50 Nuclear immunoreactivity with antibodies to HHV-8 can be seen with most Kaposi sarcomas.

Angiosarcomas may have quite variable histology.[97,130,131,133] Better differentiated tumors characteristically are highly vasoformative and have irregular vessels that dissect through surrounding stroma and normal structures (Fig. 11.51). These are lined by endothelial cells that

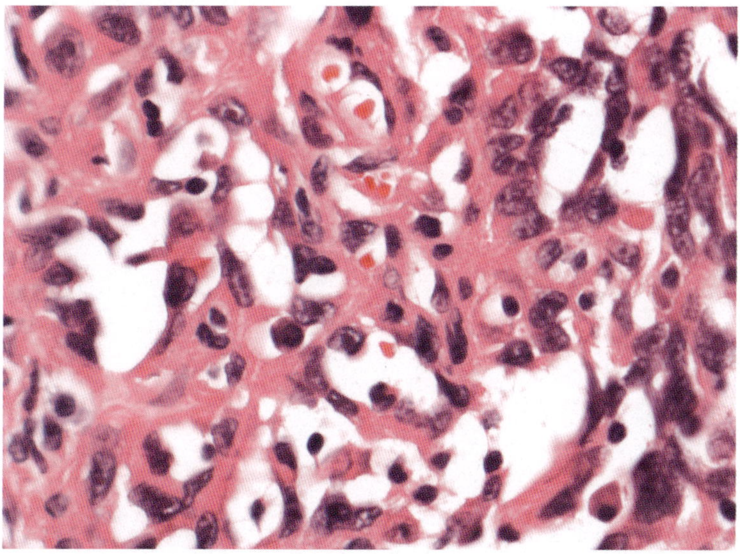

FIGURE 11.51 Irregular vessels with prominent endothelial atypia are seen in this angiosarcoma.

typically display at least moderate nuclear atypia with enlarged, pleomorphic, hyperchromatic nuclei; mitotic figures can usually be identified (eFig. 11.73). As tumors become less well-differentiated, the endothelial cells become more layered and numerous papillary growths can be found. Eventually, the vascular channels come to be harder to identify. The tumors develop a more solid appearance and the neoplastic cells themselves become more spindled. Some poorly differentiated variants will have larger, more epithelioid cells (*epithelioid angiosarcoma*) (Fig. 11.52, eFig. 11.74). These larger cells can have intracytoplasmic lumina replete with red cells.

Angiosarcomas are typically immunoreactive with antibodies to CD31, CD34, ERG, and factor VIII–related antigen (Fig. 11.53, eFig. 11.75).[130,131,133,139] It may be advisable to stain for multiple vascular antigens, as particular antigens may not be expressed by any given malignancy. Epithelioid angiosarcomas may focally be immunoreactive with antibodies to cytokeratins (eFig. 11.76).[102,140]

Distinguishing angiosarcomas from other sarcomas is generally easily accomplished using immunohistochemical stains. Although, epithelioid angiosarcomas may show focal reactivity with antibodies to cytokeratins, they will also be immunoreactive for antibodies to CD31 or other vascular antigens, thus allowing for an easy distinction from carcinoma. Angiosarcomas show much more pleomorphism than benign vascular tumors such as intravascular papillary endothelial hyperplasia or hemangioma.

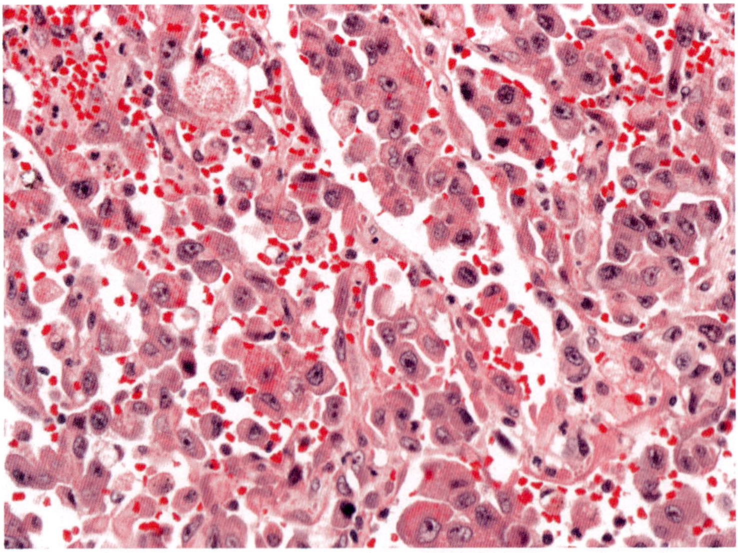

FIGURE 11.52 Some angiosarcomas may have a more epithelioid phenotype.

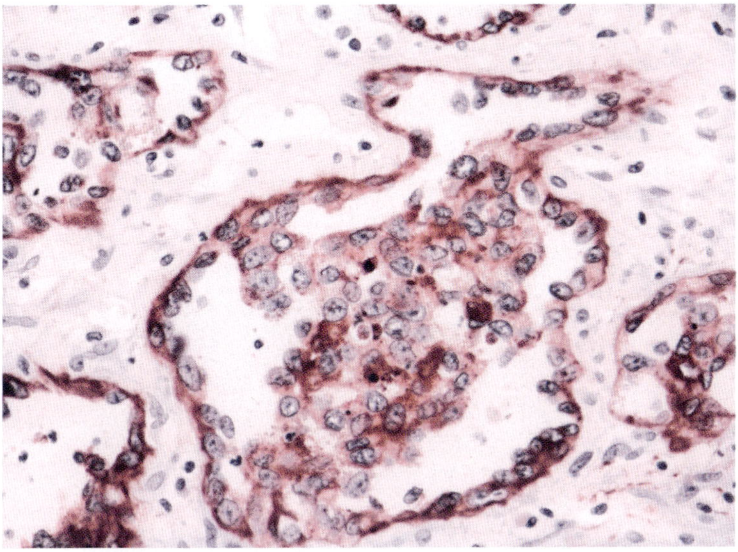

FIGURE 11.53 This epithelioid angiosarcoma showed strong immunoreactivity with antibodies to CD31.

FATTY TUMORS

Most fatty tumors have been described to involve the upper aerodigestive tract.[141–148] The majority are benign lipomas. Liposarcomas, especially well-differentiated liposarcomas or atypical lipomatous tumors, can rarely occur in this region. While lipoblastomas have been reported in the head and neck, they have only very rarely been reported in the upper aerodigestive tract.

Lipoma

Lipomas of the upper aerodigestive tract are uncommon and are usually solitary.[141–143,146,149] They more commonly involve the larynx and mouth, especially the buccal mucosa, and involvement of the sinonasal area and nasopharynx is extremely rare. The tumors are more common in men, usually arise in adults, and are, for the most part, composed of mature adipose tissue (eFig. 11.77). Other varieties of lipoma, such as *spindle cell lipoma* (i.e., *pleomorphic lipoma)* and *chondroid lipoma,* have also been reported and actually make up a higher proportion of the lipomas at these sites than at other sites within the body (Fig. 11.54, eFig. 11.78).[143] It is important to exclude well-differentiated liposarcomas, and a careful search for lipoblasts should be made. A distinction often cannot be made with a biopsy specimen, and a nonspecific diagnosis of *lipomatous neoplasm* should be used when necessary. In such cases, FISH for *MDM2* may be helpful as the gene is typically amplified in well-differentiated liposarcomas.[150] It is also important to retain spindle cell lipoma in one's

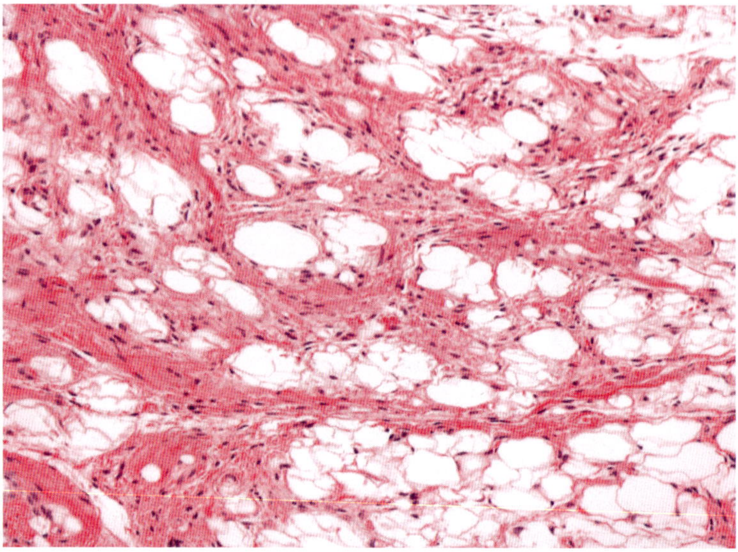

FIGURE 11.54 A spindle cell lipoma of the tongue with numerous spindled cells encircling mature adipose tissue.

differential diagnosis when looking at small biopsies of spindle cell lesions and to remember that these cells may be immunoreactive with antibodies to CD34.[151] Lipomas are cured with resection.

Liposarcoma

Liposarcomas have been reported throughout the upper aerodigestive tract, most often in the mouth and larynx.[144,145,147,148,152,153] Within the mouth, they have most commonly been identified in the tongue. In the larynx they are usually located either supraglottically or have been noted to involve the hypopharynx. Liposarcomas are malignancies of adults and they generally present as painless, slowly growing masses. Almost all liposarcomas of this area are well-differentiated liposarcomas or atypical lipomatous tumors, although both myxoid/round cell and pleomorphic liposarcomas have been described. Although most surgeries for the oral tumors have been reported as *marginal*, very few tumors have recurred. As the first surgery for most laryngeal liposarcomas tends to be even more limited, recurrence is much more common at that site.

Most atypical lipomatous tumors or well-differentiated liposarcomas are infiltrative, although they may occasionally be circumscribed or even encapsulated.[145,147,148] Histologically, they are composed of mature-appearing adipocytes that vary in size and have enlarged, hyperchromatic nuclei (Figs. 11.55 and 11.56, eFig. 11.79). Lipoblasts can be identified but can vary greatly in number from case to case (Fig. 11.57). The adipose tissue is divided into lobules by fibrous septae that often contain atypical stromal cells, present in vessel walls (Fig. 11.58, eFigs. 11.80 and 11.81). Occasional tumors have more spindled cells admixed with the

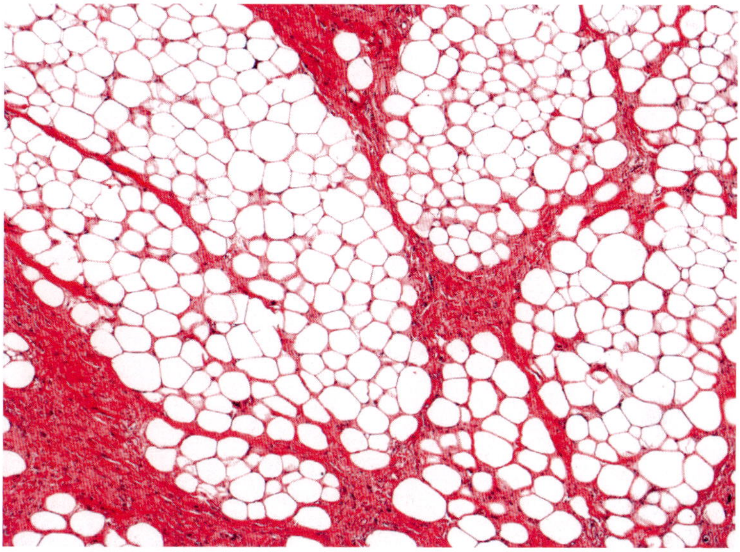

FIGURE 11.55 Well-differentiated liposarcomas have mature-appearing adipose tissue separated by fibrous bands.

adipocytes and lipoblasts. Mitotic figures are rare, and necrosis and hemorrhage are usually not seen. The adipocytes and lipoblasts usually show immunoreactivity with antibodies to S100 protein, whereas the spindled cells can be immunoreactive with antibodies to CD34.[145] FISH may be helpful because of the recurrent cytogenetic abnormalities seen with these

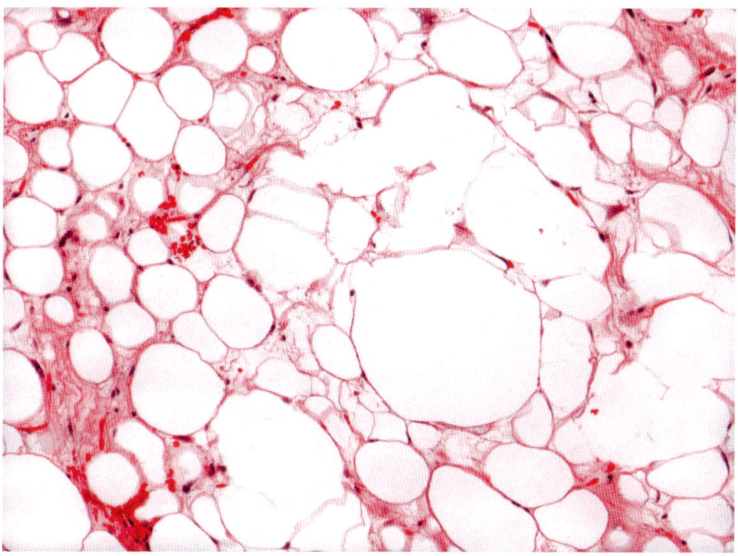

FIGURE 11.56 The adipocytes of a well-differentiated liposarcoma can vary greatly in size.

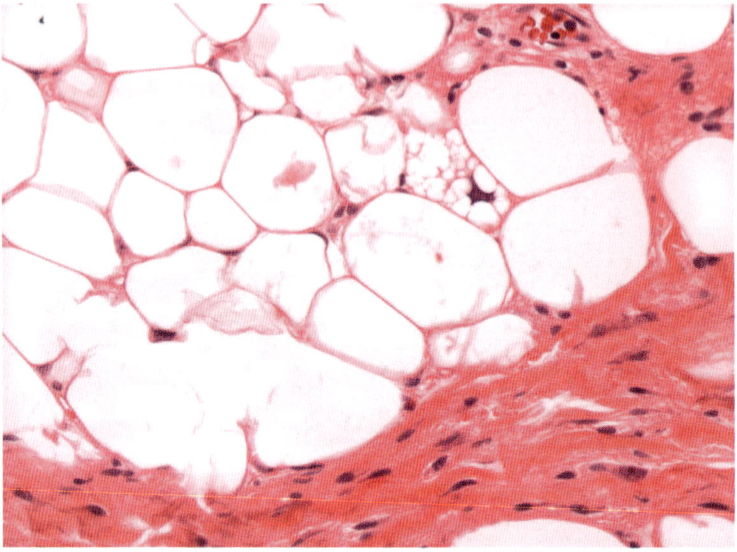

FIGURE 11.57 Rare lipoblasts can be found in most well-differentiated liposarcomas.

tumors. *MDM2* amplification is seen with most cases of well-differentiated and dedifferentiated liposarcomas. *DDIT3* and *FUS* rearrangements can be identified by FISH with most myxoid/round cell liposarcomas due to the recurrent t(12;16)(q13;p11) seen with these tumors.[154]

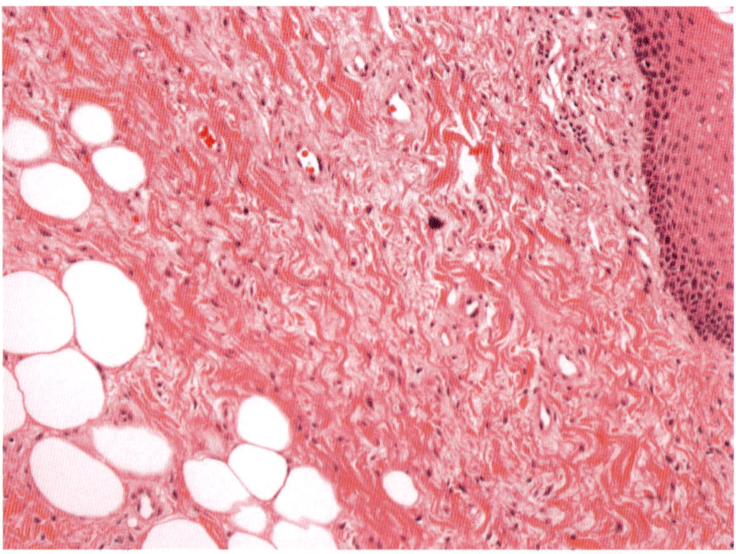

FIGURE 11.58 Atypical stromal cells may be seen in the fibrous tissue of a well differentiated liposarcoma.

OTHER TUMORS

A number of other mesenchymal tumors can involve the upper aerodigestive tract. Here we will discuss the lesions that are more common or have a propensity for involvement of the area.

(Low-Grade) Biphenotypic Sinonasal Sarcoma

Biphenotypic sinonasal sarcoma (BSS) is a low-grade sarcoma that appears to be unique to the sinonasal tract.[155–160] The tumors occur almost twice as often in women and the mean patient age at presentation is 52 years. The tumors can arise anywhere in the sinonasal tract but most often involve the nasal cavity or ethmoid sinuses. Patients typically present with nonspecific symptoms of obstruction or feeling of pressure. Local recurrence occurs in one-third to one-half of cases. Metastases have not been reported and death from tumor is very rare. The tumors have recurrent *PAX3* translocations usually with *MAML3*, less frequently with *NCOA1*, *FOXO1*, and *WWTR1*.[157,160]

Histologically, BSSs are hypercellular spindle cell proliferations with infiltrative borders (Fig. 11.59; eFig. 11.82).[157,159] Spindle cells typically extend to just beneath the surface epithelium and between seromucinous glands and invaginations of the surface epithelium. Entrapped epithelium can then appear proliferative or hyperplastic. Monotonous spindled cells are arranged in a fascicular or herringbone pattern. The nuclei are long and bland with fine chromatin and only occasional mitotic figures (1–4/hpf) are seen (Fig. 11.60). Necrosis is usually not present. Uncommonly, tumor cells may be more pleomorphic or may appear "rhabdoid."

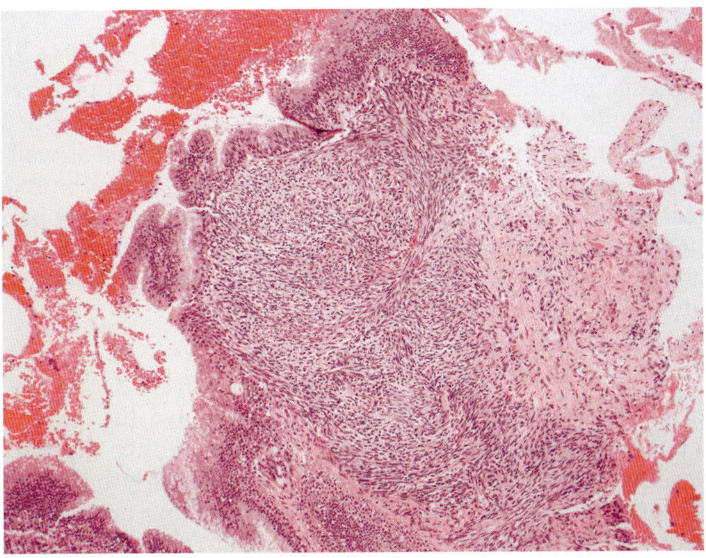

FIGURE 11.59 A fragment of a biphenotypic sinonasal sarcoma showing a hypercellular monotonous proliferation of spindle cells.

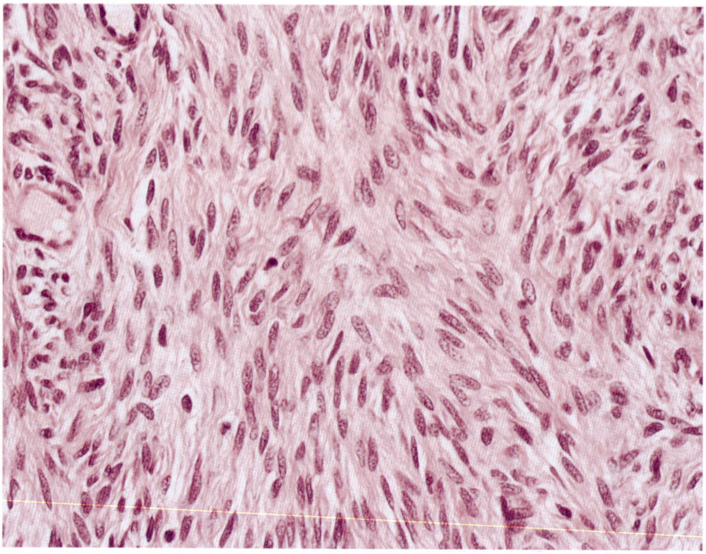

FIGURE 11.60 Biphenotypic sinonasal sarcomas are composed of bland spindle cells.

BSS was originally termed "low-grade sinonasal sarcoma with neural and myogenic differentiation" as tumor cells typically express both S100 and SMA (eFigs. 11.83 and 11.84).[155,157–159] SOX10 is not expressed; however, both desmin and MyoD1 are expressed focally in the majority of cases. PAX3 is also typically expressed secondary to the recurrent *PAX3* translocations.[156] Nuclear β-catenin and CD34 expression are seen focally in about 10% of cases.[157]

Other low-grade spindle cell neoplasms are included in the differential diagnosis for BSS. The identification of a *PAX3* translocation with low-grade spindle cell morphology would be specific for BSS; however, PAX3 expression by immunohistochemistry may work just as well for identification of the tumors. Nuclear β-catenin expression can be seen focally in some cases of BSS, whereas, in our experience, glomangiopericytomas show diffuse nuclear expression. If extrapleural solitary fibrous tumor is in the differential, STAT6 immunohistochemistry can also be used as it is specifically expressed in solitary fibrous tumors.[34]

Synovial Sarcoma

Between 5% and 10% of synovial sarcomas involve the head and neck and affect the upper aerodigestive tract through either direct extension or primary involvement.[161] They have most frequently been reported in the mouth and larynx.[162–166] The tumors arise at any age, but frequently occur in young adults. Larger tumors will appear radiographically destructive and tumors may be noted to have calcification or to be cystic. The tumor is characterized by the t(X;18)(p11;q11), which juxtaposes the *SS18* gene and either the *SSX1*, *SSX2*, or *SSX4* gene.[162,167,168] The prognosis for synovial sarcoma is similar to other sarcomas with a 5-year survival of approximately 50% to 60%.[169] Larger tumors and tumors with poorly differentiated areas do worse.

Histologically, the tumors are either biphasic, monophasic, or poorly differentiated.[163–166,170-173] Poorly differentiated areas may occur in tumors that are otherwise biphasic or monophasic. All synovial sarcomas appear cellular. Biphasic tumors have both epithelial and spindle cell components (Fig. 11.61). The proportions of these components vary from case to case and some examples may even appear predominately epithelial. The epithelial cells often line slitlike spaces and usually appear cuboidal to columnar (eFig. 11.85). They can form a single layer, be multilayered, or produce small papillary projections. The epithelial cells have a small to moderate amount of granular or finely vacuolated, lightly basophilic cytoplasm, and round to ovoid nuclei with vesicular chromatin and small nucleoli. The spindle cell component is cellular and should be reminiscent of fibrosarcoma and can even have a "herringbone" growth pattern. These areas tend to have less extracellular material than fibrosarcomas, but some synovial sarcomas have abundant myxoid or collagenous stroma. The stromal components are composed of small, immature-appearing spindle cells that usually have little cytoplasm with oval, tapered, or blunt-ended nuclei. Mitotic figures are usually plentiful and can be identified in both components. Monophasic synovial sarcomas are composed only of the stromal component and thus closely resemble fibrosarcomas (Figs. 11.62 and

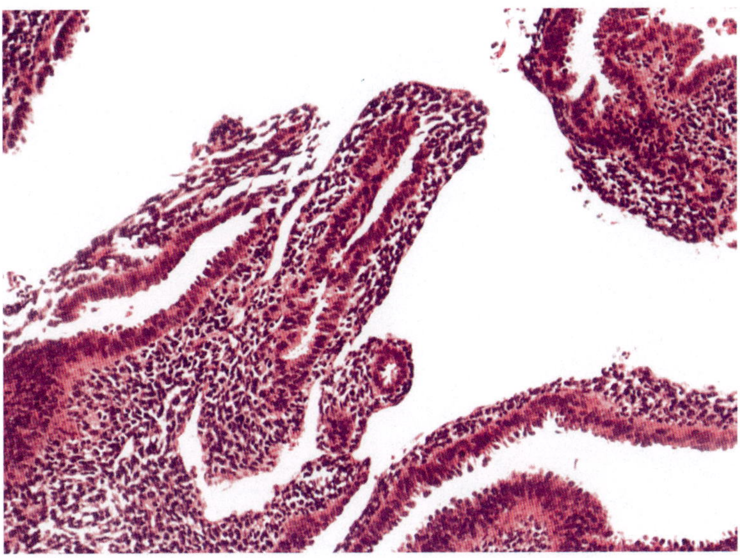

FIGURE 11.61 A biphasic synovial sarcoma with an obvious epithelial and stromal component.

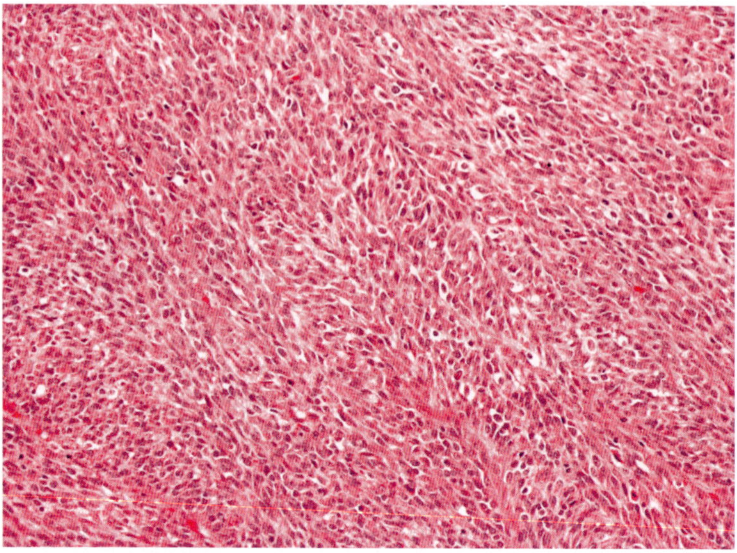

FIGURE 11.62 A monophasic synovial sarcoma is usually very cellular and often resembles a fibrosarcoma.

11.63, eFig. 11.86). Poorly differentiated tumors are more reminiscent of small blue cell tumors. They are composed of densely packed, rounded cells with little amphiphilic cytoplasm and round to oval nuclei with fine to vesicular chromatin (Fig. 11.64, eFig. 11.87).

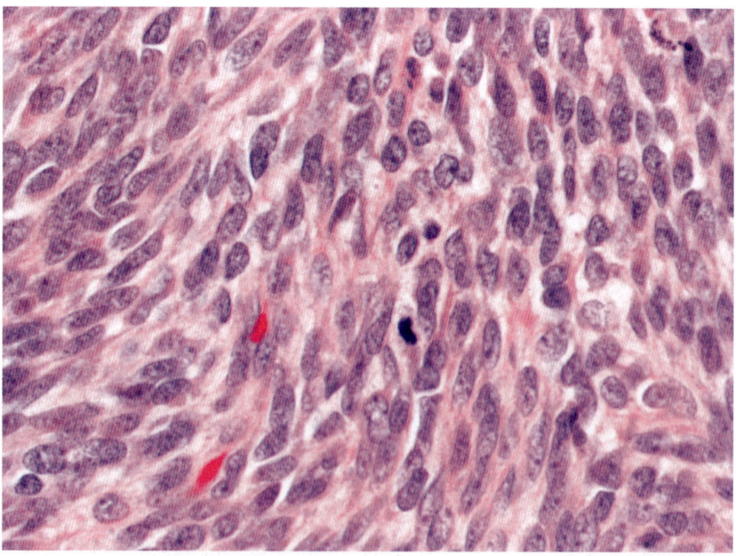

FIGURE 11.63 Monophasic synovial sarcomas may show little cellular atypia; however, abundant mitotic figures should be seen.

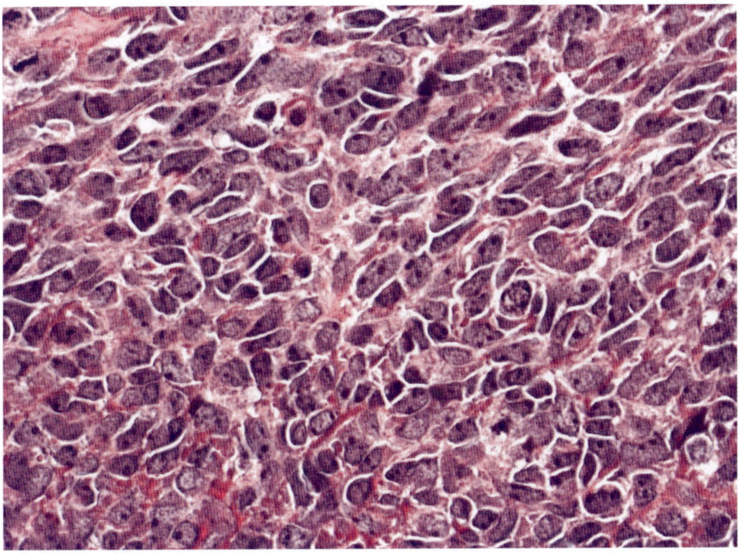

FIGURE 11.64 Poorly differentiated synovial sarcomas are composed of round, primitive-appearing cells.

By immunohistochemistry, all types of synovial sarcoma typically show immunoreactivity with antibodies to EMA and cytokeratins, although the spindle cell components do so less frequently and to a lesser degree than the epithelial components (Fig. 11.65, eFig. 11.88).[171,173,174]

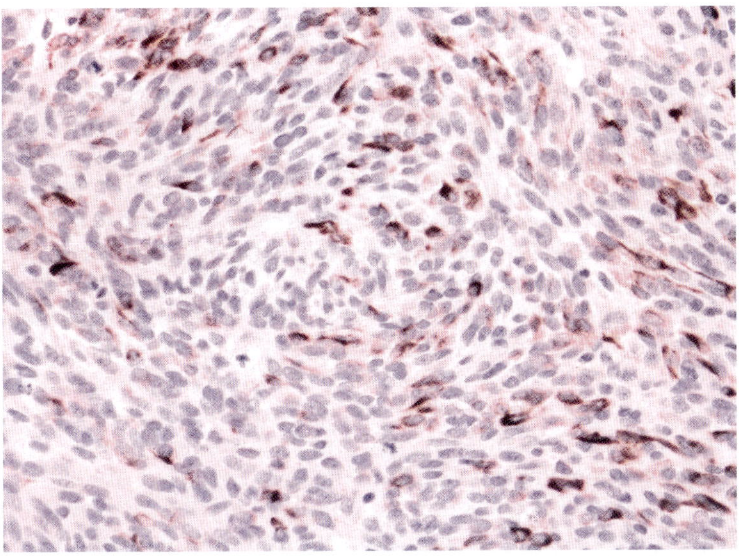

FIGURE 11.65 Immunoreactivity with antibodies to cytokeratin can be seen with most monophasic synovial sarcomas.

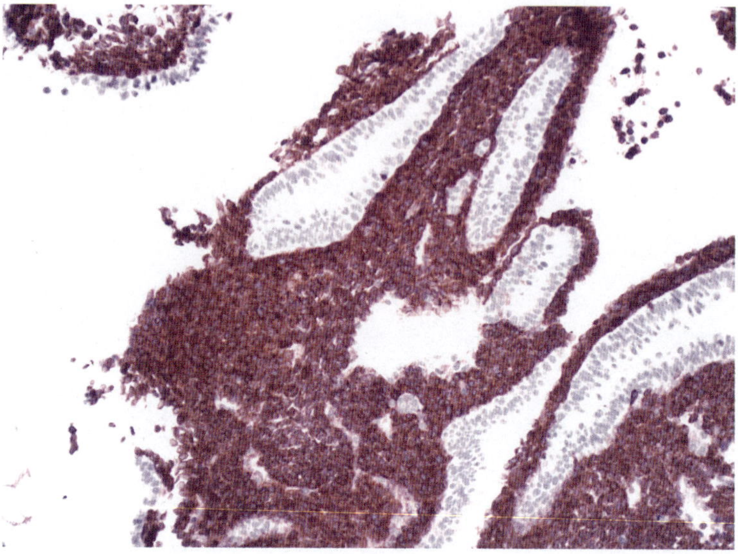

FIGURE 11.66 Strong immunoreactivity with antibodies to bcl-2 was seen in the stromal component of this synovial sarcoma.

Limited, focal immunoreactivity with antibodies to S100 protein has been noted, and tumors do not show immunoreactivity with antibodies to myogenous antigens. Both bcl-2 and CD99 (membranous) immunoreactivity have been reported in the majority of cases tested (Fig. 11.66, eFigs. 11.89 and 11.90).[151,175] The tumors are generally not immunoreactive with antibodies to CD34.

Biphasic synovial sarcomas have a distinct histologic appearance, and when immunohistochemistry is performed, it is usually just confirmatory (outside of sites such as the pleura where other biphasic malignancies are seen). The differential diagnosis for monophasic tumors is more extensive and includes malignant peripheral nerve sheath tumor, fibrosarcoma, glomangiopericytoma, and solitary fibrous tumor, among others (Table 11.5). Generally, immunohistochemistry can help to distinguish these lesions (Table 11.1). Cytokeratin or EMA immunoreactivity is seen with most synovial sarcomas and is usually not present in its mimics. CD34 immunoreactivity should be intense with most solitary fibrous tumors and glomangiopericytomas should express SMA. The differential for poorly differentiated tumors is also extensive (Table 11.6), and, again, immunohistochemistry can be very helpful. Most poorly differentiated synovial sarcomas will express cytokeratins or EMA by immunohistochemistry.[171] Antibodies to other markers, such as neuroendocrine or myogenous antigens, can also be used to distinguish these tumors. Finally, some have shown that most synovial sarcomas express TLE1, and that immunohistochemical staining for this marker can be helpful for distinguishing synovial sarcoma from its mimics.[35]

TABLE 11.5 Differential Diagnosis for Monophasic Synovial Sarcoma
Fibrosarcoma
Extrapleural solitary fibrous tumor
Malignant peripheral nerve sheath tumor
Biphenotypic sinonasal sarcoma
Glomangiopericytoma (in the sinonasal area)
Leiomyosarcoma
Low-grade myofibroblastic sarcoma

As was mentioned, synovial sarcomas classically have a t(X;18)(p11;q11).[162,167,168] This characteristic can be especially helpful for diagnosing both monophasic and poorly differentiated variants. As was mentioned previously, biopsies of soft tissue malignancies of the upper aerodigestive tract, especially those arising in children or young adults, should be triaged prior to formalin fixation and, when possible, tissue should be submitted for conventional cytogenetics and frozen. Conventional cytogenetics can identify many of the common translocations that allow for the distinction of these tumors, and frozen tissue allows for the identification of the various fusion transcripts by RT-PCR. Fluorescent in situ hybridization can be performed on formalin-fixed tissue and also can be used to identify classic rearrangements.

Alveolar Soft Part Sarcoma

Alveolar soft part sarcomas (ASPSs) are extremely rare soft tissue malignancies.[176,177] In some series, more than 10% involved the head and neck, and they are especially prone to affect the upper aerodigestive tract and tongue.[177–179] These are sarcomas of younger patients, and the mean age of diagnosis reported in most studies is in the third decade of life. Most patients present with high stage disease and do poorly. Disparate results have been published for patients with localized disease, however, and some

TABLE 11.6 Differential Diagnosis for Poorly Differentiated Synovial Sarcoma
Primitive neuroectodermal tumor
Rhabdomyosarcoma
Mesenchymal chondrosarcoma
Undifferentiated carcinoma

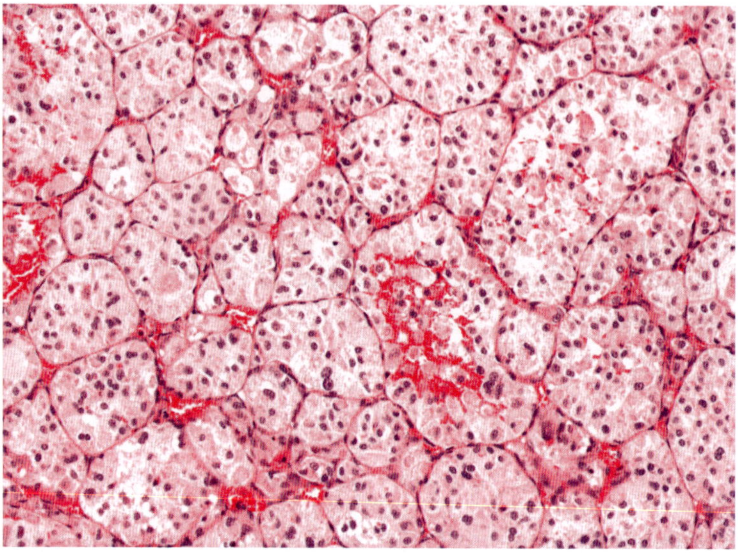

FIGURE 11.67 An alveolar soft part sarcoma with an obvious nested growth pattern.

have noted prolonged survival. These tumors have been noted to have the recurrent cytogenetic abnormality t(X;17)(p11.2;q25) which juxtaposes the *TFE3* and *ASPSCR1* genes.[180]

Grossly the tumors are firm and variegated with necrosis and hemorrhage.[178] They often appear to be encapsulated. Histologically, ASPS is composed of numerous nests of up to 50 tumor cells surrounded by thin fibrous septa and vascular channels (Fig. 11.67).[176,178] The nests appear to push into these surrounding vascular channels, and this has led some to describe a "glomeruloid" appearance. Within the center of the nests, the tumor cells become discohesive and necrotic, thus creating an alveolar appearance (eFig. 11.91). Individual tumor cells are large and have abundant, granular eosinophilic cytoplasm (Fig. 11.68). Each cell may have one or more large, pleomorphic nuclei that have vesicular chromatin and a prominent nucleolus. Mitotic figures are infrequent.

ASPSs show rather limited immunoreactivity with antibodies to vimentin and S100 protein, and with antibodies to myogenous antigens such as desmin, MyoD1 (although some have shown that antibodies to MyoD1 are nonreactive), and, sometimes, actins.[181–185] Antibodies to myogenin and myoglobin are not immunoreactive with these tumors. Some have also shown with immunohistochemistry that the TFE3 protein is overexpressed in this tumor, likely secondary to the translocation mentioned above.[180] Although usually not used, electron microscopy will reveal characteristic crystalloid structures.[186]

The tumors must be distinguished from melanoma malignant (or clear cell sarcomas, although these are unlikely to involve the upper

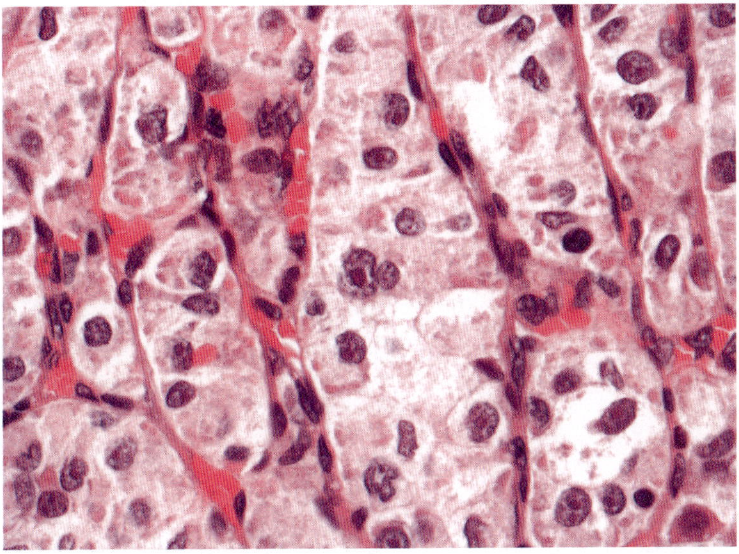

FIGURE 11.68 Alveolar rhabdomyosarcomas are composed of large cells with abundant, granular eosinophilic cytoplasm.

aerodigestive tract) and clear cell carcinomas, such as metastatic renal cell carcinoma. This can usually be accomplished with immunohistochemistry with antibodies to more specific melanocytic antigens such as HMB45 and with antibodies to cytokeratins or EMA.

Chordoma

Chordomas develop along the spinal axis and are believed by some to arise from notochordal remnants.[187–191] The tumors most often involve the sacrococcygeal areas, although up to one-quarter develop at the base of the skull. As such, projection into the nasopharynx, nasal cavity, or sinuses occurs in up to a quarter of these cases, and the tumors may be sampled through these regions.[188,192] Chordomas are more common in men and can develop at any age. In one large series of tumors involving the spheno-occipital area, the mean age at presentation was 38 years.[188] Patients with chordomas involving the base of the skull frequently present with diplopia or other visual defects. The tumors are notoriously difficult to resect in their entirety and frequently can recur, eventually leading to the death of their patients. Children with chordomas fare somewhat better, while patients with dedifferentiation within their tumors fare considerably worse.[189,193] Newer treatments using proton beam therapy, allow for increased radiation doses to the tumor while reducing doses to surrounding tissues.[194]

Grossly, chordomas are lobulated and gelatinous.[187,188] Microscopically, tumors are composed of lobules of mucoid material and neoplastic cells separated by fibrous bands (Fig. 11.69). The cellularity varies from lobule to lobule (eFig. 11.92). Tumor cells are arranged singly, in cords or in

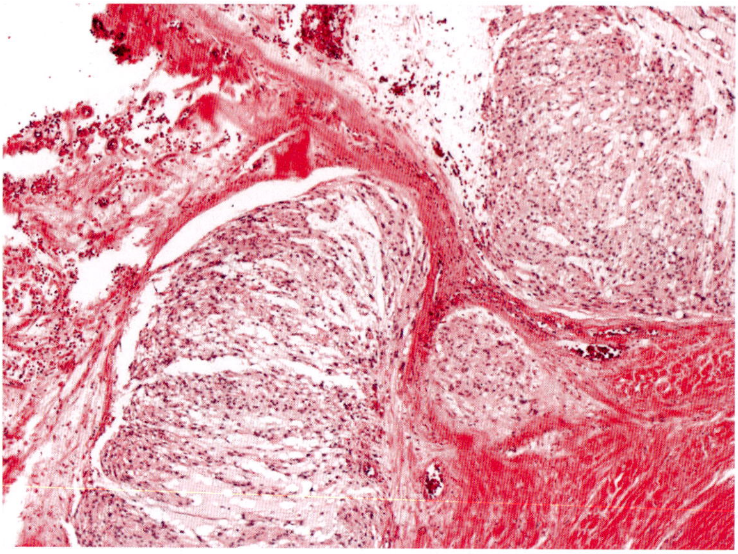

FIGURE 11.69 Chordomas are composed of lobules that are variably cellular.

sheets, and are suspended in the myxoid substance (eFig. 11.93). These cells vary in size and character. They range from smaller, more plasmacytoid cells with little or no cytoplasmic vacuolization to large, multivacuolated physaliphorous cells (Fig. 11.70, eFig. 11.94). Cellular atypia and mitotic activity vary from case to case and some examples show frank

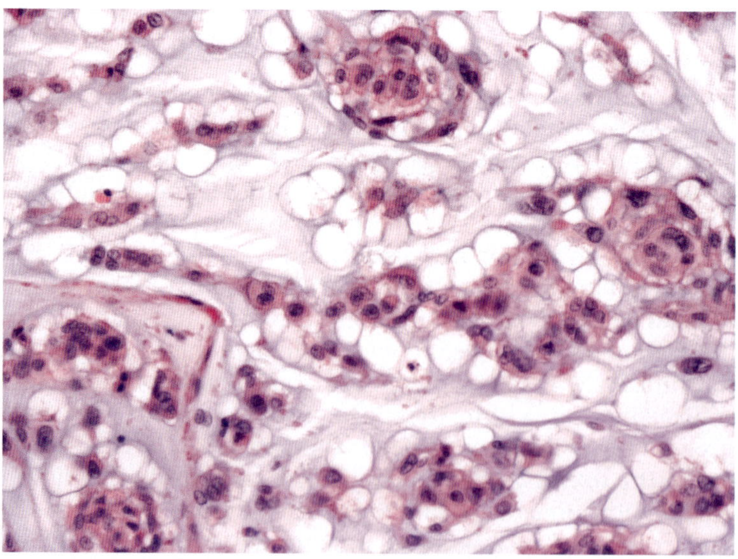

FIGURE 11.70 The neoplastic cells of chordomas often have many, large intracytoplasmic vacuoles.

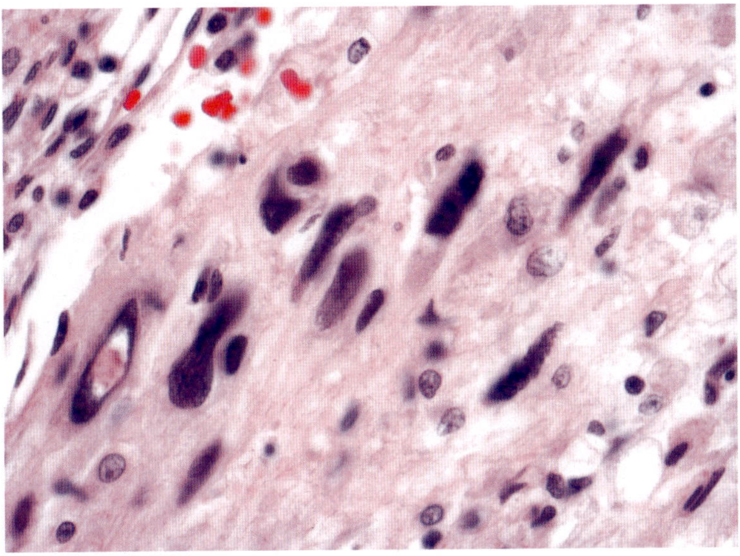

FIGURE 11.71 Cytologic atypia can be seen in some chordomas.

anaplasia with numerous mitotic figures (Fig. 11.71, eFig.11.95). In some tumors, the myxoid material focally becomes chondroid and the neoplastic cells reside in apparent lacunae (chondroid chordoma).[188,195] Areas of more obvious conventional chordoma are usually seen with these tumors. Rare chordomas are associated with areas of pleomorphic sarcoma (dedifferentiated chordoma), usually at the time of a later recurrence.[193]

The neoplastic cells of chordoma are usually immunoreactive with antibodies to cytokeratins, EMA, S100 protein, brachyury, and vimentin (eFigs. 11.96 and 11.97).[190,195,196] This unique immunoreactivity helps distinguish chordoma from both epithelial malignancies, such as mucinous carcinomas and mesenchymal neoplasms, especially cartilaginous tumors. It is typically retained in both the conventional and chondroid areas of chordomas but is diminished in dedifferentiated areas.[193]

Ectomesenchymal Chondromyxoid Tumor

Ectomesenchymal chondromyxoid tumor (EMCMT) is a rare neoplasm that develops almost exclusively in the anterior dorsum of the tongue.[197] The tumor can develop at any age, and there is no sex predilection. They do not appear to be malignant but have been noted to recur. Recently, tumors have been shown to have recurrent *RREB1-MKL2* translocations.[198]

EMCMTs are grossly rubbery with a gelatinous cut surface.[197] Histologically, the tumors are well-circumscribed and lobular and are located within the superficial muscle of the tongue. They are composed of round, fusiform, or polygonal cells that have uniform, small nuclei and moderate amounts of lightly basophilic cytoplasm. These

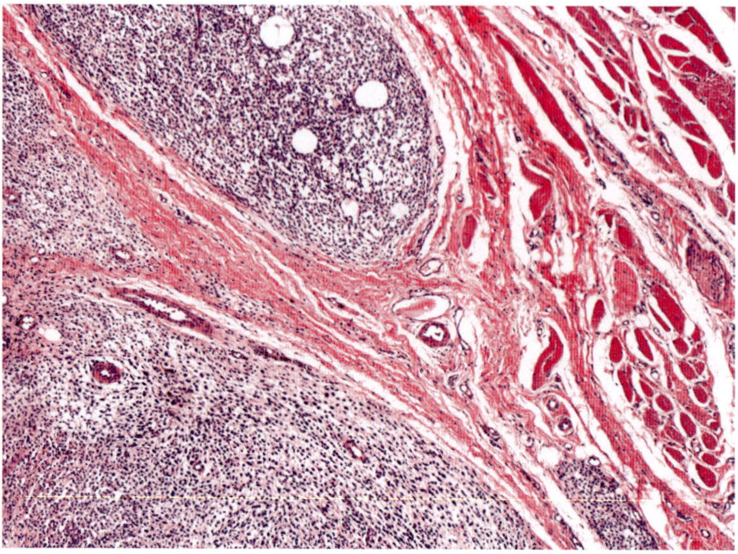

FIGURE 11.72 Lobules of small and round, uniform cells are seen with ectomesenchymal chondromyxoid tumors.

cells are arranged in cords and strands, or they can have a reticular pattern of growth with cells present in a loose, myxoid background, separated into lobules by fibrous septa (Fig. 11.72, eFig. 11.98). The nuclei are uniform, small, and round and have small, inconspicuous nucleoli (eFig. 11.99). Mitotic figures and nuclear atypia are uncommon but can be present. Chondroid and hyalinized foci are frequently seen. Immunohistochemically, tumor cells are reactive with antibodies to GFAP and cytokeratin and frequently with antibodies to S100 protein. The tumors should be differentiated from other myxoid lesions of the mouth, such as nerve sheath myxoma and neurothekeoma. Unlike those tumors, EMCMTs frequently show chondroid differentiation and are immunoreactive with antibodies to cytokeratin.

REFERENCES

1. Fletcher CD. Distinctive soft tissue tumors of the head and neck. *Mod Pathol.* 2002;15(3):324-330.
2. Fu YS, Perzin KH. Nonepithelial tumors of the nasal cavity, paranasal sinuses, and nasopharynx. A clinicopathologic study. VI. Fibrous tissue tumors (fibroma, fibromatosis, fibrosarcoma). *Cancer.* 1976;37(6):2912-2928.
3. Bouquot JE, Gundlach KK. Oral exophytic lesions in 23,616 white Americans over 35 years of age. *Oral Surg Oral Med Oral Pathol.* 1986;62(3):284-291.
4. Bouquot JE, Nikai H. Lesions of the oral cavity. In: Gnepp DR, ed. *Diagnostic Surgical Pathology of the Head and Neck.* Philadelphia: W.B. Saunders; 2001:141-238.
5. Bernstein KE, Lattes R. Nodular (pseudosarcomatous) fasciitis, a nonrecurrent lesion: clinicopathologic study of 134 cases. *Cancer.* 1982;49(8):1668-1678.

6. Hutter RV, Stewart FW, Foote FW Jr. Fasciitis. A report of 70 cases with follow-up proving the benignity of the lesion. *Cancer*. 1962;15:992-1003.
7. Montgomery EA, Meis JM. Nodular fasciitis. Its morphologic spectrum and immunohistochemical profile. *Am J Surg Pathol*. 1991;15(10):942-948.
8. Stout AP. Pseudosarcomatous fascitis in children. *Cancer*. 1961;14:1216-1222.
9. Eversole LR, Christensen R, Ficarra G, Pierleoni L, Sapp JP. Nodular fasciitis and solitary fibrous tumor of the oral region: tumors of fibroblast heterogeneity. *Oral Surg Oral Med Oral Pathol Oral Radiol Endod*. 1999;87(4):471-476.
10. Weinreb I, Shaw AJ, Perez-Ordonez B, Goldblum JR, Rubin BP. Nodular fasciitis of the head and neck region: a clinicopathologic description in a series of 30 cases. *J Cutan Pathol*. 2009;36(11):1168-1173.
11. Amary MF, Ye H, Berisha F, Tirabosco R, Presneau N, Flanagan AM. Detection of USP6 gene rearrangement in nodular fasciitis: an important diagnostic tool. *Virchows Arch*. 2013;463(1):97-98.
12. Allen PW. The fibromatoses: a clinicopathologic classification based on 140 cases. *Am J Surg Pathol*. 1977;1(3):255-270.
13. Gnepp DR, Henley J, Weiss S, Heffner D. Desmoid fibromatosis of the sinonasal tract and nasopharynx. A clinicopathologic study of 25 cases. *Cancer*. 1996;78(12): 2572-2579.
14. Bridge JA, Sreekantaiah C, Mouron B, Neff JR, Sandberg AA, Wolman SR. Clonal chromosomal abnormalities in desmoid tumors. Implications for histopathogenesis. *Cancer*. 1992;69(2):430-436.
15. Maher ER, Morson B, Beach R, Hodgson SV. Phenotypic variation in hereditary nonpolyposis colon cancer syndrome. Association with infiltrative fibromatosis (desmoid tumor). *Cancer*. 1992;69(8):2049-2051.
16. Montgomery E, Lee JH, Abraham SC, Wu TT. Superficial fibromatoses are genetically distinct from deep fibromatoses. *Mod Pathol*. 2001;14(7):695-701.
17. Bhattacharya B, Dilworth HP, Iacobuzio-Donahue C, et al. Nuclear beta-catenin expression distinguishes deep fibromatosis from other benign and malignant fibroblastic and myofibroblastic lesions. *Am J Surg Pathol*. 2005;29(5):653-659.
18. Foss RD, Ellis GL. Myofibromas and myofibromatosis of the oral region: a clinicopathologic analysis of 79 cases. *Oral Surg Oral Med Oral Pathol Oral Radiol Endod*. 2000;89(1):57-65.
19. Jones AC, Freedman PD, Kerpel SM. Oral myofibromas: a report of 13 cases and review of the literature. *J Oral Maxillofac Surg*. 1994;52(8):870-875.
20. Lingen MW, Mostofi RS, Solt DB. Myofibromas of the oral cavity. *Oral Surg Oral Med Oral Pathol Oral Radiol Endod*. 1995;80(3):297-302.
21. Montgomery E, Speight PM, Fisher C. Myofibromas presenting in the oral cavity: a series of 9 cases. *Oral Surg Oral Med Oral Pathol Oral Radiol Endod*. 2000;89(3):343-348.
22. Josephson GD, Patel S, Duckworth L, Goldstein J. Infantile myofibroma of the nasal cavity; a case report and review of the literature. *Int J Pediatr Otorhinolaryngol*. 2010;74(12):1452-1454.
23. Thompson LD, Miettinen M, Wenig BM. Sinonasal-type hemangiopericytoma: a clinicopathologic and immunophenotypic analysis of 104 cases showing perivascular myoid differentiation. *Am J Surg Pathol*. 2003;27(6):737-749.
24. Alawi F, Stratton D, Freedman PD. Solitary fibrous tumor of the oral soft tissues: a clinicopathologic and immunohistochemical study of 16 cases. *Am J Surg Pathol*. 2001;25(7):900-910.
25. Dotto JE, Ahrens W, Lesnik DJ, Kowalski D, Sasaki C, Flynn S. Solitary fibrous tumor of the larynx: a case report and review of the literature. *Arch Pathol Lab Med*. 2006;130(2):213-216.

26. Witkin GB, Rosai J. Solitary fibrous tumor of the upper respiratory tract. A report of six cases. *Am J Surg Pathol.* 1991;15(9):842-848.
27. Zukerberg LR, Rosenberg AE, Randolph G, Pilch BZ, Goodman ML. Solitary fibrous tumor of the nasal cavity and paranasal sinuses. *Am J Surg Pathol.* 1991;15(2):126-130.
28. Cox DP, Daniels T, Jordan RC. Solitary fibrous tumor of the head and neck. *Oral Surg Oral Med Oral Pathol Oral Radiol Endod.* 2010;110(1):79-84.
29. O'Regan EM, Vanguri V, Allen CM, Eversole LR, Wright JM, Woo SB. Solitary fibrous tumor of the oral cavity: clinicopathologic and immunohistochemical study of 21 cases. *Head Neck Pathol.* 2009;3(2):106-115.
30. Guillou L, Fletcher JA, Fletcher CDM, Mandahl N. Extrapleural solitary fibrous tumour and haemangiopericytoma. In: Fletcher CDM, Unni KK, Mertens F, eds. *Pathology and Genetics of Tumours of Soft Tissue and Bone.* Lyon: IARC Press; 2002:86-90.
31. Robinson DR, Wu YM, Kalyana-Sundaram S, et al. Identification of recurrent NAB2-STAT6 gene fusions in solitary fibrous tumor by integrative sequencing. *Nat Genet.* 2013;45(2):180-185.
32. Yang XJ, Zheng JW, Ye WM, et al. Malignant solitary fibrous tumors of the head and neck: a clinicopathological study of nine consecutive patients. *Oral Oncol.* 2009;45(8):678-682.
33. Mosquera JM, Fletcher CD. Expanding the spectrum of malignant progression in solitary fibrous tumors: a study of 8 cases with a discrete anaplastic component–is this dedifferentiated SFT?. *Am J Surg Pathol.* 2009;33(9):1314-1321.
34. Doyle LA, Vivero M, Fletcher CD, Mertens F, Hornick JL. Nuclear expression of STAT6 distinguishes solitary fibrous tumor from histologic mimics. *Mod Pathol.* 2014;27(3):390-395.
35. Foo WC, Cruise MW, Wick MR, Hornick JL. Immunohistochemical staining for TLE1 distinguishes synovial sarcoma from histologic mimics. *Am J Clin Pathol.* 2011;135(6):839-844.
36. Coffin CM, Watterson J, Priest JR, Dehner LP. Extrapulmonary inflammatory myofibroblastic tumor (inflammatory pseudotumor). A clinicopathologic and immunohistochemical study of 84 cases. *Am J Surg Pathol.* 1995;19(8):859-872.
37. Wenig BM, Devaney K, Bisceglia M. Inflammatory myofibroblastic tumor of the larynx. A clinicopathologic study of eight cases simulating a malignant spindle cell neoplasm. *Cancer.* 1995;76(11):2217-2229.
38. Chen YF, Zhang WD, Wu MW, Ou-Yang D, Zhang Q. Inflammatory myofibroblastic tumor of the head and neck. *Med Oncol.* 2011;28:S349-S353
39. Biron VL, Waghray R, Medlicott SA, Bosch JD. Inflammatory pseudotumours of the larynx: three cases and a review of the literature. *J Otolaryngol Head Neck Surg.* 2008;37(2):E32-E38.
40. Ong HS, Ji T, Zhang CP, et al. Head and neck inflammatory myofibroblastic tumor (IMT): evaluation of clinicopathologic and prognostic features. *Oral Oncol.* 2011;48(2):141-148.
41. Coffin CM, Patel A, Perkins S, Elenitoba-Johnson KS, Perlman E, Griffin CA. ALK1 and p80 expression and chromosomal rearrangements involving 2p23 in inflammatory myofibroblastic tumor. *Mod Pathol.* 2001;14(6):569-576.
42. Cessna MH, Zhou H, Perkins SL, et al. Are myogenin and myoD1 expression specific for rhabdomyosarcoma? A study of 150 cases, with emphasis on spindle cell mimics. *Am J Surg Pathol.* 2001;25(9):1150-1157.
43. Cessna MH, Zhou H, Sanger WG, et al. Expression of ALK1 and p80 in inflammatory myofibroblastic tumor and its mesenchymal mimics: a study of 135 cases. *Mod Pathol.* 2002;15(9):931-938.
44. Mentzel T, Dry S, Katenkamp D, Fletcher CD. Low-grade myofibroblastic sarcoma: analysis of 18 cases in the spectrum of myofibroblastic tumors. *Am J Surg Pathol.* 1998;22(10):1228-1238.

45. Montgomery E, Goldblum JR, Fisher C. Myofibrosarcoma: a clinicopathologic study. *Am J Surg Pathol.* 2001;25(2):219-228.
46. Demarosi F, Bay A, Moneghini L, Carrassi A. Low-grade myofibroblastic sarcoma of the oral cavity. *Oral Surg Oral Med Oral Pathol Oral Radiol Endod.* 2009;108(2):248-254.
47. Qiu X, Montgomery E, Sun B. Inflammatory myofibroblastic tumor and low-grade myofibroblastic sarcoma: a comparative study of clinicopathologic features and further observations on the immunohistochemical profile of myofibroblasts. *Hum Pathol.* 2008;39(6):846-856.
48. Bentz BG, Singh B, Woodruff J, Brennan M, Shah JP, Kraus D. Head and neck soft tissue sarcomas: a multivariate analysis of outcomes. *Ann Surg Oncol.* 2004;11(6):619-628.
49. Heffner DK, Gnepp DR. Sinonasal fibrosarcomas, malignant schwannomas, and "Triton" tumors. A clinicopathologic study of 67 cases. *Cancer.* 1992;70(5):1089-1101.
50. Frankenthaler R, Ayala AG, Hartwick RW, Goepfert H. Fibrosarcoma of the head and neck. *Laryngoscope.* 1990;100(8):799-802.
51. Pritchard DJ, Soule EH, Taylor WF, Ivins JC. Fibrosarcoma–a clinicopathologic and statistical study of 199 tumors of the soft tissues of the extremities and trunk. *Cancer.* 1974;33(3):888-897.
52. Kempson RL, Fletcher CDM, Evans HL, Hendrickson MR, Sibley RK. *Tumors of the Soft Tissues.* Vol 30. 3rd ed. Washington, DC: Armed Forces Institute of Pathology; 2001.
53. Bahrami A, Folpe AL. Adult-type fibrosarcoma: a reevaluation of 163 putative cases diagnosed at a single institution over a 48-year period. *Am J Surg Pathol.* 2010;34(10):1504-1513.
54. Lewis JT, Oliveira AM, Nascimento AG, et al. Low grade sinonasal sarcoma with neural and myogenic features: a clinicopathologic analysis of 28 cases. *Am J Surg Pathol.* 2012;36(4):517-525.
55. Barnes L, Kanbour A. Malignant fibrous histiocytoma of the head and neck. A report of 12 cases. *Arch Otolaryngol Head Neck Surg.* 1988;114(10):1149-1156.
56. Ferlito A, Nicolai P, Recher G, Narne S. Primary laryngeal malignant fibrous histiocytoma: review of the literature and report of seven cases. *Laryngoscope.* 1983;93(10):1351-1358.
57. Perzin KH, Fu YS. Non-epithelial tumors of the nasal cavity, paranasal sinuses and nasopharynx: a clinico-pathologic study XI. fibrous histiocytomas. *Cancer.* 1980;45(10):2616-2626.
58. Weiss SW, Enzinger FM. Malignant fibrous histiocytoma: an analysis of 200 cases. *Cancer.* 1978;41(6):2250-2266.
59. Haberal I, Samim E, Astarci M, Ozeri C. Radiation-induced malignant fibrous histiocytoma of the neck in a patient with laryngeal carcinoma. *Am J Otolaryngol.* 2001;22(2):146-149.
60. Brooks JK, Nikitakis NG, Goodman NJ, Levy BA. Clinicopathologic characterization of oral angioleiomyomas. *Oral Surg Oral Med Oral Pathol Oral Radiol Endod.* 2002;94(2):221-227.
61. Fu YS, Perzin KH. Nonepithelial tumors of the nasal cavity, paranasal sinuses, and nasopharynx: a clinicopathologic study. IV. Smooth muscle tumors (leiomyoma, leiomyosarcoma). *Cancer.* 1975;35(5):1300-1308.
62. Kleinsasser O, Glanz H. Myogenic tumours of the larynx. *Arch Otorhinolaryngol.* 1979;225(2):107-119.
63. Koutlas IG, Manivel JC. Epithelioid leiomyoma of the oral mucosa. *Oral Surg Oral Med Oral Pathol Oral Radiol Endod.* 1996;82(6):670-673.
64. McKiernan DC, Watters GW. Smooth muscle tumours of the larynx. *J Laryngol Otol.* 1995;109(1):77-79.

65. Ide F, Mishima K, Yamada H, et al. Perivascular myoid tumors of the oral region: a clinicopathologic re-evaluation of 35 cases. *J Oral Pathol Med*. 2008;37(1):43-49.

66. Kuruvilla A, Wenig BM, Humphrey DM, Heffner DK. Leiomyosarcoma of the sinonasal tract. A clinicopathologic study of nine cases. *Arch Otolaryngol Head Neck Surg*. 1990;116(11):1278-1286.

67. Montgomery E, Goldblum JR, Fisher C. Leiomyosarcoma of the head and neck: a clinicopathological study. *Histopathology*. 2002;40(6):518-525.

68. Ethunandan M, Stokes C, Higgins B, Spedding A, Way C, Brennan P. Primary oral leiomyosarcoma: a clinico-pathologic study and analysis of prognostic factors. *Int J Oral Maxillofac Surg*. 2007;36(5):409-416.

69. Kapadia SB, Meis JM, Frisman DM, Ellis GL, Heffner DK. Fetal rhabdomyoma of the head and neck: a clinicopathologic and immunophenotypic study of 24 cases. *Hum Pathol*. 1993;24(7):754-765.

70. Kapadia SB, Meis JM, Frisman DM, Ellis GL, Heffner DK, Hyams VJ. Adult rhabdomyoma of the head and neck: a clinicopathologic and immunophenotypic study. *Hum Pathol*. 1993;24(6):608-617.

71. Kodet R, Fajstavr J, Kabelka Z, Koutecky J, Eckschlager T, Newton WA Jr. Is fetal cellular rhabdomyoma an entity or a differentiated rhabdomyosarcoma? A study of patients with rhabdomyoma of the tongue and sarcoma of the tongue enrolled in the intergroup rhabdomyosarcoma studies I, II, and III. *Cancer*. 1991;67(11):2907-2913.

72. Willis J, Abdul-Karim FW, di Sant'Agnese PA. Extracardiac rhabdomyomas. *Semin Diagn Pathol*. 1994;11(1):15-25.

73. Balakumar R, Farr MRB, Fernando M, Jebreel A, Ray J, Sionis S. Adult-type rhabdomyoma of the larynx in Birt-Hogg-Dube syndrome: evidence for a real association. *Head Neck Pathol*. 2019;13(3):507-511.

74. Hicks J, Flaitz C. Rhabdomyosarcoma of the head and neck in children. *Oral Oncol*. 2002;38(5):450-459.

75. Pappo A, Barr FG, Wolden SL. Pediatric rhabdomyosarcoma: biology and results of the North American intergroup rhabdomyosarcoma trials. In: Pappo A, ed. *Pediatric Bone and Soft Tissue Sarcomas*. Berlin: Springer; 2006:103-132.

76. Pappo AS, Meza JL, Donaldson SS, et al. Treatment of localized nonorbital, nonparameningeal head and neck rhabdomyosarcoma: lessons learned from intergroup rhabdomyosarcoma studies III and IV. *J Clin Oncol*. 2003;21(4):638-645.

77. Qualman SJ, Coffin CM, Newton WA, et al. Intergroup rhabdomyosarcoma study: update for pathologists. *Pediatr Dev Pathol*. 1998;1(6):550-561.

78. Tsokos M. The diagnosis and classification of childhood rhabdomyosarcoma. *Semin Diagn Pathol*. 1994;11(1):26-38.

79. Stock N, Chibon F, Binh MB, et al. Adult-type rhabdomyosarcoma: analysis of 57 cases with clinicopathologic description, identification of 3 morphologic patterns and prognosis. *Am J Surg Pathol*. 2009;33(12):1850-1859.

80. Newton WA Jr, Gehan EA, Webber BL, et al. Classification of rhabdomyosarcomas and related sarcomas. Pathologic aspects and proposal for a new classification–an Intergroup Rhabdomyosarcoma Study. *Cancer*. 1995;76(6):1073-1085.

81. Cavazzana AO, Schmidt D, Ninfo V, et al. Spindle cell rhabdomyosarcoma. A prognostically favorable variant of rhabdomyosarcoma. *Am J Surg Pathol*. 1992;16(3):229-235.

82. Devoe K, Weidner N. Immunohistochemistry of small round-cell tumors. *Semin Diagn Pathol*. 2000;17(3):216-224.

83. Folpe AL, Hill CE, Parham DM, O'Shea PA, Weiss SW. Immunohistochemical detection of FLI-1 protein expression: a study of 132 round cell tumors with emphasis on CD99-positive mimics of Ewing's sarcoma/primitive neuroectodermal tumor. *Am J Surg Pathol*. 2000;24(12):1657-1662.

84. Morotti RA, Nicol KK, Parham DM, et al. An immunohistochemical algorithm to facilitate diagnosis and subtyping of rhabdomyosarcoma: the Children's Oncology Group experience. *Am J Surg Pathol.* 2006;30(8):962-968.
85. Sullivan LM, Atkins KA, LeGallo RD. PAX immunoreactivity identifies alveolar rhabdomyosarcoma. *Am J Surg Pathol.* 2009;33(5):775-780.
86. Davis JL, Matsumura L, Weeks DA, Troxell ML. PAX2 expression in Wilms tumors and other childhood neoplasms. *Am J Surg Pathol.* 2011;35(8):1186-1194.
87. Morgenstern DA, Hasan F, Gibson S, Winyard P, Sebire NJ, Anderson J. PAX5 expression in nonhematopoietic tissues. Reappraisal of previous studies. *Am J Clin Pathol.* 2010;133(3):407-415.
88. Oue T, Uehara S, Yamanaka H, Takama Y, Oji Y, Fukuzawa M. Expression of Wilms tumor 1 gene in a variety of pediatric tumors. *J Pediatr Surg.* 2011;46(12):2233-2238.
89. Martin SE, Temm CJ, Goheen MP, Ulbright TM, Hattab EM. Cytoplasmic p63 immunohistochemistry is a useful marker for muscle differentiation: an immunohistochemical and immunoelectron microscopic study. *Mod Pathol.* 2011;24(10):1320-1326.
90. Warren M, Hiemenz MC, Schmidt R, et al. Expanding the spectrum of dicer1-associated sarcomas. *Mod Pathol.* 2020;33(1):164-174.
91. Moon WS, Chung GH, Hong KH. Intravascular papillary endothelial hyperplasia in a vascular lesion of the paranasal sinus. *Arch Pathol Lab Med.* 2000;124(8):1224-1227.
92. Renshaw AA, Rosai J. Benign atypical vascular lesions of the lip. A study of 12 cases. *Am J Surg Pathol.* 1993;17(6):557-565.
93. Tosios K, Koutlas IG, Papanicolaou SI. Intravascular papillary endothelial hyperplasia of the oral soft tissues: report of 18 cases and review of the literature. *J Oral Maxillofac Surg.* 1994;52(12):1263-1268.
94. Fanburg-Smith JC, Michal M, Partanen TA, Alitalo K, Miettinen M. Papillary intralymphatic angioendothelioma (PILA): a report of twelve cases of a distinctive vascular tumor with phenotypic features of lymphatic vessels. *Am J Surg Pathol.* 1999;23(9):1004-1010.
95. Bridger GP, Nassar VH, Skinner HG. Hemangioma in the adult larynx. *Arch Otolaryngol.* 1970;92(5):493-498.
96. Coffin CM, Dehner LP. Vascular tumors in children and adolescents: a clinicopathologic study of 228 tumors in 222 patients. *Pathol Annu.* 1993;28(pt 1):97-120.
97. Fu YS, Perzin KH. Non-epithelial tumors of the nasal cavity, paranasal sinuses, and nasopharynx: a clinicopathologic study. I. General features and vascular tumors. *Cancer.* 1974;33(5):1275-1288.
98. Mills SE, Cooper PH, Fechner RE. Lobular capillary hemangioma: the underlying lesion of pyogenic granuloma. A study of 73 cases from the oral and nasal mucous membranes. *Am J Surg Pathol.* 1980;4(5):470-479.
99. Seikaly H, Cuyler JP. Infantile subglottic hemangioma. *J Otolaryngol.* 1994;23(2):135-137.
100. Fechner RE, Cooper PH, Mills SE. Pyogenic granuloma of the larynx and trachea. A causal and pathologic misnomer for granulation tissue. *Arch Otolaryngol.* 1981;107(1):30-32.
101. Nichols GE, Gaffey MJ, Mills SE, Weiss LM. Lobular capillary hemangioma. An immunohistochemical study including steroid hormone receptor status. *Am J Clin Pathol.* 1992;97(6):770-775.
102. Miettinen M, Wang ZF, Paetau A, et al. ERG transcription factor as an immunohistochemical marker for vascular endothelial tumors and prostatic carcinoma. *Am J Surg Pathol.* 2011;35(3):432-441.
103. Emery PJ, Bailey CM, Evans JN. Cystic hygroma of the head and neck. A review of 37 cases. *J Laryngol Otol.* 1984;98(6):613-619.
104. Apostol JV, Frazell EL. Juvenile nasopharyngeal angiofibroma. A clinical study. *Cancer.* 1965;18:869-878.

105. Hubbard EM. Nasopharyngeal angiofibromas. *AMA Arch Pathol*. 1958;65(2):192-204.
106. Neel HB III, Whicker JH, Devine KD, Weiland LH. Juvenile angiofibroma. Review of 120 cases. *Am J Surg*. 1973;126(4):547-556.
107. Sternberg SS. Pathology of juvenile nasopharyngeal angiofibroma; a lesion of adolescent males. *Cancer*. 1954;7(1):15-28.
108. Giardiello FM, Hamilton SR, Krush AJ, Offerhaus JA, Booker SV, Petersen GM. Nasopharyngeal angiofibroma in patients with familial adenomatous polyposis. *Gastroenterology*. 1993;105(5):1550-1552.
109. Guertl B, Beham A, Zechner R, Stammberger H, Hoefler G. Nasopharyngeal angiofibroma: an APC-gene-associated tumor?. *Hum Pathol*. 2000;31(11):1411-1413.
110. Chen KT, Bauer FW. Sarcomatous transformation of nasopharyngeal angiofibroma. *Cancer*. 1982;49(2):369-371.
111. Spagnolo DV, Papadimitriou JM, Archer M. Postirradiation malignant fibrous histiocytoma arising in juvenile nasopharyngeal angiofibroma and producing alpha-1-antitrypsin. *Histopathology*. 1984;8(2):339-352.
112. Beham A, Fletcher CD, Kainz J, Schmid C, Humer U. Nasopharyngeal angiofibroma: an immunohistochemical study of 32 cases. *Virchows Arch A Pathol Anat Histopathol*. 1993;423(4):281-285.
113. Hwang HC, Mills SE, Patterson K, Gown AM. Expression of androgen receptors in nasopharyngeal angiofibroma: an immunohistochemical study of 24 cases. *Mod Pathol*. 1998;11(11):1122-1126.
114. Abraham SC, Montgomery EA, Giardiello FM, Wu TT. Frequent beta-catenin mutations in juvenile nasopharyngeal angiofibromas. *Am J Pathol*. 2001;158(3): 1073-1078.
115. Eichhorn JH, Dickersin GR, Bhan AK, Goodman ML. Sinonasal hemangiopericytoma. A reassessment with electron microscopy, immunohistochemistry, and long-term follow-up. *Am J Surg Pathol*. 1990;14(9):856-866.
116. Tse LL, Chan JK. Sinonasal haemangiopericytoma-like tumour: a sinonasal glomus tumour or a haemangiopericytoma?. *Histopathology*. 2002;40(6):510-517.
117. Thompson LDR, Fanburg-Smith JC, Wenig BM. Borderline and low malignant potential tunours of soft tissues. In: Barnes L, Eveson JW, Reichart P, Sidransky D, eds. *Pathology and Genetics of Head and Neck Tumours*. Lyon: IARC Press; 2005:43-45.
118. Compagno J, Hyams VJ. Hemangiopericytoma-like intranasal tumors. A clinicopathologic study of 23 cases. *Am J Clin Pathol*. 1976;66(4):672-683.
119. el-Naggar AK, Batsakis JG, Garcia GM, Luna ML, Goepfert H. Sinonasal hemangiopericytomas. A clinicopathologic and DNA content study. *Arch Otolaryngol Head Neck Surg*. 1992;118(2):134-137.
120. Lasota J, Felisiak-Golabek A, Aly FZ, Wang ZF, Thompson LD, Miettinen M. Nuclear expression and gain-of-function beta-catenin mutation in glomangiopericytoma (sinonasal-type hemangiopericytoma): insight into pathogenesis and a diagnostic marker. *Mod Pathol*. 2015;28(5):715-720.
121. Kessaris P, Klimis T, Zanakis S. Glomus tumour of the hard palate: case report and review. *Br J Oral Maxillofac Surg*. 2001;39(6):478-479.
122. Errani C, Zhang L, Sung YS, et al. A novel WWTR1-CAMTA1 gene fusion is a consistent abnormality in epithelioid hemangioendothelioma of different anatomic sites. *Genes Chromosomes Cancer*. 2011;50(8):644-653.
123. Deyrup AT, Tighiouart M, Montag AG, Weiss SW. Epithelioid hemangioendothelioma of soft tissue: a proposal for risk stratification based on 49 cases. *Am J Surg Pathol*. 2008;32(6):924-927.
124. Weiss SW, Enzinger FM. Epithelioid hemangioendothelioma: a vascular tumor often mistaken for a carcinoma. *Cancer*. 1982;50(5):970-981.

125. Ellis GL, Kratochvil FJ III. Epithelioid hemangioendothelioma of the head and neck: a clinicopathologic report of twelve cases. *Oral Surg Oral Med Oral Pathol.* 1986;61(1):61-68.

126. Marrogi AJ, Boyd D, el-Mofty S, Waldron C. Epithelioid hemangioendothelioma of the oral cavity: report of two cases and review of literature. *J Oral Maxillofac Surg.* 1991;49(6):633-638.

127. Mohtasham N, Kharrazi AA, Jamshidi S, Jafarzadeh H. Epithelioid hemangioendothelioma of the oral cavity: a case report. *J Oral Sci.* 2008;50(2):219-223.

128. Naqvi J, Ordonez NG, Luna MA, Williams MD, Weber RS, El-Naggar AK. Epithelioid hemangioendothelioma of the head and neck: role of podoplanin in the differential diagnosis. *Head Neck Pathol.* 2008;2(1):25-30.

129. Abramson AL, Simons RL. Kaposi's sarcoma of the head and neck. *Arch Otolaryngol.* 1970;92(5):505-508.

130. Fanburg-Smith JC, Furlong MA, Childers EL. Oral and salivary gland angiosarcoma: a clinicopathologic study of 29 cases. *Mod Pathol.* 2003;16(3):263-271.

131. Favia G, Lo Muzio L, Serpico R, Maiorano E. Angiosarcoma of the head and neck with intra-oral presentation. A clinico-pathological study of four cases. *Oral Oncol.* 2002;38(8):757-762.

132. Jordan RC, Regezi JA. Oral spindle cell neoplasms: a review of 307 cases. *Oral Surg Oral Med Oral Pathol Oral Radiol Endod.* 2003;95(6):717-724.

133. Loos BM, Wieneke JA, Thompson LD. Laryngeal angiosarcoma: a clinicopathologic study of five cases with a review of the literature. *Laryngoscope.* 2001;111(7):1197-1202.

134. Mark RJ, Tran LM, Sercarz J, Fu YS, Calcaterra TC, Juillard GF. Angiosarcoma of the head and neck. The UCLA experience 1955 through 1990. *Arch Otolaryngol Head Neck Surg.* 1993;119(9):973-978.

135. Sciot R, Delaere P, Van Damme B, Desmet V. Angiosarcoma of the larynx. *Histopathology.* 1995;26(2):177-180.

136. Lamovec J, Knuutila S. Kaposi sarcoma. In: Fletcher CDM, Unni KK, Mertens F, eds. *Pathology and Genetics of Tumours of Soft Tissue and Bone.* Lyon: IARP Press; 2002:170-172.

137. Lyons LL, North PE, Mac-Moune Lai F, Stoler MH, Folpe AL, Weiss SW. Kaposiform hemangioendothelioma: a study of 33 cases emphasizing its pathologic, immunophenotypic, and biologic uniqueness from juvenile hemangioma. *Am J Surg Pathol.* 2004;28(5):559-568.

138. Heffner DK. Sinonasal angiosarcoma? Not likely (a brief description of infarcted nasal polyps). *Ann Diagn Pathol.* 2010;14(4):233-234.

139. Traweek ST, Kandalaft PL, Mehta P, Battifora H. The human hematopoietic progenitor cell antigen (CD34) in vascular neoplasia. *Am J Clin Pathol.* 1991;96(1):25-31.

140. Miettinen M, Fetsch JF. Distribution of keratins in normal endothelial cells and a spectrum of vascular tumors: implications in tumor diagnosis. *Hum Pathol.* 2000;31(9):1062-1067.

141. El-Monem MH, Gaafar AH, Magdy EA. Lipomas of the head and neck: presentation variability and diagnostic work-up. *J Laryngol Otol.* 2006;120(1):47-55.

142. Fregnani ER, Pires FR, Falzoni R, Lopes MA, Vargas PA. Lipomas of the oral cavity: clinical findings, histological classification and proliferative activity of 46 cases. *Int J Oral Maxillofac Surg.* 2003;32(1):49-53.

143. Furlong MA, Fanburg-Smith JC, Childers EL. Lipoma of the oral and maxillofacial region: site and subclassification of 125 cases. *Oral Surg Oral Med Oral Pathol Oral Radiol Endod.* 2004;98(4):441-450.

144. Gagari E, Kabani S, Gallagher GT. Intraoral liposarcoma: case report and review of the literature. *Oral Surg Oral Med Oral Pathol Oral Radiol Endod.* 2000;89(1):66-72.

145. Nascimento AF, McMenamin ME, Fletcher CD. Liposarcomas/atypical lipomatous tumors of the oral cavity: a clinicopathologic study of 23 cases. *Ann Diagn Pathol.* 2002;6(2):83-93.

146. Wenig BM. Lipomas of the larynx and hypopharynx: a review of the literature with the addition of three new cases. *J Laryngol Otol.* 1995;109(4):353-357.

147. Wenig BM, Heffner DK. Liposarcomas of the larynx and hypopharynx: a clinicopathologic study of eight new cases and a review of the literature. *Laryngoscope.* 1995;105(7 pt 1):747-756.

148. Wenig BM, Weiss SW, Gnepp DR. Laryngeal and hypopharyngeal liposarcoma. A clinicopathologic study of 10 cases with a comparison to soft-tissue counterparts. *Am J Surg Pathol.* 1990;14(2):134-141.

149. Manor E, Sion-Vardy N, Joshua BZ, Bodner L. Oral lipoma: analysis of 58 new cases and review of the literature. *Ann Diagn Pathol.* 2011;15(4):257-261.

150. Weaver J, Rao P, Goldblum JR, et al. Can MDM2 analytical tests performed on core needle biopsy be relied upon to diagnose well-differentiated liposarcoma?. *Mod Pathol.* 2010;23(10):1301-1306.

151. Suster S, Fisher C, Moran CA. Expression of bcl-2 oncoprotein in benign and malignant spindle cell tumors of soft tissue, skin, serosal surfaces, and gastrointestinal tract. *Am J Surg Pathol.* 1998;22(7):863-872.

152. Cheng J, Wang Y, Cheng A, et al. Primary liposarcoma in oral and maxillofacial region. *J Craniofac Surg.* 2011;22(5):1765-1771.

153. Davis EC, Ballo MT, Luna MA, et al. Liposarcoma of the head and neck: the University of Texas M. D. Anderson Cancer Center experience. *Head Neck.* 2009;31(1):28-36.

154. Downs-Kelly E, Goldblum JR, Patel RM, et al. The utility of fluorescence in situ hybridization (FISH) in the diagnosis of myxoid soft tissue neoplasms. *Am J Surg Pathol.* 2008;32(1):8-13.

155. Andreasen S, Bishop JA, Hellquist H, et al. Biphenotypic sinonasal sarcoma: demographics, clinicopathological characteristics, molecular features, and prognosis of a recently described entity. *Virchows Arch.* 2018;473(5):615-626.

156. Jo VY, Marino-Enriquez A, Fletcher CDM, Hornick JL. Expression of PAX3 distinguishes biphenotypic sinonasal sarcoma from histologic mimics. *Am J Surg Pathol.* 2018;42(10):1275-1285.

157. Le Loarer F, Laffont S, Lesluyes T, et al. Clinicopathologic and molecular features of a series of 41 biphenotypic sinonasal sarcomas expanding their molecular spectrum. *Am J Surg Pathol.* 2019;43(6):747-754.

158. Rooper LM, Huang SC, Antonescu CR, Westra WH, Bishop JA. Biphenotypic sinonasal sarcoma: an expanded immunoprofile including consistent nuclear beta-catenin positivity and absence of SOX10 expression. *Hum Pathol.* 2016;55:44-50.

159. Stelow EB, Bishop JA. Update from the 4th edition of the World Health Organization classification of head and neck tumours: tumors of the nasal cavity, paranasal sinuses and skull base. *Head Neck Pathol.* 2017;11(1):3-15.

160. Wang X, Bledsoe KL, Graham RP, et al. Recurrent PAX3-MAML3 fusion in biphenotypic sinonasal sarcoma. *Nat Genet.* 2014;46(7):666-668.

161. Schmidt D, Thum P, Harms D, Treuner J. Synovial sarcoma in children and adolescents. A report from the Kiel Pediatric Tumor Registry. *Cancer.* 1991;67(6):1667-1672.

162. Bridge JA, Bridge RS, Borek DA, Shaffer B, Norris CW. Translocation t(X;18) in orofacial synovial sarcoma. *Cancer.* 1988;62(5):935-937.

163. Meer S, Coleman H, Altini M. Oral synovial sarcoma: a report of 2 cases and a review of the literature. *Oral Surg Oral Med Oral Pathol Oral Radiol Endod.* 2003;96(3):306-315.

164. Nunez-Alonso C, Gashti EN, Christ ML. Maxillofacial synovial sarcoma. Light- and electron-microscopic study of two cases. *Am J Surg Pathol.* 1979;3(1):23-30.

165. Roth JA, Enzinger FM, Tannenbaum M. Synovial sarcoma of the neck: a followup study of 24 cases. *Cancer*. 1975;35(4):1243-1253.

166. Shmookler BM, Enzinger FM, Brannon RB. Orofacial synovial sarcoma: a clinicopathologic study of 11 new cases and review of the literature. *Cancer*. 1982;50(2):269-276.

167. Guillou L, Coindre J, Gallagher G, et al. Detection of the synovial sarcoma translocation t(X;18) (SYT;SSX) in paraffin-embedded tissues using reverse transcriptase-polymerase chain reaction: a reliable and powerful diagnostic tool for pathologists. A molecular analysis of 221 mesenchymal tumors fixed in different fixatives. *Hum Pathol*. 2001;32(1):105-112.

168. Sandberg AA, Bridge JA. Updates on the cytogenetics and molecular genetics of bone and soft tissue tumors. Synovial sarcoma. *Cancer Genet Cytogenet*. 2002;133(1):1-23.

169. Ferrari A, Gronchi A, Casanova M, et al. Synovial sarcoma: a retrospective analysis of 271 patients of all ages treated at a single institution. *Cancer*. 2004;101(3):627-634.

170. Crocker DW, Stout AP. Synovial sarcoma in children. *Cancer*. 1959;12:1123-1133.

171. Folpe AL, Schmidt RA, Chapman D, Gown AM. Poorly differentiated synovial sarcoma: immunohistochemical distinction from primitive neuroectodermal tumors and high-grade malignant peripheral nerve sheath tumors. *Am J Surg Pathol*. 1998;22(6):673-682.

172. Mackenzie DH. Synovial sarcoma. A review of 58 cases. *Cancer*. 1966;19(2):169-180.

173. Pelmus M, Guillou L, Hostein I, Sierankowski G, Lussan C, Coindre JM. Monophasic fibrous and poorly differentiated synovial sarcoma: immunohistochemical reassessment of 60 t(X;18)(SYT-SSX)-positive cases. *Am J Surg Pathol*. 2002;26(11):1434-1440.

174. Ordonez NG, Mahfouz SM, Mackay B. Synovial sarcoma: an immunohistochemical and ultrastructural study. *Hum Pathol*. 1990;21(7):733-749.

175. Suster S. Recent advances in the application of immunohistochemical markers for the diagnosis of soft tissue tumors. *Semin Diagn Pathol*. 2000;17(3):225-235.

176. Auerbach HE, Brooks JJ. Alveolar soft part sarcoma. A clinicopathologic and immunohistochemical study. *Cancer*. 1987;60(1):66-73.

177. Portera CA Jr, Ho V, Patel SR, et al. Alveolar soft part sarcoma: clinical course and patterns of metastasis in 70 patients treated at a single institution. *Cancer*. 2001;91(3):585-591.

178. Lieberman PH, Brennan MF, Kimmel M, Erlandson RA, Garin-Chesa P, Flehinger BY. Alveolar soft-part sarcoma. A clinico-pathologic study of half a century. *Cancer*. 1989;63(1):1-13.

179. Rekhi B, Ingle A, Agarwal M, Puri A, Laskar S, Jambhekar NA. Alveolar soft part sarcoma "revisited": clinicopathological review of 47 cases from a tertiary cancer referral centre, including immunohistochemical expression of TFE3 in 22 cases and 21 other tumours. *Pathology*. 2012;44(1):11-17.

180. Argani P, Lal P, Hutchinson B, Lui MY, Reuter VE, Ladanyi M. Aberrant nuclear immunoreactivity for TFE3 in neoplasms with TFE3 gene fusions: a sensitive and specific immunohistochemical assay. *Am J Surg Pathol*. 2003;27(6):750-761.

181. Gomez JA, Amin MB, Ro JY, Linden MD, Lee MW, Zarbo RJ. Immunohistochemical profile of myogenin and MyoD1 does not support skeletal muscle lineage in alveolar soft part sarcoma. *Arch Pathol Lab Med*. 1999;123(6):503-507.

182. Miettinen M, Ekfors T. Alveolar soft part sarcoma. Immunohistochemical evidence for muscle cell differentiation. *Am J Clin Pathol*. 1990;93(1):32-38.

183. Mukai M, Torikata C, Iri H, et al. Histogenesis of alveolar soft part sarcoma. An immunohistochemical and biochemical study. *Am J Surg Pathol*. 1986;10(3):212-218.

184. Ordonez NG, Hickey RC, Brooks TE. Alveolar soft part sarcoma. A cytologic and immunohistochemical study. *Cancer*. 1988;61(3):525-531.

185. Rosai J, Dias P, Parham DM, Shapiro DN, Houghton P. MyoD1 protein expression in alveolar soft part sarcoma as confirmatory evidence of its skeletal muscle nature. *Am J Surg Pathol*. 1991;15(10):974-981.

186. Welsh RA, Bray DM III, Shipkey FH, Meyer AT. Histogenesis of alveolar soft part sarcoma. *Cancer*. 1972;29(1):191-204.
187. Dahlin DC, Maccarty CS. Chordoma. *Cancer*. 1952;5(6):1170-1178.
188. Heffelfinger MJ, Dahlin DC, MacCarty CS, Beabout JW. Chordomas and cartilaginous tumors at the skull base. *Cancer*. 1973;32(2):410-420.
189. Hoch BL, Nielsen GP, Liebsch NJ, Rosenberg AE. Base of skull chordomas in children and adolescents: a clinicopathologic study of 73 cases. *Am J Surg Pathol*. 2006;30(7):811-818.
190. Mitchell A, Scheithauer BW, Unni KK, Forsyth PJ, Wold LE, McGivney DJ. Chordoma and chondroid neoplasms of the spheno-occiput. An immunohistochemical study of 41 cases with prognostic and nosologic implications. *Cancer*. 1993;72(10):2943-2949.
191. O'Connell JX, Renard LG, Liebsch NJ, Efird JT, Munzenrider JE, Rosenberg AE. Base of skull chordoma. A correlative study of histologic and clinical features of 62 cases. *Cancer*. 1994;74(8):2261-2267.
192. Perzin KH, Pushparaj N. Nonepithelial tumors of the nasal cavity, paranasal sinuses, and nasopharynx. A clinicopathologic study. XIV: Chordomas. *Cancer*. 1986;57(4):784-796.
193. Meis JM, Raymond AK, Evans HL, Charles RE, Giraldo AA. "Dedifferentiated" chordoma. A clinicopathologic and immunohistochemical study of three cases. *Am J Surg Pathol*. 1987;11(7):516-525.
194. Mendenhall WM, Mendenhall CM, Lewis SB, Villaret DB, Mendenhall NP. Skull base chordoma. *Head Neck*. 2005;27(2):159-165.
195. Wojno KJ, Hruban RH, Garin-Chesa P, Huvos AG. Chondroid chordomas and low-grade chondrosarcomas of the craniospinal axis. An immunohistochemical analysis of 17 cases. *Am J Surg Pathol*. 1992;16(12):1144-1152.
196. Sangoi AR, Karamchandani J, Lane B, et al. Specificity of brachyury in the distinction of chordoma from clear cell renal cell carcinoma and germ cell tumors: a study of 305 cases. *Mod Pathol*. 2011;24(3):425-429.
197. Smith BC, Ellis GL, Meis-Kindblom JM, Williams SB. Ectomesenchymal chondromyxoid tumor of the anterior tongue. Nineteen cases of a new clinicopathologic entity. *Am J Surg Pathol*. 1995;19(5):519-530.
198. Dickson BC, Antonescu CR, Argyris PP, et al. Ectomesenchymal chondromyxoid tumor: a neoplasm characterized by recurrent RREB1-MKL2 fusions. *Am J Surg Pathol*. 2018;42(10):1297-1305.

12

BONE, CARTILAGINOUS, AND JAW LESIONS THAT MAY BE SAMPLED WITH UPPER AERODIGESTIVE TRACT BIOPSIES

Numerous bony, cartilaginous, and odontogenic lesions can involve the upper aerodigestive tract. Some can involve all sights, but many show an obvious predilection for the alveolar ridge or extension into the paranasal sinuses. This is not surprising as odontogenic epithelium and rests occur throughout these sites. Furthermore bony or other lesions involving the thin bones surrounding the sinonasal tract can easily extend into the sinuses and present as masses. A discussion of all the lesions of the craniofacial bones is far beyond the scope of this monograph, however, and here we present the lesions we have encountered most frequently in upper aerodigestive tract biopsy specimens.

CHONDROID OR OSSEOUS METAPLASIA

Chondroid and osseous metaplasia occurs throughout the upper aerodigestive tract and must be distinguished from neoplasia. These metaplastic lesions typically develop in areas of chronic inflammation.[1] Metaplasia is especially prone to occur secondary to ill-fitting dentures or in areas of redundant or "flabby" alveolar ridge tissue. Most lesions have bone with overlying hyaline and fibrocartilage that blends into the surrounding fibrous tissue (Fig. 12.1, eFig. 12.1). The chondroid tissue is typically bland and resembles normal, mature cartilage. In rare cases cellular atypia may raise concerns of chondrosarcoma. Chondroid metaplasia of the true or false vocal cords also can occur, and, as was discussed in Chapter 1, cartilaginous nodules are normally seen in the anterior portion of the thyroarytenoid ligament. Finally, cartilaginous or osseous metaplasia often develops in sarcomatoid carcinomas, and one should exclude a concomitant malignancy when either is present.

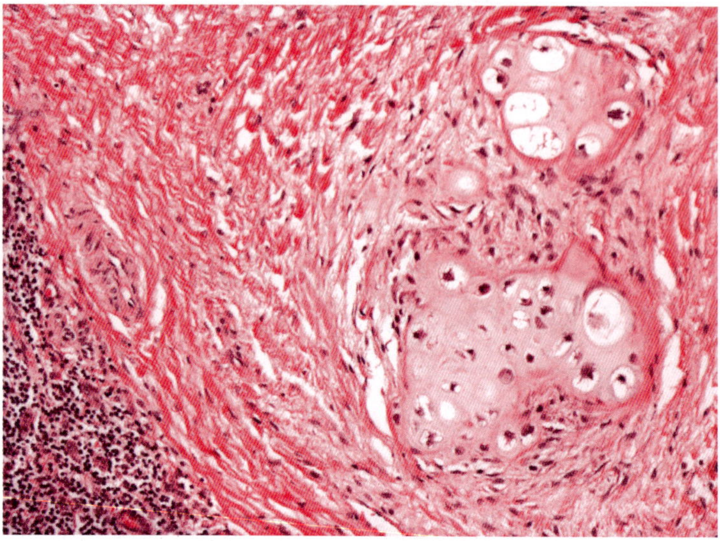

FIGURE 12.1 Chondroid metaplasia seen in peritonsillar fibrous tissue.

CHONDROMA AND OSTEOMA

Chondromas are much less common than well-differentiated chondrosarcomas and one should be wary about making this diagnosis.[2] In the upper aerodigestive tract, "chondroma" may best be used for small, circumscribed lesions that are fully excised. Indeed, it may be more prudent to diagnose lesions nonspecifically as *well-differentiated chondroid neoplasms* when only a small portion of mature-appearing cartilaginous tissue is seen in a biopsy specimen. Chondromas are composed of central, well-circumscribed hyaline cartilage devoid of cytologic atypia with rare or absent mitotic figures (eFig. 12.2). They are surrounded by a thin layer of fibrous tissue. These lesions are benign and should generally not recur after resection.

Osteomas can develop throughout the upper aerodigestive tract, often associated with adjacent bone. A unique osteoma referred to by some as a "choristoma" occurs in the dorsum of the tongue, most commonly in young to middle-aged women.[3] These vary in size, but do not generally grow to more than 2 cm. They are usually well-circumscribed and are composed of dense, mature, laminated bone (Fig. 12.2, eFig. 12.3). They do not recur after resection.

GIANT CELL REPARATIVE GRANULOMA

Giant cell reparative granuloma may be central and entirely located within mandible or maxilla.[4,5] It not infrequently, however, involves the nasal cavity or paranasal sinuses and can be sampled as a nasal or sinonasal mass. These lesions are thought to be reactive and secondary

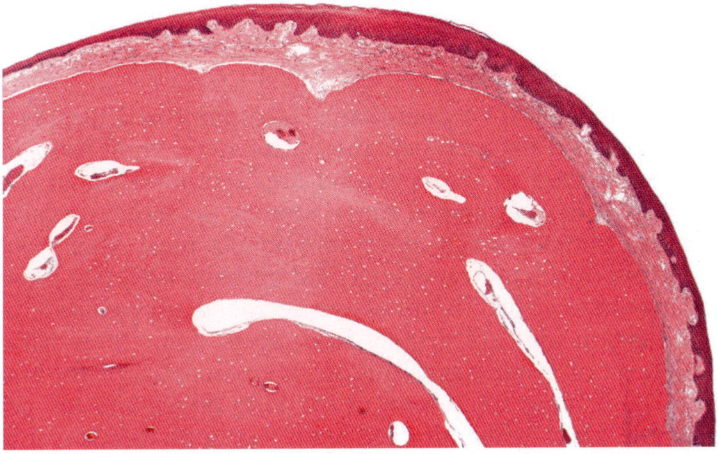

FIGURE 12.2 A well-circumscribed osteoma of the tongue made of mature bone.

to trauma, hemorrhage, or inflammation, although a neoplastic origin cannot be excluded. Patients are typically younger than 30-years. Histologically, aggregates of giant cells are seen within a fibrovascular stroma, often associated with hemorrhage (Fig. 12.3, eFig. 12.4). The giant cells tend to be smaller, with fewer nuclei than those seen with

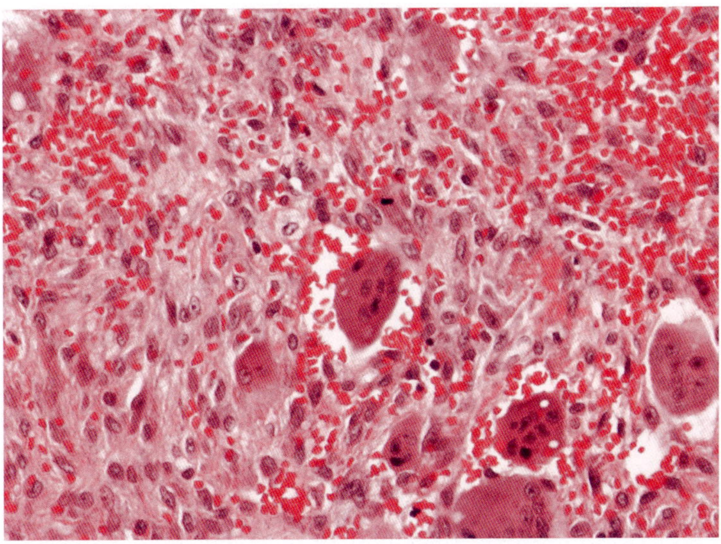

FIGURE 12.3 Giant cell reparative granuloma is characterized by numerous multinucleated giant cells within a hemorrhagic stroma.

true giant cell tumors. It has been noted that they histologically resemble solid aneurismal bone cysts. These lesions are not associated with *USP6* translocations.[6]

GIANT CELL TUMOR

Unlike giant cell reparative granuloma, true giant cell tumors are rare within the head and neck. When they arise here, they have most frequently been reported in the sphenoid and temporal bones, or within the larynx.[7,8] Within the larynx, these tumors present in adults over a wide age range and are much more common in men. Most have arisen from the thyroid or cricoid cartilages, and patients typically present with hoarseness or obstruction. Tumors have averaged approximately 4 cm in greatest dimension and are grossly infiltrative, sometimes with associated hemorrhage or cystic degeneration. Microscopically, the lesions are identical to those more often seen in the long bones and are composed of innumerable giant cells admixed with macrophages and fibroblasts (Fig. 12.4). The giant cells have numerous (often >20) bland nuclei, similar to those of the surrounding epithelioid to spindled mononuclear cells. Mitotic figure are often noted. Patients with laryngeal giant cell tumors do well, and the tumors do not recur after resection or other treatment. Malignant and aggressive giant cell tumors of the sphenoid have been reported; however, some of these may actually represent giant cell–rich osteosarcoma, as they have been noted in patients with Paget disease and in children.[8]

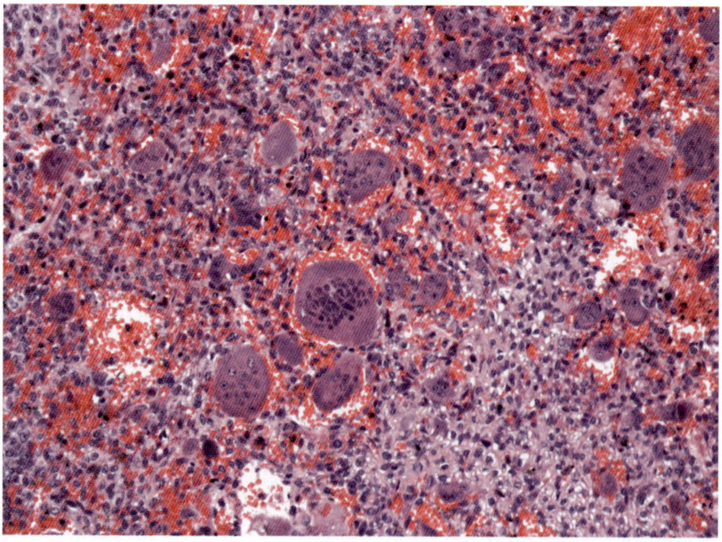

FIGURE 12.4 Large, multinucleated cells are present diffusely throughout this laryngeal giant cell tumor.

FIBRO-OSSEOUS/CEMENTIFYING LESIONS (FIBROUS DYSPLASIA, OSSIFYING/CEMENTIFYING FIBROMA, ETC.)

Fibro-osseous lesions frequently develop within the bones of the jaw. They sometimes involve the sinonasal structures or extend from the alveolar ridge (these are mentioned briefly in the discussion of fibroma within the Chapter 11). As such, they sometimes must be diagnosed with biopsy samples from the upper aerodigestive tract.

Fibrous dysplasia typically presents centrally within the jaw bones but may involve the sinonasal tract.[9] Depending on its primary site of growth, it can present with facial swelling, visual impairment, or sinonasal obstruction. When the lesions involve multiple noncontiguous bones, the disease is considered polyostotic and McCune-Albright syndrome should be excluded. The lesions typically present in children and young adults and may appear lytic, sclerotic, or mixed, depending on the age of the lesions. These are typically benign and stop growing with skeletal maturation. Classically, fibrous dysplasia is composed of intermixed, irregular fragments of woven bone with a cellular stroma. The woven bone is typically not lined by osteoblasts, and the cellular stroma is composed of bland spindled cells (Fig. 12.5, eFig. 12.5). Some osteoblastic rimming and lamellar bone formation can be seen, and one should not use that feature to exclude a diagnosis of fibrous dysplasia.

Ossifying fibromas, like most fibrous dysplasias, are also usually centrally located in the jaw bones. They too may extend into the sinonasal tract, especially certain variants, such as *juvenile psammomatoid ossifying fibroma*.[9-11] Whereas juvenile psammomatoid ossifying fibromas often

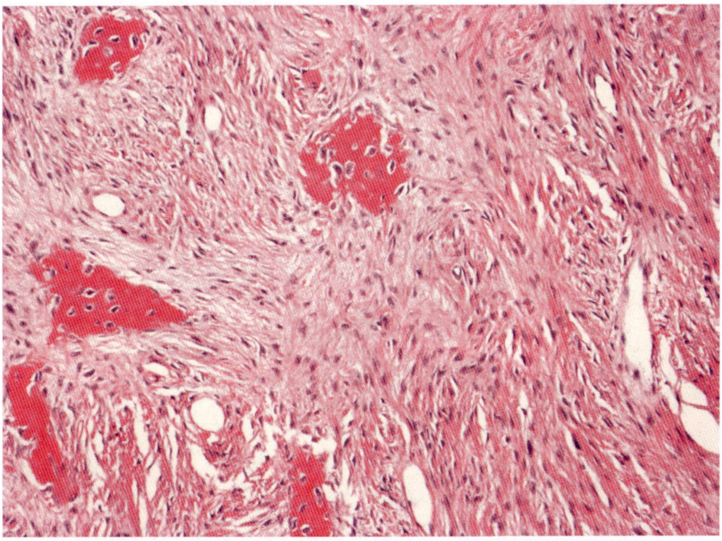

FIGURE 12.5 Woven bone admixed with a cellular stroma typifies fibrous dysplasia.

occur (as the name implies) in adolescents and young adults (although they also occur in older adults), conventional ossifying fibromas occur in patients who are, on average, in their fourth decade of life. The lesions have variable radiolucency and density, depending on the proportion of the lesion that is bony. These lesions are also benign, although juvenile psammomatoid ossifying fibroma has been noted to be locally aggressive.

Conventional ossifying fibromas are histologically similar to fibrous dysplasia with intermixed stroma and bone or cementum. The stroma varies in cellularity and is composed of bland spindled cells. Mitotic figures may be frequent. The bone and cementum form irregular ossicles, similar to those seen with fibrous dysplasia, however, more abundant osteoblastic rimming is typically seen. The radiographic features can be helpful in distinguishing these two entities, but in some instances both radiographic and microscopic features are overlapping and a diagnosis of "benign fibro-osseous lesion" is appropriate. Juvenile psammomatoid ossifying fibromas are similar and composed of bony spicules and spherules admixed with fibrous stroma. Mineralization or calcification is present as basophilic spheres (psammomalike) within the pink ossicles of bone (Fig. 12.6, eFig. 12.6).

CHONDROMYXOID FIBROMA

Chondromyxoid fibroma is a benign tumor that has been reported to involve the craniofacial bones and may present as a sinonasal or skull-based mass.[12,13] The tumors typically present in adults. Histologically,

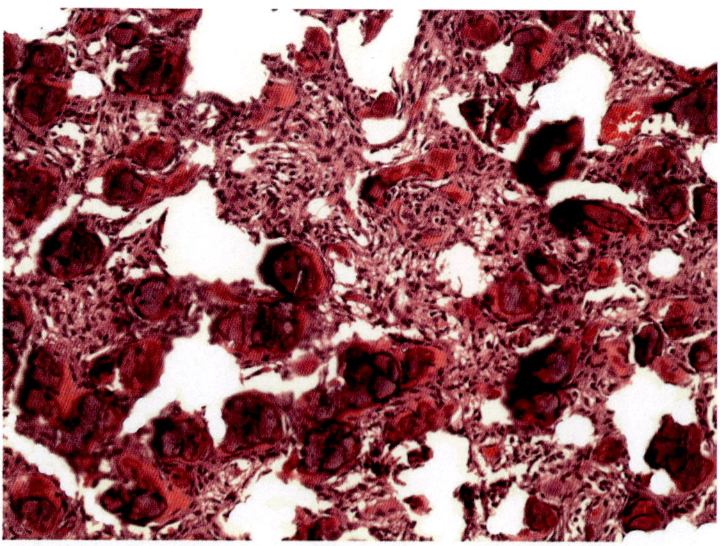

FIGURE 12.6 Spherical or "psammomatoid" areas of mineralization are seen with juvenile psammomatoid ossifying fibromas.

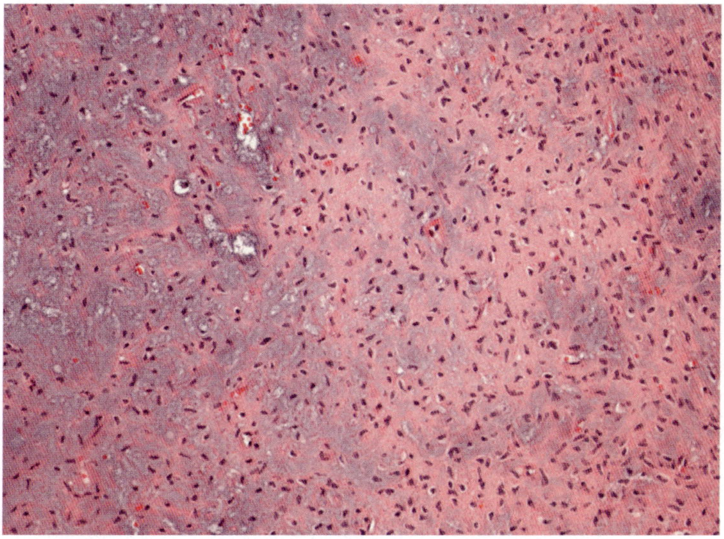

FIGURE 12.7 Bland stromal cells are present in a chondromyxoid stroma in chondromyxoid fibroma.

tumors are composed of nodules of bland spindled or stellate cells within a loosely chondroid and myxoid matrix (Fig. 12.7, eFig. 12.7). Well-formed cartilage is almost always absent. Typically, the periphery of the nodules is more cellular than the center (eFig. 12.8). Occasional giant cells can be present. These tumors should be distinguished from chondrosarcomas and chordomas. Neither chondrocytes nor physaliferous cells should be present with chondromyxoid fibroma. Tumors recur after excision in one-third of cases.[14]

CHONDROMESENCHYMAL HAMARTOMA

Chondromesenchymal hamartoma must be considered in the differential diagnosis with cartilaginous or myxoid lesions, especially of the sinonasal tract in young people. This lesion is discussed in Chapter 13.

CHONDROSARCOMA

Chondrosarcomas are the most common cartilaginous lesions of the upper aerodigestive tract and are the most common sarcomas of the larynx.[2,15,16] Most appear to arise from bone or cartilaginous tissue and then extend into adjacent soft tissues. In the sinonasal area, chondrosarcomas may arise from the nasal septum, the maxilla, and the ethmoid and sphenoid bones. In the larynx, the tumors frequently arise from the cricoid, thyroid, or arytenoid cartilages. Patients present with nonspecific symptoms secondary to mass lesions.

Well-differentiated or *low-grade chondrosarcomas* (grade 1 or 2) make up the majority of chondrosarcomas in this region, especially within the larynx.[15,16] These are malignancies of older individuals and most arise in men older than 50 years. Rare examples have been reported in children.[17] These tumors are generally infiltrative and somewhat lobular. Histologically, lobules of cartilaginous stroma are present showing differing degrees of differentiation. Some lobules are composed of well-formed hyaline cartilage, whereas others appear looser and more myxoid (Figs. 12.8 and 12.9, eFigs. 12.9–12.11); indeed, as tumors gain a more myxoid appearance, some are referred to as *myxoid chondrosarcomas*. At the periphery of the tumors, fibrocartilage can sometimes be found. The cellularity varies substantially from one tumor to another. Lower grade tumors appear similar to chondromas and have minimal cellular atypia and few mitotic figures. These lesions must be diagnosed based primarily on their infiltrative growth patterns and associated behavior. Many well-differentiated chondrosarcomas are slightly more cellular with frequent binucleated chondrocytes that have at least moderate atypia and prominent nucleoli (Fig. 12.10). Well-differentiated tumors often recur and can be locally aggressive. Even with recurrence, patients often live many years. Metastases are extremely rare in patients with low-grade chondrosarcomas unless the tumor has undergone high-grade transformation (see below).

Dedifferentiated chondrosarcomas have been described in the upper aerodigestive tract.[15,16] These tumors, by definition, are composed of areas of well-differentiated chondrosarcoma abruptly juxtaposed to

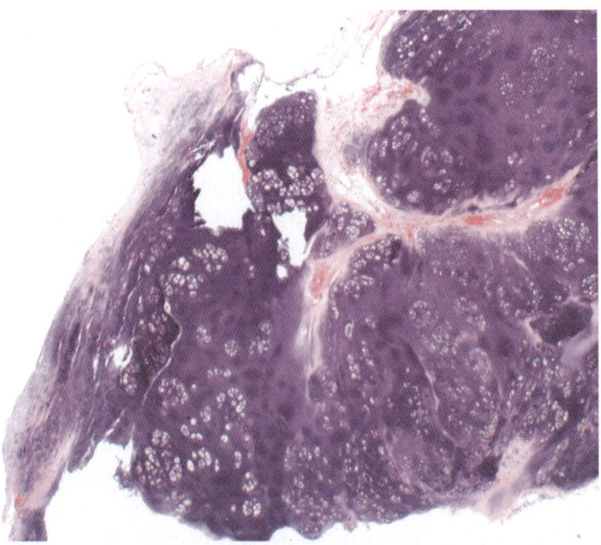

FIGURE 12.8 A biopsy of a well-differentiated chondrosarcoma may show only mature-appearing hyaline cartilage without atypia.

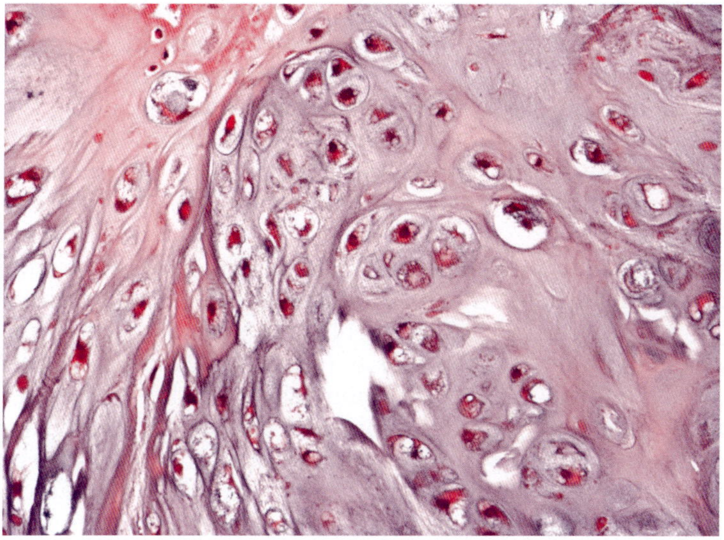

FIGURE 12.9 Low-grade chondrosarcoma having very little cytologic atypia.

undifferentiated, pleomorphic sarcomas (eFig. 12.12). These tumors, in general, have a very poor prognosis and metastasize widely. Rare cases reported in the larynx have behaved well.

Mesenchymal chondrosarcomas are uncommon chondroid malignancies that may involve the upper aerodigestive tract, especially the sinonasal area.[18] Although they may develop in patients of any age, they

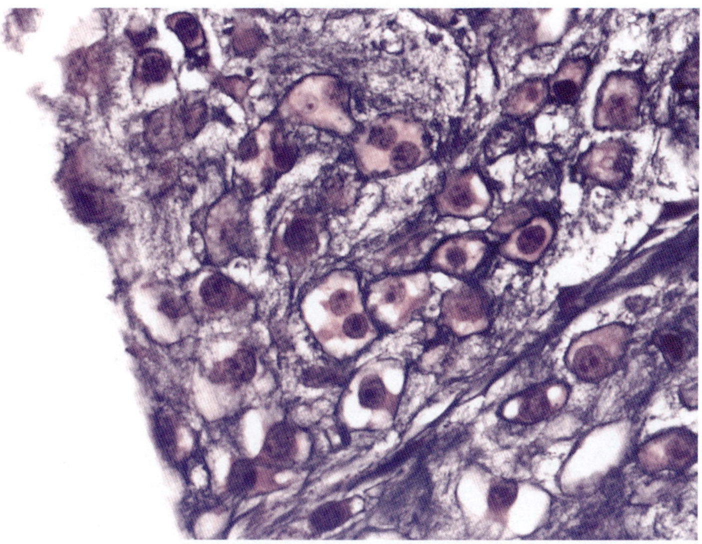

FIGURE 12.10 This low-grade chondrosarcoma is more cellular and has mild cytologic atypia.

typically occur in younger patients than do other chondrosarcomas and often arise in children. Symptoms are nonspecific and include obstruction or epistaxis. Radiographically, the lesions appear destructive and involve structures beyond the sinuses and nasal cavity, often including the periorbital tissues. Surgical resection with radiation or chemotherapy is the main treatment modality. Approximately 50% may recur and often result in the death of the patient. Metastases rarely develop long (>20 years) after the original diagnosis.

Microscopically, mesenchymal chondrosarcomas are composed of sheets of undifferentiated small, round cells that focally transition into islands of mature cartilage (Fig. 12.11).[18–20] Slitlike vascular spaces are often present within the sheets of undifferentiated cells reminiscent of glomangiopericytoma. Cell discohesion may give the tumor an alveolar appearance (eFig. 12.13). The neoplastic cells are generally round with little cytoplasm; however, spindled cells are sometimes seen. The cells have hyperchromatic nuclei with irregular contours and vesicular chromatin (eFig. 12.14). Mitotic figures usually number fewer than two per 10 high-powered fields. The lacunae of the cartilage islands contain cells similar to those in the areas of sheetlike growth, although they often appear larger and better differentiated. Hemorrhage, necrosis, and myxoid change may be present. Immunohistochemically, the neoplastic cells in the more cartilaginous areas react with antibodies to S100 protein.[21] The undifferentiated areas often show immunoreactivity with antibodies to CD99 and NSE, but should not show immunoreactivity with antibodies to myogenous antigens such as desmin or epithelial antigens such as cytokeratins.

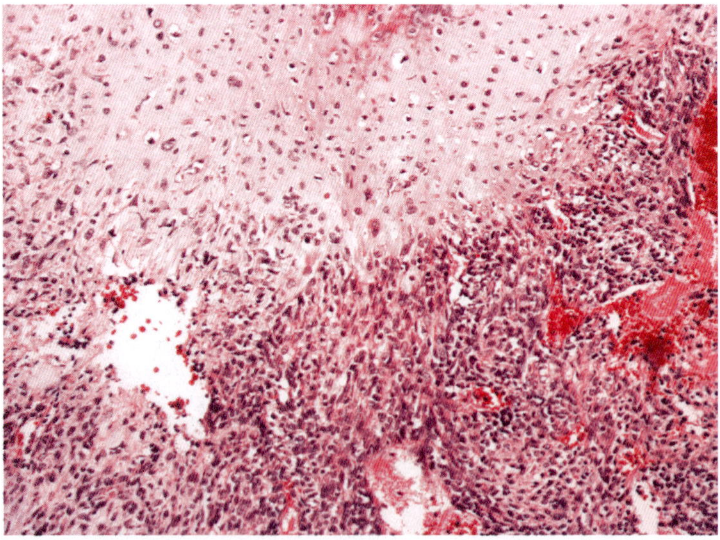

FIGURE 12.11 A mesenchymal chondrosarcoma is characterized by juxtaposed hyaline cartilage and small primitive cells.

Mesenchymal chondrosarcomas need to be distinguished from other chondrosarcomas, small round cell tumors, and even pleomorphic adenomas. The sheets of small blue cells should allow for easy distinction from other types of chondrosarcomas, whereas the presence of well-formed cartilage allows for the distinction from most other small round cell tumors. The lack of expression of myogenous antigens allows them to be distinguished from rhabdomyosarcomas. Mesenchymal chondrosarcomas have obvious immunophenotypic overlap with peripheral neuroectodermal tumors and can express NSE and CD99. Cytogenetic analysis or RT-PCR may be helpful, as mesenchymal chondrosarcomas lack the t(11;22)(q24;q12) and resultant transcript, and have been instead shown to have a *HEY1-NCOA2* fusion.[22] Because of their cartilaginous differentiation, the tumors may be confused with pleomorphic adenomas. The sheets of myoepithelial cells seen with pleomorphic adenomas should be easy to distinguish from the undifferentiated cells of mesenchymal chondrosarcomas, at least with the more generous specimens. Immunohistochemistry can be used if needed (e.g., antibodies to myoepithelial antigens such as S100 protein, SMA, cytokeratin), when small biopsy specimens raise the differential.

OSTEOSARCOMA

Most osteosarcomas sampled with upper aerodigestive tract biopsy arise from the jaws.[23-27] Most often, these arise from the mandible and the mean age of presentation is 34 years, patients being considerably older than those with long bone osteosarcomas. Upper aerodigestive tract biopsies from these lesions are usually from the mouth; however, maxillary tumors can involve the sinonasal tract. Patients may present with swelling, tooth loss, bleeding, sinonasal obstruction, and proptosis depending on the site of the tumor. Extragnathic osteosarcomas often develop secondary to preexisting conditions such as Paget disease, chronic osteomyelitis, or prior radiation therapy. They tend to be more extensive than gnathic tumors and have a worse prognosis.[25]

The histologic variability seen with osteosarcomas of long bones can be seen with gnathic and extragnathic tumors of the head and neck, although some have noted better differentiation with gnathic tumors.[27] Tumors may show extensive chondroblastic or fibroblastic differentiation and this can be all that is seen in a biopsy specimen (Fig. 12.12, eFig. 12.15). Thus one should be very hesitant about diagnosing chondrosarcoma or fibrosarcoma (or even sarcomatoid carcinoma) with a biopsy sample from the mouth when the tumor appears to involve the jaw. By definition, osteoid production must be present, but with gnathic tumors these areas may be “normalized” or very well differentiated and surrounded by bland-appearing osteoblasts (Fig. 12.13, eFig. 12.16).

As mentioned, the differential diagnosis typically includes chondroid-containing or malignant spindle cell neoplasms. Malignant osteoid

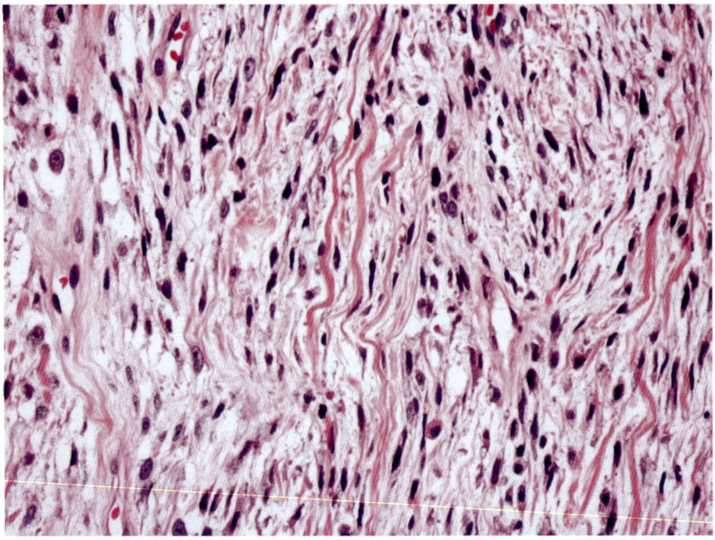

FIGURE 12.12 Fibroblastic differentiation may be all that is seen with the biopsy of a gnathic osteosarcoma.

production typically clinches a diagnosis except in cases of sarcomatoid carcinoma. Squamous differentiation or overlying squamous dysplasia obviously should lead to a diagnosis of sarcomatoid carcinoma. Furthermore, if the tumor does not involve bone and occurs at a site commonly involved by sarcomatoid carcinoma, one should be very hesitant about diagnosing

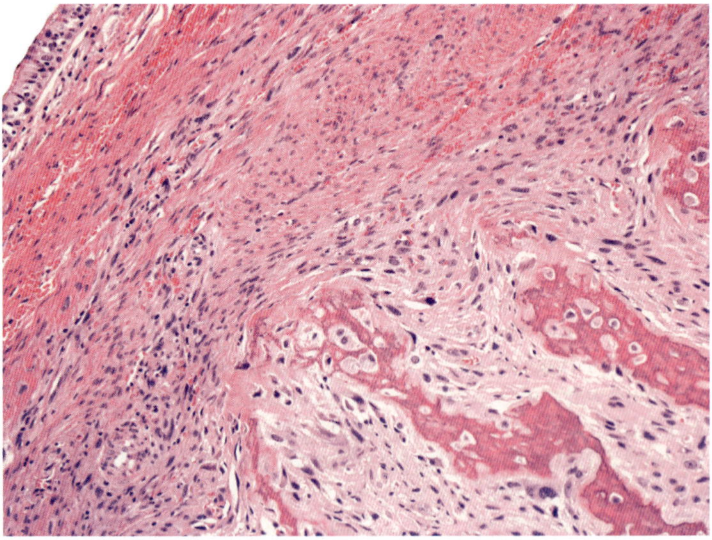

FIGURE 12.13 Atypical osteoblastic rimming and mature osteoid formation immediately below the surface epithelium of this sinonasal osteosarcoma.

the lesion as an osteosarcoma, since it has been well-documented that sarcomatoid carcinomas can produce osteoid. Even in areas of "normalization," we have noted extensive p16 immunoreactivity in some osteosarcomas, a feature that may be helpful with small biopsies for distinguishing osteosarcomas from fibro-osseous lesions (eFig. 12.17).

AMELOBLASTOMA

A myriad of odontogenic tumors can present within the jaws. The most common lesion to involve the upper aerodigestive tract, in our experience, is sinonasal ameloblastoma.[28] Here, the diagnosis is only difficult when it is not considered. These tumors occur more commonly in men and the mean age of presentation is 60 years. Patients typically present with a mass lesion and nasal obstruction but may have other nonspecific symptoms including sinusitis or epistaxis. The tumors are benign, but can recur with inadequate resection. While mandibular tumors often show *BRAF* mutation and maxillary tumors frequently have *SMO* mutations, recurrent abnormalities have not yet been identified for sinonasal lesions.[29]

Tumors are composed of nests and anastomosing cords of epithelium (eFig. 12.18). The epithelium is surrounded by a layer of columnar cells with hyperchromatic, reverse-polarized nuclei and subnuclear vacuoles (Fig. 12.14). The epithelium otherwise has a stellate reticulum–like appearance with variable degrees of squamous metaplasia and keratin formation. The surface epithelium frequently appears involved.

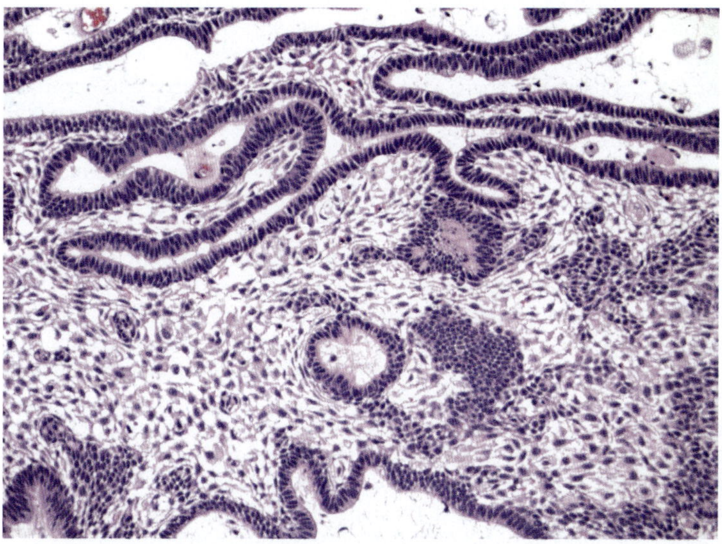

FIGURE 12.14 Columnar cells surrounding a stellate reticulum–like squamous epithelium are seen with sinonasal ameloblastoma.

The differential diagnosis includes glandular and squamous tumors. Key to recognizing ameloblastoma is the identification of a peripheral columnar cell layer. This should not be seen with squamous carcinomas, schneiderian papillomas, or salivary gland tumors. Sinonasal ameloblastomas do not have the cytologic atypia that should be seen with squamous cell carcinomas. All cells, including the columnar cells, are immunoreactive with antibodies to p63; thus biphasic staining typical of some salivary gland–type tumors is not seen.[30] Because tumors are composed of an intimate mixture of stellate and columnar epithelial cells, biphasic synovial sarcoma may also be considered. Sinonasal ameloblastomas often show more mature squamous differentiation of the stellate epithelial cells than is seen with synovial sarcoma. Furthermore, neoplastic cells are immunoreactive with antibodies to keratins throughout.

REFERENCES

1. Daley TD, Damm DD, Wysocki GP, Weir JC. Atypical cartilage in reactive osteocartilagenous metaplasia of the traumatized edentulous mandibular ridge. *Oral Surg Oral Med Oral Pathol Oral Radiol Endod.* 1997;83(1):26-29.
2. Fu YS, Perzin KH. Non-epithelial tumors of the nasal cavity, paranasal sinuses, and nasopharynx: a clinicopathologic study. 3. Cartilaginous tumors (chondroma, chondrosarcoma). *Cancer.* 1974;34(2):453-463.
3. Supiyaphun P, Sampatanakul P, Kerekhanjanarong V, Chawakitchareon P, Sastarasadhit V. Lingual osseous choristoma: a study of eight cases and review of the literature. *Ear Nose Throat J.* 1998;77(4):316-318, 320, 325.
4. Waldron CA, Shafer WG. The central giant cell reparative granuloma of the jaws. An analysis of 38 cases. *Am J Clin Pathol.* 1966;45(4):437-447.
5. Yamaguchi T, Dorfman HD. Giant cell reparative granuloma: a comparative clinicopathologic study of lesions in gnathic and extragnathic sites. *Int J Surg Pathol.* 2001;9(3):189-200.
6. Agaram NP, LeLoarer FV, Zhang L, et al. USP6 gene rearrangements occur preferentially in giant cell reparative granulomas of the hands and feet but not in gnathic location. *Hum Pathol.* 2014;45(6):1147-1152.
7. Wieneke JA, Gannon FH, Heffner DK, Thompson LD. Giant cell tumor of the larynx: a clinicopathologic series of eight cases and a review of the literature. *Mod Pathol.* 2001;14(12):1209-1215.
8. Chan J, Gannon FH, Thompson LD. Malignant giant cell tumor of the sphenoid. *Ann Diagn Pathol.* 2003;7(2):100-105.
9. Fu YS, Perzin KH. Non-epithelial tumors of the nasal cavity, paranasal sinuses, and nasopharynx. A clinicopathologic study. II. Osseous and fibro-osseous lesions, including osteoma, fibrous dysplasia, ossifying fibroma, osteoblastoma, giant cell tumor, and osteosarcoma. *Cancer.* 1974;33(5):1289-1305.
10. Wenig BM, Vinh TN, Smirniotopoulos JG, Fowler CB, Houston GD, Heffner DK. Aggressive psammomatoid ossifying fibromas of the sinonasal region: a clinicopathologic study of a distinct group of fibro-osseous lesions. *Cancer.* 1995;76(7):1155-1165.
11. Eversole LR, Leider AS, Nelson K. Ossifying fibroma: a clinicopathologic study of sixty-four cases. *Oral Surg Oral Med Oral Pathol.* 1985;60(5):505-511.
12. Keel SB, Bhan AK, Liebsch NJ, Rosenberg AE. Chondromyxoid fibroma of the skull base: a tumor which may be confused with chordoma and chondrosarcoma. A report of three cases and review of the literature. *Am J Surg Pathol.* 1997;21(5):577-582.

13. Veras EF, Santamaria IB, Luna MA. Sinonasal chondromyxoid fibroma. *Ann Diagn Pathol.* 2009;13(1):41-46.
14. Meredith DM, Fletcher CDM, Jo VY. Chondromyxoid fibroma arising in craniofacial sites: a clinicopathologic analysis of 25 cases. *Am J Surg Pathol.* 2018;42(3):392-400.
15. Casiraghi O, Martinez-Madrigal F, Pineda-Daboin K, Mamelle G, Resta L, Luna MA. Chondroid tumors of the larynx: a clinicopathologic study of 19 cases, including two dedifferentiated chondrosarcomas. *Ann Diagn Pathol.* 2004;8(4):189-197.
16. Thompson LD, Gannon FH. Chondrosarcoma of the larynx: a clinicopathologic study of 111 cases with a review of the literature. *Am J Surg Pathol.* 2002;26(7):836-851.
17. Gadwal SR, Fanburg-Smith JC, Gannon FH, Thompson LD. Primary chondrosarcoma of the head and neck in pediatric patients: a clinicopathologic study of 14 cases with a review of the literature. *Cancer.* 2000;88(9):2181-2188.
18. Knott PD, Gannon FH, Thompson LD. Mesenchymal chondrosarcoma of the sinonasal tract: a clinicopathological study of 13 cases with a review of the literature. *Laryngoscope.* 2003;113(5):783-790.
19. Bertoni F, Picci P, Bacchini P, et al. Mesenchymal chondrosarcoma of bone and soft tissues. *Cancer.* 1983;52(3):533-541.
20. Dahlin DC, Henderson ED. Mesenchymal chondrosarcoma. Further observations on a new entity. *Cancer.* 1962;15:410-417.
21. Devoe K, Weidner N. Immunohistochemistry of small round-cell tumors. *Semin Diagn Pathol.* 2000;17(3):216-224.
22. Wang L, Motoi T, Khanin R, et al. Identification of a novel, recurrent HEY1-NCOA2 fusion in mesenchymal chondrosarcoma based on a genome-wide screen of exon-level expression data. *Genes Chromosomes Cancer.* 2012;51(2):127-139.
23. Demicco EG, Deshpande V, Nielsen GP, Kattapuram SV, Rosenberg AE. Well-differentiated osteosarcoma of the jaw bones: a clinicopathologic study of 15 cases. *Am J Surg Pathol.* 2010;34(11):1647-1655.
24. Padilla RJ, Murrah VA. The spectrum of gnathic osteosarcoma: caveats for the clinician and the pathologist. *Head Neck Pathol.* 2011;5(1):92-99.
25. Nora FE, Unni KK, Pritchard DJ, Dahlin DC. Osteosarcoma of extragnathic craniofacial bones. *Mayo Clin Proc.* 1983;58(4):268-272.
26. Garrington GE, Scofield HH, Cornyn J, Hooker SP. Osteosarcoma of the jaws. Analysis of 56 cases. *Cancer.* 1967;20(3):377-391.
27. Clark JL, Unni KK, Dahlin DC, Devine KD. Osteosarcoma of the jaw. *Cancer.* 1983;51(12):2311-2316.
28. Schafer DR, Thompson LD, Smith BC, Wenig BM. Primary ameloblastoma of the sinonasal tract: a clinicopathologic study of 24 cases. *Cancer.* 1998;82(4):667-674.
29. Sweeney RT, McClary AC, Myers BR, et al. Identification of recurrent SMO and BRAF mutations in ameloblastomas. *Nat Genet.* 2014;46(7):722-725.
30. Kumamoto H, Ohki K, Ooya K. Expression of p63 and p73 in ameloblastomas. *J Oral Pathol Med.* 2005;34(4):220-226.

13

NONNEOPLASTIC LESIONS OF THE NASAL CAVITY, PARANASAL SINUSES, AND NASOPHARYNX

Most samples from the nasal cavity, paranasal sinuses, and nasopharynx are for nonneoplastic disease. Perhaps because they are so often routine (e.g., chronic sinusitis and inflammatory polyps), they may sometimes receive somewhat cursory histologic examination. That said, a variety of challenging nonneoplastic lesions occur within this region. Furthermore, the accessibility of the nasal cavity allows for biopsy and evaluation of some systemic diseases.

As with most nonneoplastic histologies, the pathologic findings are often nonspecific. The pathologist thus needs to be especially aware of clinical information in such cases. Indeed, both the clinician and pathologist may need to work together in such cases as both may be presented with nonspecific findings. With midline destructive lesions, the clinician's differential may be vast, and treatment options may vary greatly depending upon the pathologist's interpretation (Table 13.1).[1,2] When confronted with granulomatous inflammation, the pathologist's differential diagnosis may include infectious, autoimmune, iatrogenic, and even neoplastic conditions (Table 13.2).[3,4] If the pathologist is to interpret such cases correctly, he will need to be fully armed with clinical and laboratory data. Even in such cases, he may, nonetheless, be sometimes forced to give more descriptive and qualified diagnoses.

SINUSITIS

Acute sinusitis is common following upper respiratory tract infection and is often due to infection by *Streptococcus pneumoniae*, *Haemophilus influenzae*, or *Moraxella catarrhalis*. It is generally treated with antibiotics and is rarely sampled. If sampled, sinus tissue will show abundant edema and infiltration by a mixture of inflammatory cells with the predominant cell type being neutrophils.

Chronic sinusitis, on the other hand, is often sampled, as debridement is sometimes the surgical treatment of choice. The etiology of the disease is thought to be related to multiple factors including infection, allergy, and the individual patient's anatomy and physiology.

TABLE 13.1 Midline Destructive Lesions

Infectious

- Bacterial
  - Acid-fast bacilli (tuberculosis and leprosy)
  - Rhinoscleroma (Klebsiella rhinoscleromatis)
- Fungal
  - Fulminant acute invasive fungal infection
  - Chronic invasive fungal infection
  - Other
- Other infections (spirochetes, parasites, etc.)

Vasculitides

- Wegener granulomatosis
- Allergic granulomatosis and angiitis (Churg-Straus disease)
- Other (systemic lupus erythematosis, polyarteritis nodosa, etc.)

Other

- Cocaine abuse
- Sarcoidosis
- Neoplasia (especially NK/T-cell lymphoma)

NK cell, natural killer cell.

TABLE 13.2 Granulomatous Inflammatory Lesions

Infectious disease

- Mycobacterium tuberculosis or leprosy (rarely other mycobacteria)
- Fungal infection
- Rhinoscleroma
- Leishmaniasis

Vasculitides

- Wegener granulomatosis
- Allergic granulomatosis and angiitis (Churg-Straus disease)

Other

- Sarcoidosis
- Cholesterol
- Neoplasia

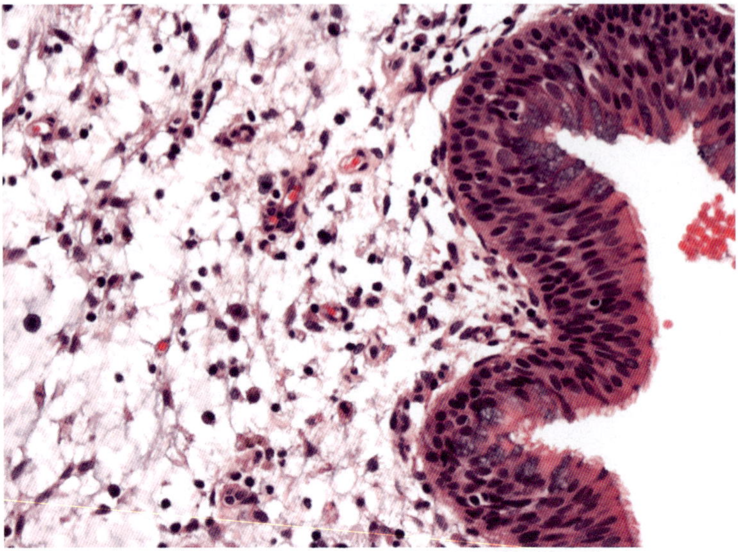

FIGURE 13.1 Chronic sinusitis with stromal edema and chronic inflammation.

Histologically, the respiratory tissue will show variable inflammation composed mostly of lymphocytes, plasma cells, and eosinophils with the relative proportions of these cells to one another varying from case to case (Fig. 13.1, eFig. 13.1).[5] Subepithelial and stromal fibrosis can be present depending on the overall chronicity of the process with epithelial hyperplasia and even polyp formation. Goblet cells may be more numerous, as may seromucinous glands. Fragments of underlying bone can have sclerotic, reactive changes.

PRIMARY CILIARY DYSKINESIA

A specific cause of chronic sinusitis is primary ciliary dyskinesia, also known as Kartagener syndrome. This disease is also associated with male sterility, chronic bronchitis, bronchiectasis, and situs inversus.[6,7] It is a genetically heterogeneous disease and typically inherited in an autosomal recessive pattern. Diagnosis requires clinical findings with anatomic and/or genetic findings, as neither anatomic nor genetic testing is entirely sensitive and specific.[8]

From the anatomic pathologic standpoint, assessment for this disease is usually twofold. Functional analysis of the cilia typically involves a wet preparation of scraped nasal epithelium with assessment of the cilia motility. Normal function should be coordinated and demonstrate both intracellular and intercellular synchrony, with cilia typically beating at a frequency of 8 to 20 Hz. Normal function excludes a diagnosis of primary ciliary dyskinesia for all practical purposes. Anatomic analysis of the cilia

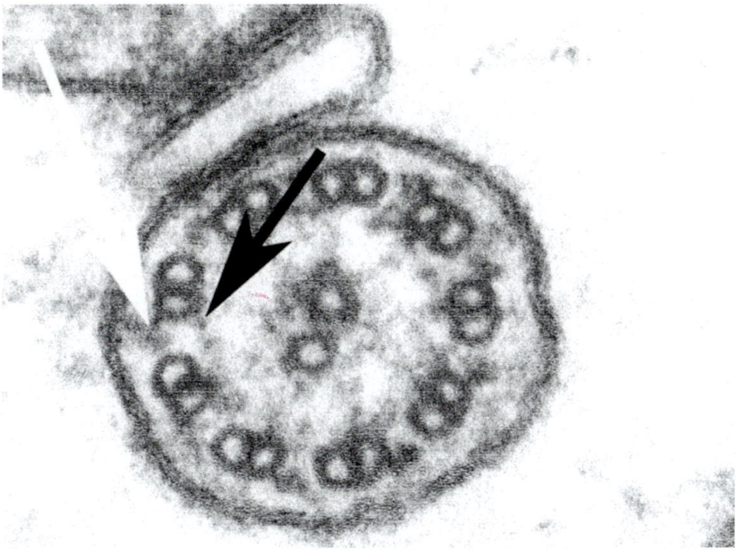

FIGURE 13.2 Electron microscopy of normal cilia showing the classic 9 + 2 microtubule configuration. Outer (white arrow) and inner (black arrow) dynein arms are seen.

is performed by electron microscopy. Normal motile cilia are composed of microtubules arranged in a 9 + 2 configuration (Fig. 13.2). Each of the nine outer doublets is attached to the adjacent doublets via nexin links, contains both inner and outer dynein arms, and has radial spokes. A description of all the variants of dysmotile cilia is beyond this book; however, the majority of dysfunction is associated with the absence of inner and/or outer dynein arms.

FUNGAL DISEASE

Fungi are the etiologic agents of a number of pathologies of the nasal cavities.[9,10] Commonly, they are related to allergic rhinitis and thus may play some role in the development of chronic sinusitis and secondary complications from such. They also play a role in a number of other sinus pathologies that can be either *noninvasive* or *invasive*.

Allergic Fungal Sinusitis

Allergic fungal sinusitis is the most common fungal disease of the sinuses. Clinically, patients with this disease are immunocompetent and may have concomitant asthma, allergic rhinitis, and nasal polyps.[11–13] The disease is suspected after a protracted history of sinusitis that has been refractory to treatments for bacterial sinusitis. It may be secondary to either hyaline molds such as *Aspergillus* or *Fusarium* species or to various dematiaceous molds.[11–14]

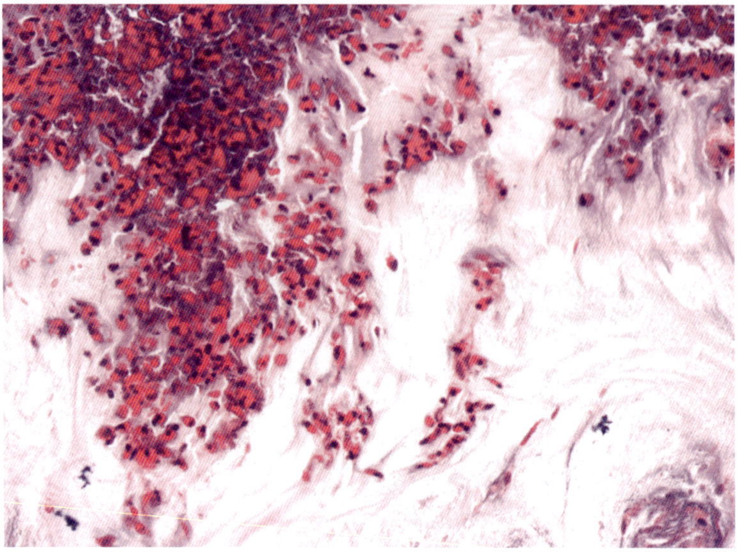

FIGURE 13.3 Mucus with numerous entrapped eosinophils.

Surgically collected specimens will grossly have tan-brown fragments of mucosa with green-brown mucoid material and have evoked for some the culinary impressions of cottage cheese and peanut butter.[9] Histologically, samples show abundant mucus with entrapped eosinophils and Charcot-Leyden crystals (*allergic mucus*) (Fig. 13.3, eFig. 13.2).[11,13] Although the fungal forms may be difficult to visualize with routine hematoxylin and eosin (H&E)–stained material, silver staining will show numerous hyphal fragments (Fig. 13.4, eFig. 13.3). The hyphal fragments often branch at 45-degree angles and may have occasional conidia.[13] Fragments of edematous and inflamed respiratory mucosa will also be present, showing changes consistent with chronic sinusitis, and should not contain organisms when viewed with special stains.

Sinus Mycetoma (Fungus Ball)

Sinus mycetomas most often occur in the maxillary sinuses of immunocompetent patients.[9,15] Patients may present with headache, facial pain, nasal obstruction, or a perceived nasty odor, and patients may even present with new-onset seizure and may sometimes have concomitant nasal polyps and sinusitis. The disease is most often caused by *Aspergillus fumigatus*.

Removed material will appear mucopurulent or cheesy.[9] On sections, a dense collection of fungal elements will be seen, devoid of allergic mucus (Fig. 13.5). Silver staining is rarely needed due to the abundance of the fungus (eFig. 13.4). The fragments of sinus tissue will show changes of chronic sinusitis, and fungi should not involve fragments of respiratory mucosa.

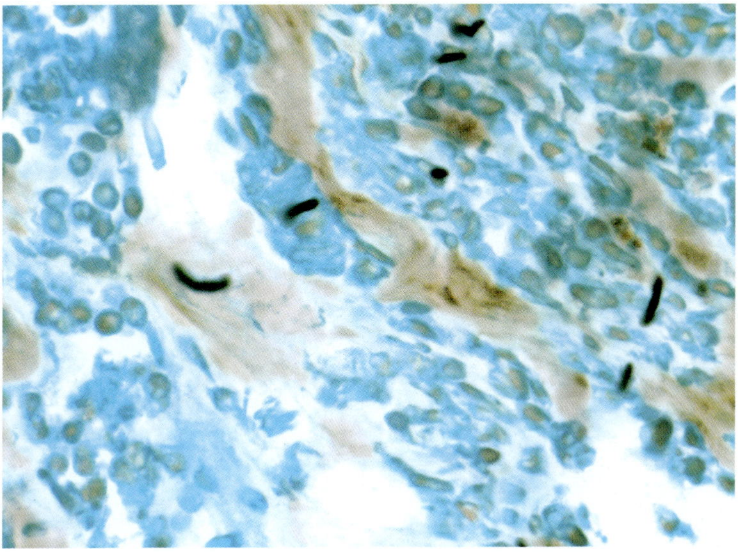

FIGURE 13.4 A silver stain shows occasional hyphal fragments.

Invasive Fungal Sinusitis

Invasive fungal sinusitis is a disease generally restricted to immunocompromised individuals, although rare instances are noted in which the disease has affected immunocompetent persons.[9,15–18] Acute or fulminant invasive fungal sinusitis may present as a painless, black, nasal septal, or palatal

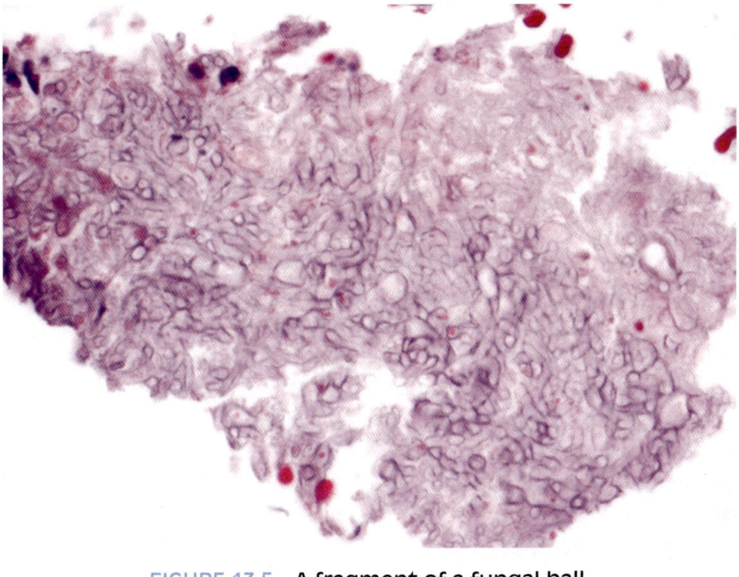

FIGURE 13.5 A fragment of a fungal ball.

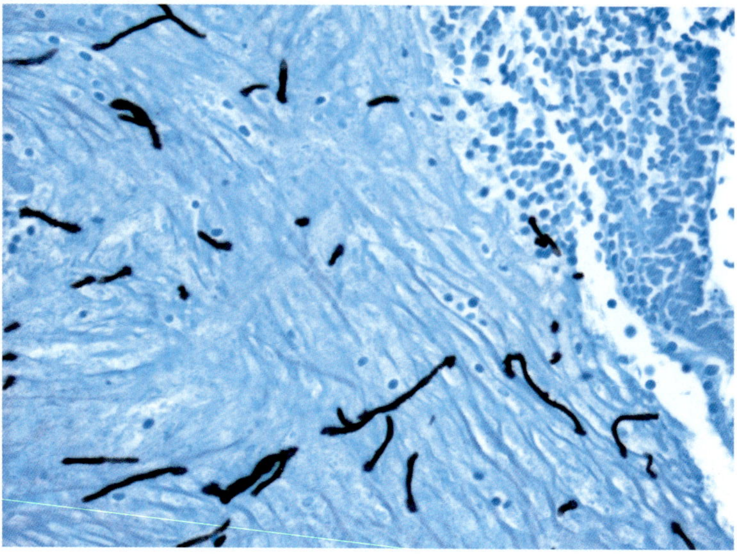

FIGURE 13.6 Invasive fungi seen with silver stain.

eschar. It is most often caused by fungi of the order Mucorales such as *Rhizopus* and *Mucor* but may also be caused by *Aspergillus* and *Fusarium* species as well as dematiaceous species.

Histologically, samples from patients with acute fungal sinusitis will show invasion of tissue by the hyphal elements often with involvement of vascular structures (Fig. 13.6, eFig. 13.5).[9,10,16] A secondary vasculitis and thrombosis with resultant hemorrhage and infarction may also be seen. Surrounding inflammation is often minimal, a reflection of the immunocompromised state of the patient. Some have suggested the use of in situ hybridization for the typing of the etiologic agents.[19]

Chronic invasive fungal sinusitis follows a more protracted course than acute invasive fungal sinusitis.[9,10] Patients are immunocompromised usually secondary to diabetes mellitus or previous treatment with corticosteroids. The disease may be associated with decreased vision and ocular immovability (orbital apex syndrome). Some believe the lesion begins as a sinus mycetoma that eventually becomes invasive due to the immunocompromised state of the patient. The disease is most often secondary to infection by *A. fumigatus*. As with acute invasive sinusitis, histologic sections show tissue and vascular invasion by hyphal elements, often with a limited inflammatory response.

Finally, paranasal granuloma or granulomatous invasive fungal sinusitis is a rare chronic fungal disease of immunocompetent patients that is associated with proptosis.[9] The disease is secondary to infection by *Aspergillus flavus*. Most reports of this lesion come from Sudan.

Histologically, tissue invasion is present which induces nonnecrotizing granulomatous inflammation with intermixed plasma cells. At the centers of these granulomata, a small amount of fibrinoid necrosis with eosinophils may be present. An associated vasculitis may also be seen.

NASAL TUBERCULOSIS

Involvement of the upper airway in tuberculosis is uncommon, and because of current chemotherapy, it is seldom considered in the differential diagnosis of nasal or pharyngeal disease.[20,21] Infection with *Mycobacterium tuberculosis* can be primary to the site or secondary to a more widespread infection. Infection creates chronic symptoms with mucorrhea and epistaxis when the nasal cavity is involved, and cervical adenopathy is often noted with involvement of the nasopharynx. A discrete mass or ulcer may be present, and some ulcers may be deep enough to lead to perforation of the nasal septum. Histologically, sections will show caseating granulomata with Langhans-type giant cells (Fig. 13.7). Special staining for acid-fast bacilli may reveal organisms. Culturing the lesion is essential for the specific diagnosis.

NASAL LEPROSY

Leprosy is an infectious, granulomatous disease that involves the skin and peripheral nerves and may sometimes involve the mucous membranes and nose.[22,23] This is especially true with lepromatous leprosy.

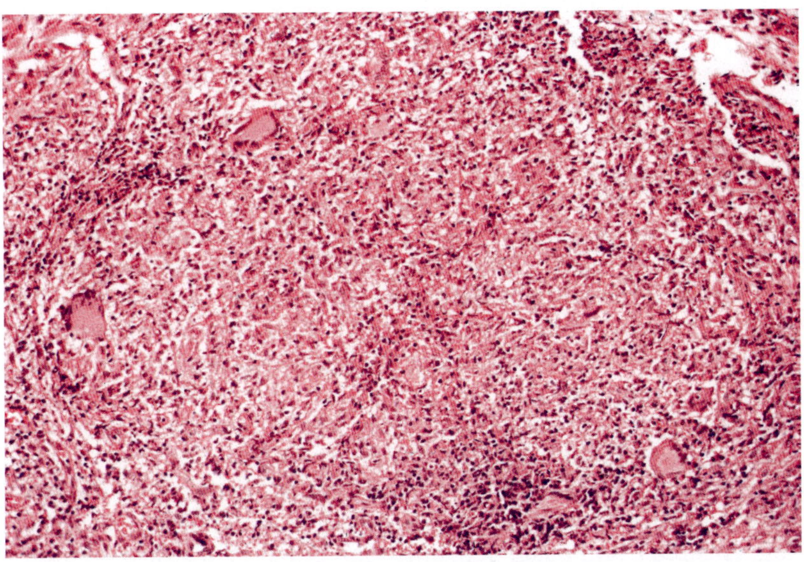

FIGURE 13.7 Necrotizing granulomatous inflammation seen with tuberculosis.

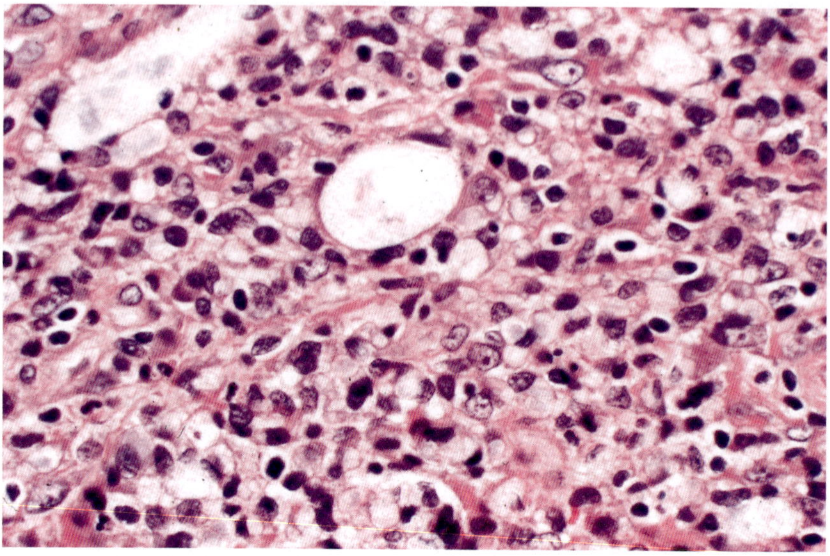

FIGURE 13.8 **Mixed inflammation with numerous macrophages seen with leprosy.**

It most often involves the inferior turbinates and septum, and crusting, obstruction, and bleeding may be noted. The typical histologic features of leprosy with epithelioid granulomata with foam cells are usually not seen with nasal samples. Investigators have noted that sections predominately show an inflammatory infiltrate rich in macrophages with admixed neutrophils, eosinophils, plasma cells, and mast cells (Fig. 13.8). Bacilli are easily identified with special stains and tend to be located within macrophages although nearly all cells may contain the organisms (eFig. 13.6).

RHINOSCLEROMA

Rhinoscleroma is a chronic, granulomatous inflammatory condition caused by infection with *Klebsiella rhinoscleromatis*.[24–27] It is endemic to Africa, Central and South America, South Central and Eastern Europe, the Middle East, and China. Sporadic cases, however, have been seen elsewhere, including in the United States.[27] The disease almost always involves the nasal cavity, although it may extend into the palate or pharynx. It is not very contagious and affects primarily immunocompetent individuals.

Clinically, patients tend to be young, in their second or third decade of life, and may present with a midfacial necrotizing lesion. Patients may also initially notice a fetid, purulent rhinorrhea with nasal obstruction, and crusting, epistaxis, and nasal deformity can occur as the disease progresses (which can happen as early diagnosis is often missed).

The histology is characterized by the particular stage–exudative, proliferative, or fibrotic (cicatricial). The early exudative phase is characterized by abundant acute and chronic inflammation with suppurative necrosis or microabscess formation. Edema and granulation tissue may be present. The proliferative or granulomatous phase shows persistent chronic inflammation with groups or even sheets of foamy macrophages (Fig. 13.9, eFig. 13.7). Plasma cells may become prominent and Russell bodies are often seen. Special staining will reveal numerous gram-negative coccobacilli consistent with *K. rhinoscheromatis* (eFig. 13.8). Overlying pseudoepitheliomatous hyperplasia may also be present. The sclerotic stage is characterized by dense sclerosis with diminished chronic inflammation. Macrophages with definitive organisms may be difficult or impossible to identify at this stage.

RHINOSPORIDIOSIS

Rhinosporidiosis is endemic to South India and Sri Lanka and is caused by the fungus, *Rhinosporidium seeberi*.[26,28] The disease usually involves the nasal cavity and is usually unilateral. Clinically, the nasal mucosa may appear polypoid, and the patient may present with obstruction, epistaxis, or rhinorrhea. The epithelium may show ulceration. Abundant acute and chronic inflammation is usually present with eosinophils and occasional giant cells. Sporangia are easily identified and are characterized by thick walls and measure from 10 to 200 μm in diameter (Fig. 13.10, eFig. 13.9).

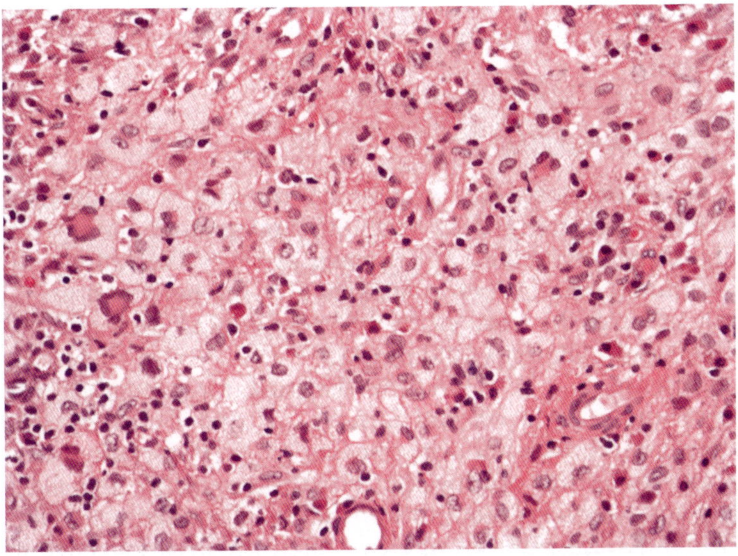

FIGURE 13.9 Sheets of foamy macrophages seen in a case of rhinoscleroma.

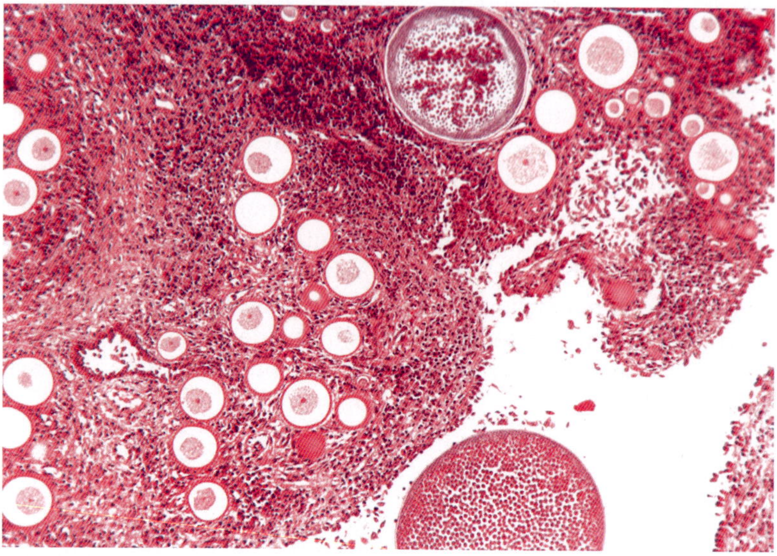

FIGURE 13.10 Numerous sporangia seen in a case of rhinosporidiosis. (Courtesy of Dr. Alan Rose, University of MN.)

LEISHMANIASIS

Nasal involvement is not uncommon in patients with cutaneous leishmaniasis, and it can sometimes be seen alone.[29,30] Other portions of the upper respiratory tract may also be involved. Lesions can appear polypoid or simply as ulcers. Biopsy typically shows epithelial ulceration. Lymphoid aggregates, plasma cells, and granulomata are typically present with multinucleated giant cells. Histiocytes containing Leishman-Donovan bodies are often seen.[29]

WEGENER GRANULOMATOSIS

Wegener granulomatosis (i.e., granulomatosis and polyangiitis) is a systemic disease characterized by vasculitis and granulomatous inflammation with tissue destruction. It generally involves the kidney, lung, and upper respiratory tract. When it does involve the head and neck, it most commonly involves the nasal cavity and paranasal sinuses, although it can involve the mouth, pharynx, and larynx.[31,32]

The disease may be difficult to diagnose for a number of reasons. Histologic features are inconstant, and the full triad of classic textbook features is present in only a minority of cases.[32,33] Furthermore, the histologic features are somewhat nonspecific. For these reasons, the diagnosis of Wegener granulomatosis requires knowledge of the patient's clinical and laboratory data, and sign-out of cases often involves language qualifiers such as "consistent with" or "suspicious for."[32,34]

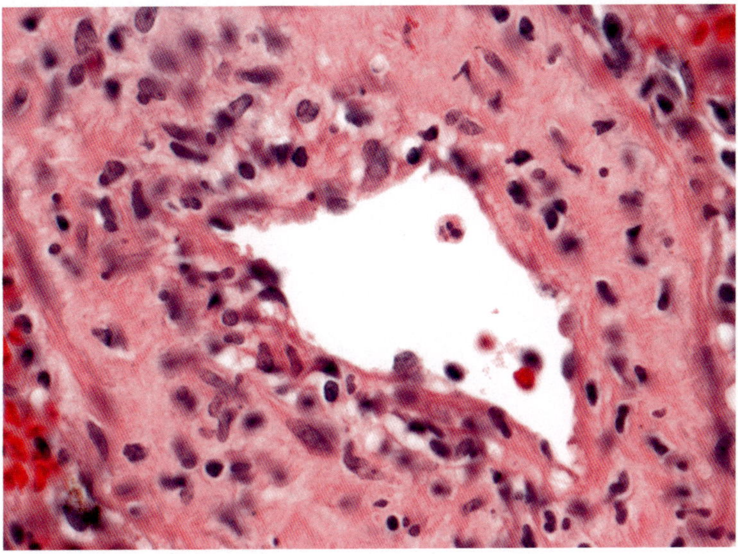

FIGURE 13.11 Mixed inflammatory vasculitis seen in Wegener's granulomatosis.

Clinically, patients may present with a myriad of symptoms. The most prevalent symptom related to nasal involvement is obstruction; however, patients may present with pain, bleeding, discharge, ulcer, or changed olfaction.[31,35] Patients will generally have antineutrophilic antibodies (c-ANCA) which, when demonstrated, can assist the pathologist with his interpretation of the biopsy material.

Patients with Wegener granulomatosis will have variable histology with both vasculitis and parenchymal damage. The vasculitis may involve vessels of any size and may be either be granulomatous or nongranulomatous with an admixture of inflammatory cells including acute and chronic inflammatory cells and giant cells (Fig. 13.11). Fibrinoid necrosis and microabscesses may be present as may fibrointimal hyperplasia (Fig. 13.12, eFig. 13.10). A leukocytoclastic vasculitis mostly involving small capillaries may also be present.[35]

Extravascular or parenchymal changes include granulomata, both small and large, sometimes with central necrosis and sometimes with central microabscesses. The granulomata are composed of palisading histiocytes and often contain multinucleated giant cells (Fig. 13.13). Areas of neutrophilic infiltration are often also present, and microabcesses can be found not included within granulomata. Areas of necrosis and eosinophilia may also be seen (eFigs. 13.11 and 13.12).

As was mentioned, the histologic features of Wegener granulomatosis are inconstant even with well-established cases. For this reason, some authors have proposed schema which combine clinical and histologic

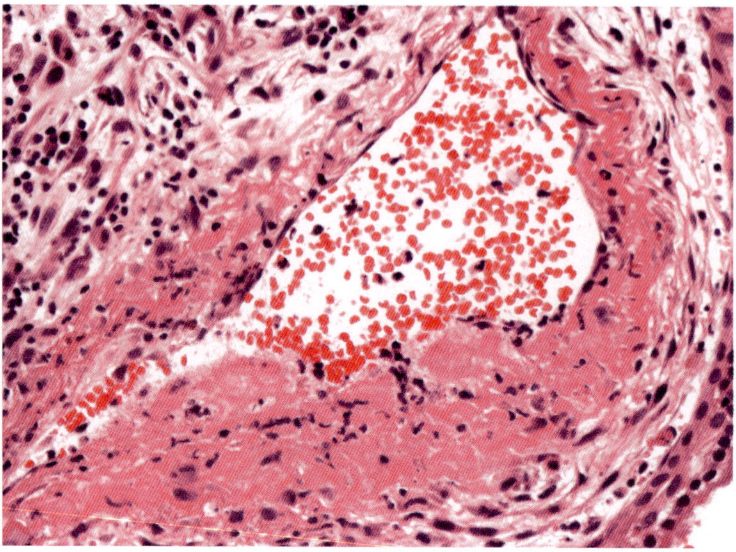

FIGURE 13.12 Fibrinoid necrosis of a vessel seen in a case of Wegener's granulomatosis.

features with a resultant diagnosis or qualified diagnosis (Table 13.3).[32] Suffice it to say, the more the number of clinical features present, including positive cANCA testing, the fewer the histologic features that are required for a definitive diagnosis. In the absence of clinical features or cANCA positivity, the diagnosis most often must be qualified.

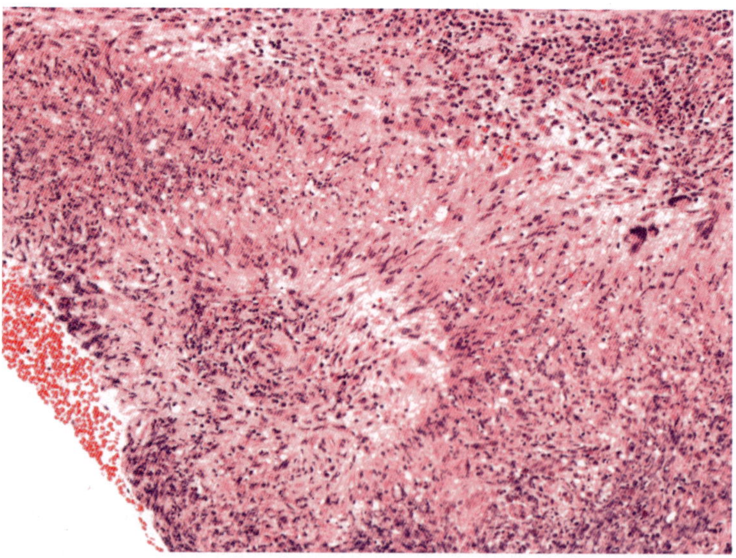

FIGURE 13.13 Palisading histiocytes seen in a case of Wegener's granulomatosis.

TABLE 13.3 Wegener Granulomatosis: Diagnosis Scheme for Head and Neck Biopsies

Granulomatous Inflammation, Necrosis, and Vasculitis	Clinical Involvement	Qualifying Terminology
All three present	Head and neck with lung and/or kidney	"Diagnostic"
Two features present	Head and neck, lung and kidney	"Diagnostic"
Two features present	Less than all three sites involved	"Probable"
One feature present	Head and neck, lung and kidney	"Suggestive"
One feature present	Head and neck and lung or head and neck and kidney	"Suspicious"
No features present	Regardless	"Nondiagnostic"

ALLERGIC GRANULOMATOSIS AND ANGIITIS (CHURG-STRAUSS SYNDROME)

Allergic granulomatosis and angiitis (Churg-Strauss syndrome) is a disseminated necrotizing vasculitis that occurs in patients who have asthma and hypereosinophilia.[36,37] Patients are usually noted to have had allergic rhinitis, fever, anemia, weight loss, and leukocytosis at some point in their illnesses. They often have both cutaneous and pulmonary manifestations, but other sites may be involved as well.

Symptoms of nasal involvement include obstruction and rhinorrhea and patients may have concomitant nasal polyps.[37] Nasal crusting is sometimes seen which may appear akin to Wegener granulomatosis. The patients are also often noted to have abnormal sinus films.

Histologically, sections will show necrotizing granulomata with peripheral palisading histiocytes (Fig. 13.14).[36,37] Abundant eosinophils are present throughout the tissue and focally form microabscesses (eFig. 13.13). Chronic inflammation with lymphocytes and plasma cells is also seen throughout the tissue. Vasculitis, although a hallmark of the disease, has not been noted in nasal biopsies.[37]

SARCOIDOSIS

Sarcoidosis is a systemic disease characterized by nonnecrotizing granulomatous inflammation. It can involve any organ system and rarely may involve the nose and paranasal sinuses.[4,38] Most patients present with symptoms of obstruction, although they may present with epistaxis or dyspnea.[4] Clinical findings include cervical and hilar lymphadenopathy,

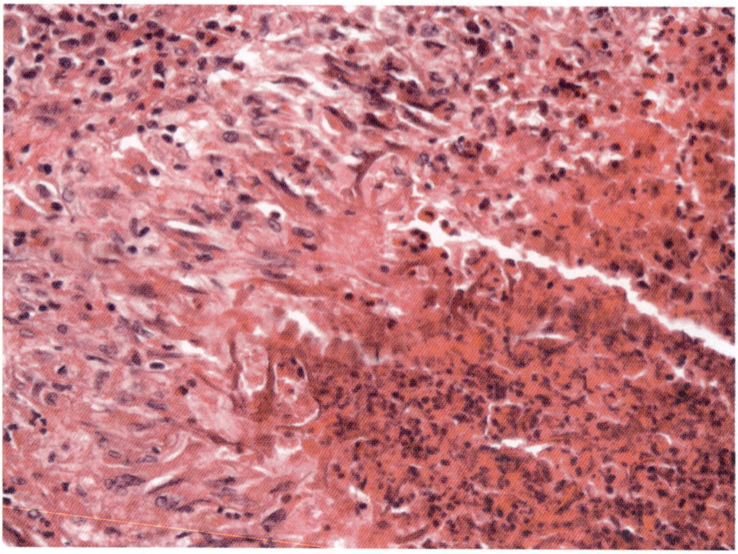

FIGURE 13.14 Necrotizing granuloma seen in a case of Churg-Strauss syndrome. (Coutesy of Dr. Mark Stoler, the University of Virginia, Charlottesville, VA.)

concomitant pulmonary and cutaneous lesions, nasal crusting, intranasal masses or nodules, and sinus thickening or opacification.[4] Histologically, parenchymal inflammation composed predominately of nonnecrotizing granulomas should be present (Fig. 13.15, eFig. 13.14).[4] Necrosis is rarely present and should be "punctate" if seen. Vasculitis and neutrophilic infiltrates should not be present.

EOSINOPHILIC ANGIOCENTRIC FIBROSIS AND IGG4-RELATED SCLEROSING LESIONS

Eosinophilic angiocentric fibrosis is a rare obstructive lesion of the upper respiratory tract.[39–42] Recent evidence suggests that the disease belongs to a family of systemic sclerosing lesions associated with increased serum levels of IgG4 such as sclerosing sialadenitis and dacryoadenitis and autoimmune pancreatitis.[43,44] Patients have presented with obstruction and mass lesions with discharge, epistaxis, and pain.[39,41] Symptoms tend to be long-standing, and patients typically do not have allergic or atopic symptoms. Nonspecific radiographic sinus opacification has been noted. Other sites of involvement, especially the lower respiratory tract, have also been noted.[43] Serum IgG4 levels may be increased.[43,44]

The lesions occur throughout the nasal cavity and sinuses and appear polypoid.[39,41] Microscopically, the lesions have an eosinophilic vasculitis which involves the capillaries and venules of the submucosal (Fig. 13.16). A spectrum of other inflammatory cells may be present, typically

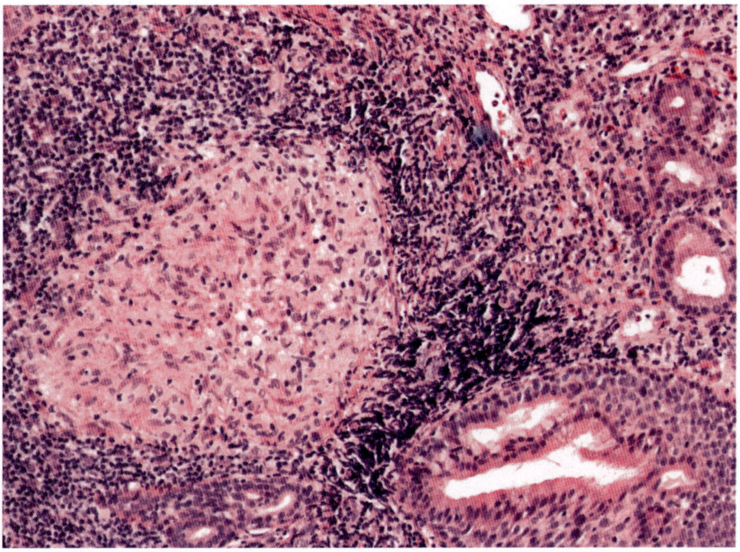

FIGURE 13.15 Noncaseating granuloma seen with nasal involvement by sarcoidosis.

with numerous plasma cells. These plasma cells are frequently immunoreactive with antibodies to IgG4. Necrosis has not been noted. A concentric, perivascular fibrosis ("onion skin type") is also present (Fig. 13.17).[39,41] Adjacent parenchyma contains a mixed inflammatory infiltrate. Granulomata, giant cells, and necrosis are not seen.

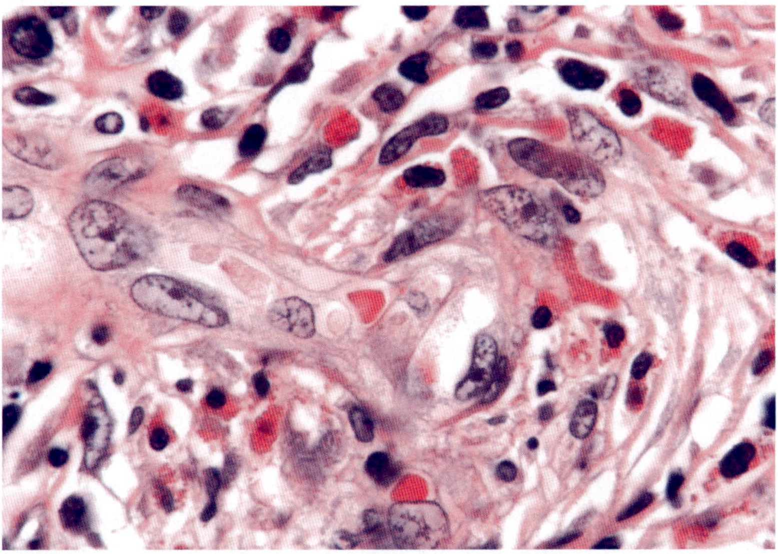

FIGURE 13.16 An eosinophilic vasculitis seen in eosinophilic angiocentric fibrosis. (Courtesy of Dr. Stefan Pambuccian, Univeristy of Minnesota.)

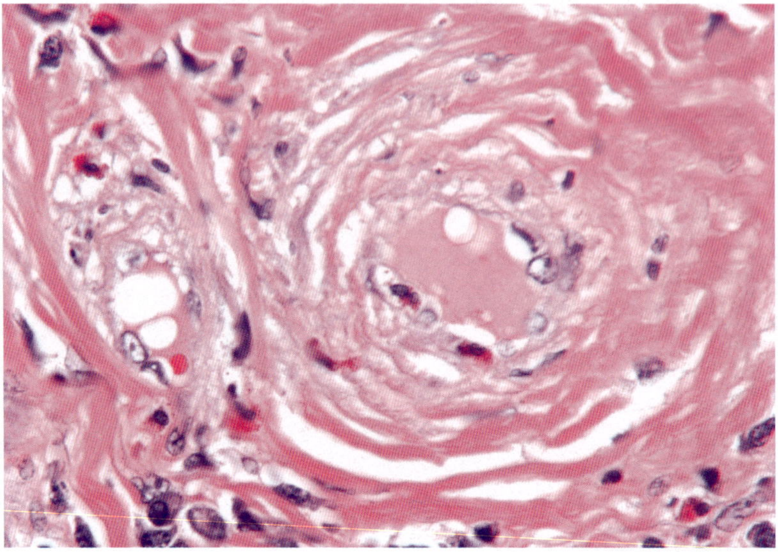

FIGURE 13.17 Angiocentric fibrosis with an "onion skin" appearance in a case of eosinophilic angiocentric fibrosis. (Courtesy of Dr. Stefan Pambuccian, University of MN.)

GRANULOMATOUS LESIONS FOLLOWING STEROID INJECTIONS

Patients who undergo corticosteroid injection of the nasal mucosa because of inflammatory disease may show a granulomatous reaction if they undergo subsequent surgery.[45] Sections will show amorphous, granular debris surrounded by palisaded histiocytes, foreign body–type giant cells, and foamy macrophages. Pathologists need to be aware of this entity so that they do not confuse it with either infectious disease or granulomatous vasculitis.

MYOSPHERULOSIS

Myospherulosis is an iatrogenic disease that can involve the sinuses, nasal cavity, and middle ear.[46–48] It results after the nasal cavity is packed with material which includes a petrolatum-based antibiotic ointment. Patients thus have histories of previous surgery for other sinonasal disease. Recurrent disease usually leads to additional surgery that demonstrates the histologic findings of myospherulosis.

Microscopically, a mild to moderate chronic or mixed inflammatory infiltrate is present.[46–48] Spaces are present within the tissue which range in diameter from a few micrometers to a millimeter in size and are often surrounded by a foreign body–type reaction (Fig. 13.18). These spaces

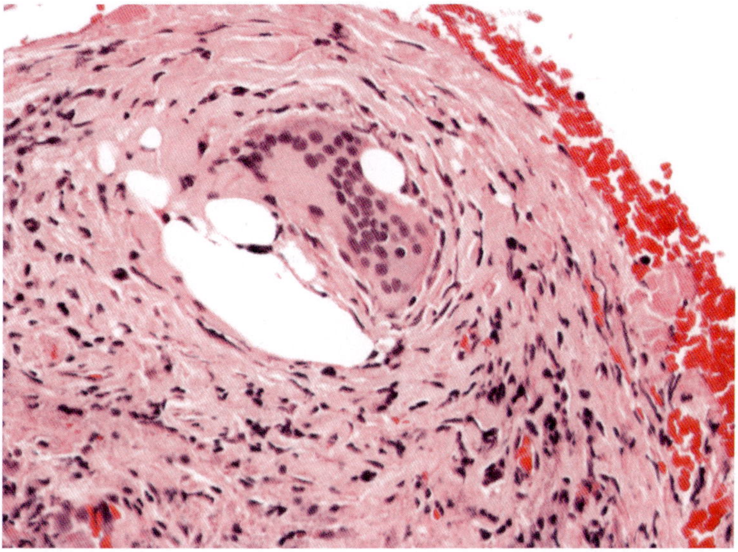

FIGURE 13.18 Spaces with surrounding foreign body–type reaction are seen with myospherulosis.

contain saclike structures that contain numerous smaller spherical structures ranging in size from 5 to 7 μm (Fig. 13.19, eFig. 13.15). The saclike structure is believed to be the foreign substance, and the small spherules are believed to be erythrocytes.[47,48] Amorphous debris may also be seen.

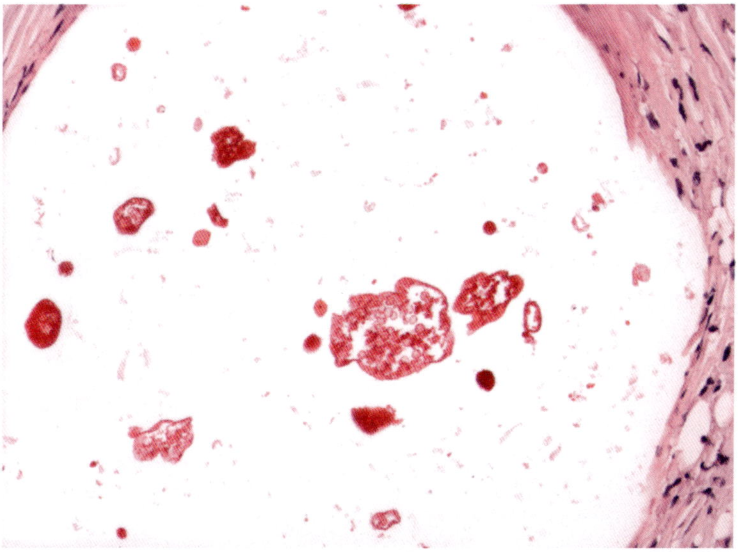

FIGURE 13.19 The spaces seen with myospherulosis can contain saclike structures.

COCAINE-INDUCED MIDLINE DESTRUCTION

Sniffing cocaine can lead to a midline nasal destructive lesion that is likely secondary to ischemic necrosis due to the vasoconstrictive effects of the drug.[49] Biopsies will show acute and chronic inflammation of variable degrees with necrosis of both the mucosa and cartilage.[49,50] Although inflammatory cells may encroach upon vascular structures, a definitive vasculitis with fibrinoid necrosis, giant cells, and granulomata should not be seen, and if present should suggest a different diagnosis.[50]

IDIOPATHIC MIDLINE DESTRUCTIVE DISEASE

Despite aggressive workup, the etiology of some midline destructive disease remains unknown. Although it is a diagnosis that should be made with caution, occasional midline destructive lesions may be identified that require the diagnosis of "idiopathic midline destructive disease."[1,2,51] Clinically, patients present with midline destructive lesions and septal perforation. Microscopically, sections should show acute and chronic inflammation without granulomata, vasculitis, or evidence of neoplasia. To exclude neoplasia, especially extranodal natural killer (NK)/T-cell lymphoma, immunohistochemistry and other ancillary studies must be performed.

MUCOCELE

Mucoceles occur most commonly in the frontal sinuses but can occur in any paranasal sinus.[52] They tend to develop in patients with histories of sinus disease or in those with previous operations or trauma at the site. They can cause visible and palpable facial swelling with associated pain and may even cause dislocation of the eye or diplopia.

The lesions are thought to develop secondary to obstruction of seromucinous gland ducts or, possibly, of the sinus outlet. Mucus then collects within the gland and the lesion expands. As it expands, it can cause bony and soft tissue destruction. Histologically, sections show a cystic cavity lined by an attenuated respiratory epithelium (Fig. 13.20, eFig. 13.16).[52] The epithelial cells may appear flattened, and cilia may be difficult to find. Squamous metaplasia may be present. The underlying stroma can be fibrotic and may contain lymphocytes, plasma cells, neutrophils, and eosinophils. With rupture, numerous foamy macrophages may be seen.

NONNEOPLASTIC POLYPS

Nonneoplastic nasal polyps are common and tend to occur in certain patients such as asthmatics and patients with cystic fibrosis. As true neoplasms may sometimes present as polypoid growths, it is important to distinguish these nonneoplastic lesions. Furthermore, there are some slight differences in the clinicopathologic features between the nonneoplastic polyps of which the pathologist should be aware (Table 13.4).

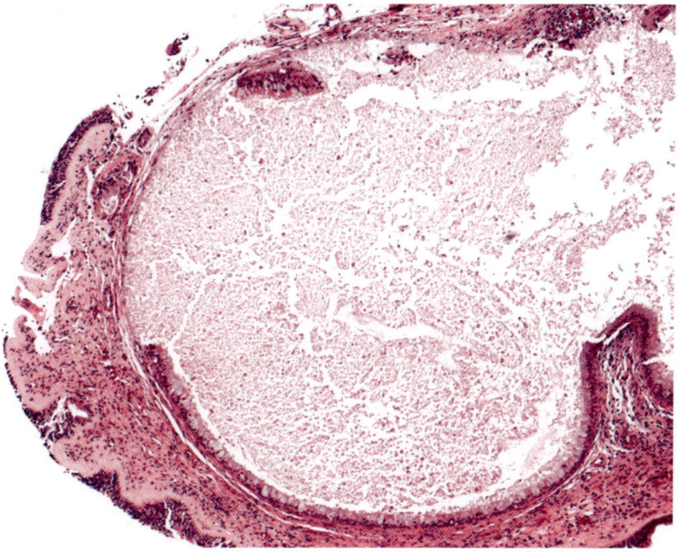

FIGURE 13.20 A mucocele.

Inflammatory Polyp

Inflammatory sinonasal polyps occur most frequently in patients with asthma and allergies. They occur more commonly in older patients and show no sexual predilection. The lesions are often multiple, tend to recur, and may involve the nasal cavity and/or paranasal sinuses. Patients present most commonly with nasal stuffiness. The polyps may range in size and tend to have short stalks, unlike antrochoanal polyps.

The polyps are lined by a ciliated respiratory epithelium which often shows squamous metaplasia. Focal erosion may also be seen. The basement membrane is also thickened, and hyaline material can extend into the subepithelial tissues. An inflammatory infiltrate is present within the stroma usually with numerous eosinophils (Fig. 13.21, eFig. 13.17). Mucous glands are prominent and can have cystic dilatation. Stroma cell atypia may be present and has led some to consider the diagnosis of sarcoma in such cases (Fig. 13.22, eFig. 13.18). Areas of stromal cell atypia can be quite cellular, and the stromal cells can be enlarged and pleomorphic and either spindled or somewhat stellate. Their nuclei are hyperchromatic and can have prominent nucleoli. No nasal polyps with such changes have behaved malignantly.

Antrochoanal Polyp

Antrochoanal polyps arise in the maxillary sinuses and extend into the choana, generally causing obstruction. They are unlike routine inflammatory polyps insomuch as they tend to be solitary, may occur at any age, and

TABLE 13.4 Nasal Polyps

	Inflammatory Polyps	Antrochoanal Polyps	Polyps Associated With Cystic Fibrosis
Patient age	>40 years old	Any age	<20 years old
Associated findings	Allergic rhinitis and sinusitis, asthma, atopy	Not associated with allergies or asthma	Cystic fibrosis
Histology	Polyps lined by ciliated respiratory epithelium with focal squamous metaplasia and erosion. Thickened basement membrane with sclerotic stroma. Mixed inflammatory infiltrate with numerous eosinophils. Stromal cell atypia may be present.	Polyps with long stalks, lined by ciliated respiratory epithelium with focal squamous metaplasia. Basement membrane is not thickened and eosinophils are less abundant.	Polyps lined by ciliated respiratory epithelium with focal squamous metaplasia. Basement membrane is not thickened, and eosinophils are not prominent. Acid mucin demonstrated cysts, mucous glands, and mucous blanket by alcian blue/ PAS stain.

PAS, periodic acid–Schiff

are not associated with asthma or allergies. An antrochoanal polyp may occur if not entirely excised.

Most antrochoanal polyps have long stalks unlike routine inflammatory polyps and tend to be larger than inflammatory polyps. The polyps are covered with a ciliated, respiratory-type epithelium and may have squamous metaplasia (Fig. 13.23). The stroma will appear edematous and will have a mixed inflammatory infiltrate; however, these polyps often contain fewer eosinophils than will be present with routine nasal polyps. As with inflammatory polyps, stromal cell atypia may occasionally be present and has no meaning.

Nasal Polyps in Patients With Cystic Fibrosis

Patients with cystic fibrosis also tend to develop nasal polyps and have sinus disease secondary to obstruction by hyperviscous mucus. The polyps occur in younger patients and can show features different from those

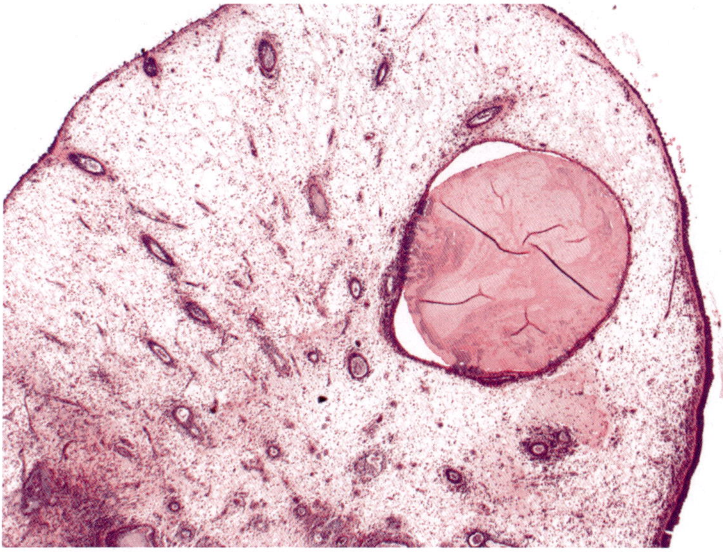

FIGURE 13.21 An inflammatory polyp with chronic inflammation.

seen in patients with asthma or allergies. Like inflammatory polyps, these polyps are covered by ciliated respiratory epithelium that is interrupted by squamous metaplasia. The basement membranes are not thickened, and the submucosa is free of any hyaline material. The stroma will show a mixed inflammatory infiltrate with edema; however, eosinophils may be difficult to find. The mucous glands may appear somewhat hyperplastic.

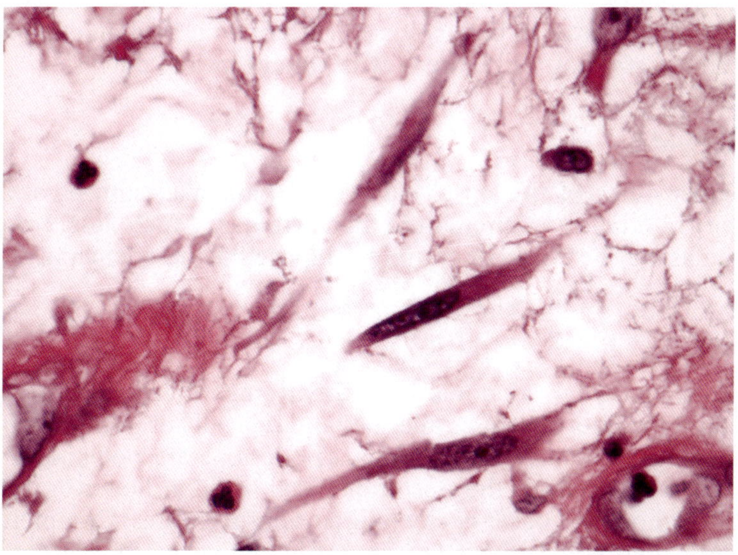

FIGURE 13.22 Stromal atypia can be seen with inflammatory polyps.

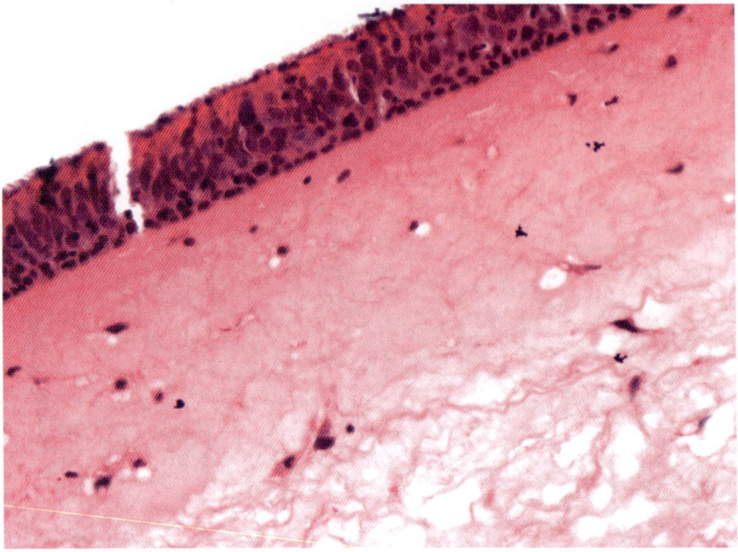

FIGURE 13.23 Antrochoanal polyps usually have less inflammation than inflammatory polyps.

Rarely, patients with cystic fibrosis may present with nasal polyps.[53] As inflammatory polyps present mostly in older individuals, the main differential for a nonneoplastic polyp in a young person is an antrochoanal polyp. There are some histologic differences, however, and some have shown that special mucin stains may be helpful for diagnosing these lesions. With alcian blue/periodic acid–Schiff (PAS) stain, the mucous blanket, glands, and cysts stain a purplish blue color consistent with acid mucins, whereas a purplish red staining will be seen with other types of polyps.

HAMARTOMA

Most hamartomas of the nasal cavity and paranasal sinuses are purely respiratory epithelial adenomatoid hamartomas. Much less commonly, hamartomas may be mixed or entirely composed of mesenchymal elements.

Respiratory Epithelial Adenomatoid Hamartoma and Seromucinous Hamartoma

Respiratory epithelial adenomatoid hamartomas mostly occur in older, adult men.[54] Patients may have allergies and typically present with obstruction, bleeding, or recurrent infections. The lesions are polypoid and rubbery and usually involve the posterior nasal septum; however, they may occur throughout the nasal cavity and paranasal sinuses. Complete resection affords a cure with these lesions. Although generally not considered neoplastic, some recent evidence suggests the contrary.[55]

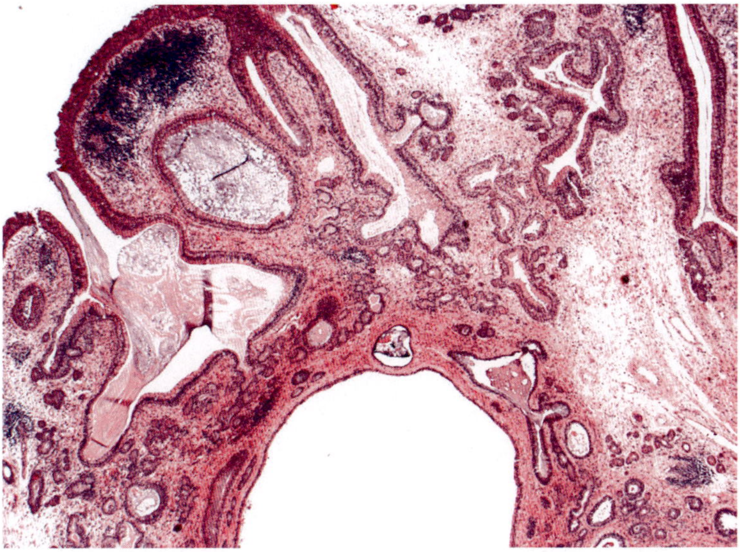

FIGURE 13.24 Respiratory epithelial adenomatoid hamartoma with numerous bland glandular structures.

The polypoid lesions are composed of bland glandular structures lined by ciliated columnar cells (Fig. 13.24, eFigs. 13.19 and 13.20).[54] The glands usually appear to empty onto the surface. Occasional mucus cells are usually seen intermixed with the columnar cells. Focally, the glands may be distended by mucus and focal squamous metaplasia or atrophic change may be seen. The stroma between the glands usually shows chronic inflammation and may appear sclerotic or hyalinized. The number of seromucinous glands varies, but they should be organized in a lobular architecture. Tumors composed predominately of small seromucinous glands have been termed "seromucinous hamartomas."[56]

Nasal Chondromesenchymal Hamartoma

Nasal chondromesenchymal hamartomas are almost always seen in children.[57] The tumors are mostly found in the nasal cavity, but often also involve the sinuses. Patients usually present with a mass and may have difficulty breathing or recurrent infection. The lesions are often described as well-circumscribed and do not recur if completely excised. The tumors are associated with *DICER1* mutations, and patients with familial pleuropulmonary blastoma are at increased risk for these lesions.[58–61] As additional somatic mutations of *DICER1* have been seen in some tumors arising in patients with germline *DICER1* mutations, these lesions may be truly neoplastic.

Histologically, the lesions are composed of a variety of mesenchymal element and often have a lobular architecture (Fig. 13.25, eFigs. 13.21 and 13.22). The most prominent tissue is hyaline cartilage. The intervening

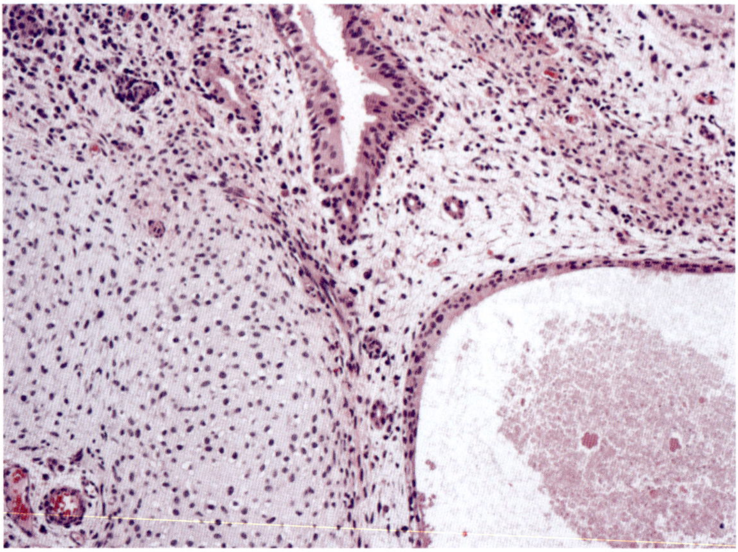

FIGURE 13.25 Chondroid tissue seen in a case of nasal chondromesenchymal hamartoma.

stroma is composed of bland spindled cells and can appear either hypercellular or myxoid. Osteoclast-like giant cells can be present as can vascular proliferation. The perivascular tissue may appear hyalinized.

Hairy Polyp

Hairy polyps are likely not neoplasms but instead represent a developmental abnormality of the first or second branchial cleft and are thus considered by some to be accessory auricles.[62] The lesions predominately present in infants, but may occasionally be detected in older children and adolescents. The tumors present most frequently in the nasopharynx but may also present in the oropharynx or middle ear and eustachian tube. Symptoms are secondary to local mass effect. The lesions are grossly polypoid. Histologically, they are covered by a dermis with keratinizing, stratified squamous epithelium and appendages (Fig. 13.26, eFig. 13.23). The underlying soft tissue consists of adipose tissue with admixed fibrous tissue. Mature cartilage and bone may also be present. Lesions resembling hairy polyps, seen outside of the pharynx, are generally classified as dermoids.

HETEROTOPIC GLIAL TISSUE AND ENCEPHALOCELES

Nonneoplastic glial tissue can be found external to the nose or within the nasal cavity, and it can be in continuity with the central nervous system (CNS) (encephalocele) or separate from the CNS (glial heterotopia).[63,64]

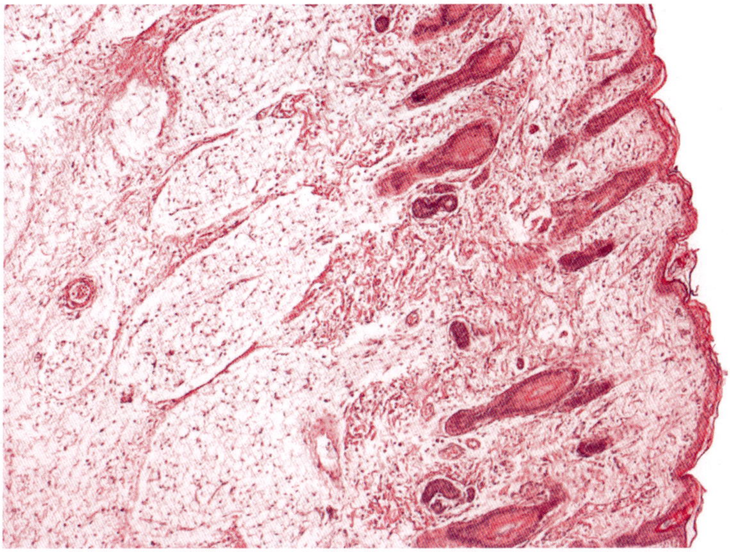

FIGURE 13.26 A hairy polyp lined by a stratified squamous epithelium.

Radiology is important for this distinction as both clinical and pathologic features of these entities are similar. Patients usually present as children, although the lesions can be identified at any age. Most patients present with obstructive and mass symptoms, although a myriad of symptoms have been described including drainage, sinusitis, and chronic otitis media. Histologically, cases are composed predominately of glial tissue with or without occasional neurons (Fig. 13.27, eFig. 13.24). Ependymal, choroid plexus, and leptomeningeal components are generally not seen. The glial tissue can be difficult to appreciate; however, gemistocytic astrocytes, which are often present, can usually be readily identified. Immunostaining with antibodies to S100 protein or glial fibrillary acidic protein can be helpful as both will highlight the glial component (eFig. 13.25). It has been noted that adult examples will have more abundant fibrosis.[63,64]

LYMPHOID HYPERPLASIA

Lymphoid hyperplasia can form mass lesions throughout the upper aerodigestive tract, especially in the nasopharynx and nose.[65,66] By definition, the lesions are composed of nonneoplastic lymphocytes. Thus, a mixture of lymphocytes is usually seen within a background architecture that usually contains reactive, expanded germinal centers and expanded interfollicular areas. As the lesions often present as masses, it is sometimes prudent to exclude lymphoma with ancillary studies such as immunohistochemistry, flow cytometry, and molecular testing for clonal gene rearrangements.

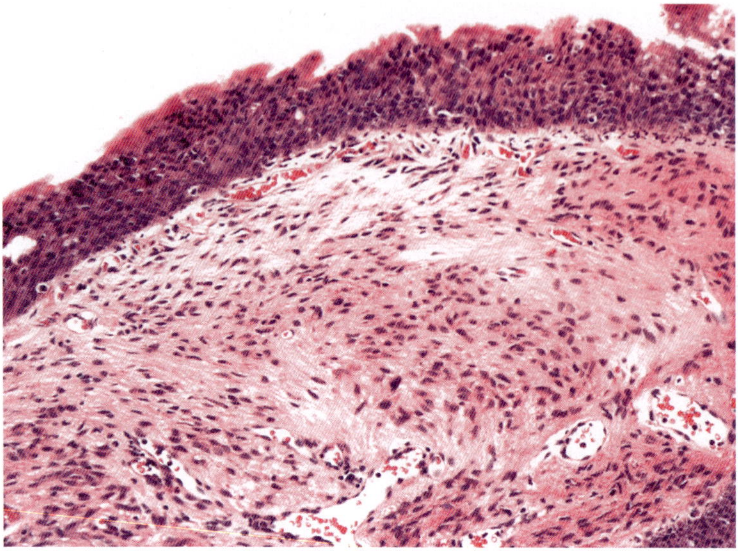

FIGURE 13.27 Subepithelial glial tissue seen with glial heterotopia.

OTHER

The nasal cavity may be involved in a vast array of infectious and systemic pathologies including lupus, amyloidosis, and infectious entities such as yaws and glanders. The histologic findings for these diseases are often nonspecific and recapitulated pathology seen at other sites of the body. Of note, localized amyloidosis may be associated with low-grade B-cell lymphomas, specifically extranodal marginal zone lymphoma or extramedullary plasmacytoma.

REFERENCES

1. Crissman JD, Weiss MA, Gluckman J. Midline granuloma syndrome: a clinicopathologic study of 13 patients. *Am J Surg Pathol*. 1982;6:335-346.
2. Tsokos M, Fauci AS, Costa J. Idiopathic midline destructive disease (IMDD): a subgroup of patients with the "midline granuloma" syndrome. *Am J Clin Pathol*. 1982;77:162-168.
3. Coup AJ, Hopper IP. Granulomatous lesions in nasal biopsies. *Histopathology*. 1980;4:293-308.
4. McCaffrey TV, McDonald TJ. Sarcoidosis of the nose and paranasal sinuses. *Laryngoscope*. 1983;93:1281-1284.
5. Stierna P, Carlsoo B. Histopathological observations in chronic maxillary sinusitis. *Acta Otolaryngol*. 1990;110:450-458.
6. Carlen B, Stenram U. Primary ciliary dyskinesia: a review. *Ultrastruct Pathol*. 2005;29:217-220.
7. Leigh MW, Pittman JE, Carson JL, et al. Clinical and genetic aspects of primary ciliary dyskinesia/Kartagener syndrome. *Genet Med*. 2009;11:473-487.

8. Lucas JS, Davis SD, Omran H, Shoemark A. Primary ciliary dyskinesia in the genomics age. *Lancet Respir Med.* 2020;8:202-216.
9. deShazo RD, Chapin K, Swain RE. Fungal sinusitis. *N Engl J Med.* 1997;337:254-259.
10. Brandwein M. Histopathology of sinonasal fungal disease. *Otolaryngol Clin North Am.* 1993;26:949-981.
11. Katzenstein AL, Sale SR, Greenberger PA. Allergic Aspergillus sinusitis: a newly recognized form of sinusitis. *J Allergy Clin Immunol.* 1983;72:89-93.
12. Waxman JE, Spector JG, Sale SR, Katzenstein AL. Allergic Aspergillus sinusitis: concepts in diagnosis and treatment of a new clinical entity. *Laryngoscope.* 1987;97:261-266.
13. Torres C, Ro JY, el-Naggar AK, Sim SJ, Weber RS, Ayala AG. Allergic fungal sinusitis: a clinicopathologic study of 16 cases. *Hum Pathol.* 1996;27:793-799.
14. Friedman GC, Hartwick RW, Ro JY, Saleh GY, Tarrand JJ, Ayala AG. Allergic fungal sinusitis. Report of three cases associated with dematiaceous fungi. *Am J Clin Pathol.* 1991;96:368-372.
15. Corey JP, Romberger CF, Shaw GY. Fungal diseases of the sinuses. *Otolaryngol Head Neck Surg.* 1990;103:1012-1015.
16. McGill TJ, Simpson G, Healy GB. Fulminant aspergillosis of the nose and paranasal sinuses: a new clinical entity. *Laryngoscope.* 1980;90:748-754.
17. Morgan MA, Wilson WR, Neel HB III, Roberts GD. Fungal sinusitis in healthy and immunocompromised individuals. *Am J Clin Pathol.* 1984;82:597-601.
18. Drakos PE, Nagler A, Or R, et al. Invasive fungal sinusitis in patients undergoing bone marrow transplantation. *Bone Marrow Transplant.* 1993;12:203-208.
19. Montone KT, LiVolsi VA, Lanza DC, et al. In situ hybridization for specific fungal organisms in acute invasive fungal rhinosinusitis. *Am J Clin Pathol.* 2011;135:190-199.
20. Waldman SR, Levine HL, Sebek BA, Parker W, Tucker HM. Nasal tuberculosis: a forgotten entity. *Laryngoscope.* 1981;91:11-16.
21. Waldron J, Van Hasselt CA, Skinner DW, Arnold M. Tuberculosis of the nasopharynx: clinicopathological features. *Clin Otolaryngol Allied Sci.* 1992;17:57-59.
22. McDougall AC, Rees RJ, Weddell AG, Kanan MW. The histopathology of lepromatous leprosy in the nose. *J Pathol.* 1975;115:215-226.
23. Pollack JD, Pincus RL, Lucente FE. Leprosy of the head and neck. *Otolaryngol Head Neck Surg.* 1987;97:93-96.
24. Berger SA, Pollock AA, Richmond AS. Isolation of Klebsiella ozaenae and Klebsiella rhinoscleromatis in a general hospital. *Am J Clin Pathol.* 1977;67:499-502.
25. Meyer PR, Shum TK, Becker TS, Taylor CR. Scleroma (Rhinoscleroma). A histologic immunohistochemical study with bacteriologic correlates. *Arch Pathol Lab Med.* 1983;107:377-383.
26. Batsakis JG, el-Naggar AK. Rhinoscleroma and rhinosporidiosis. *Ann Otol Rhinol Laryngol.* 1992;101:879-882.
27. Andraca R, Edson RS, Kern EB. Rhinoscleroma: a growing concern in the United States? Mayo Clinic experience. *Mayo Clin Proc.* 1993;68:1151-1157.
28. Jimenez JF, Young DE, Hough AJ Jr. Rhinosporidiosis. A report of two cases from Arkansas. *Am J Clin Pathol.* 1984;82:611-615.
29. Daneshbod Y, Oryan A, Davarmanesh M, et al. Clinical, histopathologic, and cytologic diagnosis of mucosal leishmaniasis and literature review. *Arch Pathol Lab Med.* 2011;135:478-482.
30. Amato VS, Tuon FF, Imamura R, Abegao de Camargo R, Duarte MI, Neto VA. Mucosal leishmaniasis: description of case management approaches and analysis of risk factors for treatment failure in a cohort of 140 patients in Brazil. *J Eur Acad Dermatol Venereol.* 2009;23:1026-1034.

31. McDonald TJ, DeRemee RA, Kern EB, Harrison EG Jr. Nasal manifestations of Wegener's granulomatosis. *Laryngoscope*. 1974;84:2101-2112.
32. Devaney KO, Travis WD, Hoffman G, Leavitt R, Lebovics R, Fauci AS. Interpretation of head and neck biopsies in Wegener's granulomatosis. A pathologic study of 126 biopsies in 70 patients. *Am J Surg Pathol*. 1990;14:555-564.
33. Del Buono EA, Flint A. Diagnostic usefulness of nasal biopsy in Wegener's granulomatosis. *Hum Pathol*. 1991;22:107-110.
34. Colby TV, Tazelaar HD, Specks U, DeRemee RA. Nasal biopsy in Wegener's granulomatosis. *Hum Pathol*. 1991;22:101-104.
35. Matsubara O, Yoshimura N, Doi Y, Tamura A, Mark EJ. Nasal biopsy in the early diagnosis of Wegener's (pathergic) granulomatosis. Significance of palisading granuloma and leukocytoclastic vasculitis. *Virchows Arch*. 1996;428:13-19.
36. Chumbley LC, Harrison EG Jr, DeRemee RA. Allergic granulomatosis and angiitis (Churg-Strauss syndrome). Report and analysis of 30 cases. *Mayo Clin Proc*. 1977;52:477-484.
37. Olsen KD, Neel HB III, Deremee RA, Weiland LH. Nasal manifestations of allergic granulomatosis and angiitis (Churg-Strauss syndrome). *Otolaryngol Head Neck Surg*. 1980;88:85-89.
38. Postma D, Fry TL, Malenbaum BT. The nose, minor salivary glands, and sarcoidosis. *Arch Otolaryngol*. 1984;110:28-30.
39. Roberts PF, McCann BG. Eosinophilic angiocentric fibrosis of the upper respiratory tract: a mucosal variant of granuloma faciale? A report of three cases. *Histopathology*. 1985;9:1217-1225.
40. Altemani AM, Pilch BZ, Sakano E, Altemani JM. Eosinophilic angiocentric fibrosis of the nasal cavity. *Mod Pathol*. 1997;10:391-393.
41. Thompson LD, Heffner DK. Sinonasal tract eosinophilic angiocentric fibrosis. A report of three cases. *Am J Clin Pathol*. 2001;115:243-248.
42. Jain R, Robblee JV, O'Sullivan-Mejia E, et al. Sinonasal eosinophilic angiocentric fibrosis: a report of four cases and review of literature. *Head Neck Pathol*. 2008;2:309-315.
43. Deshpande V, Khosroshahi A, Nielsen GP, Hamilos DL, Stone JH. Eosinophilic angiocentric fibrosis is a form of IgG4-related systemic disease. *Am J Surg Pathol*. 2011;35:701-706.
44. Moteki H, Yasuo M, Hamano H, Uehara T, Usami S. IgG4-related chronic rhinosinusitis: a new clinical entity of nasal disease. *Acta Otolaryngol*. 2011;131:518-526.
45. Wolff M. Granulomas in nasal mucous membranes following local steroid injections. *Am J Clin Pathol*. 1974;62:775-782.
46. McClatchie S, Warambo MW, Bremner AD. Myospherulosis: a previously unreported disease?. *Am J Clin Pathol*. 1969;51:699-704.
47. Kyriakos M. Myospherulosis of the paranasal sinuses, nose and middle ear. A possible iatrogenic disease. *Am J Clin Pathol*. 1977;67:118-130.
48. Rosai J. The nature of myospherulosis of the upper respiratory tract. *Am J Clin Pathol*. 1978;69:475-481.
49. Sercarz JA, Strasnick B, Newman A, Dodd LG. Midline nasal destruction in cocaine abusers. *Otolaryngol Head Neck Surg*. 1991;105:694-701.
50. Trimarchi M, Gregorini G, Facchetti F, et al. Cocaine-induced midline destructive lesions: clinical, radiographic, histopathologic, and serologic features and their differentiation from Wegener granulomatosis. *Medicine (Baltimore)*. 2001;80:391-404.
51. Rodrigo JP, Suarez C, Rinaldo A, et al. Idiopathic midline destructive disease: fact or fiction. *Oral Oncol*. 2005;41:340-348.
52. Natvig K, Larsen TE. Mucocele of the paranasal sinuses. A retrospective clinical and histological study. *J Laryngol Otol*. 1978;92:1075-1082.

53. Wiatrak BJ, Myer CM III, Cotton RT. Cystic fibrosis presenting with sinus disease in children. *Am J Dis Child.* 1993;147:258-260.
54. Wenig BM, Heffner DK. Respiratory epithelial adenomatoid hamartomas of the sinonasal tract and nasopharynx: a clinicopathologic study of 31 cases. *Ann Otol Rhinol Laryngol.* 1995;104:639-645.
55. Ozolek JA, Hunt JL. Tumor suppressor gene alterations in respiratory epithelial adenomatoid hamartoma (REAH): comparison to sinonasal adenocarcinoma and inflamed sinonasal mucosa. *Am J Surg Pathol.* 2006;30:1576-1580.
56. Weinreb I, Gnepp DR, Laver NM, et al. Seromucinous hamartomas: a clinicopathological study of a sinonasal glandular lesion lacking myoepithelial cells. *Histopathology.* 2009;54:205-213.
57. McDermott MB, Ponder TB, Dehner LP. Nasal chondromesenchymal hamartoma: an upper respiratory tract analogue of the chest wall mesenchymal hamartoma. *Am J Surg Pathol.* 1998;22:425-433.
58. Dehner LP, Messinger YH, Schultz KA, Williams GM, Wikenheiser-Brokamp K, Hill DA. Pleuropulmonary blastoma: evolution of an entity as an entry into a familial tumor predisposition syndrome. *Pediatr Dev Pathol.* 2015;18:504-511.
59. Schultz KA, Yang J, Doros L, et al. DICER1-pleuropulmonary blastoma familial tumor predisposition syndrome: a unique constellation of neoplastic conditions. *Pathol Case Rev.* 2014;19:90-100.
60. Stewart DR, Best AF, Williams GM, et al. Neoplasm risk among individuals with a pathogenic germline variant in DICER1. *J Clin Oncol.* 2019;37:668-676.
61. Stewart DR, Messinger Y, Williams GM, et al. Nasal chondromesenchymal hamartomas arise secondary to germline and somatic mutations of DICER1 in the pleuropulmonary blastoma tumor predisposition disorder. *Hum Genet.* 2014;133:1443-1450.
62. Heffner DK, Thompson LD, Schall DG, Anderson V. Pharyngeal dermoids ("hairy polyps") as accessory auricles. *Ann Otol Rhinol Laryngol.* 1996;105:819-824.
63. Penner CR, Thompson L. Nasal glial heterotopia: a clinicopathologic and immunophenotypic analysis of 10 cases with a review of the literature. *Ann Diagn Pathol.* 2003;7:354-359.
64. Theaker JM, Fletcher CD. Heterotopic glial nodules: a light microscopic and immunohistochemical study. *Histopathology.* 1991;18:255-260.
65. Rimarenko S, Schwartz IS. Polypoid nasal pseudolymphoma. *Am J Clin Pathol.* 1985;83:507-509.
66. Shahab I, Osborne BM, Butler JJ. Nasopharyngeal lymphoid tissue masses in patients with human immunodeficiency virus-1. Histologic findings and clinical correlation. *Cancer.* 1994;74:3083-3088.

14

NONNEOPLASTIC LESIONS OF THE ORAL CAVITY

A vast array of nonneoplastic lesions arise in the mouth including traumatic, infectious, inflammatory, and autoimmune processes, among others. Given its location and its embryology, it is not surprising that this region can be affected by both cutaneous and gastrointestinal processes. Furthermore, it is the wet, moist, crushing portal of entry for food, drink, and air, and thus is often traumatized and infected. This chapter will discuss many of the nonneoplastic lesions that can be sampled within the oral cavity, along with differential diagnoses and the ancillary methods that are useful to distinguish these entities.

HETEROTOPIC TISSUES AND CHORISTOMAS

Because of the mouth's location, its local relationship with other structures and role in embryogenesis, it can be involved by a number of heterotopic tissues or choristomas (Table 14.1). *Heterotopic glial tissue*, which most commonly involves the sinonasal area, can be present within the mouth, most often in the tongue (lingual glial choristoma).[1] As in the sinonasal area (Chapter 13), these lesions are composed of mature glial tissue, mostly astrocytes with some ganglion cells. It is unclear whether such tissue represents true heterotopia or, instead, a monodermic form of a mature teratoma. Regardless, the lesions do not recur following excision.

Lingual thyroid tissue can be present in the posterior dorsal region of the tongue at the foramen cecum, whence the normal thyroid migrates in utero.[2] Here, the thyroid tissue usually presents as a painless mass. Sometimes patients are hypothyroid, whereas larger masses cause obstruction. Histologically, lingual thyroids are composed of mature-appearing follicular thyroid tissue, intermixed to some degree with the skeletal muscle of the tongue (Fig. 14.1). Conventional thyroid neoplasia can develop in lingual thyroid tissue and should be excluded. *Thyroglossal dust cysts* are also found at this site and will present as painful nodules when infected. Histologically, they are lined by ciliated columnar or squamous-type epithelium with varying degrees of acute and chronic inflammation present (eFig. 14.1). Mature-appearing thyroid follicular tissue can be present but

TABLE 14.1 Heterotopic Tissues of the Mouth

Glial tissue
Enteric duplication cysts
Lingual thyroid and thyroglossal duct cysts
Sebaceous gland tissue (Fordyce granules)
Branchial cleft remnant (hairy polyps, etc.)

is not always seen. As with lingual thyroid tissue, conventional thyroid neoplasia should be excluded.

Heterotopic gastrointestinal epithelium or *enteric duplication cysts* are found in the oral cavity, usually in the tongue or in the floor of the mouth. Most often these present as superficial or deep swellings within the tongue; there is, however, a report of child who would squirt others with a brown fluid from one of these lesions that connected to his tongue's surface via a sinus tract.[3] The cysts are lined by an enteric, glandular epithelium that is often intermixed with columnar, ciliated, and squamous epithelium (Fig. 14.2, eFig. 14.2).[4] Fundic-type epithelium with parietal cells is frequently seen. We have seen rare duplication cysts here associated with enteric-type adenocarcinomas.

Ectopic sebaceous glands or *Fordyce granules* are found sometimes within the mouth.[5] These lesions clinically appear as small, yellow papules, usually within the buccal mucosa (some consider the smaller buccal lesions to be normal). They vary considerably in number. Histologically, the

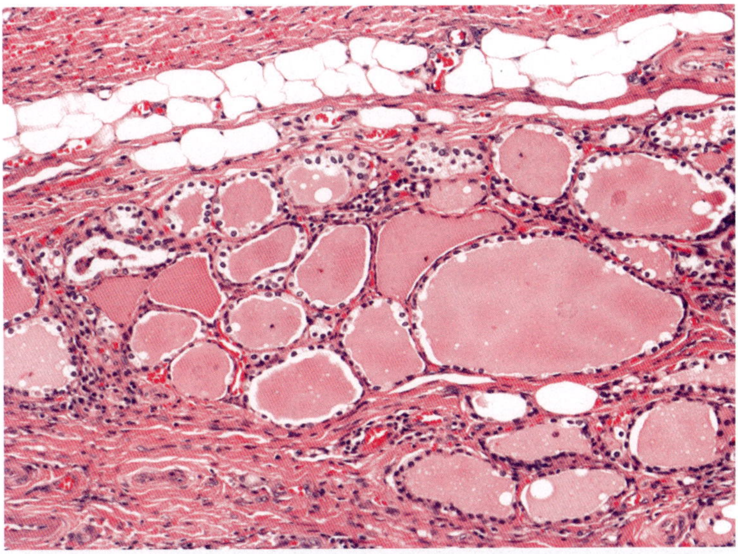

FIGURE 14.1 Lingual thyroid tissue.

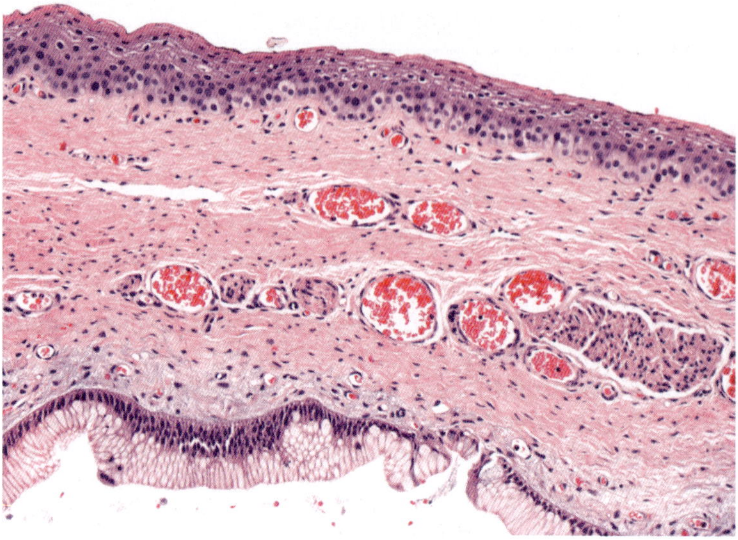

FIGURE 14.2 An enteric cyst immediately beneath the surface epithelium of the tongue.

papules are composed of sebaceous glands located within or immediately beneath the surface epithelium (Fig. 14.3). When present below the epithelium, ductal connections to the surface are usually not seen. Some have suggested that the formation of these lesions is related to inherited defects of mismatch repair proteins (hereditary nonpolyposis colon cancer).[6]

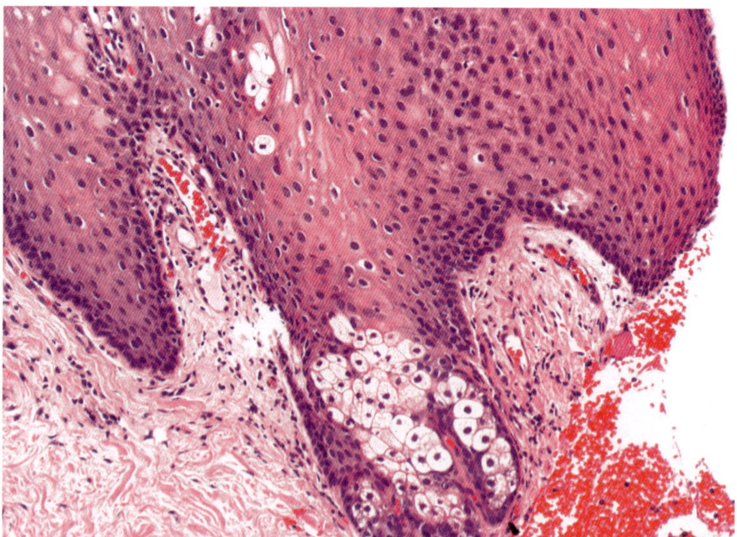

FIGURE 14.3 Fordyce granule.

Other possible choristomas include osteomas and chondromas of the mouth (discussed in Chapter 12). The vestigial organ of Chievitz found in the area of the retromolar trigone was discussed in Chapter 1. Mass-forming, apparent tonsillar tissue can be present throughout the mouth.

OTHER POSSIBLE CONGENITAL ABNORMALITIES

Other disparate congenital abnormalities afflict the mouth. These often present as mass lesions; however, some present secondary to disease to which the lesion has predisposed the patient (e.g., hemorrhage secondary to persistent caliber arteries and median rhomboid glossitis secondary to candidiasis). Awareness of these lesions and their clinical features helps pathologists to distinguish them from other disease processes.

Palatal and *gingival cysts* can frequently be seen in infants and clinically appear as small (approximately 1 mm) yellow-white cysts at the mid-palatal raphe at the junction of the hard and soft palate and along the alveolar ridge, respectively.[7] Palatal cysts are composed of nests of epithelium surrounding keratin. Gingival cysts are similar; however, nests of odontogenic epithelium are frequently noted within the surrounding stroma.

Median rhomboid glossitis is believed by some to be a congenital lesion, the result of persistent tuberculum impar anterior to the foramen cecum.[8] This theory, however, is debated and others believe it to be an atrophic change secondary to the relative decreased vascularity of the area, especially as the lesions are not noted in children.[8] These are midline, rhomboid-shaped, flat, and erythematous areas of squamous epithelium anterior to the circumvallate papillae, devoid of papillae. Histologically, the lesions may or may not be keratotic and resemble pseudoepitheliomatous hyperplasia (Fig. 14.4, eFig. 14.3). Chronic inflammation is present to some degree in the surrounding stroma. This lesion is frequently associated with infection by *Candida* and some patients improve with antifungal therapy.[9] In such cases, keratosis is typically seen and fungus can be identified by special stains (e.g., GMS or PAS staining) (eFig. 14.4).

Some arteries in the lower lip fail to reduce in size as they approach the surface near the vermillion border.[10] These have been termed *caliber persistent arteries*. These arteries are sometimes associated with ulceration of the surface epithelium and can, when traumatized, bleed significantly. Rarely, they are associated with squamous cell carcinoma, perhaps secondary to the chronic ulcer.

TRAUMA AND IATROGENIC PROCESSES

Not uncommonly, the mouth is traumatized. Acute traumatic lesions are seldom sampled as their etiologies are rarely in question. Chronic traumatic lesions often have a nonspecific clinical appearance and may be sampled. The most common of these lesions is likely the traumatic

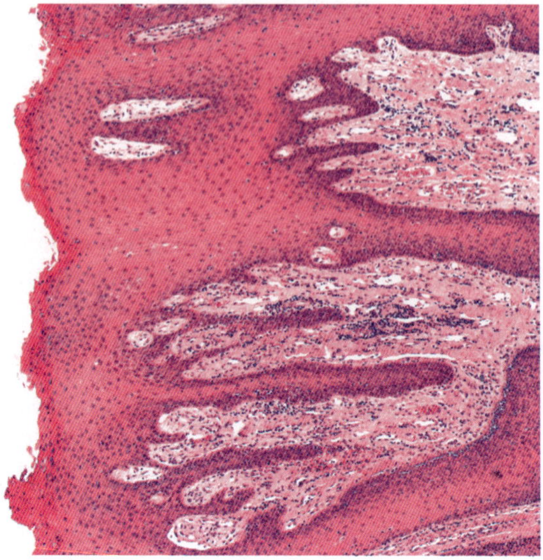

FIGURE 14.4 **Median rhomboid glossitis.**

fibroma. These fibromas along with their numerous alternative designations are discussed in Chapter 11. Osseous and cartilaginous metaplasias, secondary to chronic trauma or inflammation are also discussed in Chapter 12.

Inflammatory papillary hyperplasia and fibrous hyperplasia are both believed to be secondary to chronic trauma.[11] *Inflammatory papillary hyperplasia* is associated with denture use and most often involves the hard palate. Some have suggested that infection with *Candida* may play a role in the development of this condition.[12] Clinically, patients present with numerous, red papillary or verrucoid lesions. Microscopically, numerous papillary growths are covered by thickened and parakeratotic squamous epithelium with some degree of pseudoepitheliomatous hyperplasia, often with the formation of small keratinous cysts (Fig. 14.5).[11] The stromal tissue is usually edematous and contains a lymphoplasmacellular infiltrate (eFig. 14.5). Calcification or even cartilaginous or osseous metaplasia can be present. The underlying seromucinous glands may be atrophic and fibrotic. Small mucoid pools can be seen, which, together with the pseudoepitheliomatous hyperplasia and keratinous cysts, can lead one to consider mucoepidermoid carcinoma in the differential diagnosis.

The diagnosis of *fibrous hyperplasia* is generally used to connote traumatic fibrous lesions of the mouth and is synonymous with oral fibroma. These lesions can show a vast range of reactive histologic changes. Aside from cartilaginous and osseous metaplasia, calcification, and cementum formation, discussed in Chapter 12, some lesions will have many multinucleated giant cells (peripheral giant cell granuloma). These are often quite numerous and resemble osteoclasts.[13]

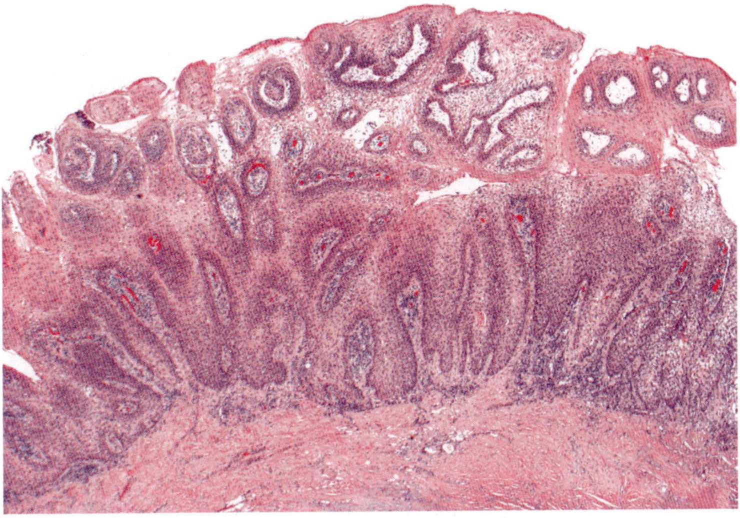

FIGURE 14.5 Inflammatory papillary hyperplasia of the palate.

Traumatic ulcerative granuloma is an uncommon lesion that can be clinically confused with malignancy. This lesion has acquired a number of appellations, mostly reflecting its presumed etiology and histology (e.g., *eosinophilic ulcer*, *oral traumatic granuloma*, *ulcerative eosinophilic granuloma*, and *Riga-Fede disease*).[14–18] It develops rapidly in either sex and at any age and is believed to be secondary to trauma, particularly crush injury. Although the lesions frequently involve the lateral or dorsal portion of the tongue, they arise at all locations within the mouth.[17,18] Most cases clinically present as ulcers; however, some are raised and exophytic.[15]

The surface of the traumatic ulcerative granulomas is typically covered by a fibrinopurulent exudate (Fig. 14.6).[14–16,18] A dense mixed inflammatory infiltrate, rich in eosinophils, extends deep into the submucosa and is intermingled with skeletal muscle fibers (eFig. 14.6). Other inflammatory cells include lymphocytes, macrophages, and neutrophils. Occasionally larger, atypical mononuclear cells are present (Fig. 14.7). These large cells frequently react with antibodies to CD30, a feature suggesting these lesions are lymphoproliferative disorders (eFig. 14.7).[19] Molecular studies have been mixed regarding clonality, with T-cell receptor rearrangement seen in some cases.[20,21] Nonetheless, the behavior of these lesions, when limited to the mucosa, is benign.

Because of their growth pattern and histologic features, traumatic eosinophilic granulomas must be distinguished from malignancies. Most often, anaplastic large cell lymphomas or Langerhan histiocytosis is considered in the differential diagnosis. Aside from the clinical presentations, these lesions can usually be distinguished by immunohistochemistry. The atypical mononuclear cells do not react with antibodies to S100 protein or

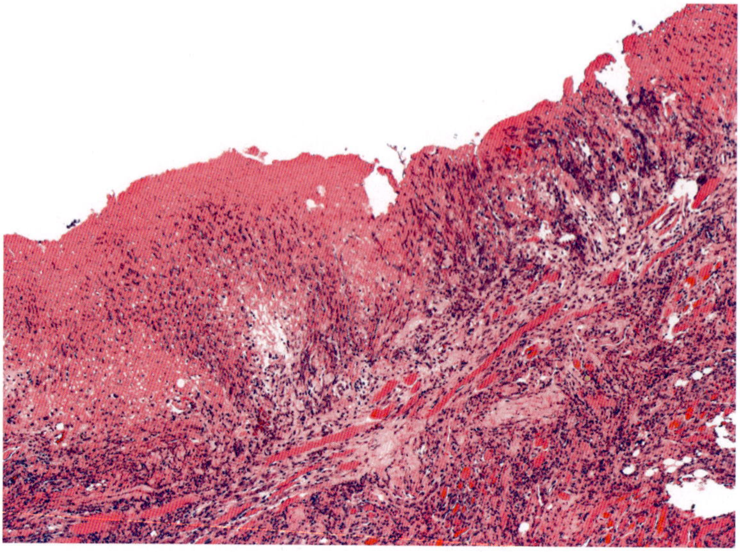

FIGURE 14.6 A traumatic ulcerative granuloma.

CD1a as would the neoplastic cells of Langerhan histiocytosis. They also do not react with antibodies to anaplastic lymphoma kinase (ALK1).

Gingival fibromatosis or *hyperplasia* can result from the use of certain drugs, including phenytoin, cyclosporine, and nifedipine, among others.[22,23] These apparently reactive conditions form within a few months of therapy

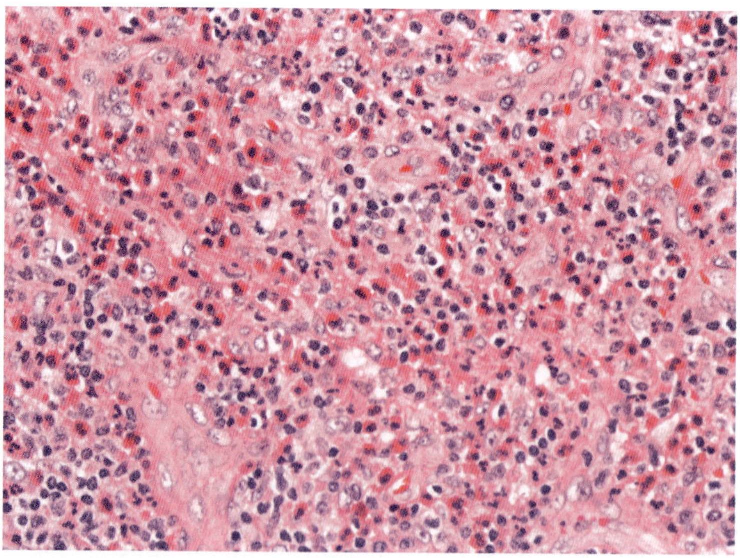

FIGURE 14.7 Eosinophils with occasional large lymphocytes seen in a traumatic ulcerative granuloma.

with the inciting medication and may be related to individual patient's dental hygiene. Clinically, the lesions begin with enlargement of the interdental papillae. These growths eventually become lobular and extend both labially and lingually. In advanced disease, teeth are often covered and displaced by the lesions. Histologically, the squamous epithelium is hyperplastic, with some degree of keratosis and elongated rete pegs. Fibroblasts proliferate within the underlying connective tissue and produce abundant collagen.

Patients who receive allogeneic bone marrow transplants, or, uncommonly, those who receive solid organ transplants or even blood transfusions, can develop graft-versus-host disease.[24] *Acute graft-versus-host disease* develops within days to weeks of bone marrow transplantation. Clinically, patients present with variable erythema that can progress to widespread blistering. The lesions progress histologically from focal basal cell vacuolar change to basal cell dyskeratosis to subepithelial cleft formation to the formation of bullae. A mononuclear perivascular infiltrate of variable degree is seen within the upper lamina propria and exocytosis is usually present, especially as the histologic changes worsen.

Chronic graft-versus-host disease develops in about half of adults and about 20% of children months to years after bone marrow transplantation.[24–26] Clinically, the lesions often appear similar to those of oral lichen planus with linear white stria or ulcers. Patients also typically are noted to have xerostomia. A lichenoid infiltrate of mononuclear cells is present with exocytosis, basal cell vacuolization, cell death, and, with worse cases, bullae (Fig. 14.8, eFig. 14.8). The seromucinous glands have prominent chronic inflammation, with degeneration and fibrosis. They are sometimes cystically dilated.

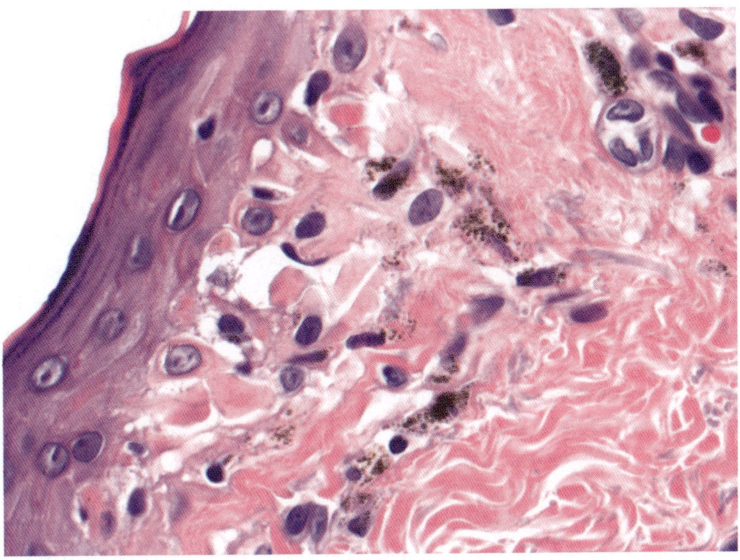

FIGURE 14.8 Chronic graft-versus-host disease with basal cell vacuolization and necrosis.

Other traumatic or iatrogenic lesions have also been reported. Some authors have shown that adipose tissue from the buccal pad can herniate into the mouth with trauma and erroneously be diagnosed as a lipoma (*traumatic pseudolipoma*).[27] *Mucositis* secondary to chemotherapy or radiation therapy is rarely biopsied and is instead usually diagnosed clinically.[28] It is associated with ulceration and nonspecific histologic features (see Chapter 4). *Thermal injury* of the mouth is common but rarely sampled. The histology is similar to that seen with burns of other squamous covered surfaces and depends on the burn's severity. Necrosis of the epithelium and subepithelial tissue can be seen with the formation of subepithelial bullae.

INFECTIOUS DISEASE

The mouth can be involved by a great variety of infectious diseases, especially in patients who are for one reason or another immunocompromised. Infectious lesions may appear inflammatory or ulcerative. They can also mimic neoplastic masses or neoplastic intraepithelial proliferations (e.g., leukoplakia). Ancillary testing is usually helpful for identifying causative agents. The role of human papillomavirus in oral pathology has been discussed in chapters dealing with squamous neoplasia (Chapters 2–5).

Hairy leukoplakia secondary to infection by Epstein-Barr virus (EBV) most frequently occurs in immunocompromised individuals; however, it can occasionally develop in patients who appear to be immunocompetent.[29-31] Clinically, these lesions are white, broad, and flat to slightly raised. The surface typically appears corrugated or "hairy." While the lesions most often involve the lateral or ventral surfaces of the tongue, they can develop anywhere within the mouth. Unlike infections secondary only to *Candida* (i.e., thrush), abrasion will not dislodge the plaque material.[30]

Histologically, the squamous epithelium is acanthotic with parakeratosis (eFig. 14.9).[30,31] Individual superficial squamous cells have optically clear cytoplasm with somewhat compressed, darkened nuclei (Fig. 14.9). Within these cells, the chromatin often appears marginated and intranuclear inclusions are commonly seen. The squamous epithelium is often not inflamed, and only mild chronic inflammation is present in the lamina propria. In situ hybridization for EBV-encoded RNA is helpful as the affected squamous epithelium will contain virus. Staining for fungal or bacterial organisms may demonstrate secondary colonization of the superficial epithelium.

Other herpes viruses can infect the oral mucosa including the herpes simplex viruses (*HSV1* and *HSV2*) and *varicella zoster*, as well as *cytomegalovirus*.[32] Infections associated with simplex viruses and varicella cause painful vesicles which eventually ulcerate. Primary infections with HSV-1 manifest as a gingivostomatitis. Most reactivations in immunocompetent patients are labial, although intraoral recurrences also develop. Immunocompromised patients can have severe intraoral disease either at

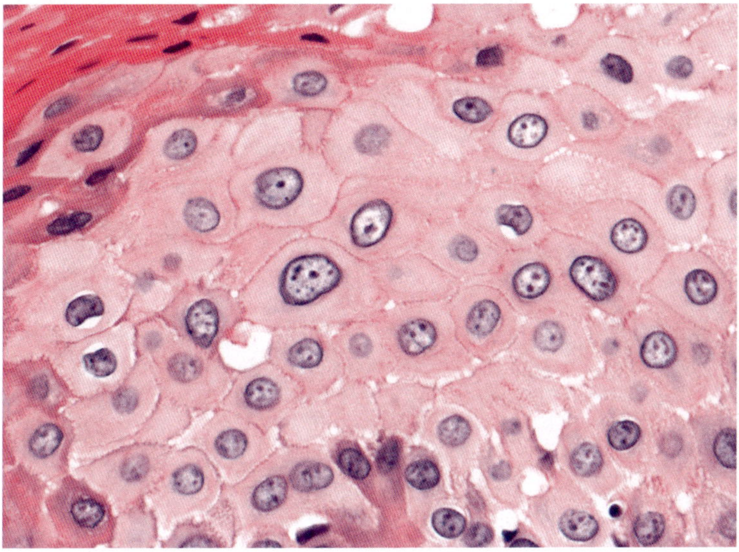

FIGURE 14.9 The cytoplasm of the squamous cells in hairy leukoplakia will appear glassy.

the time of primary infection or at the time of reactivation. The histology of these lesions is similar to that seen in other squamous epithelia. The mucosa will be eroded and ulcerated with a diffuse mixed inflammatory infiltrate. Telltale signs of herpes infection include single and multinucleated epithelial cells with Cowdry type A and B intranuclear inclusions (Fig. 14.10).[32] Ductal cells of the minor salivary glands can also be infected. Immunohistochemistry with antibodies to specific types of herpes viruses will confirm the diagnosis, if needed. The large intranuclear and intracytoplasmic inclusions of cytomegalovirus are typically found within lesional endothelial cells, as this virus does not usually infect squamous epithelium (eFig. 14.10).[32]

The oral cavity can be involved by all stages of *syphilis*.[33] Primary chancres measure between 1 and 2 cm and most often involve the lips, tongue, or gingiva. They may be painful due to secondary infection. The squamous epithelium will be eroded or atrophic, and an underlying dense lymphoplasmacytic infiltrate is commonly present. An obliterative endarteritis and neuritis is sometimes seen with occasional granulomas and foci of necrosis (eFigs. 14.11 and 14.12). Secondary syphilis develops 4 to 6 weeks after the primary lesion. Symptoms are nonspecific and include a fever with a generalized rash and lymphadenopathy. During this period, a white mucous patch or broad-based verrucal plaque (condyloma latum) can develop. Biopsy of these lesions will show epithelial hyperplasia and keratosis, again with a subepithelial lymphoplasmacytic infiltrate and possible concomitant vasculitis and neuritis (Figs. 14.11 and 14.12). With tertiary syphilis, nodular, ulcerative lesions or gumma sometimes develop

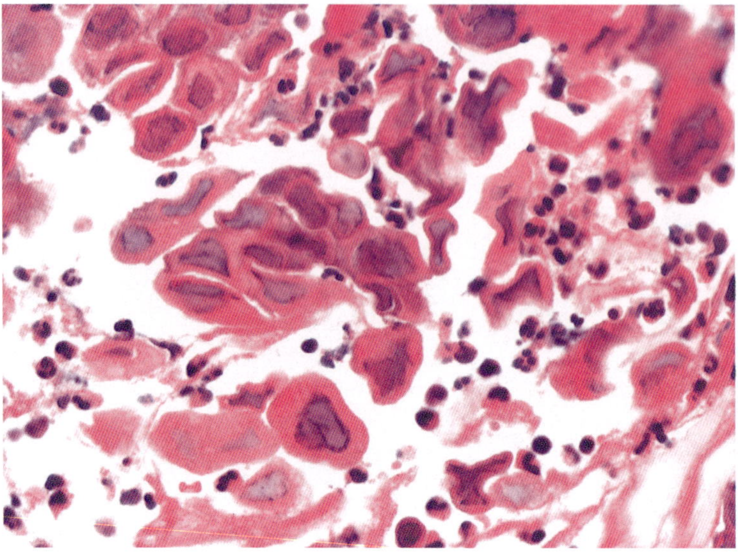

FIGURE 14.10 Characteristic intranuclear inclusions seen in lingual herpes.

on the mucous membranes. Healing of glossal gummas can lead to an atrophic glossitis that is believed to be a risk factor for the development of squamous cell carcinoma.

As with other sites in the upper aerodigestive tract, the mouth can be infected by *Mycobacterium tuberculosis*.[33] Lesions in the mouth are almost

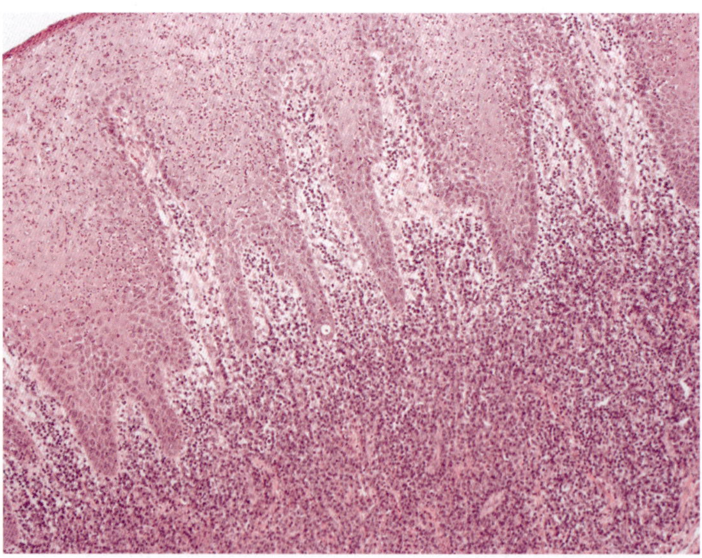

FIGURE 14.11 Oral condyloma latum with pseudoepitheliomatous hyperplasia and a dense plasma cell infiltrate.

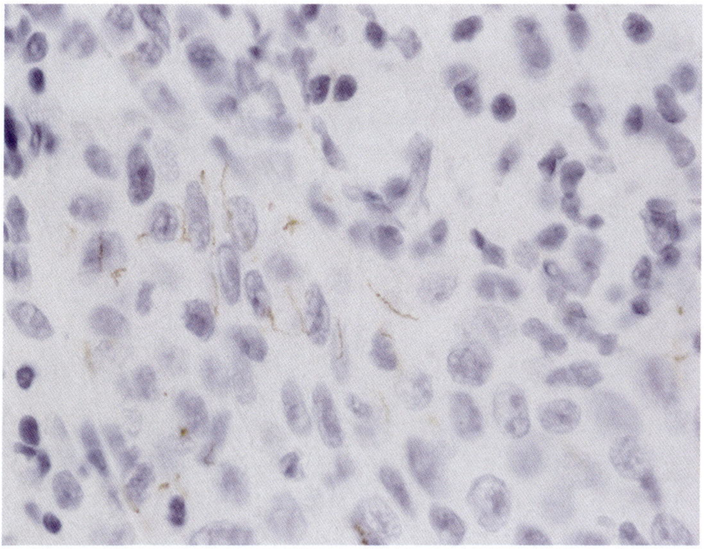

FIGURE 14.12 *Treponema pallidum* identified by immunohistochemistry in a case of oral syphilis.

always associated with rapidly progressive pulmonary infections. Within the mouth, the mid-dorsum of the tongue is the most commonly affected site. The histologic findings are somewhat nonspecific with ulceration of the surface, a mixed inflammatory infiltrate, and epithelioid granulomas. Necrosis is frequently not present and organisms are usually not identified even with the use of histochemical stains. Correct diagnosis hinges on the recognition of the patient's concomitant pulmonary disease.

Although not commonly biopsied, the mouth is involved in *lepromatous leprosy* in more than 20% of cases.[34,35] Changes are often both clinically and histologically nonspecific. Patients may have macules, papules, or fissures. Biopsies typically show nonspecific lymphoplasmacytic inflammation without granulomas or identifiable bacilli. Occasional histiocytic infiltrates or granulomas are rarely seen that, when stained, will contain bacilli. It is interesting to note that these can sometimes be identified in clinically normal-appearing tissues by special stain (e.g., Fite stain). Tuberculoid or borderline leprosy may also involve the mouth.[36]

Candidiasis or *thrush* is the most common oral fungal infection. Patients with oral candidiasis are often immunocompromised; however, the disease has long been recognized in immunocompetent individuals, especially neonates and persons receiving antibiotic therapy.[32] These lesions can present with a semiadherent, white, creamy plaque (pseudomembranous form), erythema (atrophic form), or leukoplakia (hyperplastic form). Pseudomembranes can usually be removed by brushing the lesion, leaving an erythematous, bleeding surface. The hyperplastic variety most often involves the buccal mucosa bilaterally. Histologically, candidiasis is usually

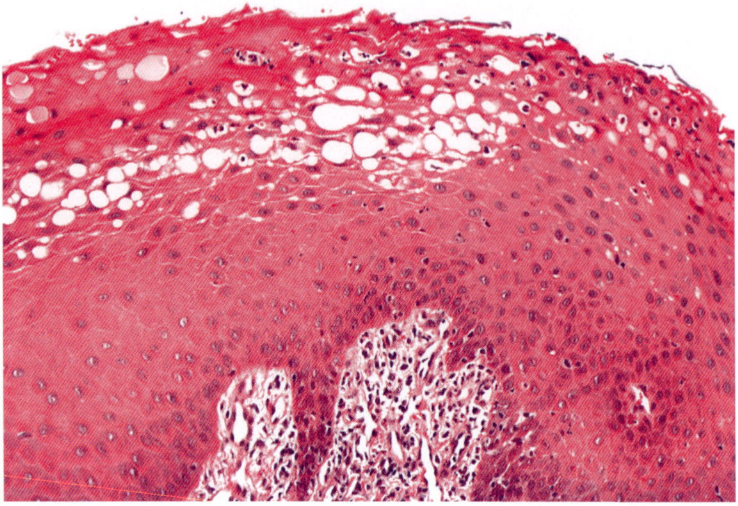

FIGURE 14.13 Superficial infection of the tongue with *Candida*.

characterized by a thickened and parakeratotic squamous epithelium containing numerous pseudohyphae and yeast forms consistent with *Candida* (Fig. 14.13, eFigs. 14.13 and 14.14).[32] Some degree of epithelial infiltration with neutrophils is often seen but it is not universally present.

Other fungal diseases involve the mouth, almost always in immunocompromised patients. *Cryptococcus* has been noted within the stromal tissues with little accompanying inflammation.[32] Oral *histoplasmosis* has been diagnosed with the yeast seen within large foamy macrophages in the stromal tissues.[32] *Paracoccidioidomycosis* is uncommon in the United States but can be seen in patients from Mexico and Central or South America.[37] It is a deep mycosis that, when presenting orally, is characterized by an erythematous, finely granular lesion with pinpoint hemorrhages. Some lesions have been noted to resemble mulberries. Histologically, the lesions have pseudoepitheliomatous hyperplasia with intraepithelial microabcesses, subepithelial granulomatous inflammation, and numerous neutrophils and plasma cells. Yeast forms may be found within the microabcesses with multinucleated giant cells. Rarely, the "pilot wheel" form may be seen with numerous yeasts budding from a central organism.

NONINFECTIOUS INFLAMMATORY CONDITIONS

The oral mucosa is frequently involved by noninfectious inflammatory conditions that present with nonspecific clinical features. Many lesions appear white, vesicular, or ulcerated. Vesicular or blistering lesions, when they involve the gingivae, often lead clinically to desquamative gingivitis (Table 14.2).[38] Chronic disease leads to glossal fissuring or even to the

TABLE 14.2 Causes of Desquamative Gingivitis

Pemphigus (vulgaris, drug-induced, etc.)
Lichen planus
Bullous pemphigoid
Systemic or discoid lupus erythematosis
Erythema multiforme
Graft-versus-host disease
Herpes virus infections
Epidermolysis bullosa

so-called scrotal tongue. The histologic findings are also often nonspecific. For example, lichen planus shares many histologic features with chronic graft-versus-host disease and lupus erythematosis. A number of diseases present with either intraepithelial or subepithelial bullae or with caseating or noncaseating granulomatous inflammation (Table 14.3). Clinical history and ancillary testing is often needed to make a specific diagnosis. Even with both, nonspecific diagnoses must sometimes be rendered.

Noncaseating granulomas can be found in many cases of *Crohn disease* and help to distinguish this idiopathic inflammatory bowel disease from other processes. Oral lesions associated with the disease include a number of entities and can sometimes proceed the diagnosis of the inflammatory bowel disease.[39,40] These lesions include aphthae, ulcers, swelling

TABLE 14.3 Oral Diseases With Granulomatous Inflammation

Infection
Tuberculosis
Leprosy
Atypical mycobacterium
Mycosis (although *Candida* is the cause of most oral mycoses, those that induce an actual granulomatous reaction are more likely to be atypical organisms (e.g., *Histoplasma*, *Paracoccidioides*, etc.)
Syphilis
Crohn disease
Sarcoidosis
Wegener granulomatosis
Orofacial granulomatosis (granulomatous cheilitis and Melkersson-Rosenthal syndrome)
Foreign body reaction

of the lips and cheeks, fissuring of the lips, gingivitis, erythema, and scaling. Most disease involves either the lips or buccal mucosa; the palate and tongue are rarely involved. Affected individuals can have secondary malabsorption and develop atrophic glossitis secondary to iron, folate, or vitamin B_{12} deficiency. Biopsy of the lesions can show nonspecific histologic features together with occasional noncaseating granulomas (eFig. 14.15).[33] The latter are often located deeply and may not be seen on biopsy.

The term *orofacial granulomatosis* is used for lesions that clinically and histologically resemble those seen in Crohn disease, while the patients lack evidence of inflammatory bowel disease (Fig. 14.14, eFig. 14.16).[33,41] Other causes of granulomatous inflammation, such as sarcoidosis, mycobacterial or fungal infections, and foreign body reactions, should also be excluded before this diagnosis is rendered. Orofacial granulomatosis is sometimes secondary to inciting food agents such as cinnamon and improves with their withdrawal. When limited to the lips, the lesions are termed *cheilitis granulomatosis* (eFig. 14.17).[42,43] Patients with this disease are more frequently young women and present with episodic swelling of the lips. *Melkersson-Rosenthal syndrome* is characterized by facial nerve palsy, a fissured tongue, and labial swelling secondary to granulomatous inflammation.[44,45] This disease is more frequently diagnosed in young women and typically shows broader symptomatology than the originally described triad with frequent swelling of the buccal mucosa, gingiva, and even the eyelids.

Recurrent aphthous ulcers of the mouth are extremely common in some populations, especially in white, affluent women.[46] Patients develop recurrent shallow, rounded ulcers at intervals generally ranging from days to months. Most are considered to be minor aphthae, are less than 5 mm

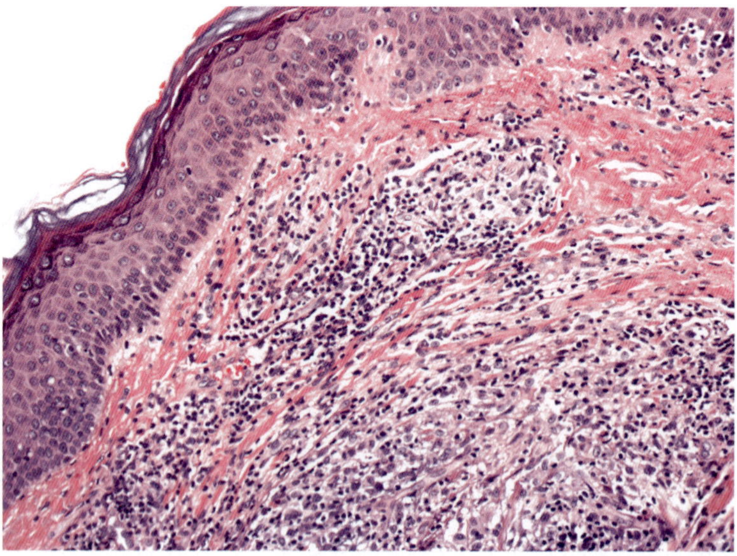

FIGURE 14.14 Orofacial granulomatous.

in size, and typically present on the labial or buccal mucosa or on the floor of the mouth; however, larger aphthae can rarely develop as can numerous coalescing aphthae. These lesions follow a benign course and clinical symptoms of more aggressive disease such as those seen with Behcet disease should not be present.

Aphthous ulcers show variable histologic features depending upon when they are sampled.[46] Prior to ulceration, lymphocytes migrate into the squamous epithelium and edema develops both within the keratinocytes and stroma. Eventually, a vasculitis develops primarily affecting small vessels and capillaries. Ulcerated lesions are covered by fibrinous exudates and characteristically have dense mixed inflammatory infiltrates with neutrophils, lymphocytes, and plasma cells (Fig. 14.15). Vasculitis is usually seen, predominately affecting the smaller vessels.

Behcet disease typically presents with recurrent oral aphthous ulcers with other systemic manifestations, including genital ulcers and eye disease.[47] Additional symptoms include skin lesions and vasculitis with thrombosis and resultant ischemia. The disease presents in both sexes at any age and most frequently comes to clinical attention when the patient is in his or her third decade of life. Frequently, the disease runs a chronic and unpredictable course, and most patients develop some chronic morbidity, most often blindness. Men and those patients diagnosed at younger ages fare worse.[47] Although large vessel vasculitis and thrombosis are typical of the disease, Behcet disease is diagnosed clinically based on a myriad of symptoms. The histologic changes seen with these aphthous ulcers are nonspecific and similar to those described above.

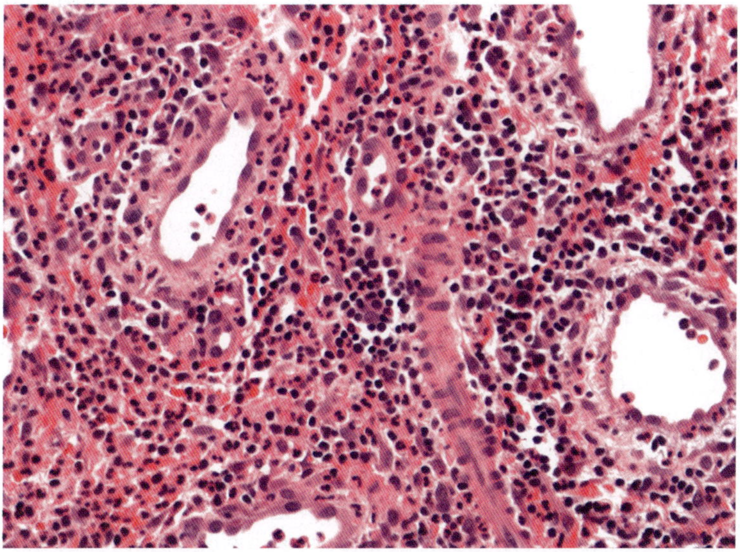

FIGURE 14.15 An intense acute inflammatory infiltrate seen at the base of an aphthous ulcer.

Benign migratory stomatitis or *geographic tongue* is an odd inflammatory condition of the tongue that is typically painless.[48–50] These lesions are usually multiple and variably sized. They grossly appear as well-demarcated erythematous areas that are surrounded by a raised yellow-white circinate border. They typically occur on the anterior two-thirds of the dorsum of the tongue; however, they can occur anywhere within the mouth (migratory stomatitis). Individual lesions heal, but new ones quickly develop in other areas. Although benign and usually only associated with minor sensitivity to some foods, these lesions can be troubling to the patients who may also have glossal fissuring.

Histologically, the squamous epithelium of geographic tongue appears atrophic at the center of the lesions with loss of filiform papillae.[50] A mixed inflammatory infiltrate is seen within the underlying lamina propria with exocytosis of neutrophils and small microabcesses (eFig. 14.18). At the periphery of the lesions and corresponding with the yellow-white border, hyperkeratosis and acanthosis is seen.

Erythema multiforme is an acute inflammatory disorder affecting the skin and mucous membranes.[51,52] The disease can vary in severity and can range from a mild, self-limited cutaneous variant with little mucosal involvement to a severe variant with extensive mucocutaneous necrosis (*Stevens-Johnson syndrome*). It most commonly affects young, sometimes genetically predisposed individuals between the ages of 20 and 40 years after an exposure to an exogenous trigger. Possible triggers include infectious agents, foods, drugs, or even other immune processes. The disease is usually self-limited, but recurrences develop in up to 25% of patients. Clinically, patients with erythema multiforme have macules or erythematous papules that often assume a targetoid appearance. Mucous membrane involvement includes macules, blisters, and ulcers. When the mouth is affected, the most severe disease is seen anteriorly, and the lips are frequently cracked and crusted.

When the epithelium is intact, an interphase and spongiotic mucositis is present with basal cell vacuolization and necrosis (Fig. 14.16).[51,52] The lamina propria is typically edematous with a perivascular chronic lymphocytic infiltrate, intermixed with neutrophils and eosinophils. In more severe lesions, widespread basal cell necrosis produces bullous change (eFigs. 14.19 and 14.20). Eventually, complete necrosis of the squamous epithelium may be present raising a possibility of *toxic epidermal necrolysis*.

Lichen planus is a frequently mucosal chronic inflammatory disorder that more commonly affects women and usually presents in a patient's fourth or fifth decade of life.[53,54] Lesions can vary significantly in clinical appearance. Most appear as linear, white keratotic stria (reticular), but erosive or bullous lesions also occur. These more severe lesions frequently involve the gingiva and are one of the causes of desquamative gingivitis. It is unclear if the disease is truly a complication of infectious disease, but it has been noted in association with hepatitis C infection.[55,56] Many believe lichen planus to carry increased risk for the development of oral squamous cell carcinoma.[57–59]

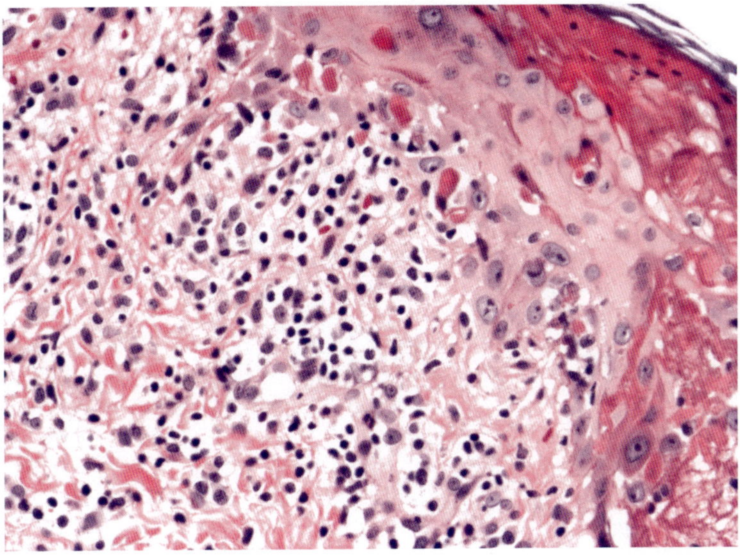

FIGURE 14.16 Erythema multiforme with an interphase chronic inflammatory infiltrate.

Histologically, lichen planus is characterized by a band of chronic inflammatory cells within the superficial lamina propria that extends into the overlying squamous epithelium (Fig. 14.17).[53,57] Civatte bodies (necrotic, dyskeratotic squamous cells) are usually present, and dissolution of the basal epithelium is typically seen (Fig. 14.18, eFig. 14.21).

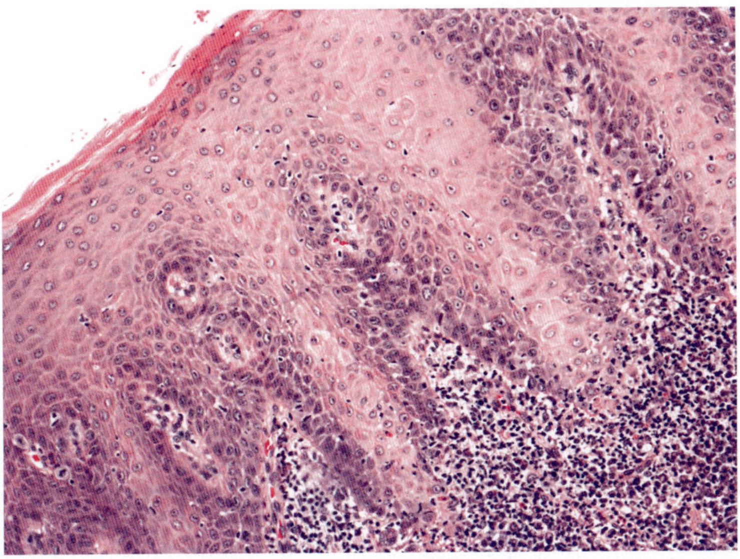

FIGURE 14.17 Lichen planus.

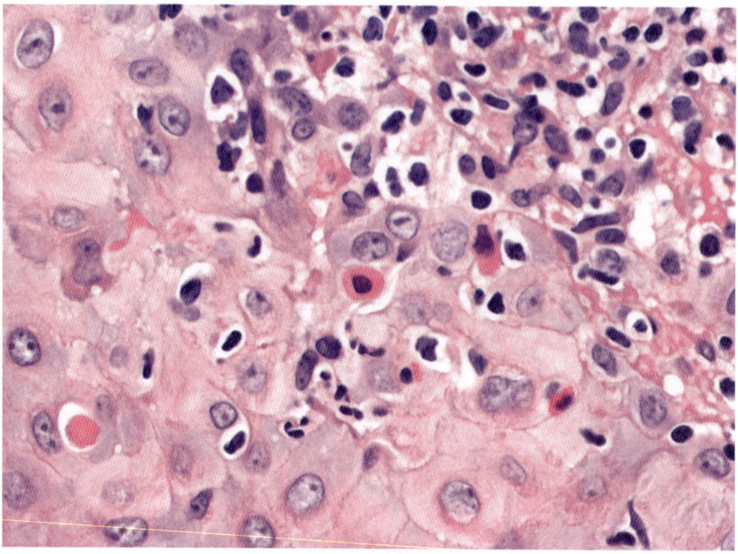

FIGURE 14.18 Civatte bodies seen in a case of lichen planus.

The epithelium itself may range from atrophic to acanthotic; parakeratosis or orthokeratosis are almost always present. Acanthotic epithelium is frequently associated with irregular, "sawtooth" rete ridges. Finally, a band of fibrin is often present just beneath the basal squamous epithelium. For a definitive diagnosis, clinical and pathologic features are usually necessary.[60]

Within the upper aerodigestive tract, frequently within the mouth, patients develop a mucositis characterized by a dense plasma cell infiltrate (*mucinous membrane plasmacytosis* or *idiopathic lymphoplasmacytic mucositis*).[61,62] The lesions typically appear cobblestone or warty but can also simply appear as thickenings and fissurings of the mucosa. Multiple areas within the upper aerodigestive tract are often involved, either through direct extension or multifocal involvement. Patients are older and most cases present during or after the fifth decade of life.

Histologically, the squamous epithelium appears psoriasiform with parakeratosis, elongation of the rete ridges, and suprapapillary thinning.[61–63] A diffuse plasma cell infiltrate is present within the underlying stroma with intermixed lymphocytes and neutrophils (Fig. 14.19). Exocytosis is seen with rare aggregates of neutrophils within the epithelium (eFig. 14.22). Immunohistochemistry should be performed with these lesions and will show polyclonal staining, excluding the diagnosis of extraosseous plasmacytoma.

The *pemphigoids* are immune-mediated subepithelial blistering diseases usually associated with autoantibodies to components of hemidesmosomes.[64,65] The mucous membranes are predominately affected by cicatricial or mucous membrane pemphigoid. The disease may actually

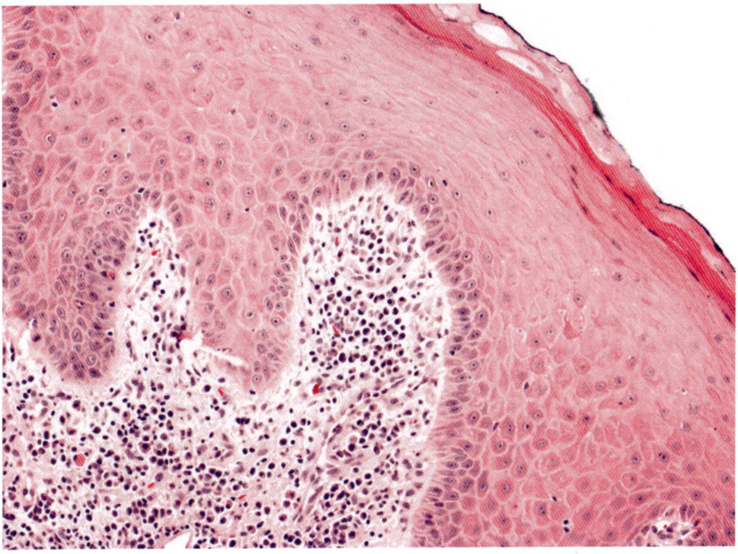

FIGURE 14.19 A subepithelial plasma cell infiltrate seen with idiopathic lymphoplasmacytic mucositis.

include multiple entities, as patients present with lesions only in the mouth or with involvement of other mucosal surfaces, such as the conjunctivae or skin. Typical presenting symptoms include pain, bleeding, or peeling of the oral mucosa. Vesicles or bullae form anywhere within the mouth but are usually present within the gingivae, hard and soft palates, buccal mucosa, or tongue.[66]

Histologically, the lesions show junctional separation at the level of the basement membrane (Fig. 14.20, eFig. 14.23; Table 14.4).[64] Eosinophils, lymphocytes, and neutrophils are seen within the vesicles and the lamina propria. Direct immunofluorescence of perilesional specimens will show linear deposits of IgG and C3 along the basement membrane (eFig. 14.24). Indirect immunofluorescence can be used to determine a patient's amount of antibody. Immunofluorescence can also be used to exclude genetic defects of hemidesmosome proteins that also present with subepithelial vesicles (e.g., epidermolysis bullosa).

Pemphigus is a group of autoimmune diseases characterized by epithelial blistering most often secondary to autoantibodies to components of desmosomes.[65,67] Pemphigus vulgaris is the specific disease most commonly affecting the oral mucosa, likely because it is often secondary to antibodies to desmoglein 3, a protein preferentially expressed in the desmosomes of the oral squamous epithelium. Patients are older and there tends to be regional differences in presentation, suggesting a genetic basis for the disease. Some cases are related to neoplasia (frequently hematopoietic) or drug therapy (paraneoplastic pemphigus or drug-induced pemphigus).[67,68] Patients present with vesiculobullous disease and ulcers of the oral and

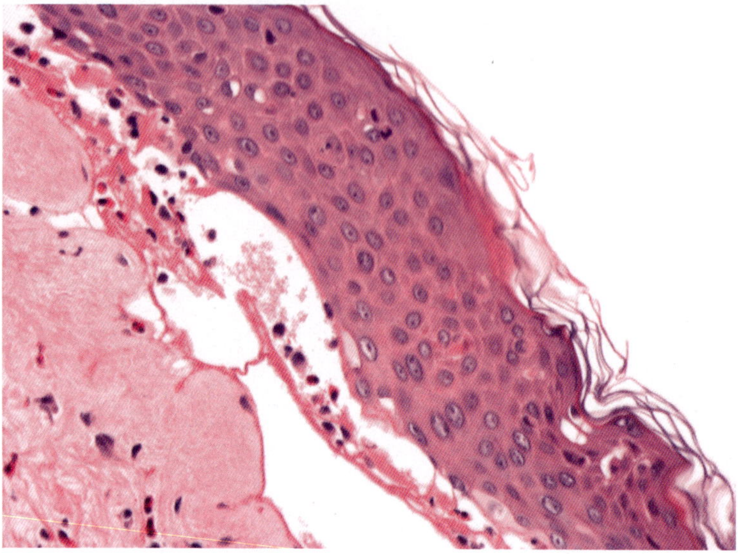

FIGURE 14.20 **Mucous membrane pemphigoid.**

gingival mucosa. Other sites, such as the conjunctiva, genitals, esophagus, larynx, and skin, are also affected. Previously, the disease frequently led to the death because of either dehydration or secondary infection; however, current therapy allows many patients to achieve remission from their disease.

The various forms of *pemphigus* show slightly different histologic features. Pemphigus vulgaris is characterized by intraepithelial acantholysis and splitting, usually just above the basal layer of epithelial cells (Fig. 14.21; Table 14.4). Acantholytic cells float within the blister.

TABLE 14.4 Pemphigoid and Pemphigus of the Mouth

	Pemphigoid	Pemphigus
Most common variant to affect the mouth	Cicatricial or mucous membrane pemphigoid	Pemphigus vulgaris
Autoantibody	Against component of hemidesmosome, usually against BP1 or BP2	Against component of desmosome, usually IgG against DG3
Location of bullae	Subepithelial	Intraepithelial, usually above basal keratinocytes
Direct immunofluorescence	Linear IgG and C3 along the basement membrane	Intercellular IgG and C3 within the squamous epithelium

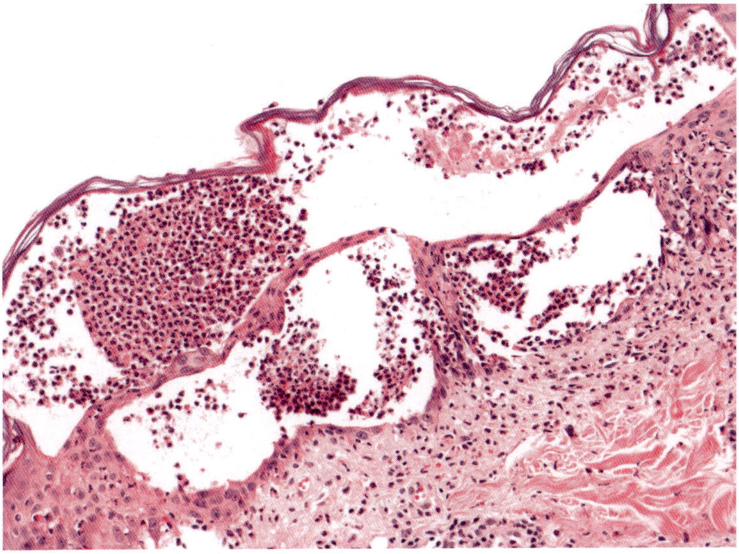

FIGURE 14.21 Intraepithelial bullae in a case of pemphigus vulgaris.

Ulceration with acute inflammation and a fibrinous exudate is typically present. The bullae often contain inflammatory cells including neutrophils, eosinophils, lymphocytes, and plasma cells that typically extend into the lamina propria (eFig. 14.25). By direct immunofluorescence, intercellular deposits of IgG and C3 can be seen (eFig. 14.26).[28] Indirect immunofluorescence can be used to determine the patient's antibody titer.

Oral lesions develop in patients with *lupus erythematosis*, both when they have systemic disease and when they have disease primarily limited to the skin.[69] Clinically, the oral lesions vary considerably. Some patients present with white, plaquelike lesions, some with erythematous lesions, and some with vesicles or ulcers. Many patients have multiple lesions that show a combination of these features.

Biopsies of lupus erythematosis typically show parakeratosis or hyperkeratosis, frequently with "keratin plugging."[70] The epithelium is often hyperplastic with alternative areas of atrophy, thus forming irregular fingerlike or "sawtooth" rete ridges.[71] A lymphoplasmacytic infiltrate is present within the lamina propria and extends into the epithelium (eFig. 14.27). Basal cell degeneration is usually seen, sometimes with subepithelial vesicle formation and subbasal fibrin deposition.[69] The inflammatory infiltrate may be dense in the upper lamina propria and often extends deeply. In areas where the inflammatory infiltrate is less dense, a perivascular distribution is often noted (Fig. 14.22, eFig. 14.28). Edema can usually be seen within the lamina propria. Direct immunofluorescence will demonstrate a granular, subepithelial deposition of immunoglobulin and C3.[72]

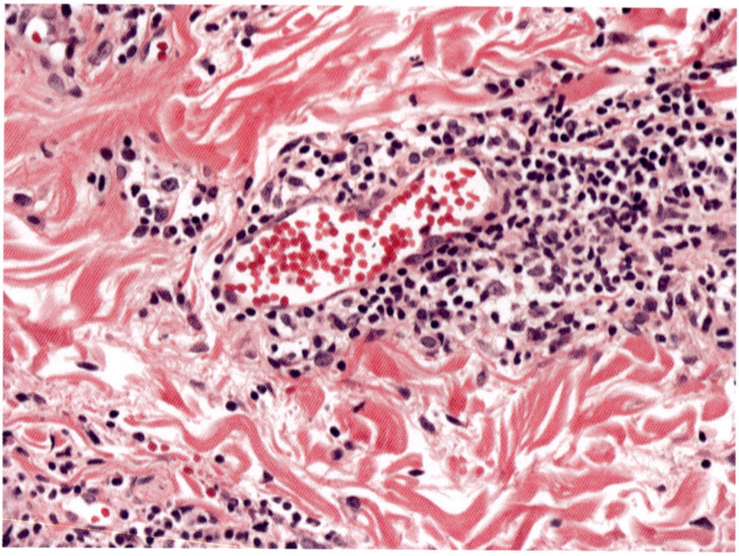

FIGURE 14.22 A deep perivascular infiltrate can be seen with lupus erythematosis.

While the clinical context is usually very helpful, some lesions may be hard to distinguish from lichen planus. Histologically, features supportive of a diagnosis of lupus include edema, subepithelial vesicle formation, a deep or perivascular inflammatory infiltrate, and keratin plugging.[70,71] Lichen planus is also much less likely to show subepithelial granular deposits of immunoglobulin or C3.[72]

Sjogren syndrome is a systemic autoimmune disease that preferentially affects women.[73] Patients present with dry eyes and mouth. Diagnostic testing for the disease includes the objective assessment of lacrimal activity (Schirmer test) and testing for autoantibodies (anti-SS-A/Ro, anti-SS-B/La, ANA, or IgM rheumatoid factor). Patients also frequently note the presence of swollen and tender salivary glands. The diagnosis requires the presence of a number of clinical and pathologic features.[73,74]

The use of biopsy of the minor salivary glands for the diagnosis of Sjogren syndrome is somewhat controversial, and studies have shown varying degrees of sensitivity and specificity for the test.[74,75] Multiple salivary gland lobules should be present for the biopsy to be considered adequate.[73,74] Polymorphous lymphocytes should be present as aggregates and may be either periductal (when primary) or perivascular (when secondary) (Fig. 14.23, eFig. 14.29). Current diagnostic systems, such as the Greenspan system, quantify the foci of lymphoid aggregates (defined as more than 50 lymphocytes).

Other inflammatory conditions affecting the mouth include systemic diseases that more frequently present in other regions of the upper aerodigestive tract, such as *sarcoidosis* and *Wegener granulomatosis*.[33,76] Sarcoidosis is again a diagnosis of exclusion, and other etiologies of

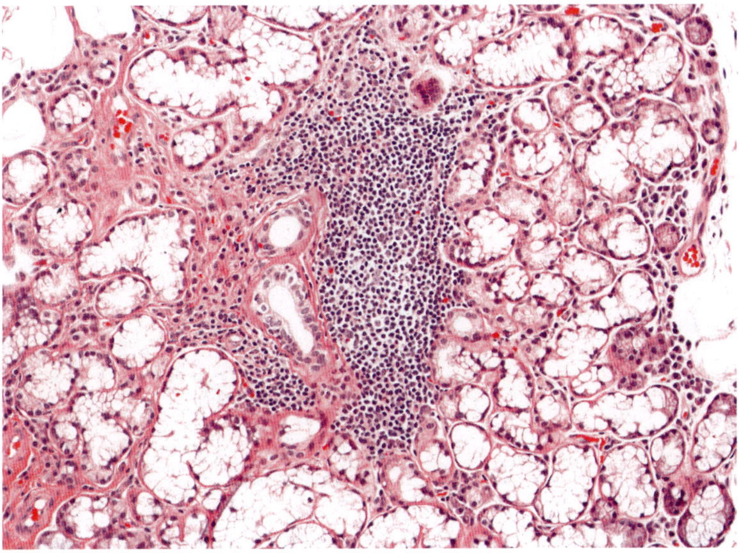

FIGURE 14.23 A periductal lymphoid infiltrate is seen in a biopsy from a patient suspected to have Sjogren syndrome.

noncaseating granulomas should be excluded. The diagnosis of Wegener granulomatosis presents the same challenges that it does with samples from the sinonasal tract (see Chapter 13). Oral lesions associated with Wegener granulomatosis include swelling, ulcers, and palatal perforation. Rarely, a proliferative gingivitis can be seen characterized by a mottled, red and purple granular surface (strawberry gingivitis).[33] The histologic triad of vasculitis, necrosis, and granulomatous inflammation though diagnostic is rarely seen. Foreign body reactions secondary to endogenous and exogenous materials such as amalgam filling and toothpaste are rarely encountered (Fig. 14.24, eFig. 14.30).[33]

OTHER LESIONS

Oral focal mucinosis occurs in both men and women at any age.[77] The lesions occur anywhere throughout the mouth and typically present as rounded papules of variable duration. Frequently, they are clinically believed to be traumatic fibromas. Microscopically, these lesions are characterized by well-circumscribed myxoid change within the stroma that can extend to and flatten the overlying squamous epithelium (Fig. 14.25, eFig. 14.31).

Mucoceles appear clinically akin to oral focal mucinosis or traumatic fibromas although they rarely are destructive. Histologically, they appear similar to those described in the sinonasal area (Chapter 13). A circumscribed mucinous lake is surrounded by a single layer of mucinous epithelium that is focally attenuated or even entirely lost (Fig. 14.26, eFig. 14.32).

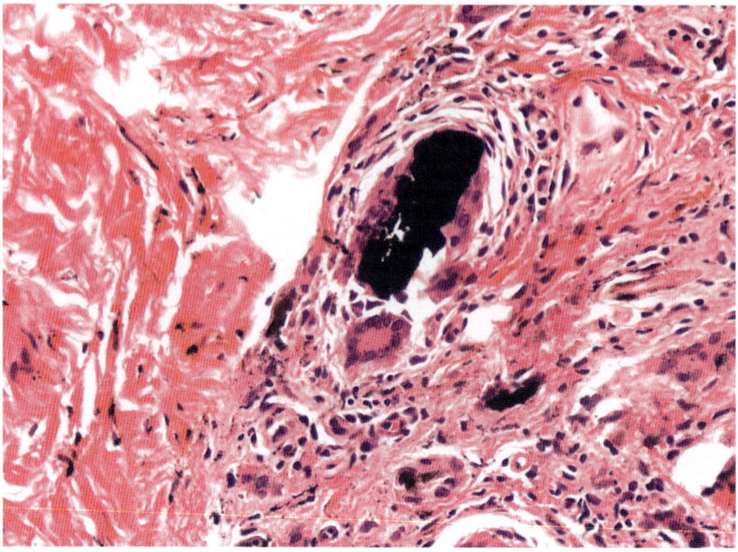

FIGURE 14.24 A foreign body reaction seen in an amalgam tattoo.

Chronic inflammation, fibrosis, and foreign body reaction surround the mucus. Low-grade mucoepidermoid carcinomas should be excluded through examination of the surrounding epithelium.

White sponge nevus is a soft, white spongy plaque that typically develops in the mouth, often bilaterally on the buccal mucosa, although anatomic sites throughout the body can be involved.[78] Clinically, the

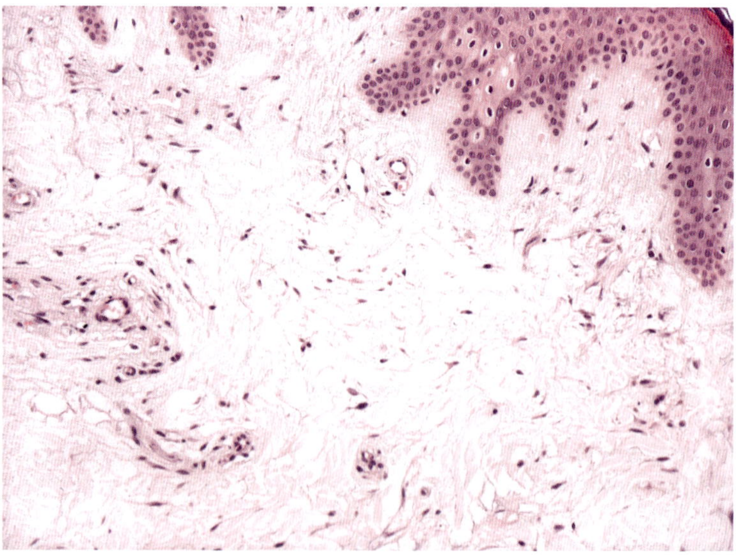

FIGURE 14.25 Oral focal mucinosis.

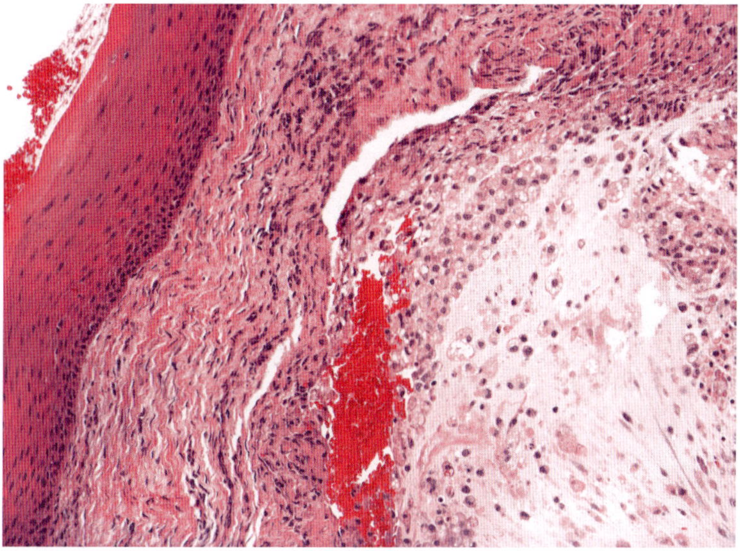

FIGURE 14.26 A small subepithelial mucocele of the lip.

lesions are often mistaken for leukoplakia. Histologically, there is squamous hyperplasia with hyperkeratosis. The suprabasal squamous cells are vacuolated and sometimes contain keratohyaline granules. These lesions are associated with mutations of the genes encoding CK4 and CK13.[79,80]

Leukoedema is yet another gray-white lesion of the mouth that should be distinguished from leukoplakia and lichen planus.[81] Although its definitive etiology is not known, many believe it to be secondary to local irritation. The lesions preferably involve the buccal mucosa, occur at any age, and are more common in African Americans. Histologically, the squamous epithelium is thickened and parakeratosis may be seen. The rete pegs are elongated and irregular. Intracellular edema was noted originally as a defining feature of this process.

Verruciform xanthomas are exophytic, rough lesions that are usually solitary and measure less than 2 cm in size.[82,83] They develop anywhere within the mouth and are most frequently noted to involve the gingiva, hard palate, or tongue. They may occur at any age and are frequently noted to have been present for extended periods of time. Neither sex is preferentially affected. Histologically, these lesions have a verrucoid, papillary, or nodular architecture. The squamous epithelium is typically thickened with keratosis and parakeratosis (Fig. 14.27, eFig. 14.33). Numerous foamy histiocytes are present immediately beneath the squamous epithelium within the connective tissue papillae. These may extend deeper into the lamina propria and are intermixed with other inflammatory cells.

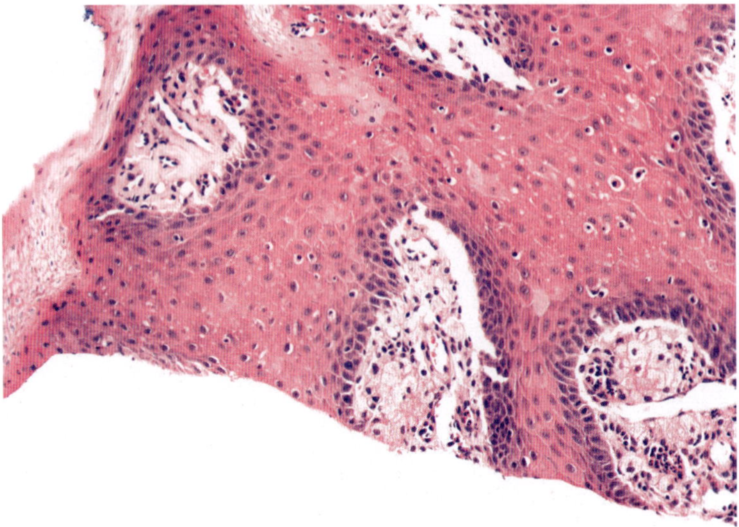

FIGURE 14.27 Verruciform xanthoma.

CONCLUSION

Although this chapter has attempted to review the most common nonneoplastic lesions sampled of the mouth, many of the various dermatologic and congenital lesions that rarely affect the mouth have gone undescribed. Readers should peruse more exhaustive dermatopathologic textbooks on these processes when they are needed.

REFERENCES

1. Takamizawa S, Inoue T, Ono Y, et al. A case report of glial choristoma of the tongue. *J Pediatr Surg*. 2006;41:e13-e15.
2. Baughman RA. Lingual thyroid and lingual thyroglossal tract remnants. A clinical and histopathologic study with review of the literature. *Oral Surg Oral Med Oral Pathol*. 1972;34:781-799.
3. Lipsett J, Sparnon AL, Byard RW. Embryogenesis of enterocystomas-enteric duplication cysts of the tongue. *Oral Surg Oral Med Oral Pathol*. 1993;75:626-630.
4. Chai RL, Ozolek JA, Branstetter BF, Mehta DK, Simons JP. Congenital choristomas of the oral cavity in children. *Laryngoscope*. 2011;121:2100-2106.
5. Daley TD. Intraoral sebaceous hyperplasia. Diagnostic criteria. *Oral Surg Oral Med Oral Pathol*. 1993;75:343-347.
6. De Felice C, Parrini S, Chitano G, Gentile M, Dipaola L, Latini G. Fordyce granules and hereditary non-polyposis colorectal cancer syndrome. *Gut*. 2005;54:1279-1282.
7. Jorgenson RJ, Shapiro SD, Salinas CF, Levin LS. Intraoral findings and anomalies in neonates. *Pediatrics*. 1982;69:577-582.
8. Baughman R. Median rhomboid glossitis: a developmental anomaly?. *Oral Surg Oral Med Oral Pathol*. 1971;31:56-65.

9. Kolokotronis A, Kioses V, Antoniades D, Mandraveli K, Doutsos I, Papanayotou P. Median rhomboid glossitis. An oral manifestation in patients infected with HIV. *Oral Surg Oral Med Oral Pathol.* 1994;78:36-40.
10. Miko TL, Molnar P, Vereckei L. Interrelationships of calibre persistent artery, chronic ulcer and squamous cancer of the lower lip. *Histopathology.* 1983;7:595-599.
11. Bhaskar SN, Beasley JD, Cutright DE. Inflammatory papillary hyperplasia of the oral mucosa: report of 341 cases. *J Am Dent Assoc.* 1970;81:949-952.
12. Poulopoulos A, Belazi M, Epivatianos A, Velegraki A, Antoniades D. The role of Candida in inflammatory papillary hyperplasia of the palate. *J Oral Rehabil.* 2007;34:685-692.
13. Bonetti F, Pelosi G, Martignoni G, et al. Peripheral giant cell granuloma: evidence for osteoclastic differentiation. *Oral Surg Oral Med Oral Pathol.* 1990;70:471-475.
14. Bhaskar SN, Lilly GE. Traumatic granuloma of the tongue (human and experimental). *Oral Surg Oral Med Oral Pathol.* 1964;18:206-218.
15. Tang TT, Glicklich M, Hodach AE, Oechler HW, McCreadie SR. Ulcerative eosinophilic granuloma of the tongue. A light- and electron-microscopic study. *Am J Clin Pathol.* 1981;75:420-425.
16. el-Mofty SK, Swanson PE, Wick MR, Miller AS. Eosinophilic ulcer of the oral mucosa. Report of 38 new cases with immunohistochemical observations. *Oral Surg Oral Med Oral Pathol.* 1993;75:716-722.
17. Sklavounou A, Laskaris G. Eosinophilic ulcer of the oral mucosa. *Oral Surg Oral Med Oral Pathol.* 1984;58:431-436.
18. Elzay RP. Traumatic ulcerative granuloma with stromal eosinophilia (Riga-Fede's disease and traumatic eosinophilic granuloma). *Oral Surg Oral Med Oral Pathol.* 1983;55:497-506.
19. Cepeda LT, Pieretti M, Chapman SF, Horenstein MG. CD30-positive atypical lymphoid cells in common non-neoplastic cutaneous infiltrates rich in neutrophils and eosinophils. *Am J Surg Pathol.* 2003;27:912-918.
20. Hirshberg A, Amariglio N, Akrish S, et al. Traumatic ulcerative granuloma with stromal eosinophilia: a reactive lesion of the oral mucosa. *Am J Clin Pathol.* 2006;126:522-529.
21. Sciallis AP, Law ME, Inwards DJ, et al. Mucosal CD30-positive T-cell lymphoproliferations of the head and neck show a clinicopathologic spectrum similar to cutaneous CD30-positive T-cell lymphoproliferative disorders. *Mod Pathol.* 2012;25:983-992.
22. Butler RT, Kalkwarf KL, Kaldahl WB. Drug-induced gingival hyperplasia: phenytoin, cyclosporine, and nifedipine. *J Am Dent Assoc.* 1987;114:56-60.
23. Dongari A, McDonnell HT, Langlais RP. Drug-induced gingival overgrowth. *Oral Surg Oral Med Oral Pathol.* 1993;76:543-548.
24. Hood AF, Farmer ER: Interphase dermatitis. In: Hood AF, Farmer ER, eds. *Pathology of the Skin.* New York: McGraw-Hill; 2000:202-204.
25. Piboonniyom SO, Treister N, Pitiphat W, Woo SB. Scoring system for monitoring oral lichenoid lesions: a preliminary study. *Oral Surg Oral Med Oral Pathol Oral Radiol Endod.* 2005;99:696-703.
26. Nicolatou-Galitis O, Kitra V, Van Vliet-Constantinidou C, et al. The oral manifestations of chronic graft-versus-host disease (cGVHD) in paediatric allogeneic bone marrow transplant recipients. *J Oral Pathol Med.* 2001;30:148-153.
27. Brooke RI, MacGregor AJ. Traumatic pseudolipoma of the buccal mucosa. *Oral Surg Oral Med Oral Pathol.* 1969;28:223-225.
28. Scully C, Sonis S, Diz PD. Oral mucositis. *Oral Dis.* 2006;12:229-241.
29. Dias EP, Rocha ML, Silva Junior A, et al. Oral hairy leukoplakia. Histopathologic and cytopathologic features of a subclinical phase. *Am J Clin Pathol.* 2000;114:395-401.

30. Sciubba J, Brandsma J, Schwartz M, Barrezueta N. Hairy leukoplakia: an AIDS-associated opportunistic infection. *Oral Surg Oral Med Oral Pathol.* 1989;67:404-410.
31. Piperi E, Omlie J, Koutlas IG, Pambuccian S. Oral hairy leukoplakia in HIV-negative patients: report of 10 cases. *Int J Surg Pathol.* 2010;18:177-183.
32. de Faria PR, Vargas PA, Saldiva PH, Bohm GM, Mauad T, de Almeida OP. Tongue disease in advanced AIDS. *Oral Dis.* 2005;11:72-80.
33. Eveson JW. Granulomatous disorders of the oral mucosa. *Semin Diagn Pathol.* 1996;13:118-127.
34. Chimenos Kustner E, Pascual Cruz M, Pinol Dansis C, Vinals Iglesias H. Rodriguez de Rivera Campillo ME, Lopez Lopez J: lepromatous leprosy: a review and case report. *Med Oral Patol Oral Cir Bucal.* 2006;11:E474-E479.
35. de Abreu MA, Michalany NS, Weckx LL, Neto Pimentel DR, Hirata CH, de Avelar Alchorne MM. The oral mucosa in leprosy: a clinical and histopathological study. *Braz J Otorrinolaringol.* 2006;72:312-316.
36. Alfieri N, Fleury RN, Opromolla DV, Ura S, de Campos I. Oral lesions in borderline and reactional tuberculoid leprosy. *Oral Surg Oral Med Oral Pathol.* 1983;55:52-57.
37. Almeida OP, Jacks J Jr, Scully C. Paracoccidioidomycosis of the mouth: an emerging deep mycosis. *Crit Rev Oral Biol Med.* 2003;14:377-383.
38. Casiglia J, Woo SB, Ahmed AR. Oral involvement in autoimmune blistering diseases. *Clin Dermatol.* 2001;19:737-741.
39. Plauth M, Jenss H, Meyle J. Oral manifestations of Crohn's disease. An analysis of 79 cases. *J Clin Gastroenterol.* 1991;13:29-37.
40. Dupuy A, Cosnes J, Revuz J, Delchier JC, Gendre JP, Cosnes A. Oral Crohn disease: clinical characteristics and long-term follow-up of 9 cases. *Arch Dermatol.* 1999;135: 439-442.
41. Leao JC, Hodgson T, Scully C, Porter S. Review article: orofacial granulomatosis. *Aliment Pharmacol Ther.* 2004;20:1019-1027.
42. El-Hakim M, Chauvin P. Orofacial granulomatosis presenting as persistent lip swelling: review of 6 new cases. *J Oral Maxillofac Surg.* 2004;62:1114-1117.
43. van der Waal RI, Schulten EA, van der Meij EH, van de Scheur MR, Starink TM, van der Waal I. Cheilitis granulomatosa: overview of 13 patients with long-term follow-up–results of management. *Int J Dermatol.* 2002;41:225-229.
44. Zimmer WM, Rogers RS III, Reeve CM, Sheridan PJ. Orofacial manifestations of Melkersson-Rosenthal syndrome. A study of 42 patients and review of 220 cases from the literature. *Oral Surg Oral Med Oral Pathol.* 1992;74:610-619.
45. Greene RM, Rogers RS III. Melkersson-Rosenthal syndrome: a review of 36 patients. *J Am Acad Dermatol.* 1989;21:1263-1270.
46. Jurge S, Kuffer R, Scully C, Porter SR. Mucosal disease series. Number VI. Recurrent aphthous stomatitis. *Oral Dis.* 2006;12:1-21.
47. Escudier M, Bagan J, Scully C. Number VII Behcet's disease (Adamantiades syndrome). *Oral Dis.* 2006;12:78-84.
48. Shulman JD, Carpenter WM. Prevalence and risk factors associated with geographic tongue among US adults. *Oral Dis.* 2006;12:381-386.
49. Littner MM, Dayan D, Gorsky M, Moskona D, Harel-Raviv M. Migratory stomatitis. *Oral Surg Oral Med Oral Pathol.* 1987;63:555-559.
50. Jainkittivong A, Langlais RP. Geographic tongue: clinical characteristics of 188 cases. *J Contemp Dent Pract.* 2005;6:123-135.
51. Al-Johani KA, Fedele S, Porter SR. Erythema multiforme and related disorders. *Oral Surg Oral Med Oral Pathol Oral Radiol Endod.* 2007;103:642-654.
52. Farthing P, Bagan JV, Scully C. Mucosal disease series. Number IV. Erythema multiforme. *Oral Dis.* 2005;11:261-267.

53. Vincent SD, Fotos PG, Baker KA, Williams TP. Oral lichen planus: the clinical, historical, and therapeutic features of 100 cases. *Oral Surg Oral Med Oral Pathol.* 1990;70:165-171.
54. Parashar P. Oral lichen planus. *Otolaryngol Clin North Am.* 2011;44:89-107, vi.
55. de Mattos Camargo Grossmann S, de Aguiar MC, Teixeira R, do Carmo MA. Oral lichen planus and chronic hepatitis C: a controversial association. *Am J Clin Pathol.* 2007;127:800-804.
56. Lodi G, Scully C, Carrozzo M, Griffiths M, Sugerman PB, Thongprasom K. Current controversies in oral lichen planus: report of an international consensus meeting. Part 1. Viral infections and etiopathogenesis. *Oral Surg Oral Med Oral Pathol Oral Radiol Endod.* 2005;100:40-51.
57. Ingafou M, Leao JC, Porter SR, Scully C. Oral lichen planus: a retrospective study of 690 British patients. *Oral Dis.* 2006;12:463-468.
58. Lodi G, Scully C, Carrozzo M, Griffiths M, Sugerman PB, Thongprasom K. Current controversies in oral lichen planus: report of an international consensus meeting. Part 2. Clinical management and malignant transformation. *Oral Surg Oral Med Oral Pathol Oral Radiol Endod.* 2005;100:164-178.
59. van der Meij EH, Mast H, van der Waal I. The possible premalignant character of oral lichen planus and oral lichenoid lesions: a prospective five-year follow-up study of 192 patients. *Oral Oncol.* 2007;43(8):742-748.
60. van der Meij EH, van der Waal I. Lack of clinicopathologic correlation in the diagnosis of oral lichen planus based on the presently available diagnostic criteria and suggestions for modifications. *J Oral Pathol Med.* 2003;32:507-512.
61. Ferreiro JA, Egorshin EV, Olsen KD, Banks PM, Weiland LH. Mucous membrane plasmacytosis of the upper aerodigestive tract. A clinicopathologic study. *Am J Surg Pathol.* 1994;18:1048-1053.
62. Bharti R, Smith DR. Mucous membrane plasmacytosis: a case report and review of the literature. *Dermatol Online J.* 2003;9:15.
63. Brix WK, Nassau SR, Patterson JW, Cousar JB, Wick MR. Idiopathic lymphoplasmacellular mucositis-dermatitis. *J Cutan Pathol.* 2010;37:426-431.
64. Bagan J, Lo Muzio L, Scully C. Mucosal disease series. Number III. Mucous membrane pemphigoid. *Oral Dis.* 2005;11:197-218.
65. Said S, Golitz L. Vesiculobullous eruptions of the oral cavity. *Otolaryngol Clin North Am.* 2011;44:133-160, vi.
66. Lamey PJ, Rees TD, Binnie WH, Rankin KV. Mucous membrane pemphigoid. Treatment experience at two institutions. *Oral Surg Oral Med Oral Pathol.* 1992;74:50-53.
67. Black M, Mignogna MD, Scully C, Number. Pemphigus vulgaris. *Oral Dis.* 2005;11:119-130.
68. Kaplan I, Hodak E, Ackerman L, Mimouni D, Anhalt GJ, Calderon S. Neoplasms associated with paraneoplastic pemphigus: a review with emphasis on non-hematologic malignancy and oral mucosal manifestations. *Oral Oncol.* 2004;40:553-562.
69. Shklar G, McCarthy PL. Histopathology of oral lesions of discoid lupus erythematosus. A review of 25 cases. *Arch Dermatol.* 1978;114:1031-1035.
70. Schiodt M. Oral discoid lupus erythematosus. III. A histopathologic study of sixty-six patients. *Oral Surg Oral Med Oral Pathol.* 1984;57:281-293.
71. Karjalainen TK, Tomich CE. A histopathologic study of oral mucosal lupus erythematosus. *Oral Surg Oral Med Oral Pathol.* 1989;67:547-554.
72. Schiodt M, Holmstrup P, Dabelsteen E, Ullman S. Deposits of immunoglobulins, complement, and fibrinogen in oral lupus erythematosus, lichen planus, and leukoplakia. *Oral Surg Oral Med Oral Pathol.* 1981;51:603-608.
73. Fox RI. Sjogren's syndrome. *Lancet.* 2005;366:321-331.
74. Soto-Rojas AE, Kraus A. The oral side of Sjogren syndrome. Diagnosis and treatment. A review. *Arch Med Res.* 2002;33:95-106.

75. Bamba R, Sweiss NJ, Langerman AJ, Taxy JB, Blair EA. The minor salivary gland biopsy as a diagnostic tool for Sjogren syndrome. *Laryngoscope*. 2009;119:1922-1926.
76. Allen CM, Camisa C, Salewski C, Weiland JE. Wegener's granulomatosis: report of three cases with oral lesions. *J Oral Maxillofac Surg*. 1991;49:294-298.
77. Tomich CE. Oral focal mucinosis. A clinicopathologic and histochemical study of eight cases. *Oral Surg Oral Med Oral Pathol*. 1974;38:714-724.
78. Kamalamma MK, Prabhu SR, Shetty JN, Rao NR. The white sponge nevus. *Oral Surg Oral Med Oral Pathol*. 1970;30:51-54.
79. Rugg EL, McLean WH, Allison WE, et al. A mutation in the mucosal keratin K4 is associated with oral white sponge nevus. *Nat Genet*. 1995;11:450-452.
80. Richard G, De Laurenzi V, Didona B, Bale SJ, Compton JG. Keratin 13 point mutation underlies the hereditary mucosal epithelial disorder white sponge nevus. *Nat Genet*. 1995;11:453-455.
81. Archard HO, Carlson KP, Stanley HR. Leukoedema of the human oral mucosa. *Oral Surg Oral Med Oral Pathol*. 1968;25:717-728.
82. Zegarelli DJ, Aegarelli-Schmidt EC, Zegarelli EV. Verruciform xanthoma. A clinical, light microscopic, and electron microscopic study of two cases. *Oral Surg Oral Med Oral Pathol*. 1974;38:725-734.
83. Nowparast B, Howell FV, Rick GM. Verruciform xanthoma. A clinicopathologic review and report of fifty-four cases. *Oral Surg Oral Med Oral Pathol*. 1981;51:619-625.

15

NONNEOPLASTIC LESIONS OF THE LARYNX

The larynx is most often biopsied because of suspicion of malignancy. Many biopsies will be diagnosed as conventional squamous cell carcinomas; however, nonneoplastic pathologies can also involve the larynx (Table 15.1). This chapter reviews the various infectious and inflammatory processes that can involve the larynx, as well as nonneoplastic polyps and cysts.

CONTACT ULCER

Contact ulcer or "laryngeal granuloma" is a relatively common lesion that typically involves the posterior portion of one or both sides of the larynx. The descriptor "contact" emphasizes the traumatic etiology for most of the lesions which includes, but is not limited to, endotracheal intubation, acid reflux (peptic contact ulcer), and vocal cord abuse related to shouting, coughing, etc.[1–6] Patients tend to be older than 30 years and most are men. Most patients present with hoarseness and may be noted to have low-pitched voices and frequent coughing. Occasional patients may present with severe pain. The posterior vocal cords are usually ulcerated; however, some lesions can have a marked nodular or polypoid appearance simulating neoplasia.[2,5,6] Although the epithelium is frequently ulcerated and covered with a fibrinous exudate (Fig. 15.1, eFig. 15.1), lesions can be covered by a proliferative epithelium or even pseudoepitheliomatous hyperplasia. Abundant granulation tissue is seen either at the ulcer site or immediately beneath the squamous epithelium and comprises the bulk of the lesion (Fig. 15.2, eFig. 15.2). Occasional atypical stromal cells may be seen; however, stromal mitotic figures are rare (eFig. 15.3).[6] The granulation tissue is composed of numerous capillaries and a mixed inflammatory infiltrate. It should not have the lobular growth pattern typical of lobular capillary hemangiomas that are found in the mouth and sinonasal area. Indeed, true lobular capillary hemangiomas or pyogenic granulomas of the larynx either do not occur or are extremely rare.[7]

TABLE 15.1 Nonneoplastic Disease of the Larynx

Traumatic
Contact ulcer
Vocal cord polyps
Infectious
Fungal
Mycobacterial
Bacterial
Autoimmune
Rheumatoid arthritis
Systemic lupus erythematosis
Relapsing polychondritis
Sjogren syndrome
Wegener granulomatosis
Crohn disease
Vesiculobullous disease
Deposition
Gout
Amyloid
Other
Cysts (laryngocele, saccular cysts, and ductal cysts)
Foreign body reactions (e.g., Teflon)
Sarcoid
Eosinophilic angiocentric fibrosis
Involvement by tracheopathia osteoplastica
Hamartoma

FOREIGN BODY REACTION

Foreign body reactions within the larynx are most often iatrogenic.[5,8–11] The most extensively studied reaction is that secondary to Teflon injection.[5,8,11] Teflon or polytetrafluoroethylene is a synthetic substance that can be injected into a paralyzed vocal cord to restore glottic competence. In general, this induces a localized foreign body giant cell reaction that is walled off by fibrous tissue. Occasionally, the material may infiltrate into surrounding tissues. The resultant foreign body reaction may form a mass that bulges into the larynx. Histologically, clusters and

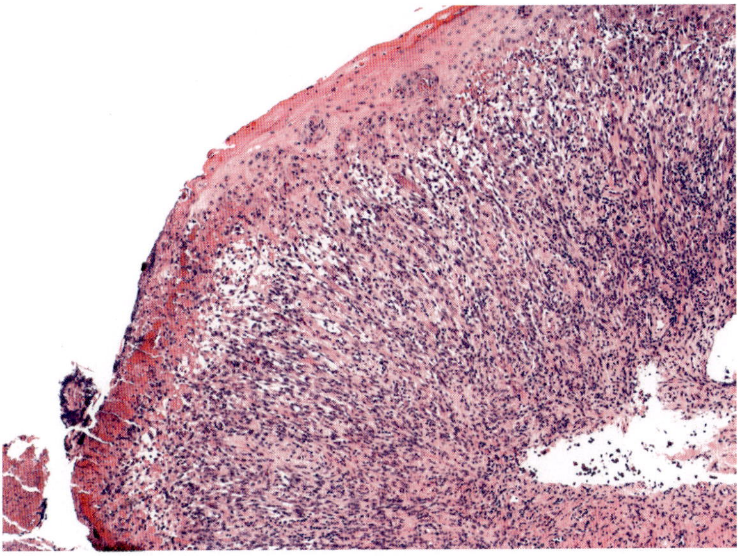

FIGURE 15.1 A contact ulcer with eroded epithelium and a fibrinous exudate.

sheets of multinucleated foreign body–type giant cells that contain birefringent clear material are present with intermixed chronic inflammation and fibrosis (Fig. 15.3, eFigs. 15.4 and 15.5). Other material, including silicone, Gore-Tex, and titanium, may be used for vocal cord

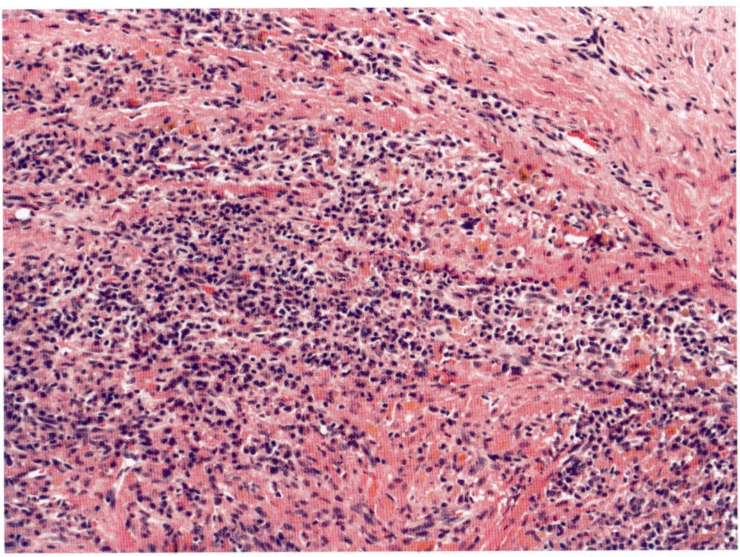

FIGURE 15.2 Abundant chronic inflammation can be seen within the stroma of a contact ulcer.

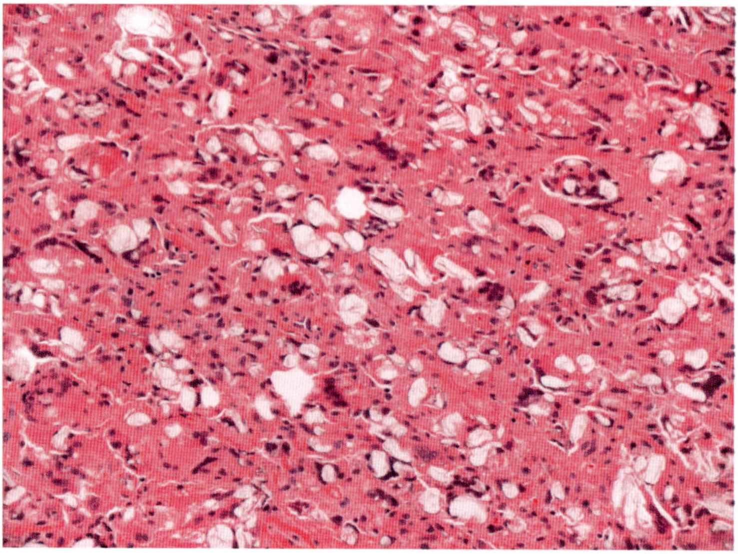

FIGURE 15.3 Foreign body giant cells with foreign material are observed in this reaction to Teflon.

medialization.[9,10] These foreign materials are generally not absorbed and induce surrounding fibrosis and chronic inflammation with a variable foreign body reaction.

INFECTIOUS DISEASE

The larynx may be infected by a great host of organisms that more commonly involve the lungs or sinonasal area. Many of these entities present as mass lesions and an infectious etiology is often unsuspected. Pathologists, however, should be well aware of these lesions as the correct diagnosis can spare a patient unnecessary treatment.

Tuberculosis

Patients with long-standing tuberculosis frequently are noted to have laryngeal involvement in advanced disease.[12] Since the advent of effective antituberculosis treatments, laryngeal involvement has only seldom been reported, and when reported, it has been described as a mimic of laryngeal carcinoma.[12-16] As such, patients are older, usually in their fifth or sixth decades of life, and typically present with hoarseness and a solitary laryngeal mass that frequently involves the vocal cords. Only rarely do patients have more developed pulmonary symptoms (although pulmonary disease may be present). Grossly, the lesions are sometimes ulcerated and can appear granular and nodular. Laryngeal disease shares the

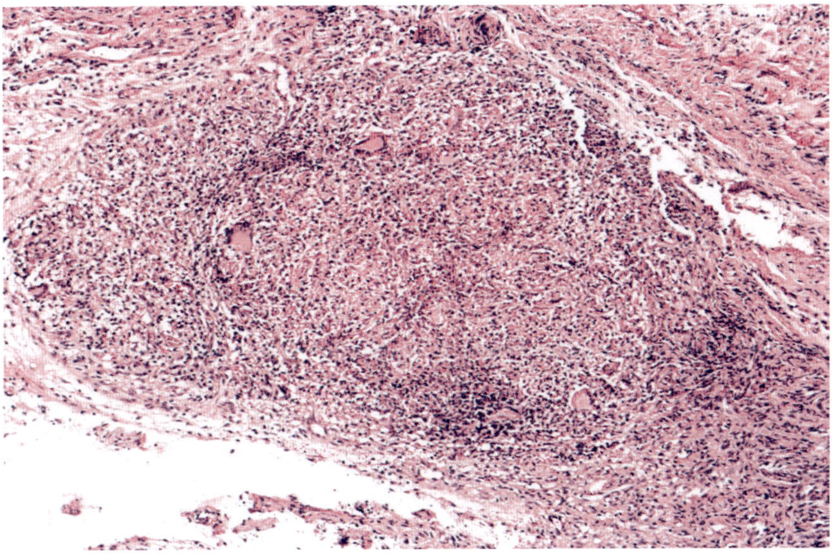

FIGURE 15.4 Laryngeal tuberculosis appears similar to tuberculosis seen at other sites in the body with necrotizing granulomatous inflammation.

histologic features of tuberculosis found elsewhere with caseating granulomatous inflammation and Langhans giant cells (Fig. 15.4, eFig. 15.6).[15] Histochemical and immunohistochemical staining for acid-fast bacilli can sometimes be helpful given the differential that must be considered (Table 15.2).

TABLE 15.2 Granulomatous Disease of the Larynx
Tuberculosis
Leprosy
Histoplasmosis
Blastomycosis
Coccidiomycosis
Candidiasis
Rhinoscleroma
Sarcoidosis
Wegener granulomatosis
Foreign body reaction (e.g., Teflon)
Amyloidosis
Necrobiosis (e.g., rheumatoid nodules)
Crohn disease

Leprosy

The larynx is the second most common site in the head and neck after the sinonasal area to be involved by leprosy.[15] Within the larynx, the lesions are painless and develop supraglottically and then progress to the glottis. The lesions may appear nodular and ulcerated, and infection can eventually lead to laryngeal stenosis. Histologically, the process is similar to that noted in the nasal area and is usually composed of a mixture of chronic inflammatory cells and large, foamy macrophages. *Myocobacterium leprae* (Hansen bacillus) may be identified by histochemical staining for acid-fast bacilli.

Fungal Infections

Fungal infections of the larynx are uncommon, are frequently associated with widespread disease, and are most often found in immunocompromised patients. Laryngeal *histoplasmosis* may present as either multiple nodular or ulcerated lesions.[15,17] These may also appear somewhat granular and verrucoid. Patients frequently have involvement of the vocal cords with concomitant disease within the mouth.[17] The microscopic appearance is variable. A mixture of acute and chronic inflammation is usually present with numerous large macrophages with abundant granular cytoplasm. Some cases may have well-formed caseating granulomatous inflammation and others may be devoid of granulomata. The overlying epithelium is often ulcerated; however, marked pseudoepitheliomatous hyperplasia may be present and should not be confused with squamous cell carcinoma. Although the organisms can frequently be seen on routine, hematoxlin and eosin (H&E)–stained material, silver or periodic acid–Schiff (PAS) staining also can be used to highlight their presence (Fig. 15.5, eFig. 15.7).

Extrapulmonary involvement by blastomycosis is common. When it affects the larynx, patients typically present with hoarseness, with or without coexistent pulmonary or cutaneous lesions.[15,18,19] Laryngeal blastomycosis is typically described as erythematous, irregular, and granular lesions that may also appear verrucoid. Histologically, these lesions are characterized by pseudoepitheliomatous hyperplasia with mixed acute and chronic inflammation. Langhans giant cells are usually seen, together with intraepithelial microabscesses and granulomata, some of which may be suppurative (Fig. 15.6). The causative organism, *Blastomyces dermatitidis*, can usually be identified with H&E-stained material, or with silver or PAS stain. It characteristically demonstrates broad-based budding (eFigs. 15.8 and 15.9).

Rarely, *Coccidioides immitis* can involve the larynx.[20,21] Patients with laryngeal infection almost always have coexistent pulmonary disease. For an unknown reason, most reported cases have affected blacks. Patients typically present with hoarseness and a sore throat. Grossly, the lesions most often involve the cords and typically appear granular and nodular. Frequently, the differential diagnosis included squamous cell carcinoma or tuberculosis. Histologically, pseudoepitheliomatous hyperplasia is often

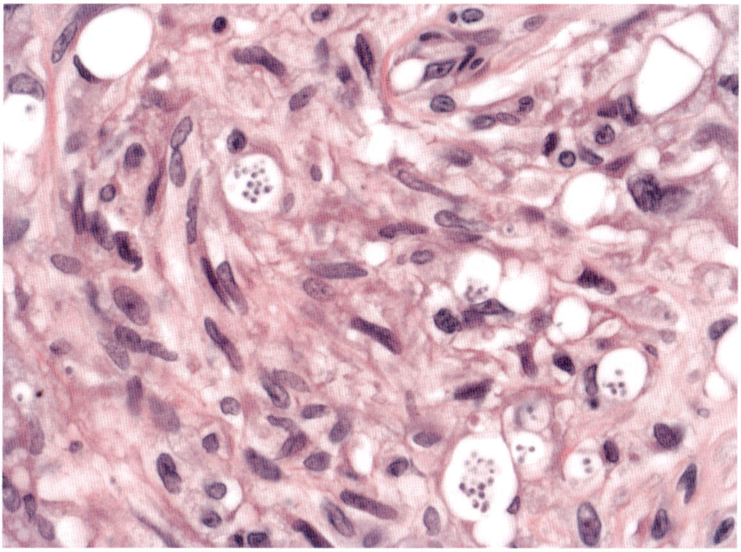

FIGURE 15.5 Intracellular organisms consistent with Histoplasma are seen in this case of laryngeal infection.

seen with mixed inflammation and giant cells, with or without well-formed granulomata. The characteristic spherules and endospores of the organisms can be seen both by conventional H&E stain and with silver or PAS stains.

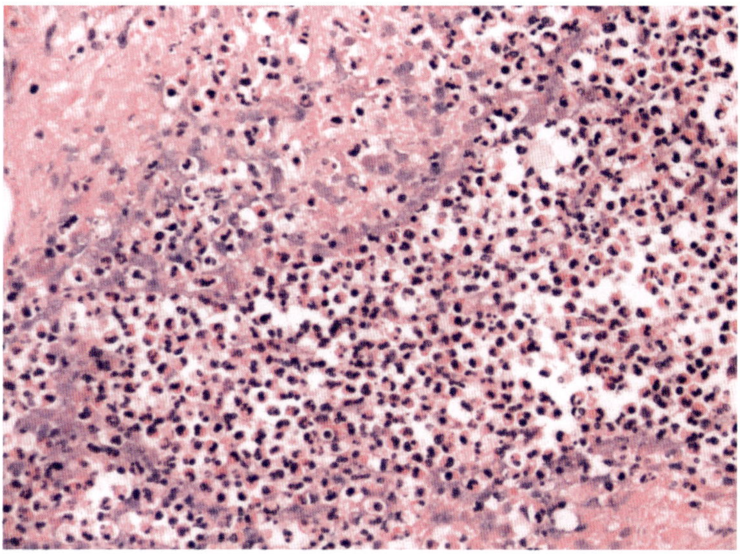

FIGURE 15.6 This case of laryngeal blastomycosis has numerous suppurative granulomata.

Other fungal organisms may also involve the larynx and infections secondary to *Cryptococcus neoformans*, *Candida albicans*, *Aspergillus* spp., *Rhinosporidium seeberi*, and *Paracoccidioides* have been reported (Fig. 15.7, eFig. 15.10).[22-26] Each of these may be seen in immunocompromised patients with or without more widespread disease. Occasionally, they may present in apparently immunocompetent patients without evidence of disease elsewhere. Patients typically present with hoarseness and have granular and sometimes exophytic lesions involving the larynx. As with other fungal infections, pseudoepitheliomatous hyperplasia is often present (eFig. 15.11). A mixed inflammatory infiltrate is typically seen that can involve the epithelium. Fungal organisms may be identified on routine and special stains. A mucicarmine stain can be used to highlight the capsule of *C. neoformans* (eFig. 15.12).

Bacterial Infections

Bacterial infection of the supraglottic larynx and hypopharynx is now rare, thanks to vaccination for *Haemophilus influenzae* and *Corynebacterium diphtheriae*.[27,28] Patients with infection by *H. influenzae* typically present with fever and difficulty breathing. Abundant edema is seen within the supraglottic larynx, especially involving the epiglottis.[28] Tissue is rarely reviewed histologically but will show abundant acute inflammation. Patients with diphtheria have ulceration of the oral cavity, pharynx, and larynx with pseudomembrane formation. Histologically, the pseudomembranes contain fibrin, neutrophils, cell debris, and bacteria. The underlying stromal tissues are edematous with acute inflammation.[27]

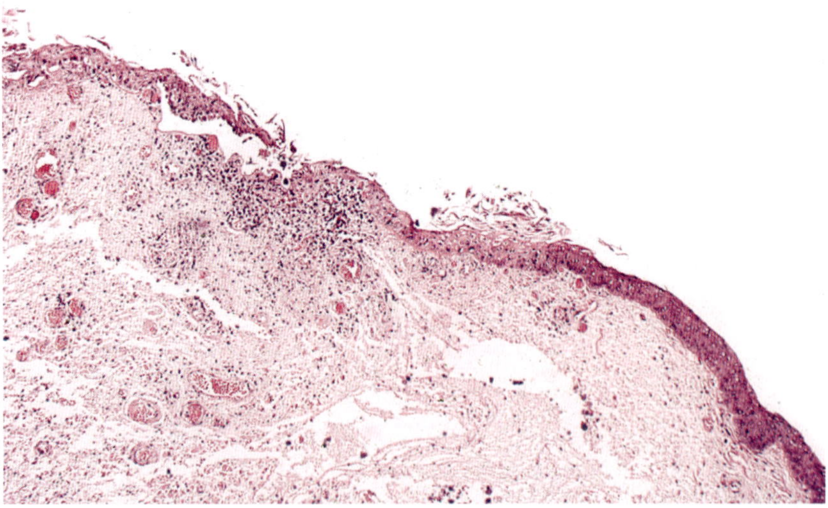

FIGURE 15.7 Surface erosion with numerous pseudohyphae is seen in this case of laryngeal candidiasis.

Secondary and tertiary syphilis can rarely involve the larynx.[15,23] Secondary syphilis is characterized by maculopapular erythema or condyloma latum. Histologically, secondary syphilis is characterized by a thinned epithelium or, conversely, epithelial hyperplasia (condyloma latum) with a dense lymphoplasmacytic infiltrate, sometimes with granulomas. Tertiary syphilis is characterized by gummas, destructive and painless necrotic lesions. Histologically, these are characterized by necrotizing, granulomatous inflammation. A lymphoplasmacytic vasculitis may be noted in both secondary and tertiary forms of disease. Spirochetes may be identified in earlier lesions with silver stains (Warthin-Starry, Dieterle, etc.).

The larynx is rarely involved by rhinoscleroma secondary to infection by *Klebsiella rhinoscleromatis*.[15,29,30] Patients usually also have sinonasal disease; however, isolated laryngeal infection has been reported. The histologic features are similar to those of the sinonasal area (described in Chapter 13), and the disease is thought to proceed through exudative, proliferative, and sclerotic phases.

Rare cases of laryngeal infection secondary to *Actinomyces* have been reported.[15,31] Histologically, these lesions characteristically have sulfur granules (basophilic clusters of bacterial with a peripheral, more eosinophilic zone of radiating filaments) surrounded by acute inflammation and granulation tissue.

SARCOIDOSIS

Between 1% and 5% of patients with sarcoidosis will have symptomatic involvement of their larynges.[15,32,33] Rarely, the larynx may be the solely involved structure. Clinically, the supraglottic larynx is most frequently affected and the lesions may appear edematous, granular, or even nodular.[33] The histologic features are classic for sarcoid with numerous noncaseating granulomata with occasional Schaumann or asteroid bodies (Fig. 15.8, eFigs. 15.13 and 15.14). Some have noted that a lymphoid infiltrate is more prominent with sarcoidosis of the larynx.[32] Although central punctuate necrosis may be seen, more extensive necrosis should lead one to favor an infectious etiology. A vasculitis should not be seen with sarcoid, and if identified should lead one to consider Wegener granulomatosis.

AUTOIMMUNE DISEASE

Systemic autoimmune disease, such as rheumatoid arthritis and systemic lupus erythematosis, can involve larynx as can autoimmune disease that primarily affects mucosa and skin. While involvement of the larynx usually only occurs in well-developed disease, it can sometimes represent the initial presentation of the disease. Because such cases are rare, other disease is usually suspected clinically.

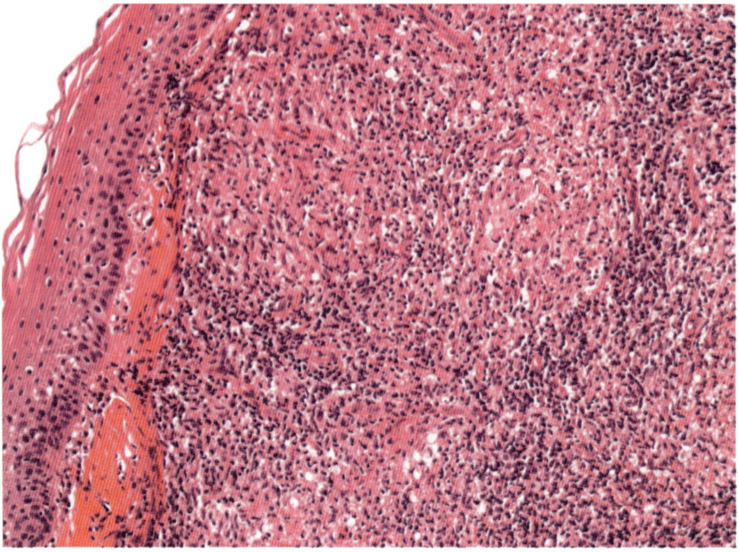

FIGURE 15.8 Laryngeal sarcoidosis appears similar to sarcoidosis seen at other sites in the body, with numerous noncaseating granulomata.

Rheumatoid Arthritis and Rheumatoid Nodules

Up to one-quarter of patients with rheumatoid arthritis have involvement of the larynx, and a characteristic synovitis can be demonstrated in biopsy specimens of the cricothyroid and cricoarytenoid joints.[34] Rheumatoid nodules may involve the larynx, and it is these lesions that are most likely to be sampled by biopsy.[35] Nodules may develop throughout the larynx, and symptoms depend on their location. The lesions have the typical appearance of necrobiotic collagen nodules with central fibrinoid necrosis surrounded by palisading histiocytes with some lymphocytes and occasional multinucleated giant cells (Fig. 15.9, eFigs. 15.15 and 15.16). Rheumatoid nodules may also be seen in patients who have other autoimmune diseases such as systemic lupus erythematosus.[36]

Wegener Granulomatosis

Wegener granulomatous involves the upper or lower respiratory tract, and laryngeal disease occurs in up to 25% of affected patients.[5,15,37,38] Laryngeal involvement may progress to subglottic stenosis.[38] The histologic features are similar to those seen elsewhere and are discussed in depth in the chapter discussing nonneoplastic disease of the nose and paranasal sinuses (Chapter 13). Although necrosis, vasculitis, and granulomata are considered diagnostic of the disease, the three are seldom seen together in biopsy specimens.[37] In fact, many cases will show only nonspecific acute and chronic inflammation. Testing for antineutrophil cytoplasmic antibodies

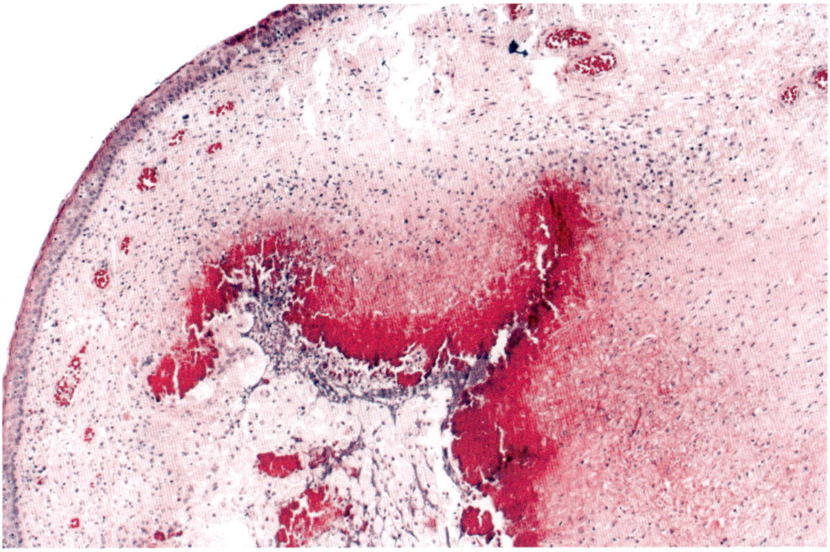

FIGURE 15.9 A subepithelial necrobiotic collagen nodule was seen in this patient with long-standing rheumatoid arthritis.

(ANCA) may be especially helpful for arriving at the correct diagnosis, as cytoplasmic ANCA (c-ANCA) staining correlates well with a diagnosis of Wegener granulomatosis.[39]

Relapsing Polychondritis

Relapsing polychondritis is a rheumatic disease characterized by episodic and progressive inflammation of cartilage.[40,41] It may involve multiple structures throughout the body, but most frequently affects the external ear, joints, eye, respiratory tract, nose, and inner ear. Patients typically present with bilateral, erythematous swellings and can have a variable clinical course. Attacks may be severe and last up to a month with eventual collapse of the involved cartilage. Involvement of laryngeal cartilages and the epiglottis can lead to severe airway compromise as the cartilaginous support of the airway fails. The diagnosis of relapsing polychondritis is generally based on clinical criteria; however, histologic findings are also often a requirement. Histologically, the cartilage usually shows a loss of basophilia or metachromasia with perichondrial acute and chronic inflammation (Fig. 15.10).[40,41] Cartilage destruction and its replacement by fibrous tissue are also seen. Although the histologic features are somewhat specific, one should keep in mind that this is not a diagnosis that should be made out of the correct clinical context.

Other Autoimmune Disease

A number of other autoimmune diseases affect the larynx. As was mentioned above, *systemic lupus erythematosus* can be associated with

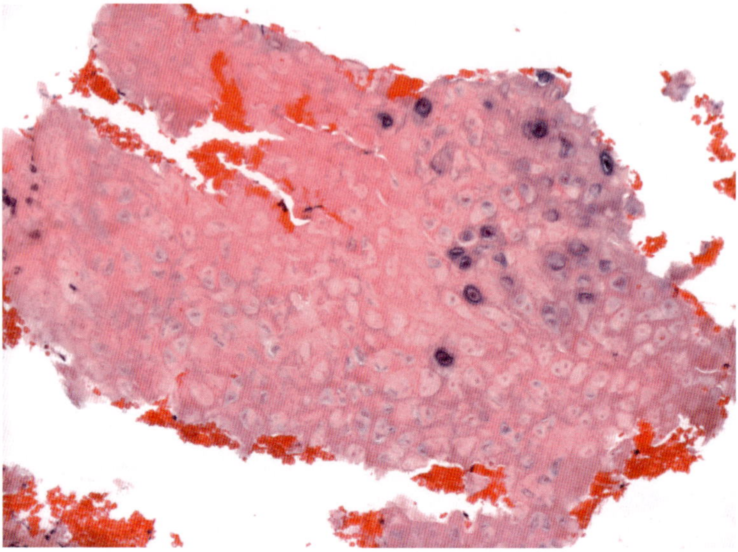

FIGURE 15.10 A fragment of necrotic cartilage is seen in this biopsy of the epiglottis in a patient with relapsing polychondritis.

laryngeal rheumatoid nodules. Diffuse acute and chronic inflammation may also be seen with hematoxylin bodies and lupus erythematosus (LE) cells, and although less common, a vasculitis with fibrinoid necrosis may also be seen.[23,42] *Sjogren syndrome* may also involve the larynx and, as with lupus, can be associated with rheumatoid nodules.[43,44] The disease may also be associated with more conventional-appearing vocal cord polyps possibly secondary to a lack of secretions. An intense infiltrate composed of lymphocytes and plasma cells can also be seen with the disease. *Bullous pemphigoid* and *pemphigus vulgaris* may both involve the larynx.[23,45,46] The histologic features are similar to those in the mouth and are discussed in the previous chapter. Finally, *Crohn disease* rarely involves the upper aerodigestive tract and larynx.[47] It is histologically characterized by nonspecific chronic inflammation. Rarely, noncaseating granulomata may be seen.

GOUTY TOPHI

Patients with long-term hyperuricemia eventually develop soft tissue deposits of crystallized uric acid. Rarely, these have been reported in the larynx.[48–50] Patients typically complain of hoarseness and dysphagia and are noted clinically to have mass lesions, often involving the cords; limited mobility is also usually noted. Histologically, pseudoepitheliomatous hyperplasia may be present overlying deposits of an amorphous negatively birefringent crystalline material that is surrounded by a foreign body–type reaction (Fig. 15.11, eFig. 15.17).

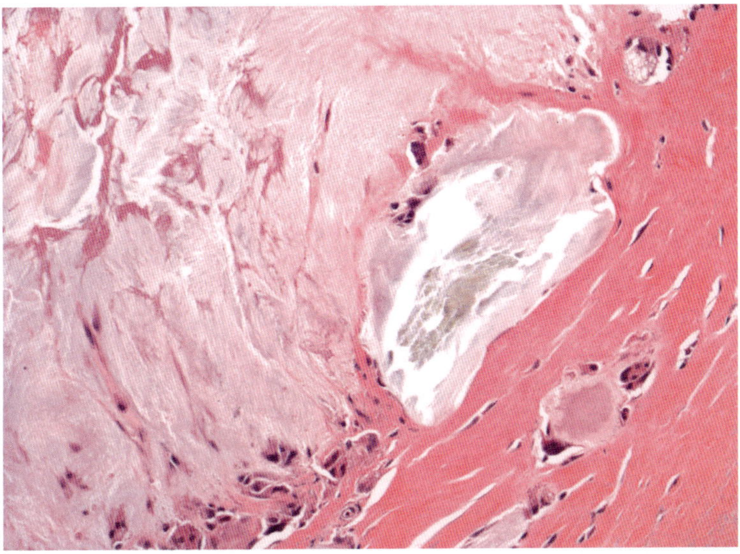

FIGURE 15.11 Deposited material can be seen with most gouty tophi.

EOSINOPHILIC ANGIOCENTRIC FIBROSIS

Eosinophilic angiocentric fibrosis can involve the larynx, and rare cases have been reported to cause breathing difficulties.[51] Like the cases in the nasal cavities or paranasal sinuses, these lesions have abundant fibrosis that appears to wrap around small blood vessels (see Chapter 13). Numerous eosinophils are seen with occasional lymphocytes. This is considered to be an IGg4-related sclerosing disease.[52]

VOCAL CORD POLYPS

Vocal cord polyps or singer's nodules occur equally in men and women and can be found at any age (some have noted the lesions to be more common in men).[53–55] The patients present with hoarseness and often have been noted to have abused their voices. Polyps are usually unilateral and are located on the anterior third of the vocal cord. They are generally small, less than 5 mm in size. Histologically, the overlying squamous epithelium is most often intact and smooth. Occasionally, it may appear hyperplastic or atrophic. The underlying stroma is paucicellular because of edema or, less commonly, fibrin deposition (Fig. 15.12 and 15.13, eFigs. 15.18 and 15.19). Rarely the stroma may appear hyaline or myxoid (eFig. 15.20).[53] Dilated vessels are frequently seen. A mild amount of chronic inflammation is often present and hemosiderin-laden macrophages may be seen. Occasional cases have been noted to have atypical stromal cells.[5]

Vocal cord nodules are similar histologically to vocal cord polyps; however, they tend to be bilateral and occur slightly more posteriorly at the

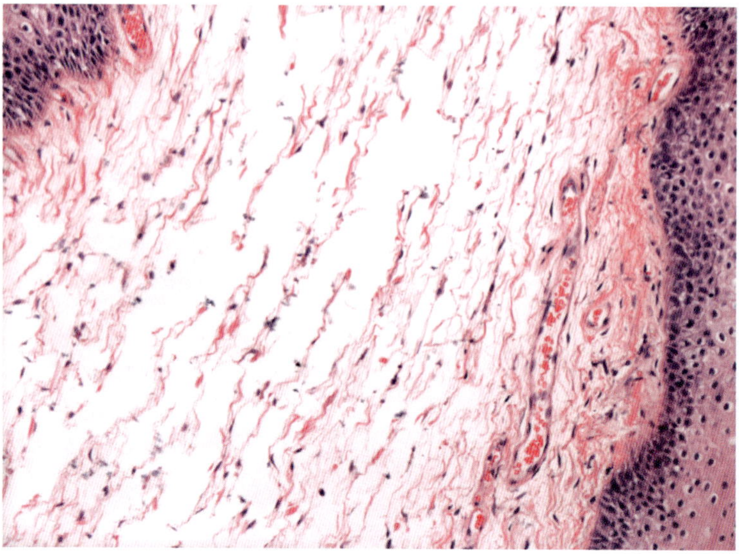

FIGURE 15.12 Stromal edema is commonly seen with vocal cord polyps.

border of the anterior and middle third of the vocal cord.[53] *Reinke edema* may be either unilateral or bilateral and usually is described as a sessile swelling.[53] Both lesions share the histologic features typical of vocal cord polyps.

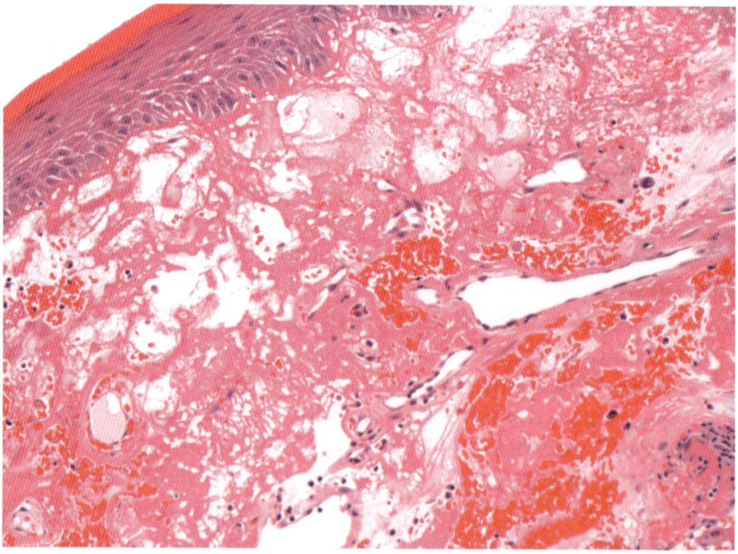

FIGURE 15.13 Some vocal cord polyps will have fibrinous material within their stroma.

NONNEOPLASTIC CYSTS

Nonneoplastic cysts of the larynx include laryngoceles, saccular cysts, and ductal cysts.[56–59] Oncocytic cystadenomas of the larynx do also occur and were discussed in Chapter 6; however, they may simply represent one end of the spectrum of ductal cysts. Although laryngoceles and saccular cysts have a similar histology, they occur in slightly different clinical situations.

Laryngoceles are cystic dilatations of the saccule of Morgagni.[56,58] They communicate with the larynx and are air-filled. Some laryngoceles are internal and as such are limited to the larynx.[58] These extend from the saccule posterosuperiorly into the area of the false cord and aryepiglottic fold. External laryngoceles extend through the opening in the thyrohyoid membrane into the soft tissues of the neck.[58] Laryngoceles are less common than saccular cysts and develop in either sex at any age. Patients present with hoarseness or cough and, when the lesion extends into the neck, a mass. Interestingly, enlarged saccules can frequently be demonstrated in patients who play breath-powered musical instruments. Histologically, laryngoceles are lined by a columnar, ciliated epithelium and may be surrounded by chronic inflammation (Fig. 15.14, eFigs. 15.21 and 15.22). Focally, the epithelium can appear more oncocytic (Fig. 15.15).

Saccular cysts also occur at the laryngeal saccule; however, they do not communicate with the larynx and are filled with mucin.[57,58] Saccular cysts are either lateral and extend posterosuperiorly into the false cord and aryepiglottic fold or are anterior and extend medially and posteriorly and thus protrude into the laryngeal lumen. Lateral saccular cysts may

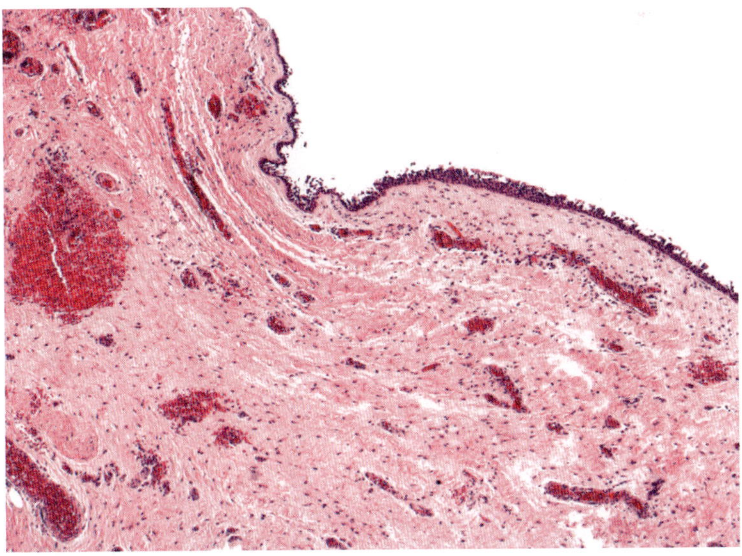

FIGURE 15.14 Laryngoceles have fibrous walls with some degree of chronic inflammation.

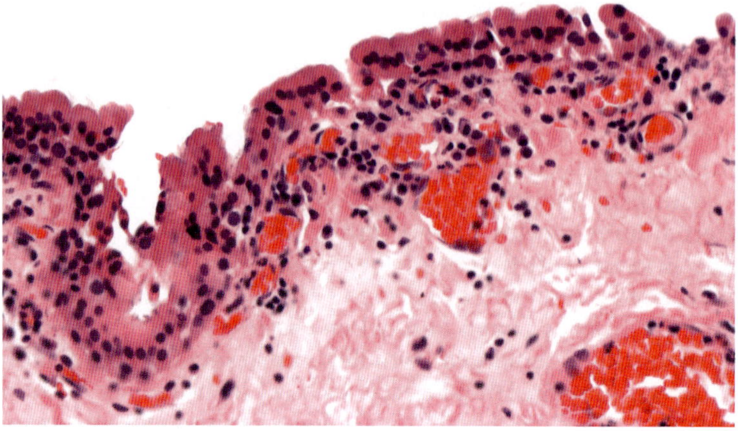

FIGURE 15.15 Some laryngoceles have more oncocytic-appearing epithelium.

also extend through the thyrohyoid membrane. Like laryngoceles, saccular cysts can occur at any age and may even be congenital. The cysts are generally lined by a ciliated, columnar epithelium that may have squamous or oncocytic metaplasia (Fig. 15.16, eFig. 15.23).

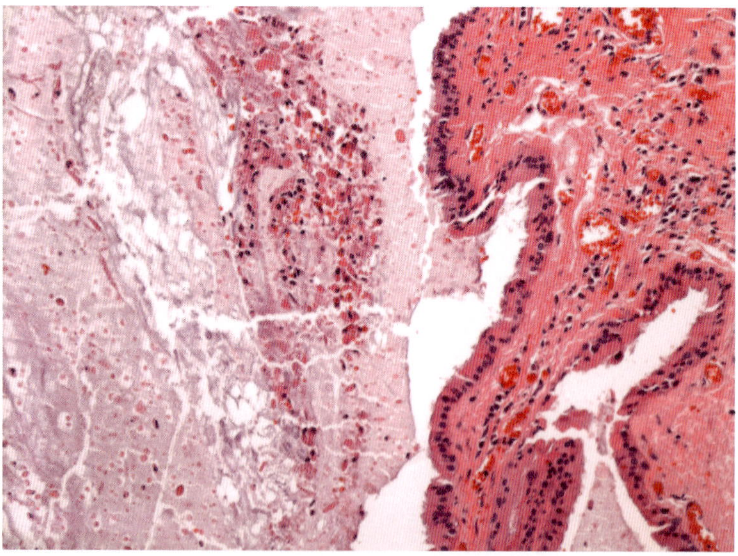

FIGURE 15.16 This saccular cyst is filled with mucus and lined by an oncocytic epithelium.

Ductal cysts occur throughout the larynx and are thought to result from the retention of mucus within the ducts of the submucosal seromucinous glands.[57,59] These cysts are much more common than saccular cysts. They are lined by a columnar or cuboidal mucinous epithelium that can have squamous or oncocytic metaplasia. As these frequently involve the supraglottic larynx, they are often associated with tonsillar tissue.[59]

AMYLOID DEPOSITION

Amyloid deposition within the larynx may be localized or secondary to systemic disease.[60–66] It may be the result of a familial condition, a primary disorder, or secondary to an underlying disease state or tumor. In the upper aerodigestive tract, amyloid deposits may be associated with plasmacytomas, especially when they are found in the nasopharynx.[64] Patients vary widely in age, with the mean age at presentation in the fourth or fifth decades of life. Laryngeal amyloidosis is usually a localized phenomenon and is composed of amyloid light chain (AL).[61–63,66] Patients typically present with progressive hoarseness. The lesions are usually supraglottic or transglottic and range from firm elevated, smooth lesions to polypoid masslike lesions that have a tan-yellow to red-grey cut surface. Histologically, these lesions characteristically have abundant amorphous, eosinophilic material deposited extracellularly (Fig. 15.17, eFigs. 15.24 and 15.25). The material may show a more periglandular or perivascular deposition.[63,66] Scattered lymphocytes and plasma cells are

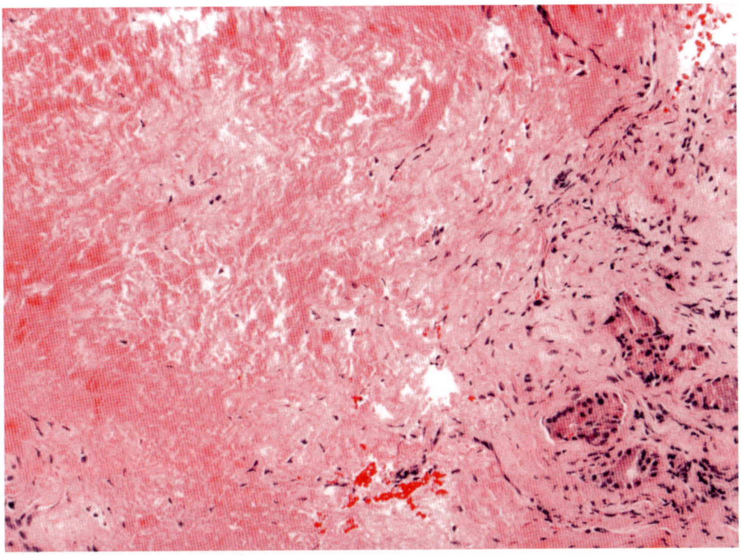

FIGURE 15.17 Amorphous eosinophilic material can be seen adjacent to seromucinous glands in this case of laryngeal amyloidosis.

often noted with occasional macrophages and rare giant cells. Congo red or methyl violet histochemical staining can be used to confirm the diagnosis of amyloid (eFig. 15.26). Light chain restriction can sometimes be demonstrated in the plasma cell population and predicts recurrent disease.[66] The diagnosis should obviously instigate further workup for systemic causes of amyloid deposition.

LARYNGEAL INVOLVEMENT BY TRACHEOPATHIA OSTEOPLASTICA

Tracheopathia osteoplastica is a bizarre condition that most commonly affects men older than 50 years.[67,68] The etiology of this condition is not understood and some believe it to be the result of ecchondrosis and exostosis from the cartilage rings, while others believe that it represents a metaplastic condition. Patients may present with hemoptysis, cough, hoarseness, or wheezing. The mucosa will appear cobblestone as hard, irregular nodules project into the laryngeal and tracheal lumina. Histologically, islands of hyaline cartilage and lamellar bone are present immediately beneath the epithelium. These lesions are actually interconnected by fibrous tissue and form a ring that entirely encircles the lumina. The overlying epithelium usually shows squamous metaplasia and may be ulcerated.

SUBGLOTTIC STENOSIS

Subglottic laryngeal stenosis is most often acquired; however, occasional cases may be congenital.[5,69–71] Causes include trauma, prolonged intubation, burns, surgery, radiotherapy, infection, autoimmune disease, neoplasia, sarcoid, amyloidosis, and, possibly, gastroesophageal reflux.[5] Some cases, however, are considered to be idiopathic. All age groups and both sexes may be affected. Patients usually have difficulty breathing, and children may be noted to have feeding abnormalities or abnormal crying. The larynx will appear markedly narrowed. This narrowing may be asymmetric and can give the impression of a mass lesion.[5] Histologically, sections usually show a nonspecific fibrosis with dense eosinophilic collagen, fibroblasts, and variable chronic inflammatory infiltrate (Fig. 15.18, eFig. 15.27). Clinical history may be helpful for determining the etiology of the disease.

LARYNGEAL HAMARTOMA

Hamartomas of the larynx are extremely rare.[72] They appear somewhat reminiscent of respiratory epithelial adenomatoid hamartomas of the nasal cavity with a disorganized proliferation of respiratory epithelium, seromucinous glands, smooth muscle, and cartilage (see Chapter 13).

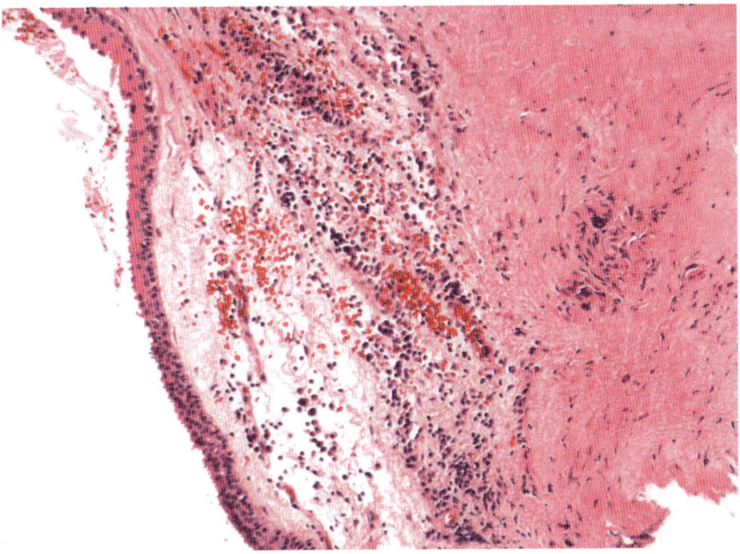

FIGURE 15.18 **Subglottic stenosis characteristically has nonspecific histologic features with fibrosis and chronic inflammation.**

REFERENCES

1. Barton RT. Observation on the pathogenesis of laryngeal granuloma due to endotracheal anesthesia. *N Engl J Med*. 1953;248:1097-1099.
2. Holinger PH, Johnston KC. Contact ulcer of the larynx. *Jama*. 1960;172:511-515.
3. Miko TL. Peptic (contact ulcer) granuloma of the larynx. *J Clin Pathol*. 1989;42:800-804.
4. Ward PH, Zwitman D, Hanson D, Berci G. Contact ulcers and granulomas of the larynx: new insights into their etiology as a basis for more rational treatment. *Otolaryngol Head Neck Surg*. 1980;88:262-269.
5. Wenig BM, Devaney K, Wenig BL. Pseudoneoplastic lesions of the oropharynx and larynx simulating cancer. *Pathol Annu*. 1995;30(pt 1):143-187.
6. Wenig BM, Heffner DK. Contact ulcers of the larynx. A reacquaintance with the pathology of an often underdiagnosed entity,. *Arch Pathol Lab Med*. 1990;114:825-828.
7. Fechner RE, Cooper PH, Mills SE. Pyogenic granuloma of the larynx and trachea. A causal and pathologic misnomer for granulation tissue,. *Arch Otolaryngol*. 1981;107:30-32.
8. Schmidt PJ, Wagenfeld D, Bridger MW, vanNostrand AW, Briant TD. Teflon injection of the vocal cord: a clinical and histopathologic study. *J Otolaryngol*. 1980;9:297-302.
9. Stein J, Eliachar I, Myles J, Munoz-Ramirez H, Strome M. Histopathologic study of alternative substances for vocal fold medialization. *Ann Otol Rhinol Laryngol*. 2000;109:221-226.
10. Ustundag E, Boyaci Z, Keskin G, Kaur A, Ozkarakas H. Soft tissue response of the larynx to silicone, Gore-Tex, and irradiated cartilage implants. *Laryngoscope*. 2005;115:1009-1014.
11. Varvares MA, Montgomery WW, Hillman RE. Teflon granuloma of the larynx: etiology, pathophysiology, and management. *Ann Otol Rhinol Laryngol*. 1995;104:511-515.
12. Bull TR. Tuberculosis of the larynx. *Br Med J*. 1966;2:991-992.
13. Bailey CM, Windle-Taylor PC. Tuberculous laryngitis: a series of 37 patients. *Laryngoscope*. 1981;91:93-100.

14. Hunter AM, Millar JW, Wightman AJ, Horne NW. The changing pattern of laryngeal tuberculosis. *J Laryngol Otol.* 1981;95:393-398.
15. Pillsbury HC III, Sasaki CT. Granulomatous diseases of the larynx. *Otolaryngol Clin North Am.* 1982;15:539-551.
16. Thaller SR, Gross JR, Pilch BZ, Goodman ML. Laryngeal tuberculosis as manifested in the decades 1963-1983. *Laryngoscope.* 1987;97:848-850.
17. Bennett DE. Histoplasmosis of the oral cavity and larynx. A clinicopathologic study. *Arch Intern Med.* 1967;120:417-427.
18. Blair PA, Gnepp DR, Riley RS, Sprinkle PM. Blastomycosis of the larynx. *South Med J.* 1981;74:880-882.
19. Dumich PS, Neel HB III. Blastomycosis of the larynx. *Laryngoscope.* 1983;93:1266-1270.
20. Platt MA. Laryngeal coccidioidomycosis. *J Am Med Assoc.* 1977;237:1234-1235.
21. Ward PH, Berci G, Morledge D, Schwartz H. Coccidioidomycosis of the larynx in infants and adults. *Ann Otol Rhinol Laryngol.* 1977;86:655-660.
22. Benson-Mitchell R, Tolley N, Croft CB, Gallimore A. Aspergillosis of the larynx. *J Laryngol Otol.* 1994;108:883-885.
23. Brandwein MS, Kapadia SB, Gnepp DR. Nonsquamous pathology of the larynx, hypopharynx, and trachea. In: Gnepp DR, ed. *Diagnostic Surgical Pathology of the Head and Neck*. Philadelphia: W. B. Saunders; 2001:239-323.
24. Ganesan S, Harar RP, Dawkins RS, Prior AJ. Invasive laryngeal candidiasis: a cause of stridor in the previously irradiated patient. *J Laryngol Otol.* 1998;112:575-578.
25. Kheir SM, Flint A, Moss JA. Primary aspergillosis of the larynx simulating carcinoma. *Hum Pathol.* 1983;14:184-186.
26. Smallman LA, Stores OP, Watson MG, Proops DW. Cryptococcosis of the larynx. *J Laryngol Otol.* 1989;103:214-215.
27. Goutas N, Simopoulou S, Papazoglou K, Agapitos E. A fatal case of diphtheria. *Pediatr Pathol.* 1994;14:391-395.
28. Senior BA, Radkowski D, MacArthur C, Sprecher RC, Jones D. Changing patterns in pediatric supraglottitis: a multi-institutional review, 1980 to 1992. *Laryngoscope.* 1994;104:1314-1322.
29. Jay J, Green RP, Lucente FE. Isolated laryngeal rhinoscleroma. *Otolaryngol Head Neck Surg.* 1985;93:669-673.
30. Gaafar HA, Gaafar AH, Nour YA. Rhinoscleroma: an updated experience through the last 10 years. *Acta Otolaryngol.* 2011;131:440-446.
31. Brandenburg JH, Finch WW, Kirkham WR. Actinomycosis of the larynx and pharynx. *Otolaryngology.* 1978;86:ORL-739-742.
32. Devine KD. Sarcoidosis and sarcoidosis of the larynx. *Laryngoscope.* 1965;75:533-569.
33. Neel HB III, McDonald TJ. Laryngeal sarcoidosis: report of 13 patients. *Ann Otol Rhinol Laryngol.* 1982;91:359-362.
34. Bridger MW, Jahn AF, van Nostrand AW. Laryngeal rheumatoid arthritis. *Laryngoscope.* 1980;90:296-303.
35. Sorensen WT, Moller-Andersen K, Behrendt N. Rheumatoid nodules of the larynx. *J Laryngol Otol.* 1998;112:573-574.
36. Schwartz IS, Grishman E. Rheumatoid nodules of the vocal cords as the initial manifestation of systemic lupus erythematosus. *J Am Med Assoc.* 1980;244:2751-2752.
37. Devaney KO, Travis WD, Hoffman G, Leavitt R, Lebovics R, Fauci AS. Interpretation of head and neck biopsies in Wegener's granulomatosis. A pathologic study of 126 biopsies in 70 patients. *Am J Surg Pathol.* 1990;14:555-564.
38. Hoare TJ, Jayne D, Rhys Evans P, Croft CB, Howard DJ. Wegener's granulomatosis, subglottic stenosis and antineutrophil cytoplasm antibodies. *J Laryngol Otol.* 1989;103:1187-1191.

39. Merkel PA, Polisson RP, Chang Y, Skates SJ, Niles JL. Prevalence of antineutrophil cytoplasmic antibodies in a large inception cohort of patients with connective tissue disease. *Ann Intern Med.* 1997;126:866-873.
40. Batsakis JG, Manning JT. Relapsing polychondritis. *Ann Otol Rhinol Laryngol.* 1989;98:83-84.
41. Damiani JM, Levine HL. Relapsing polychondritis–report of ten cases. *Laryngoscope.* 1979;89:929-946.
42. Smith GA, Ward PH, Berci G. Laryngeal lupus erythematosus. *J Laryngol Otol.* 1978;92:67-73.
43. Barrs DM, McDonald TJ, Duffy J. Sjogren's syndrome involving the larynx: report of a case. *J Laryngol Otol.* 1979;93:933-936.
44. Prytz S. Vocal nodules in Sjogren's syndrome. *J Laryngol Otol.* 1980;94:197-203.
45. Block LJ, Caldarelli DD, Holinger PH, Pearson RW. Pemphigus of the air and food passages. *Ann Otol Rhinol Laryngol.* 1977;86:584-587.
46. Frangogiannis NG, Gangopadhyay S, Cate T. Pemphigus of the larynx and esophagus. *Ann Intern Med.* 1995;122:803-804.
47. Gianoli GJ, Miller RH. Crohn's disease of the larynx. *J Laryngol Otol.* 1994;108:596-598.
48. Goodman M, Montgomery W, Minette L. Pathologic findings in gouty cricoarytenoid arthritis. *Arch Otolaryngol.* 1976;102:27-29.
49. Guttenplan MD, Hendrix RA, Townsend MJ, Balsara G. Laryngeal manifestations of gout. *Ann Otol Rhinol Laryngol.* 1991;100:899-902.
50. Marion RB, Alperin JE, Maloney WH. Gouty tophus of the true vocal cord. *Arch Otolaryngol.* 1972;96:161-162.
51. Fageeh NA, Mai KT, Odell PF. Eosinophilic angiocentric fibrosis of the subglottic region of the larynx and upper trachea. *J Otolaryngol.* 1996;25:276-278.
52. Deshpande V, Khosroshahi A, Nielsen GP, Hamilos DL, Stone JH. Eosinophilic angiocentric fibrosis is a form of IgG4-related systemic disease. *Am J Surg Pathol.* 2011;35:701-706.
53. Dikkers FG, Nikkels PG. Benign lesions of the vocal folds: histopathology and phonotrauma. *Ann Otol Rhinol Laryngol.* 1995;104:698-703.
54. Kambic V, Radsel Z, Zargi M, Acko M. Vocal cord polyps: incidence, histology and pathogenesis. *J Laryngol Otol.* 1981;95:609-618.
55. Kleinsasser O. Pathogenesis of vocal cord polyps. *Ann Otol Rhinol Laryngol.* 1982;91:378-381.
56. Canalis RF, Maxwell DS, Hemenway WG. Laryngocele–an updated review. *J Otolaryngol.* 1977;6:191-199.
57. DeSanto LW, Devine KD, Weiland LH. Cysts of the larynx–classification. *Laryngoscope.* 1970;80:145-176.
58. Holinger LD, Barnes DR, Smid LJ, Holinger PH. Laryngocele and saccular cysts. *Ann Otol Rhinol Laryngol.* 1978;87:675-685.
59. Newman BH, Taxy JB, Laker HI. Laryngeal cysts in adults: a clinicopathologic study of 20 cases. *Am J Clin Pathol.* 1984;81:715-720.
60. Bartels H, Dikkers FG, van der Wal JE, Lokhorst HM, Hazenberg BP. Laryngeal amyloidosis: localized versus systemic disease and update on diagnosis and therapy. *Ann Otol Rhinol Laryngol.* 2004;113:741-748.
61. Berg AM, Troxler RF, Grillone G, et al. Localized amyloidosis of the larynx: evidence for light chain composition. *Ann Otol Rhinol Laryngol.* 1993;102:884-889.
62. Godbersen GS, Leh JF, Hansmann ML, Rudert H, Linke RP. Organ-limited laryngeal amyloid deposits: clinical, morphological, and immunohistochemical results of five cases. *Ann Otol Rhinol Laryngol.* 1992;101:770-775.

63. Lewis JE, Olsen KD, Kurtin PJ, Kyle RA. Laryngeal amyloidosis: a clinicopathologic and immunohistochemical review. *Otolaryngol Head Neck Surg*. 1992;106:372-377.

64. Michaels L, Hyams VJ. Amyloid in localised deposits and plasmacytomas of the respiratory tract. *J Pathol*. 1979;128:29-38.

65. Pribitkin E, Friedman O, O'Hara B, et al. Amyloidosis of the upper aerodigestive tract. *Laryngoscope*. 2003;113:2095-2101.

66. Thompson LD, Derringer GA, Wenig BM. Amyloidosis of the larynx: a clinicopathologic study of 11 cases. *Mod Pathol*. 2000;13:528-535.

67. Smid L, Lavrencak B, Zargi M. Laryngo-tracheo-bronchopathia chondro-osteoplastica. *J Laryngol Otol*. 1992;106:845-848.

68. Young RH, Sandstrom RE, Mark GJ. Tracheopathia osteoplastica: clinical, radiologic, and pathological correlations. *J Thorac Cardiovasc Surg*. 1980;79:537-541.

69. Benjamin B, Jacobson I, Eckstein R. Idiopathic subglottic stenosis: diagnosis and endoscopic laser treatment. *Ann Otol Rhinol Laryngol*. 1997;106:770-774.

70. Grillo HC, Mark EJ, Mathisen DJ, Wain JC. Idiopathic laryngotracheal stenosis and its management. *Ann Thorac Surg*. 1993;56:80-87.

71. Jindal JR, Milbrath MM, Shaker R, Hogan WJ, Toohill RJ. Gastroesophageal reflux disease as a likely cause of "idiopathic" subglottic stenosis. *Ann Otol Rhinol Laryngol*. 1994;103:186-191.

72. Zapf B, Lehmann WB, Snyder GG III. Hamartoma of the larynx: an unusual cause for stridor in an infant. *Otolaryngol Head Neck Surg*. 1981;89:797-799.

16

PATHOLOGY OF THE EAR

Like the sinonasal tract, the ear has a rather complicated anatomy with multiple types of epithelium, adnexa, and close proximity to disparate structures. The different portions of the ear are affected by both similar and diverse pathologic processes. The auricle is covered by skin and is extensively sun-exposed. Not surprisingly, it frequently develops cutaneous malignancies. The inner and middle ear are involved by many of the same malignancies that affect the upper aerodigestive tract. In addition, distinct neoplasms such as middle ear adenoma and endolymphatic sac tumor are unique to these structures. This chapter discusses both nonneoplastic and neoplastic disease of the ear.

NONNEOPLASTIC DISEASE

Nonneoplastic diseases of the ear are more common than actual neoplasia; however, they are infrequently sampled and thus seldom seen by pathologists. While the infectious lesions are by far the most frequent of the nonneoplastic conditions, it is most important that pathologists recognize the lesions of the ear that form masses and mimic neoplasms. Some of these disease processes are specific to the ear, such as chondrodermatitis nodularis chronica helicis.

Congenital Abnormalities and Choristomas

Congenital abnormalities of the ear usually present in childhood. *Accessory tragi* arise from remnants of the first branchial cleft.[1] These pedunculated lesions are typically less than 1 cm in size and most often are located just anterior to the true tragus. The lesions are either solitary or multiple and are sometimes bilateral. While they are generally not associated with other congenital abnormalities, some patients are also found to have midline abnormalities such as cleft lip or palate. Histologically, accessory tragi have all the components of the normal external ear. They are covered by a stratified squamous epithelium and the underlying dermis is replete with appendages (Fig. 16.1, eFig. 16.1).[1] The stroma contains fibroadipose tissue and mature hyaline cartilage.

Other anomalies of the first branchial cleft include *cysts*, *sinuses*, and *fistulas*.[2] Each usually occurs anterior to the tragus, similar to an accessory

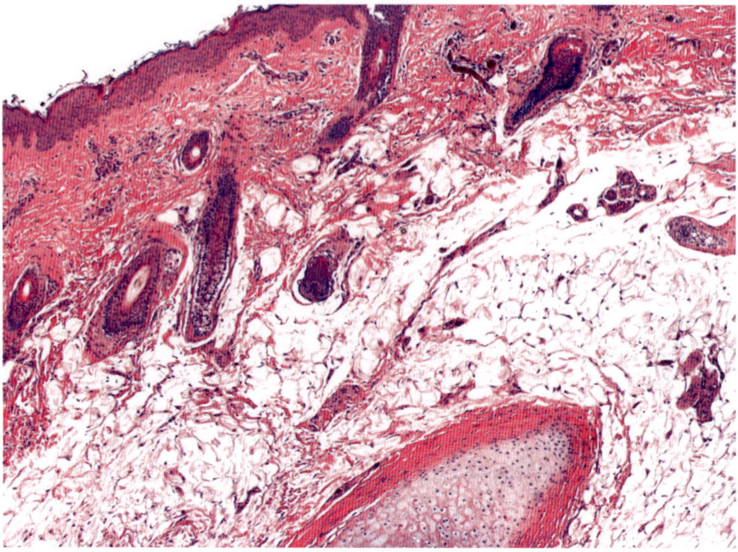

FIGURE 16.1 An accessory tragus.

tragus; however, their locations vary much more widely. Indeed, these lesions frequently involve the parotid gland and can be confused clinically with parotid tumors. Sinuses and fistulas often drain into the external ear canal or even the middle ear. First branchial cleft cysts, sinuses, or fistulas are akin to other branchial cleft abnormalities and are lined by ciliated columnar or stratified squamous epithelium surrounded by adnexal structures and lymphoid tissue.[2] Unlike other branchial cleft abnormalities, first branchial cleft cysts sometimes contain cartilage. These remnants are frequently infected at the time of their discovery, and the epithelium is sometimes denuded or necrotic; abundant acute inflammation will then be present.

Both *glial* and *salivary gland choristomas* are found in the middle ear.[3–9] It has been noted by some that true glial choristomas may actually be very rare at these sites, and that most reported glial choristomas actually represent either encephaloceles or extruded brain tissue presenting as a middle ear lesion after other local disease processes such as cholesteatomas have led to the destruction of intervening temporal bone.[3] Choristomas present in the middle ear behind an intact tympanic membrane and are histologically composed of either glial tissue or salivary gland tissue. The glial choristomas are composed of predominately astrocytes and neurofibrils.[3,8] Salivary gland choristomas have a mixture of mucinous and serous glands with ducts (Fig. 16.2).[6,7,9] Some amount of adipose tissue is often noted.

Congenital cholesteatomas resemble their acquired counterparts described below.[10–14] They present in younger patients than acquired cholesteatomas and are much less common, representing less than 5% of

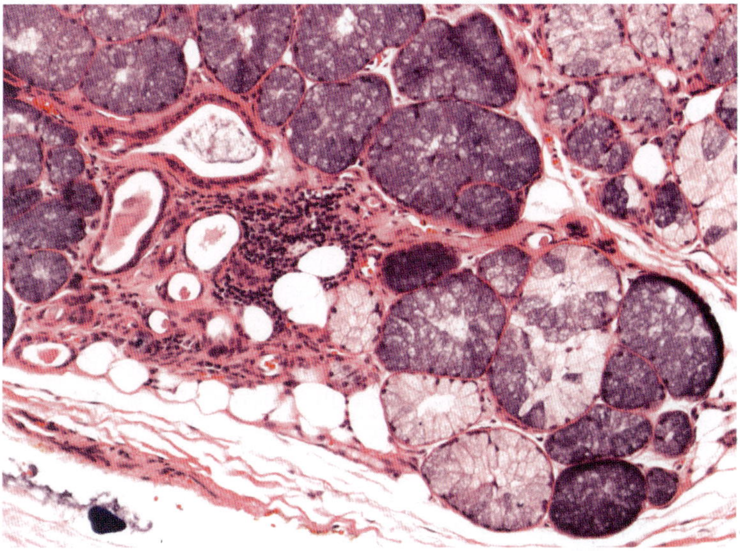

FIGURE 16.2 Salivary gland choristoma found in a middle ear biopsy of a cholesteatoma.

cholesteatomas. An intact tympanic membrane is usually but not universally present. The lesions are discovered either incidentally during otologic examination or because of unilateral hearing loss. Some believe that these lesions develop from epidermoid remnants found in the middle ear. Regardless, they are histologically identical to acquired cholesteatomas, and samples are composed of fragments of stratified squamous epithelium and keratin. A foreign body reaction is sometimes seen.

Infectious Disease

Infections of the external and middle ear are relatively common, but histologic sampling rarely is performed. They can be caused by a variety of organisms including viruses, bacteria, and fungi. Most disease is self-limited, although severe life-threatening infections sometimes develop, especially in immunocompromised patients.

Abscesses or *furuncles* of the external ear are usually associated with sebaceous glands and hair follicles and thus present within the auricle or outer canal.[15,16] These are red, inflamed nodules that may be exquisitely painful. Although they are most often secondary to infection by *Staphylococcus aureus*, a number of bacteria can be linked etiologically to these pustules. Histologically, pockets of neutrophils and debris are surrounded by abundant acute and chronic inflammation, typically with some degree of fibrosis and granulomatous inflammation. Involved pilosebaceous units are usually seen.

Otitis externa, both benign and "malignant," is most often caused by infection with *Pseudomonas aeruginosa*.[15,17–19] Both forms of disease represent variants of cellulitis. The benign or more common form develops most often in the lateral portion of the external auditory canal and may be secondary to predisposing factors such as local trauma and disruption of the ceruminal barrier. The disease develops most often in tropical climates and in humid weather. Swimming is a risk factor for the development of the disease. The "malignant" or necrotizing form is much more aggressive and typically involves the more medial portion of the external auditory canal. It occurs in older patients, many of whom are immunocompromised secondary to diabetes mellitus. These infections may spread along tissue and fascial planes, along cranial nerves and vessels, and eventually involve the parotid gland, surrounding bone or brain. Thrombophlebitis of the cavernous sinus even develops in some cases. Histologically, the findings correspond to the extent of the infection. Edema and acute and chronic inflammation are seen throughout the involved soft tissue. Ulceration, necrotizing vasculitis, and tissue necrosis are all seen as the process worsens.

As with otitis externa, *otitis media* is very unlikely to be sampled. This extremely common disease of childhood presents with ear pain and bulging, erythematous, or exudative tympanic membranes on otologic examination.[16] Recurrent and chronic infections secondary to blockage of the eustachian tubes sometimes lead to complications, including cholesteatoma.[20] Causative agents include bacteria, such as *Streptococcus pneumoniae*, *Haemophilus influenzae*, and *Moraxella catarrhalis,* along with various upper respiratory tract viruses.[16] Sampling shows a nonspecific acute and chronic inflammatory infiltrate within the epithelial and stromal tissues. Rarely, *Mycobacterium tuberculosis* infects the middle ear and, when sampled, a granulomatous reaction is seen.[21] Finally, it should be noted that otitis media in adults is frequently associated with neoplasia.

Viral infections sometimes involve the external ear and tympanic membrane (myringitis). The ear canal and tympanic membrane can be involved by *Varicella zoster* (Ramsay-Hunt syndrome) and *Herpes simplex virus*.[19,22] The clinical and pathologic findings are identical to those seen at other sites. The telltale nuclear inclusions within the squamous cells of the vesicles or ulcerated areas should lead one to the correct diagnosis. Occasional hemorrhagic vesicles can be seen on the external tympanic membrane in cases of influenza.[16]

Fungi rarely infect the squamous epithelium of the external ear (*otomycoses*).[15,22-24] Most of these infections are caused by *Aspergillus* or *Candida* species. In general, these infections present as typical cases of otitis externa, and it is estimated that 2% of cases of otitis externa are caused by fungi. Histologically, the squamous epithelium is thickened with parakeratosis and focal collections of intraepithelial neutrophils (Fig. 16.3). Hyphal and yeast forms are then found within the parakeratotic plaques. Subepithelial chronic inflammation is also typically noted. The fungi should not extend into the subepithelial tissues in uncomplicated cases of otomycosis. Deeper infections by a number of organisms such as cryptococcus and blastomyces are rare but have been reported.

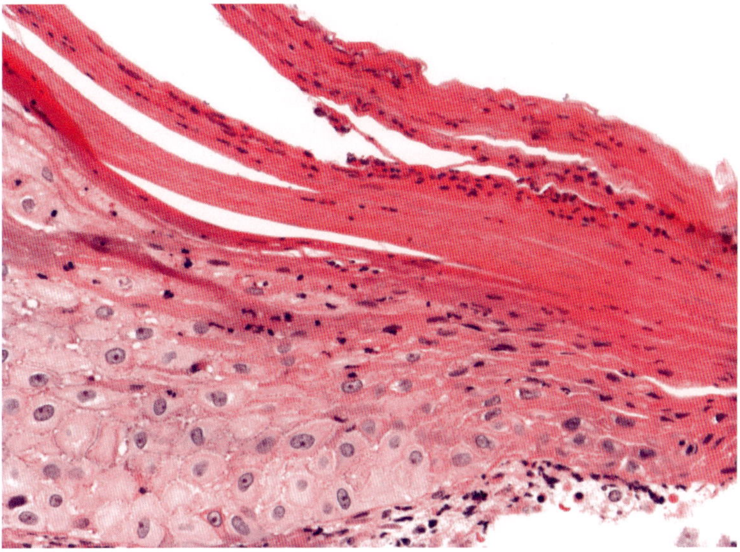

FIGURE 16.3 Parakeratotic plaque with intraepithelial neutrophils seen in a patient with otomycosis.

Inflammatory and Reactive Conditions and Other Abnormalities

The lengthy designation *chondrodermatitis nodularis chronica helicis* describes a painful, inflammatory lesion of the external ear.[25–27] The lesion occurs somewhat more frequently in older men and typically involves the outer portion of the helix, but any portion of the auricle may be involved. It most often presents as a painful, solitary nodule that is less than 1 cm in size. A surface crust is typically seen, and clinicians often believe the lesions are malignant prior to biopsy. The pathogenesis of the condition is uncertain. Most believe it to arise from localized ischemia related to chronic conditions such as sun damage and repeated pressure-related trauma. This process is benign and is typically cured by limited local resection.

Histologically, the centrally ulcerated and crusted area is surrounded by thickened and parakeratotic squamous epithelium.[25–27] The fibrinous debris of the ulcer base extends centrally to the perichondrium and auricular cartilage and is surrounded by granulation tissue and acute and chronic inflammation. Some degree of erosion of the cartilage is often seen with surrounding necrosis and basophilia (Fig. 16.4, eFigs. 16.2 and 16.3). Reactive changes such as stromal cellular atypia and fibrosis can be seen.

Idiopathic cystic chondromalacia, also known as pseudocyst of the auricle, typically presents as a swelling of the auricle in young to middle-aged adults.[28,29] Although any portion of the auricle can be involved, the helix is the most commonly affected site. The pathogenesis of these lesions

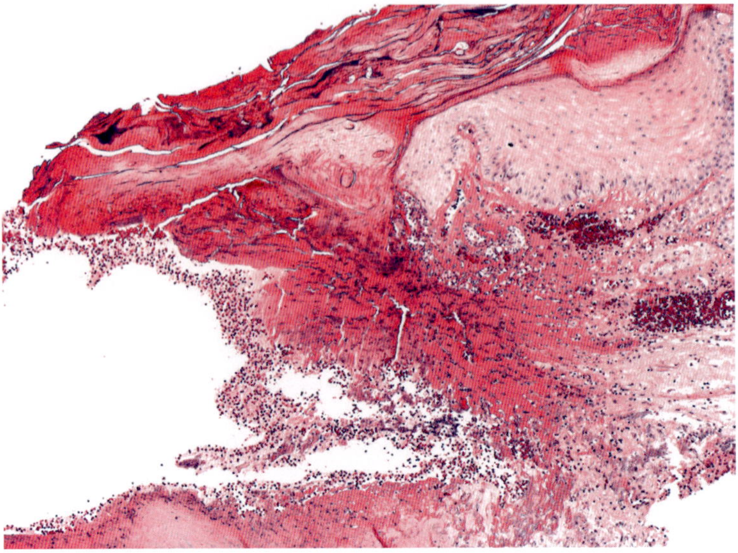

FIGURE 16.4 An ulcer extends to the auricular cartilage in this case of chondrodermatitis nodularis chronica helicis.

is unknown, but as with chondrodermatitis nodularis chronica helicis, trauma may play some role. Histologically, these are pseudocystic spaces within the auricular cartilage with surrounding normal cartilage, degenerated cartilage, or granulation tissue (Fig. 16.5, eFig. 16.4).

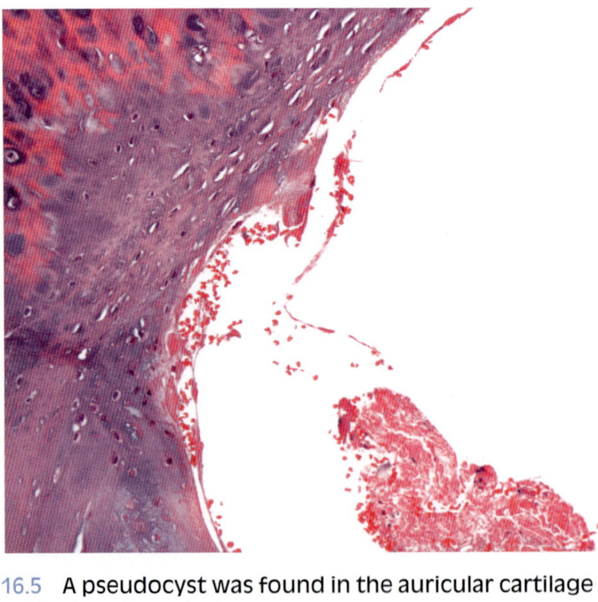

FIGURE 16.5 A pseudocyst was found in the auricular cartilage consistent with idiopathic cystic chondromalacia.

As was discussed in the chapter describing nonneoplastic disease of the larynx (Chapter 15), *relapsing polychondritis* is a rheumatic disease characterized by episodic and progressive inflammation of cartilage.[30,31] The ears are often affected and involvement is typically bilateral. Diagnosis requires a combination of clinical and pathologic findings. Histologically, the cartilage will typically appear necrotic or degenerated with surrounding acute and chronic inflammation.

Kimura disease is a chronic inflammatory condition that frequently involves the head and neck at or just behind the ear.[32–36] Patients are more often men, and the disease appears to be much more common in Asian populations. The lesions typically present as painless masses averaging 2.5 cm in size and located deep to the dermis with associated regional lymphadenopathy and parotid involvement. Although the pathogenesis is unknown, patients are frequently noted to have peripheral eosinophilia and elevated serum concentrations of IgE.

Histologic sections of Kimura disease usually show some degree of residual lymph node architecture with follicular hyperplasia and well-formed mantle zones (Fig. 16.6).[32–35] The inflammatory infiltrate most often extends into the perinodal soft tissues and capsular and stromal fibrosis are typically present. Eosinophilic folliculolysis is usually seen with necrosis and proteinaceous debris noted within the germinal centers. Abundant eosinophils are also present in the interfollicular areas, sinusoids, and perinodal tissue, and these frequently aggregate into small eosinophilic microabscesses (eFigs. 16.5 and 16.6). An increased number

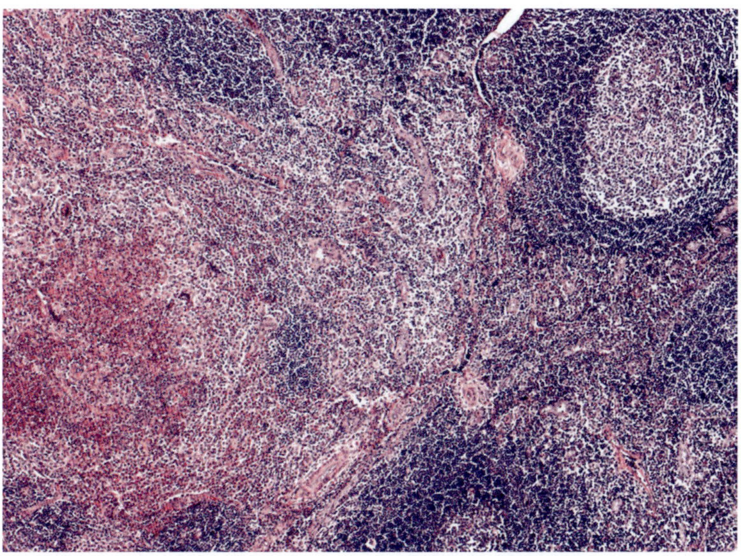

FIGURE 16.6 Kimura disease with follicular hyperplasia, fibrosis, and an eosinophilic abscess.

of vessels is frequently noted, as is a postcapillary venular proliferation. Immunohistochemistry supports the diagnosis of a reactive process and testing for Epstein-Barr virus is usually negative.

Kimura disease should be distinguished from angiolymphoid hyperplasia with eosinophilia (epithelioid/histiocytoid hemangioma) as the two are distinct clinicopathologic entities (Table 16.1).[32–35] Kimura disease occurs more frequently in Asians and men, more often is deep to the dermis, and is associated with adenopathy and salivary gland involvement, increased serum IgE levels, and peripheral eosinophilia. Angiolymphoid hyperplasia with eosinophilia occurs equally in all races, is more common in women, presents as a superficial papule, and is not associated with peripheral eosinophilia, increased serum IgE levels, or adenopathy. In Kimura disease, the vascular component is much less prominent than it is in angiolymphoid hyperplasia with eosinophilia, and the endothelial cells are typically flattened rather than epithelioid.

Keloids of the ear resemble those seen throughout the rest of the body, both clinically and pathologically.[37,38] As such, they develop more frequently in black individuals and often arise after local trauma, such as ear piercing. They present as firm, pink nodules, usually covered by an intact epithelium. The histologic features are rather distinct with thick, eosinophilic bands of collagen present throughout the dermal tissue, often obliterating adnexal structures and flattening the surface epithelium (Fig. 16.7, eFig. 16.7). As such, the lesions appear quite hypocellular and are composed predominately of collagen with occasional intermixed fibroblasts.

TABLE 16.1 Clinicopathologic Features of Kimura Disease and Angiolymphoid Hyperplasia With Eosinophilia

	Kimura Disease	Angiolymphoid Hyperplasia with Eosinophilia
Patients	More likely to affect Asians and men	No racial predilection; occurs slightly more often in women
Clinical	Associated with peripheral eosinophilia and elevated IgE levels	Not associated with peripheral eosinophilia or elevated IgE levels
Gross	Deep, subcutaneous lesions with local adenopathy and salivary gland involvement	Superficial dermal papules that may itch or bleed; no local adenopathy or salivary gland involvement
Histology	Inflammatory infiltrate with follicular hyperplasia and eosinophils, fibrosis and postcapillary venular proliferation	Abundant vascular proliferation with plump, epithelioid endothelial cells; background lymphoplasmacellular infiltrate with eosinophils and fibrosis

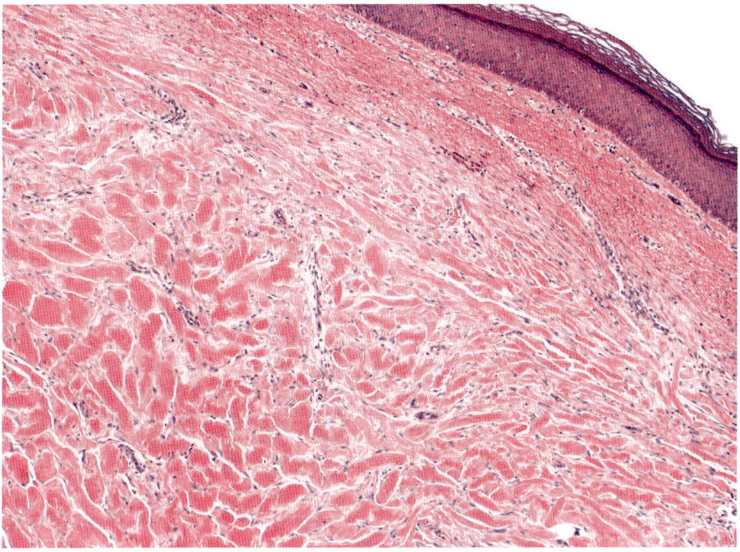

FIGURE 16.7 A keloid.

Keratin accumulation in the external ear canal can cause obstruction either secondary to the keratin itself or secondary to the body's response to the keratin. Some individuals apparently have impaired lateral extrusion of external canal keratin, which then accumulates and plugs the canal (*keratosis obturans*).[39] The keratin in such cases actually accumulates to such a degree as to widen the canal and cause pressure ulceration of the surrounding epithelium. Secondary infections are common. The histologic features are as unexciting as one would expect. There is abundant keratinous debris, sometimes with cholesterol clefts, inflammation, and evidence of epithelial ulceration (Fig. 16.8; eFig. 16.8). Keratinous cysts of the external ear can also cause obstruction. As with the more common middle ear lesions, they are called *cholesteatomas* here.[39] Histologically, they are cystic structures, lined by a bland, stratified squamous epithelium. With rupture of these cysts or through ear canal trauma, keratin can come into contact with the stroma and abundant foreign body reaction can be formed (*keratin granulomas*).[39,40] These further lead to obstruction of the canal and can cause hearing loss and pain.

Acquired cholesteatomas of the middle ear are nonneoplastic masses caused by the production of keratin by stratified squamous epithelium.[11,13,27,41,42] Given the small volume of the middle ear, one can imagine that very small lesions easily result in clinical problems. Acquired cholesteatomas are distinguished from congenital cholesteatomas through assessment of the tympanic membrane. As acquired cholesteatomas are believed to result from severe otitis media or, rarely, trauma, and entry of squamous epithelium from the external ear into the middle ear, they are typically associated with ruptured tympanic membranes. Clinically, acquired cholesteatomas appear white and pearly. Histologically, they are composed

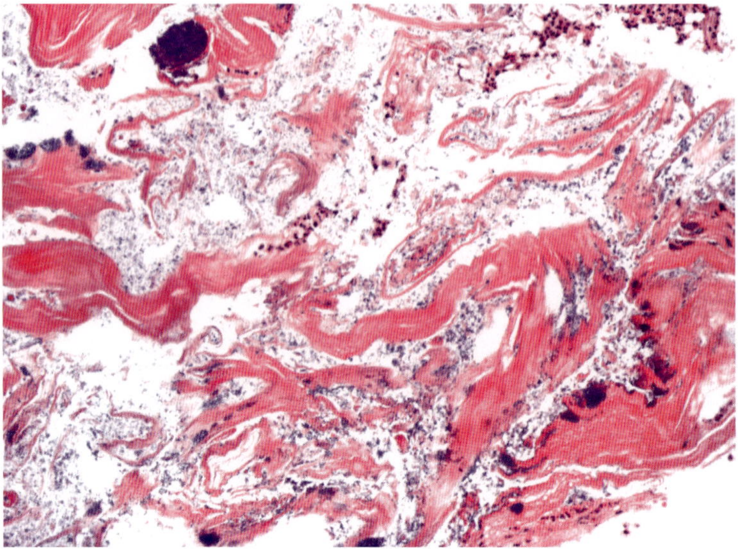

FIGURE 16.8 Abundant keratin was removed from the external auditory canal of a patient with apparent keratosis obturans.

of keratin and stratified squamous epithelium that is sometimes fragmented (Fig. 16.9). They occasionally present as intact cystic structures (eFig. 16.9). Calcification, inflammation, and foreign body reaction are also commonly present.

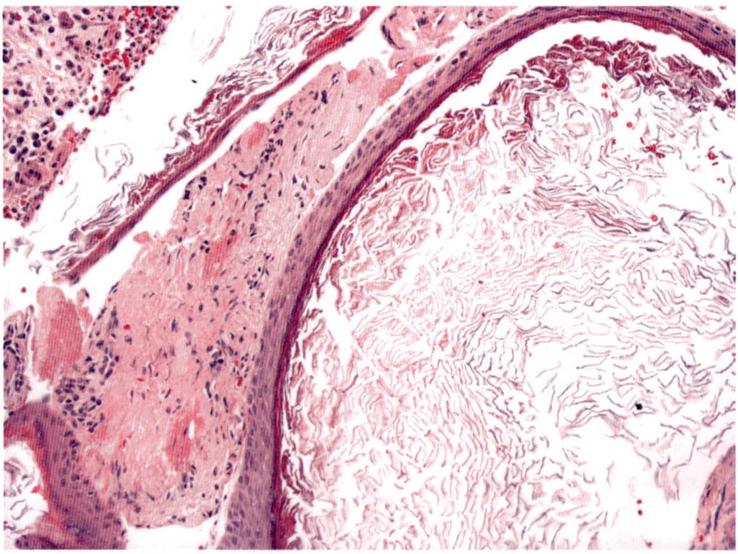

FIGURE 16.9 Resections of acquired cholesteatomas show fragmented squamous epithelium and keratinous debris.

Chronic otitis media is sometimes associated with middle ear *cholesterol granulomas*.[43] These yellow, nodular lesions are believed to be secondary to hemorrhage. Histologically, they are composed of red blood cells, hemosiderin-laden macrophages, cholesterol clefts, and a foreign body reaction. It is important that these lesions not be mislabeled as cholesteatomas as they are not locally aggressive.

Chronic otitis media is also associated with the formation of an *inflammatory polyp* (*aural polyp*) of the middle ear.[44] These nonneoplastic lesions frequently extend through the tympanic membrane into the external auditory canal. They are polypoid masses of granulation tissue and inflamed stroma (Fig. 16.10, eFig. 16.10). Edema, fibrosis, foreign body reaction, hemosiderin-laden macrophages, and cholesterol granulomas all may be present within the body of the polyp. The surface epithelium is often eroded but if present is either ciliated columnar or squamous. Inflammatory polyps may be associated with cholesteatomas or neoplasms.

Most masses composed of mature bone within the ear canal are classified as *osteomas* or as bony *exostoses*.[45,46] External ear osteomas are more common in men, occur over a broad age range, and present as solitary, pedunculated bony lesions attached to underlying bone. Bony exostoses are broad-based, often bilateral lesions of the external auditory canal that are also more common in men and often present with obstructive hearing loss. Both lesions are composed of mature, lamellar bone present beneath the intact squamous epithelium of the canal (Fig. 16.11, eFig. 16.11). Osteomas have been noted to have larger interlamellar spaces. These lesions are difficult to confuse with other entities although some have noted that lesions such as fibrous dysplasia should be excluded.

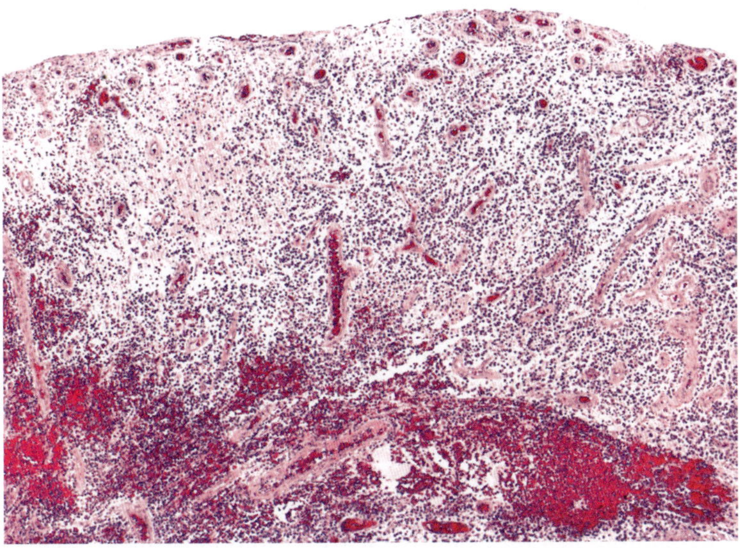

FIGURE 16.10 Aural polyps are composed of granulation tissue.

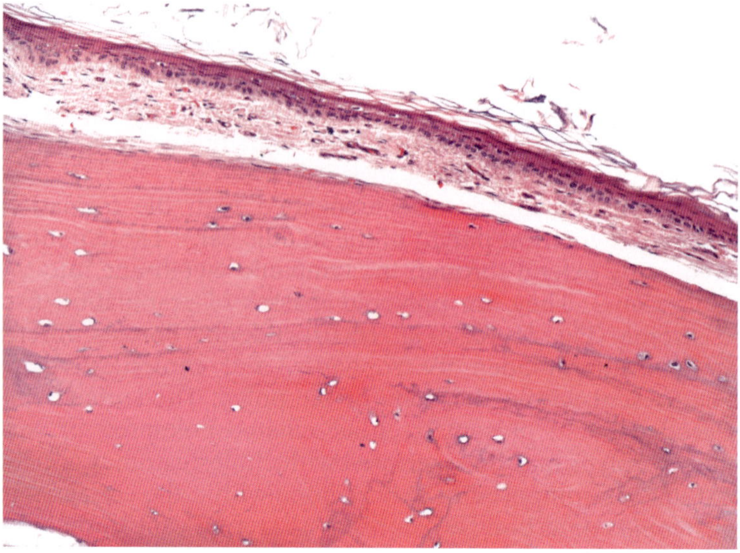

FIGURE 16.11 An osteoma of the external auditory canal.

Many other inflammatory processes affect various or all portions of the ear. The auricle can be easily traumatized, sometimes chronically such as with the ear pieces of glasses *(spectacle frame acanthoma* or *granuloma fissuratum*).[47] Chronic trauma also sometimes leads to calcification or ossification of the ear lobe (*petrified auricle*).[48] *Malakoplakia* and *xanthomas* have been reported in the ear.[49,50] IgG4-related sclerosing lesions have been reported in the ear.[51] Ulcers secondary to cold and humid weather (*chilblains*) have been reported.[52] Elastic nodules can form on the external ear secondary to severe sun damage.[53] The external auditory canal may exhibit a foreign body reaction to any of the many things that are placed within it and *myospherulosis*, akin to that seen in the sinonasal area, has been seen.[54,55] Finally, systemic processes, such as *sarcoidosis* and *Wegener granulomatosis*, sometimes involve portions of the ear.[56]

NEOPLASTIC DISEASE

As mentioned in the chapter introduction, neoplasms of the ear include dermal-type tumors, neoplasms also seen in biopsies of the upper aerodigestive tract, and occasional pathologic entities specific to the area. A nice summary of the frequencies of these neoplasms, based on the Armed Forces Institute of Pathology (AFIP) experience, was originally published in the second edition of the AFIP fascicle concerning neoplasms of the upper aerodigestive tract and ear (Tables 16.2 and 16.3).[57] Most of the lesions in this area are biopsied prior to definitive surgical resection and thus correct diagnosis is essential.

TABLE 16.2 Neoplasms of the External Ear[57]

Neoplasm	Percentage
Squamous cell carcinoma	34
Basal cell carcinoma	31
Melanocytic neoplasia	11
Osteoma	3
Ceruminous neoplasia, benign	3
Ceruminous neoplasia, malignant	3
Atypical fibroxanthoma	1
Others	14

External Ear and External Auditory Canal

The majority of neoplasms arising in the external ear and auditory canal occur on the auricle and are dermal in nature. Because of its location and exophytic nature, the auricle is subject to abundant sun exposure. As such, most of the neoplasia that develops here is secondary to sun damage and is identical to sun damage–induced dermal neoplasia elsewhere.

Seborrheic keratoses are not uncommonly found on the external ear or within the ear canal.[58,59] They appear here, like elsewhere, as brown irregular patches that look to have been "stuck on" to the skin of older adults. These lesions can vary in size but are usually approximately 1 cm. Occasionally, they appear somewhat atypical and raise clinical concerns for melanoma. These are, however, benign tumors that only rarely recur after surgical removal. Histologically, the epidermis in thickened; the bases of the lesions are smooth and do not extend more deeply than the

TABLE 16.3 Neoplasms of the Middle Ear and Temporal Bone[57]

Neoplasm	Percentage
Schwannoma	41
Paraganglioma	15
Middle ear adenoma	9
Squamous cell carcinoma	5
Metastasis	5
Langerhans cell histiocytosis	2
Rhabdomyosarcoma	2
Choristoma	1
Others	20

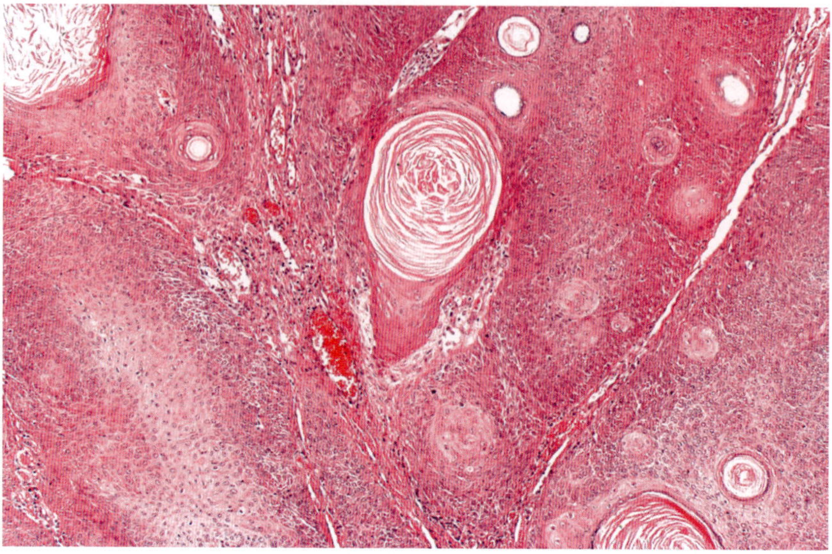

FIGURE 16.12 Frequent pseudohorn cysts are seen in most seborrheic keratoses.

surrounding uninvolved epidermis. The epithelium is composed of proliferating and bland basal cells, and invaginations of the surface keratin lend the lesions their well-known pseudohorn cysts (Fig. 16.12). Inflamed lesions may show more individual cell keratinization and some lesions have basilar pigmentation.

Squamous cell carcinomas of the ear often develop on the auricle and are related to actinic damage.[60–63] Many thus develop in older, fair-skinned men. Some squamous cell carcinomas of the ear develop in the external auditory canal. While these also occur in older individuals, they appear to be not related to sun damage and may instead be associated with chronic otitis externa. They have been found to be more common in women. Symptoms depend on the location of the tumor. Tumors appear as painful mass lesions that are sometimes ulcerated. Those of the external auditory canal often present with otorrhea.

Squamous cell carcinomas share the same histologic features regardless of site (see Chapter 4).[60–62] Those of the ear show variable differentiation or maturation with infiltrating irregular nests of atypical squamous cells (Fig. 16.13, eFig. 16.12). Squamous cell variants are also seen associated with the ear, especially spindle cell or sarcomatoid carcinomas (see Chapter 5). Those with a basaloid morphology are better termed "basal cell carcinomas" when they occur in sun-exposed skin (see below). Background actinic change with solar elastosis will be seen with those tumors originating in sun-exposed skin. As with squamous cell carcinomas seen at other sites, the differential diagnosis includes benign squamoproliferative processes, especially those lesions associated with pseudoepitheliomatous hyperplasia. Careful attention to architectural and cytologic

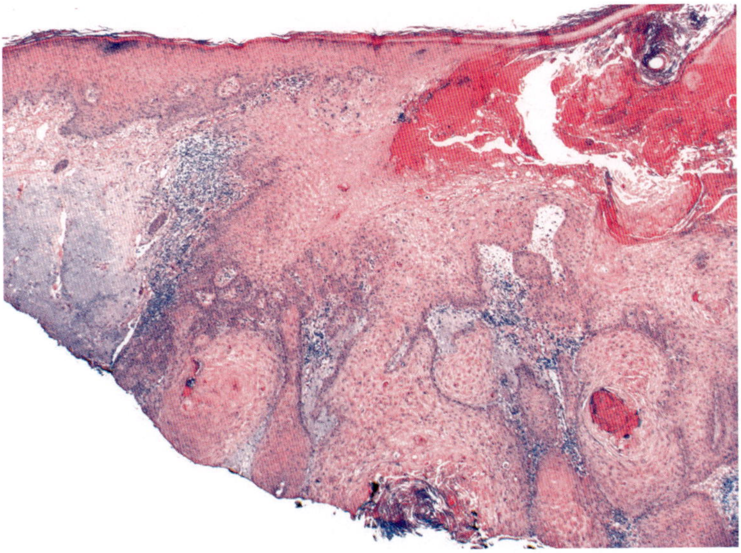

FIGURE 16.13 A well-differentiated squamous cell carcinoma of the sun-damaged external ear extending to the deep margin of the biopsy.

atypia should allow for the distinction of most of these lesions. Spindle cell carcinomas need to be distinguished from melanomas and mesenchymal neoplasms. This distinction often rests with the use of immunohistochemistry and has been discussed in Chapter 5.

Invasive malignancies arising from the epidermis that maintain a basaloid phenotype are diagnosed as *basal cell carcinomas*.[61,64,65] These lesions are actually much more common than squamous cell carcinomas of the skin. (Basal cell carcinomas are much less common in the external auditory canal, however.) As with their more conventional cutaneous counterparts, they are related to sun damage and occur most frequently in fair-skinned elderly men. Basal cell carcinomas present as raised, nodular, erythematous masses than can be ulcerated. Some variants, e.g., the morphealike variant, present as plaquelike lesions.

The histologic features of basal cell carcinomas are well known to pathologists. Most tumors have a nodular growth pattern with infiltrating, smoothly contoured nests of basaloid cells that focally are attached to the overlying epidermis (Fig. 16.14). Nuclear palisading is frequently seen at the periphery of these nests and separation clefts are often formed between the neoplastic cells and the surrounding dermis. The surrounding dermal tissue usually shows an obvious desmoplastic reaction, and some degree of chronic inflammation is frequently present. The morphealike form, which may represent up to one-third of the basal cell carcinomas of the external ear, appears much more desmoplastic (eFig. 16.13). Rather than nests of basaloid cells, the neoplastic cells are arranged in thin cords that weave their way through the desmoplastic dermal stroma. The individual

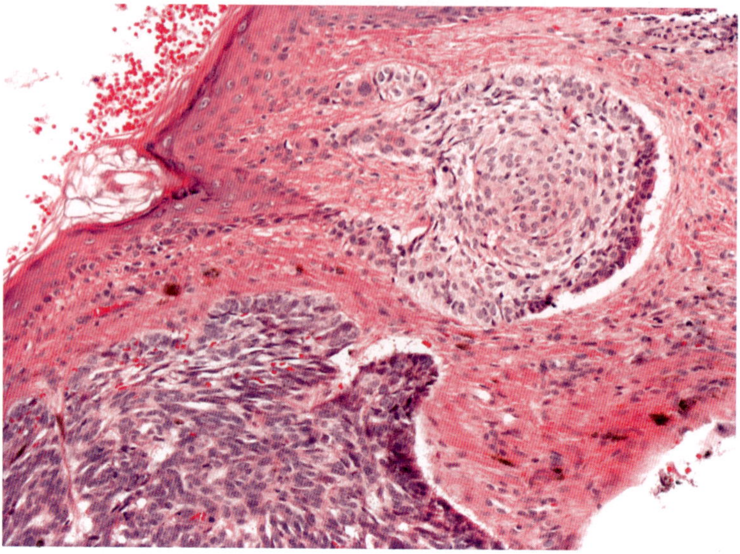

FIGURE 16.14 Nests of basaloid cells connected to the epidermis and peripheral clefting characterize the basal cell carcinoma of the external ear.

neoplastic cells of basal cell carcinomas are small and monotonous with high nuclear to cytoplasmic ratios (eFig. 16.14). The nuclei have vesicular chromatin and prominent nucleoli are not commonly seen. Features of high-grade malignancy such as tumor necrosis and abundant mitotic activity are not seen. As with other neoplasms associated with sun damage, actinic change and solar elastosis are frequently present in the surrounding uninvolved skin.

Virtually all forms of *melanocytic neoplasia*, including *benign nevi*, *malignant lentigo*, and *malignant melanoma*, may involve the external ear.[61,66–70] Given its abundant exposure to the sun, it is not surprising that malignant melanomas are common at this site. Indeed, 10% of all head and neck melanomas occur on the external ear. The patient age range is wide, but most individuals with malignant melanoma of the external ear are older adults; the mean age of presentation is 50 years. Melanomas present as atypical pigmented macules or nodules and up to one-third present with regional metastases. Most lesions arise in the helix although the external auditory canal has rarely been involved.

Although all varieties of melanoma have been found to involve the external ear, superficial spreading and nodular melanoma are the two most common variants seen in this location.[68,71] Superficial spreading melanomas are characterized by atypical melanocytes that first spread radially through the epidermis and at the dermal-epidermal junction and eventually grow vertically (Fig. 16.15). Transepidermal migration of atypical melanocytes is an early feature of this malignancy. Nodular melanomas are composed of malignant melanocytes showing a vertical

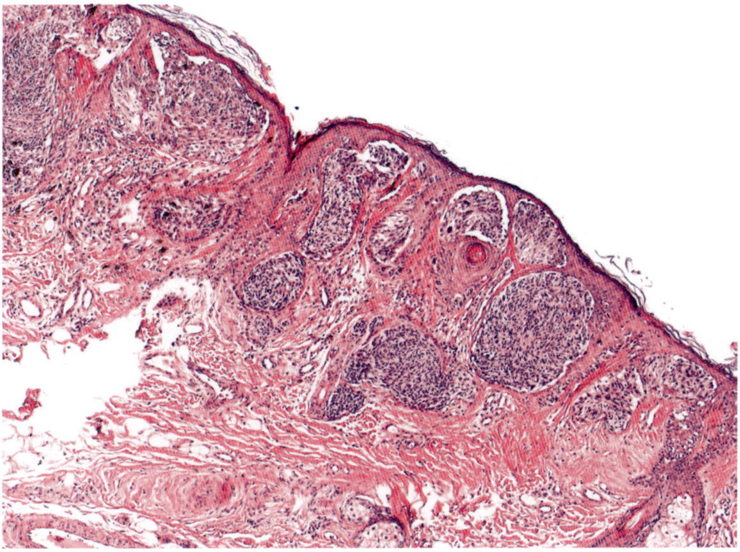

FIGURE 16.15 A superficial spreading melanoma of the ear with radial growth.

pattern of growth deep into the dermis without a concomitant radial growth component (eFig. 16.15). The malignant melanocytes are usually enlarged compared to benign melanocytes and have an epithelioid or somewhat spindled shape (Fig. 16.16, eFigs. 16.16 and 16.17). The amount of cytoplasm can vary greatly from case to case and cell to cell, as can its character. The neoplastic cells frequently have atypical,

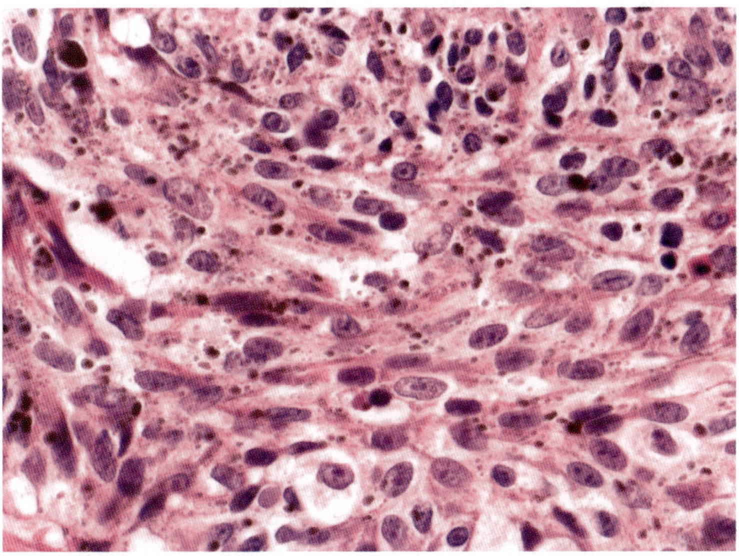

FIGURE 16.16 Pigmented, atypical spindled cells in a case of malignant melanoma.

enlarged nuclei with prominent nucleoli and occasional mitotic figures. Other variants of melanoma can also be seen in the ear including spindle cell and desmoplastic melanomas and have histologic features reflective of their designations.

The reporting of melanomas is an art unto itself. Clark level, Breslow thickness, the presence of ulceration, the histologic subtype, mitotic counts, inflammatory response, the presence of regression, the presence of satellite lesions, and the presence of vascular invasion all should be recorded.[68,72] Distinguishing the tumors from other neoplasms and malignancies is obviously very important and can be assisted with immunohistochemistry. The most sensitive immunohistochemical stain for malignant melanoma remains antibody to S100 protein.[73] Other antigens frequently expressed include SOX10, HMB45, and Melan-A, among others. Melanomas typically should not react with antibodies to epithelial antigens, such as cytokeratins, or with antibodies to CD45 (leukocyte common antigen). Melanomas must also be distinguished from benign nevi or other melanocytic tumors. It has been noted that compound nevi of the auricle frequently show some atypical features; however, careful histologic assessment usually allows for accurate distinction.[70]

Atypical fibroxanthoma (AFX) is an uncommon dermal malignancy that develops in sun-exposed skin.[74–78] Not surprisingly, AFX occurs more frequently in older patients with lighter skin, many of whom have had other cutaneous cancers. The tumors most frequently involve the head and neck, and nearly 25% develop on the external ear. Patients typically present with a single, firm nodule or ulcer with an average size of 1.2 cm. Although most AFXs are believed to be secondary to sun exposure, occasionally patients report having received radiation therapy to the affected area. AFXs are considered to be malignant, but they infrequently recur (<10%) and patients do not die from the disease. Metastasis is very uncommon (<5%).

Atypical fibroxanthomas are located mostly within the dermis but can extend into the subcutaneous adipose tissue.[74–78] The tumors abut the epidermis and ulceration is often seen. Surrounding skin shows evidence of sun damage with degeneration of the collagen and actinic changes. The tumors are circumscribed and cellular, composed of spindled and polygonal, foamy cells present in different proportions from case to case. The spindled cells are often present in a storiform arrangement, whereas the foamy cells are interspersed throughout the lesion or present as aggregates (Fig. 16.17). Marked nuclear and cellular pleomorphism is present and is a hallmark of AFX (eFigs. 16.18 and 16.19). Nuclei typically have vesicular chromatin and prominent nucleoli. Bizarre mononucleated and multinucleated cells are usually present in variable numbers, whereas Touton-type giant cells are notably uncommon. Mitotic figures are frequent and bizarre, multipolar forms are usually found. Fibrosis, myxoid change, and large areas of necrosis are not usually seen and intratumoral inflammation is limited.

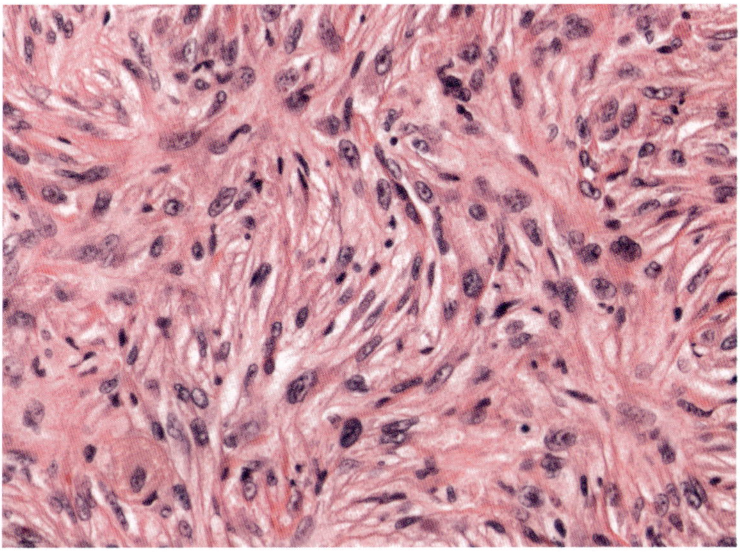

FIGURE 16.17 This atypical fibroxanthoma had atypical spindled cells arranged in a storiform architecture.

Because of histologic overlap with other poorly differentiated malignancies of the skin, namely squamous cell carcinomas and malignant melanomas, immunohistochemistry should be used to distinguish these lesions.[79,80] Almost all AFXs show no immunoreactivity with antibodies to keratins, S100 protein, or other markers of melanocytic differentiation, such as HMB-45. Aside from vimentin immunoreactivity, these tumors are frequently immunoreactive with antibodies to CD10 and SMA.[81–84] P63 immunoreactivity is uncommon.

Angiolymphoid hyperplasia with eosinophilia, also known as *histiocytoid hemangioma* and *epithelioid hemangioma*, is a benign vascular tumor that preferentially involves the external ear.[34,35,54,85–87] The lesions occur anywhere in the skin throughout the body, however, and may also involve the oral cavity. Patients vary in age and the peak incidence occurs in the third to fifth decades of life; women are more often affected. Clinically, the lesions present as painful or itchy, red-purple nodules that are often ulcerated. Although the lesions do not metastasize, they recur after resection in approximately 30% of cases and do not regress without therapy.

As noted above in the section on nonneoplastic lesions, histologically these tumors show some resemblance to Kimura disease. However, both clinical and histologic features usually allow for the distinction of these lesions (Table 16.1). Angiolymphoid hyperplasia with eosinophilia is characterized by lobules of capillaries that are lined by plump epithelioid (histiocytoid) endothelial cells that have eosinophilic, vacuolated cytoplasm and round to oval nuclei with vesicular chromatin and occasional nucleoli

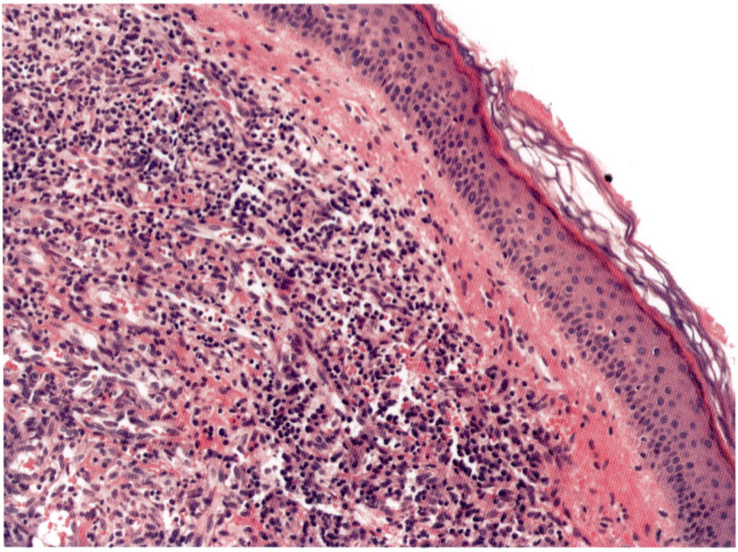

FIGURE 16.18 Angiolymphoid hyperplasia of the ear with abundant chronic inflammation.

(Figs. 16.18 and 16.19, eFig. 16.20).[4,34,35,54,85–87] Mitotic figures are uncommon. As with lobular capillary hemangiomas, the capillaries often appear compressed and distinct lumina are sometimes not seen. Larger vessels are frequently noted adjacent to or within the lobules of capillaries.

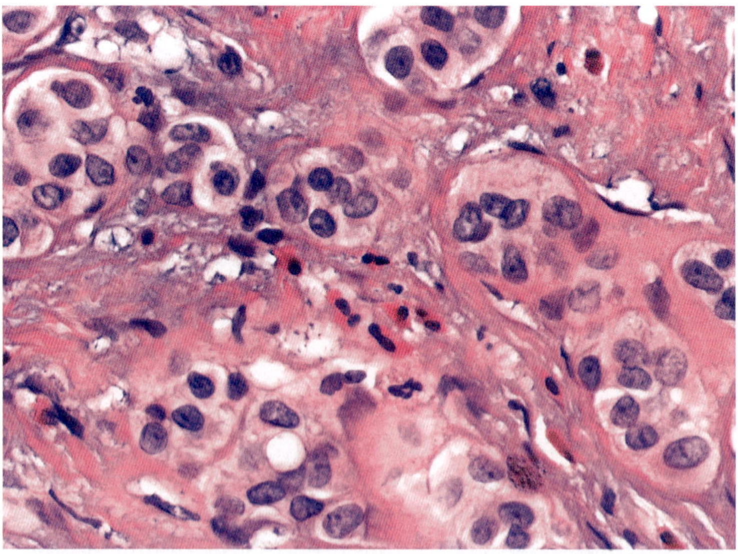

FIGURE 16.19 Epithelioid of "histiocytoid" endothelial cells with numerous eosinophils seen in a case of angiolymphoid hyperplasia with eosinophilia.

The inflammatory infiltrate contains numerous lymphocytes, plasma cells, and eosinophils. Germinal center formation is sometimes seen, usually at the periphery of the lesions. Immunohistochemically, the lesional cells react with antibodies to endothelial antigens (ERG, FVIII, CD31, CD34) as would be expected.

Squamous papillomas and *fibroepithelial polyps* are benign potentially neoplastic lesions of the external ear.[88] Papillomas are arborizing papillary fibrovascular structures that are covered by a bland stratified squamous epithelium (Fig. 16.20). Fibroepithelial polyps are less complex lesions with more abundant central stromal tissue. Both lesions are generally solitary and rarely recur after removal. *Aural papillomatosis* is rare.

Several neoplasms of the ear show a ceruminous phenotype (Table 16.4).[89-98] The most common of these, and the most common neoplasm of the external auditory canal, is the *ceruminous adenoma* or "ceruminoma." These tumors develop in patients of either sex over a wide age range, but most patients tend to be older with a mean age in the sixth decade of life. Individuals usually present with a grossly observable mass, although some report hearing changes. The tumors are slow growing and it has been noted that many wait for a considerable time before seeking treatment for their symptoms.

Ceruminous adenomas, as well as other ceruminous neoplasms, develop in the outer half to the outer third of the external auditory canal, where the bulk of the normal ceruminous glands are found.[90,97] Adenomas are polypoid tumors that measure, on average, about 1 cm in greatest

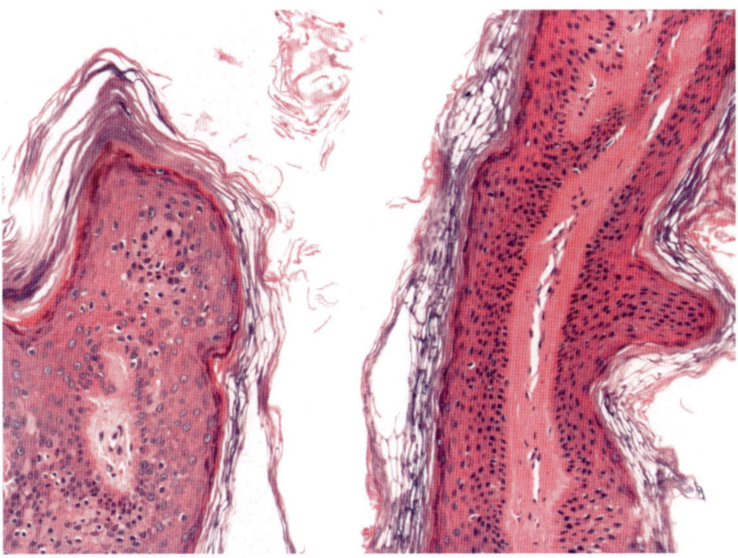

FIGURE 16.20 Papillary cores lined by bland squamous epithelium were seen with this squamous papilloma of the external auditory canal.

TABLE 16.4 WHO Classification of Ceruminous Neoplasia
Adenoma
Pleomorphic adenoma (chondroid syringoma)
Syringocystadenoma papilliferum
Cylindroma
Adenocarcinoma
Adenoid cystic carcinoma
Mucoepidermoid carcinoma

dimension. The lesions recur in about 10% of cases; however, as the name implies, metastases do not develop and patients do not die from these tumors.

Microscopically, ceruminous adenomas are circumscribed but not encapsulated.[90,97] They are predominately composed of glandular structures with occasional cystically dilated spaces and rare solid or papillary structures (Fig. 16.21). The glandular structures have an inner epithelial lining surrounded by basal or myoepithelial cells and a basement membrane (Fig. 16.22, eFig. 16.21). The epithelial or luminal cells have abundant eosinophilic cytoplasm, many with apical caps. Many of these cells also contain a golden-yellow-brown lipofuscin pigment similar to that seen within nonneoplastic ceruminous glands. Some degree of nuclear stratification is often seen and nucleoli are sometimes present; however,

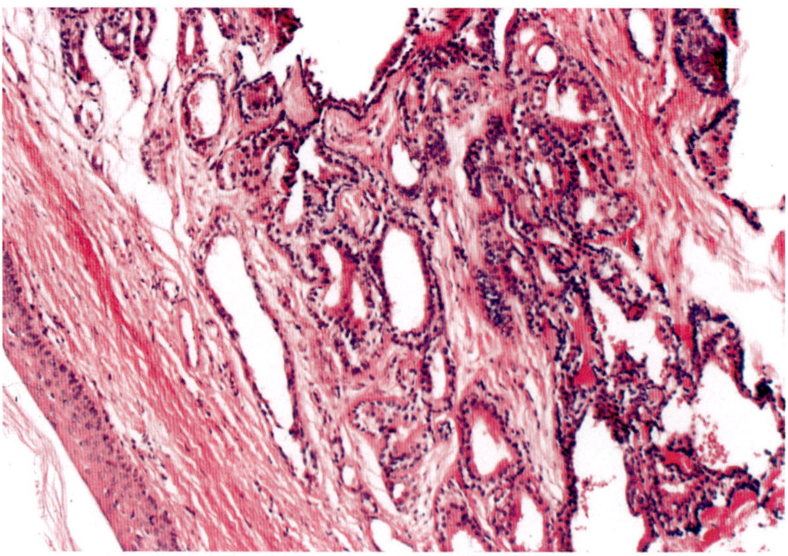

FIGURE 16.21 A ceruminous adenoma.

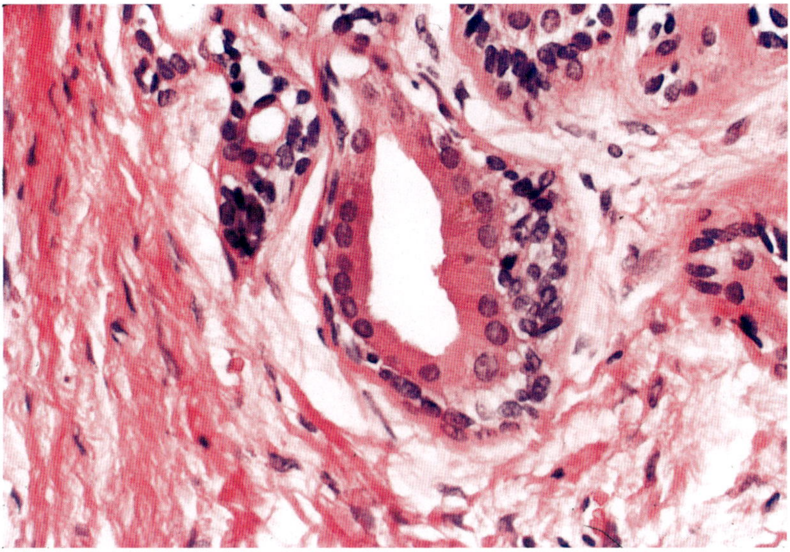

FIGURE 16.22 The glands of ceruminous adenomas are surrounded by basal cells.

tumor cells frequently show little cytologic atypia and mitotic figures are not easily identified. Occasional cases will have prominent background sclerosis and inflammation. Surface ulceration and involvement are also infrequently noted. By immunohistochemistry, antibodies to a broad spectrum of cytokeratins will highlight both the luminal and basal cells while antibodies to CK7 and CD117 highlight the epithelial cells, and antibodies to S100 and p63 label the basal cells.[97]

Ceruminous adenocarcinomas that are not better classified as adenoid cystic carcinomas or mucoepidermoid carcinomas are extremely rare.[77,93,97–99] They occur in either sex and, as with adenomas, over a wide age range. These tumors present with symptoms secondary to mass effect; however, they are more likely than adenomas to present with pain, probably due to invasion of adjacent nerves. Ceruminous adenocarcinomas are much more locally aggressive than adenomas. They relentlessly recur, but metastases are exceedingly rare. Unlike ceruminous adenomas, adenocarcinomas infiltrate surrounding soft tissue and bone (Fig. 16.23). These tumors have variable cytologic atypia and should show some evidence of ceruminous differentiation (eFig. 16.22). The glands frequently lack a basal cell layer histologically, and this can be confirmed with immunohistochemistry, although areas of the tumor may show definite biphasic growth with obvious basal cells (eFig. 16.23).[97,99] Lower grade tumors typically retain a more distinct apocrine phenotype. With these tumors, metastatic adenocarcinoma must be excluded.

Both benign and malignant ceruminous tumors sometimes resemble salivary gland–type tumors. Benign tumors are most often *mixed tumors* (*ceruminous pleomorphic adenomas*).[91,92,97] These clinically and

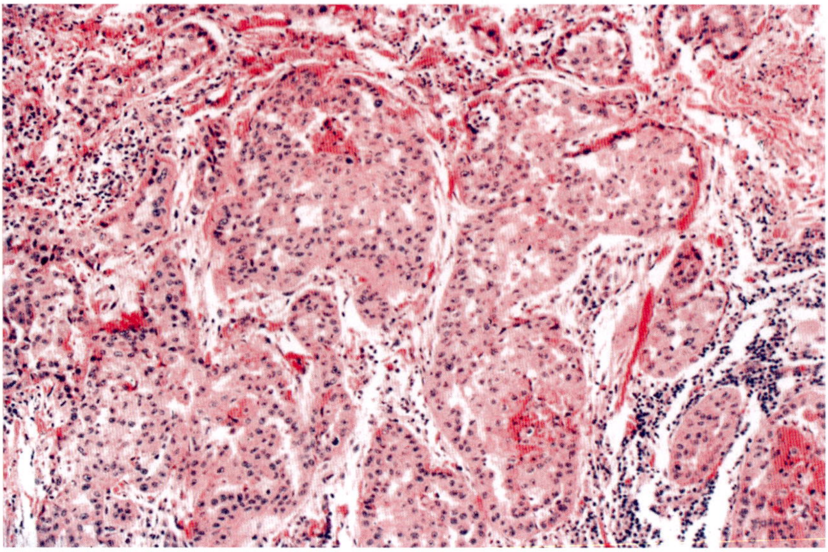

FIGURE 16.23 A ceruminous adenocarcinoma with infiltrating glands lined by oncocytic epithelial cells.

grossly have the same features as conventional ceruminous adenomas. Microscopically, they resemble mixed tumors seen at other sites and vary in their proportions of epithelial cells, myoepithelial cells, and stroma (Fig. 16.24, eFig, 16.24). Some of these tumors will have areas more

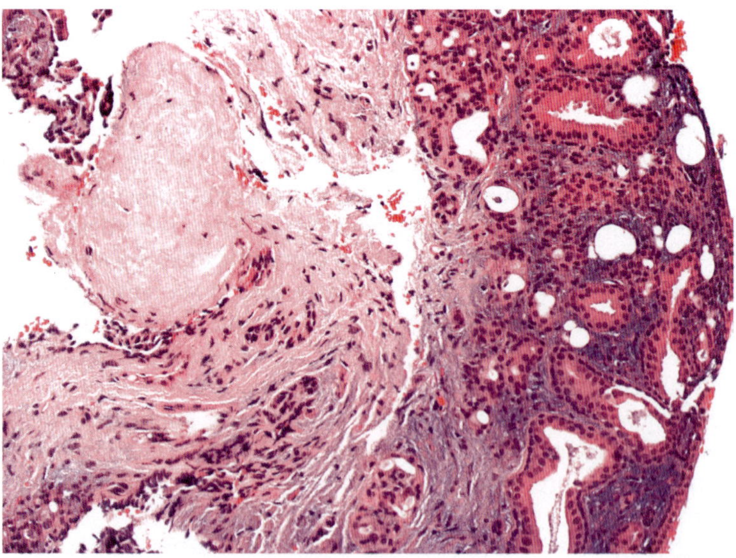

FIGURE 16.24 A pleomorphic adenoma of the ear with ceruminous-appearing glandular structures.

typical of conventional ceruminous adenomas or adenocarcinomas (carcinoma ex pleomorphic adenoma). Rarely, benign ceruminous tumors will have an appearance similar to *syringocystadenoma papilliferum*.[94] These lesions are both exophytic and endophytic with surface papillary growth covered by squamous and glandular epithelium. Papillary invaginations into the underlying stroma are also seen, again lined by squamous and glandular epithelium (eFig. 16.25). This glandular epithelium often has two layers of cells with both surface apocrine cells and underlying basal cells.

Adenoid cystic carcinomas of the ceruminous glands are actually more common than non–salivary-type ceruminous gland adenocarcinomas.[92,95,97] As with other ceruminous neoplasms, these tumors occur over a wide age range and relatively equally in both sexes. Because of the well-known tendency for adenoid cystic carcinomas to invade nerves, patients with these lesions are more likely to present with pain than are patients with other ceruminous neoplasms. Ceruminous adenoid cystic carcinomas are aggressive and frequently recur, often over a protracted period of time. As with adenoid cystic carcinomas at other sites, distant (lung) metastases eventually develop in many patients. Adenoid cystic carcinomas often appear grossly polypoid, but they may occasionally appear as a nonspecific area of ulceration. Histologically, they are identical to adenoid cystic carcinomas seen elsewhere (see Chapter 6) and will have a tubular, cribriform, solid, or mixed growth patterns, frequently with extensive perineural infiltration (Fig. 16.25, eFig. 16.26).

Rarely, *mucoepidermoid carcinomas* have been reported in the external ear canal.[96] The few of these that have been described had numerous

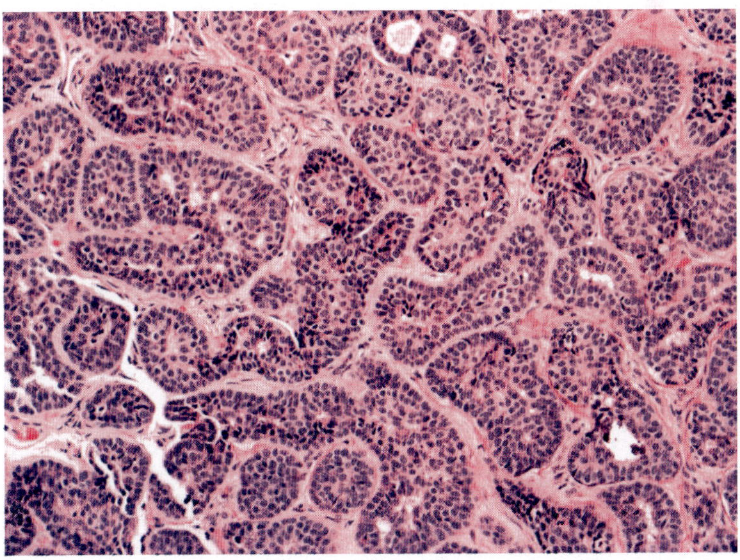

FIGURE 16.25 An adenoid cystic carcinoma of the ear.

glandular spaces and clear cells with intracellular and extracellular mucus. Intermixed epidermoid cells were also present. While these mucoepidermoid carcinomas tend to be solid, severe cytologic atypia, mitotic figures, necrosis, and perineural invasion are usually not seen.

Most cutaneous neoplasia has been reported on the external ear.[61] Other malignant lesions related to sun exposure, such as Merkel cell carcinomas occur here, as do the ever-expanding plethora of cutaneous adnexal tumors (Fig. 16.26, eFig. 16.27). Vascular neoplasms ranging from benign lobular capillary hemangiomas to high-grade angiosarcomas and Kaposi sarcoma occur here as well. The diagnostic approach to neoplasms of the external ear is in large part an exercise in dermatopathology.

Middle Ear and Temporal Bone Neoplasia

Papillomas identical to schneiderian papillomas of the sinonasal tract rarely are found within the middle ear.[100,101] These tumors occur in adults over a wide age range. Affected patients present with pain and hearing loss, often secondary to a ruptured tympanic membrane. Papillomas are usually treated conservatively and recurrence is common. All variants occur; however, as in the sinonasal tract, most are exophytic or endophytic lesions lined by transitional/schneiderian-type epithelium with mucous cells and intraepithelial inflammatory microcysts (Fig. 16.27, eFig. 16.28). These tumors, when endophytic or inverted, need to be distinguished from squamous cell carcinomas. Unlike squamous malignancies, little cytologic atypia is usually present and irregular infiltrating nests should not be seen. Distinction from aggressive papillary tumors, discussed below, may be

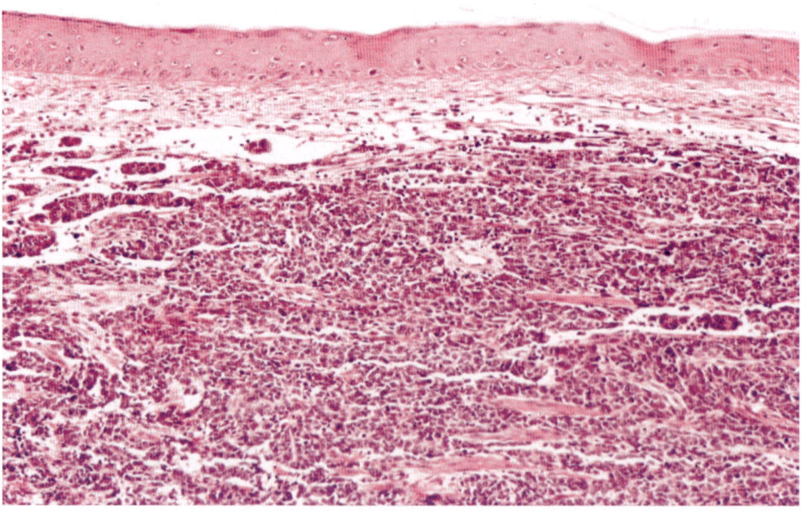

FIGURE 16.26 Merkel cell carcinomas sometimes involve the ear.

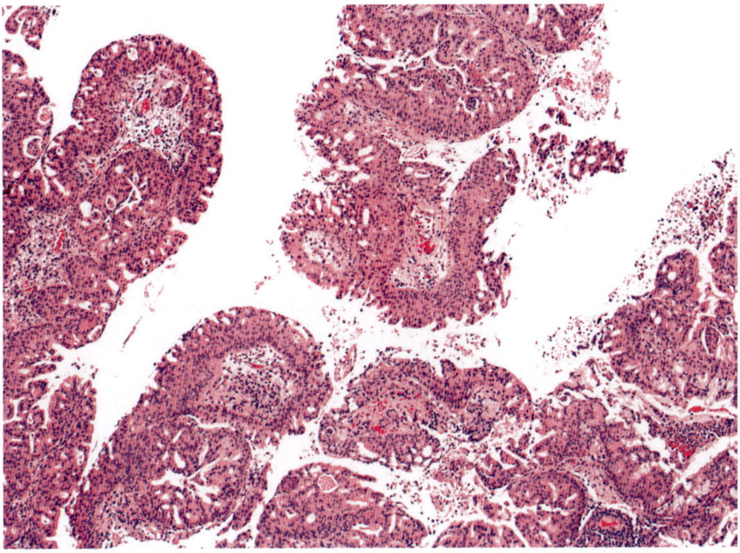

FIGURE 16.27 Middle ear schneiderian papillomas are identical to those of the sinonasal tract.

more difficult and there may be some histologic overlap between these lesions and what some have described as aggressive papillary tumor.

Squamous cell carcinomas are the fourth most common malignancy of the middle ear and temporal bone, occurring at a frequency of about half that of middle ear adenoma.[57,61] Patients are older and the average age is 60 years. No sex predilection is present. Individuals frequently present with ear pain and discharge. Hearing impairment is universal and facial nerve palsy is common. The prognosis for these tumors is poor, likely related to the anatomic location of the tumor that renders surgical resection difficult or impossible. The histologic features are identical to squamous cell carcinomas encountered elsewhere, and bony invasion is frequently seen.

There has been some debate in the literature regarding the nomenclature used to diagnose *middle ear adenomas*.[102–111] Furthermore, some authors have argued that a distinct carcinoid tumor may also exist at this site. We agree with the WHO that the designation of *middle ear adenoma* is suitable for these lesions, in spite of their frequent neuroendocrine phenotype.[112] We do not designate tumors from this site as carcinoids.

Middle ear adenomas occur in patients of either sex and at any age; the mean age of presentation is 45 years.[106,108,110] Most patients complain of hearing loss. Other common symptoms include the identification of a mass, pain, balance problems, and tinnitus. Patients have often endured symptoms for a considerable amount of time (multiple years) prior to their diagnosis. Recurrences after surgical resection develop in approximately 20% of patients, but the tumors do not metastasize or cause death.

Middle ear adenomas are small tumors and are usually removed piecemeal. The average aggregate dimension of received tumor is less than 1 cm.[110] The tumors most often fill the middle ear cavity and only rarely extend into bone or out of the middle ear. Microscopically, they are characteristically cellular and unencapsulated and display a variety of growth patterns including glandular, trabecular, solid, and organoid patterns (Fig. 16.28, eFig. 16.29).[106,108,110] Tumor cells are usually cuboidal to columnar; however, flattened, plasmacytoid, and spindled cells are occasionally found (Fig. 16.29, eFigs. 16.30 and 16.31). These cells have a moderate amount of eosinophilic homogenous to granular cytoplasm and round to oval nuclei with finely granular chromatin. Necrosis, severe cytologic atypia, and nucleoli are only rarely present. In areas with a glandular architectural pattern, two cell layers are often seen with the basal layer appearing more cuboidal and the luminal cells, flattened. Rare cases will demonstrate pagetoid spread of the neoplastic cells within the surface epithelium of the middle ear.

Immunohistochemically, most middle ear adenomas react with antibodies to pankeratin, CK7 and CAM 5.2.[104,110,111] Immunoreactivity with antibodies to CK20 is uncommon. Most are also immunoreactive with antibodies to neuroendocrine antigens, especially chromogranin. It is interesting to note that in areas where two cell layers can be appreciated, the basal cells are more likely to react with antibodies to neuroendocrine antigens, whereas the luminal cells are more likely to be immunoreactive with antibodies to CK7.

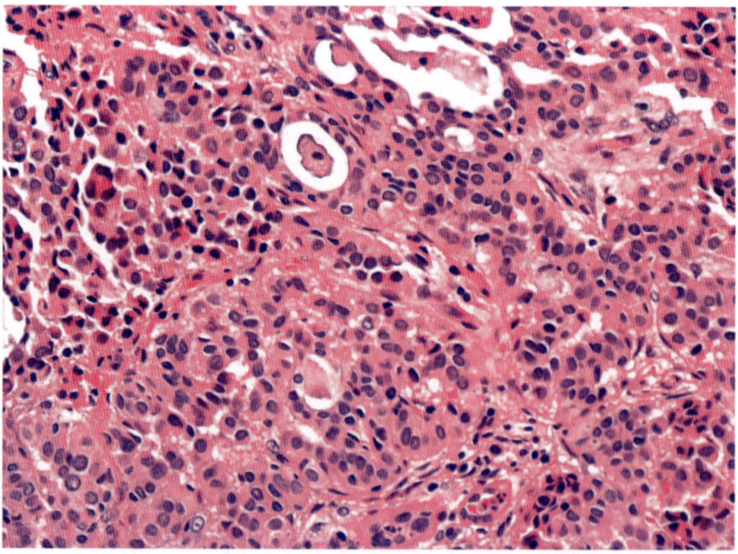

FIGURE 16.28 Glandular and solid growth patterns are seen with this middle ear adenoma.

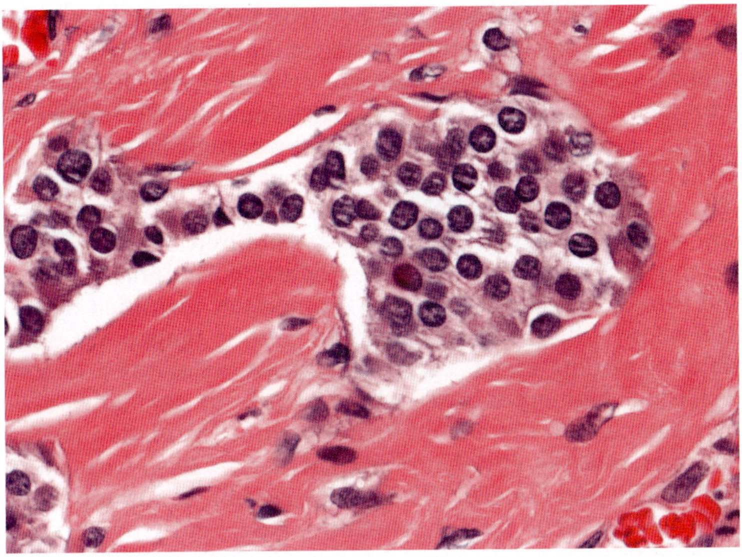

FIGURE 16.29 Middle ear adenomas are composed of neoplastic cells with round nuclei and granular chromatin.

The WHO currently allows for the distinction of *endolymphatic sac tumors* and *aggressive papillary tumors of the middle ear*.[113,114] This is in spite of the fact that the literature has consistently confused the two tumors in their morphologies and both have been described to have germline or sporadic mutations of the *VHL* gene.[115–125] That some of these tumors appear to occur in the middle ear and do not appear to involve the endolymphatic sac suggests to us that epithelium of the middle ear may also give rise to tumors that histologically and immunophenotypically recapitulate the endolymphatic sac of the inner ear. A variety of other names have been applied to this tumor, and these usually incorporate the words papillary or endolymphatic. Nomenclature is further confused due to the intermediate behavior of these tumors. Here we will discuss endolymphatic sac tumors with a note about "aggressive papillary tumor" at the end.

Endolymphatic sac tumors occur slightly more often in women and develop over a wide age range.[115,116,120,123,126] Symptoms include a neural hearing loss, vertigo, tinnitus, ataxia, and facial nerve palsy. The tumors do not metastasize (hematogenously), but they are often very locally aggressive. They frequently recur and cause death in approximately 10% of cases secondary to involvement of vital structures. Between 10% and 15% of these tumors arise in patients with von Hippel-Lindau disease. Such tumors occur at a younger age than sporadic tumors, are more common in women, and tend to be bilateral. Because of this association, and the risk that von Hippel-Lindau disease carries for other neoplasms, it is recommended that all patients with these tumors be screened for the syndrome.

Endolymphatic sac tumors produce lytic lesions of the temporal bone and are usually between 4 and 6 cm in size at the time of diagnosis.[115,116,118,120] Many examples extend into the posterior cranial cavity, and some actually cause radiographic shifting of the brain. Histologically, the tumors are papillary and cystic with both components lined by a single layer of low-cuboidal or flattened cells (Fig. 16.30). These cells may focally appear columnar or, conversely, they may be extremely attenuated (eFigs. 16.32 and 16.33). The epithelium forms small cysts containing eosinophilic material that appears not to be mucus. Neoplastic cells have lightly eosinophilic or clear cytoplasm and intracytoplasmic glycogen is sometimes identified by PAS stain. The nuclei show little pleomorphism and mitotic figures are uncommon. The underlying stroma varies significantly in its cellularity and some areas appear sclerotic. Numerous small blood vessels or capillaries are present within this stroma with occasional foci of hemosiderin-laden macrophages. Immunohistochemically, endolymphatic sac tumors react with antibodies to pankeratin, PAX8 and CA IX.[127] They show variable immunoreactivity with antibodies to EMA, S100 protein, vimentin, NSE, and synaptophysin. They do not react with antibodies to thyroglobulin, CD10 or RCC.

Endolymphatic sac tumors should be distinguished from papillary choroid plexus tumors.[115,128] These lesions appear clinically distinct, as choroid plexus papillary tumors most often involve the ventricular spaces and are usually not locally invasive, especially into bone. Choroid plexus papillary tumors show less histologic variability and are usually immunoreactive with antibodies to S100 protein and transthyretin, unlike aggressive papillary tumors. Choroid plexus papillary tumors are not associated with von Hippel-Lindau disease.

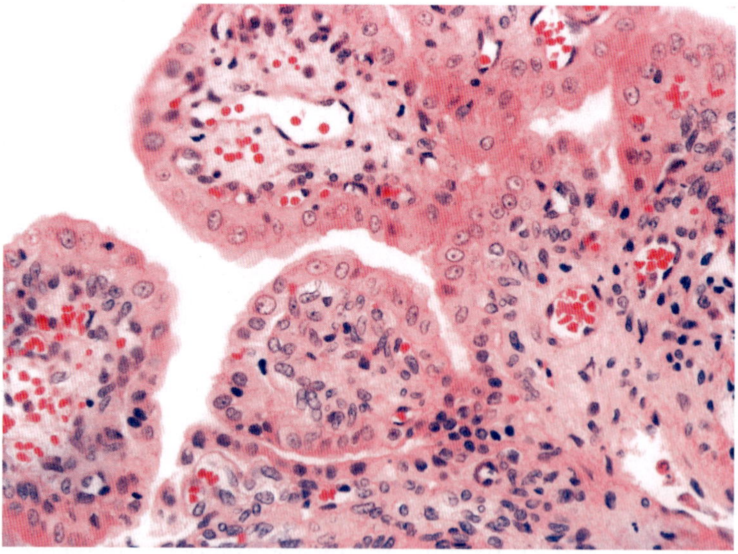

FIGURE 16.30 Endolymphatic sac tumors are composed of papillae lined by a single layer of epithelial cells with little atypia.

Finally, a note about *aggressive papillary tumor*. This diagnosis has been widely used in the literature synonymously with *endolymphatic sac tumor*. If the diagnosis is to be used, it should be used for a papillary tumor morphologically and immunohistochemically distinct from endolymphatic sac tumor.

One of the largest reported series of *jugulotympanic paragangliomas* was recorded in the second series fascicle of the upper aerodigestive tract.[129] The patients were predominately women and the mean age was 50 years, although the tumors occurred over a broad age range. Symptoms included conductive hearing loss, tinnitus, vertigo, pain, facial nerve palsy, and bleeding. As with paragangliomas at other sites, these tumors sometimes occur in familial syndromes (see Chapter 8). At this site, they are usually located near the jugular bulb (85%). Some occur in the middle ear space (12%) or, rarely, in the external year, possibly associated with Arnold nerve.

Most jugulotympanic paragangliomas are very small and measure only 2 to 3 mm in size.[129–133] They are extremely vascular and bleed easily when manipulated. These tumors histologically resemble paragangliomas found elsewhere (see Chapter 8) with nests and sheets of spindled to epithelioid cells and a delicate intervening vasculature (eFigs. 16.34 and 16.35). In our experience, cell nests (zellballen) are often not as well formed as in paragangliomas from other locations (Fig. 16.31). This can add to the diagnostic confusion. The tumors should be distinguished from epithelial and other neural tumors that can occur in this area. Immunoreactivity with antibodies to neuroendocrine antigens such as synaptophysin, chromogranin, or NSE; staining of sustentacular cells with antibodies to S100

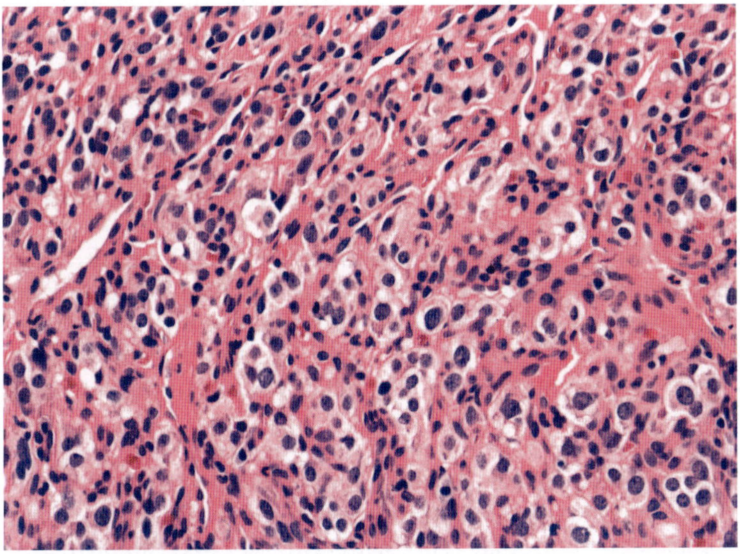

FIGURE 16.31 Jugulotympanic paragangliomas show less well-defined nesting when compared to paragangliomas at other sites.

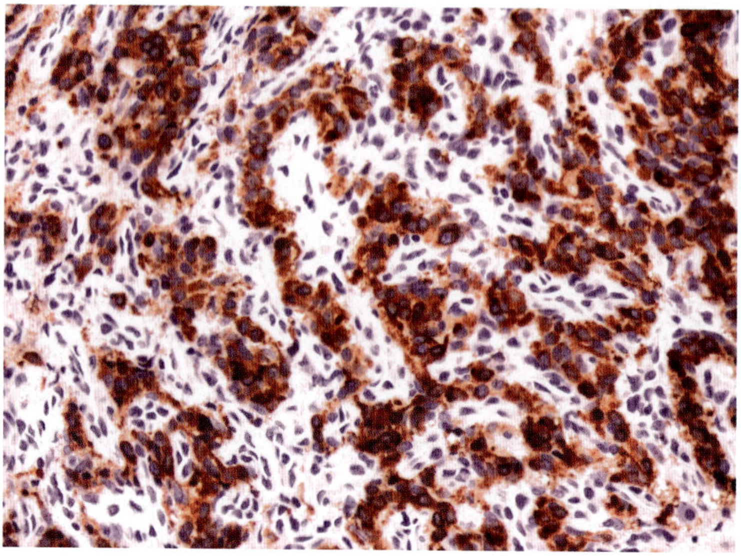

FIGURE 16.32 A chromogranin immunostain highlights many of the neoplastic cells of the jugulotympanic paraganglioma.

protein; and lack of reactivity with keratin antibodies confirm the diagnosis of paraganglioma and exclude other tumors included in the differential diagnosis (Fig. 16.32, eFig. 16.36).

The most common tumor of the middle ear and temporal bone is the *vestibular schwannoma*.[57] These usually arise unilaterally in patients older than 40 years, although patients with neurofibromatosis type 2 develop bilateral tumors at a younger age.[129,134–137] Indeed, the presence of bilateral disease establishes a diagnosis of neurofibromatosis, type 2. The tumors arise from the superior vestibular branch of the eighth cranial nerve end extend out of the temporal bone either cranially or peripherally. Patients present with hearing loss and balance problems. Although cases associated with neurofibromatosis type 2 are found to have mutations of the *MERLIN* or *SCHWANNOMIN* gene, sporadic cases have not been found to have these changes.

Histologically, vestibular schwannomas resemble schwannomas seen at other sites (see Chapter 8).[136] They are circumscribed, encapsulated, and often somewhat lobulated. As with schwannomas elsewhere, Antoni type "A" and "B" areas are present, with Verocay bodies and hyalinized vessels (Fig. 16.33, eFigs. 16.37 and 16.38). Degenerative changes with hemorrhage, necrosis, myxoid change, and prominent nuclear atypia may be seen and do not connote malignancy (eFig. 16.39). Indeed, malignant peripheral nerve sheath tumors at this site are extremely rare. Immunohistochemically, these tumors can easily be distinguished from meningiomas. Schwannomas react with antibody to S100 protein, whereas meningiomas do not, but instead react with antibodies to EMA. The vast

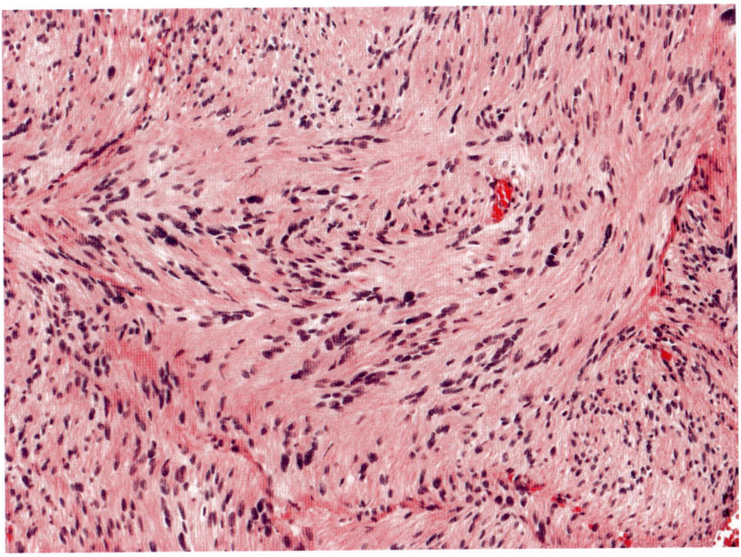

FIGURE 16.33 Schwannomas of the temporal bone often show predominantly cellular areas.

majority of neoplastic cells in a schwannoma are not reactive with antibodies to CD34. It is interesting to note that the proliferation index of familial tumors has been found to be higher than that of sporadic tumors, based on Ki-67 immunostaining.[138]

Meningiomas occasionally involve the middle year and may also affect the temporal bone and external auditory canal.[139–143] They more frequently occur in women and present at any age with a mean age at presentation of 50 years. Symptoms are nonspecific and include hearing loss, chronic infection, headache, mass, nerve palsy, vertigo, and tinnitus. Patients frequently have had the symptoms for extended periods of time. Although most of the tumors involve the middle ear, approximately 10% involve either the external auditory canal or temporal bone alone. Nearly one-third of patients develop recurrences after attempted complete excision, and the 5-year survival rate is 80%.

The mean size of meningiomas occurring in the middle ear is 1.2 cm and specimens are usually received as fragments of firm, gray-white to pink tissue.[140,141,143] Histologically, most are meningothelial, with whorled or nested neoplastic cells that have indistinct cell borders and round to oval nuclei with fine chromatin (Fig. 16.34, eFig. 16.40). Intranuclear pseudoinclusions are seen in most cases. The tumors frequently show an infiltrative growth pattern and approximately 30% of cases are found to infiltrate into bone. Psammoma bodies are also seen in approximately one-third of cases. Atypical meningiomas at this site are very rare. It has also been noted that more than 25% of these cases have concomitant cholesteatomas. Immunohistochemically, the neoplastic meningothelial cells

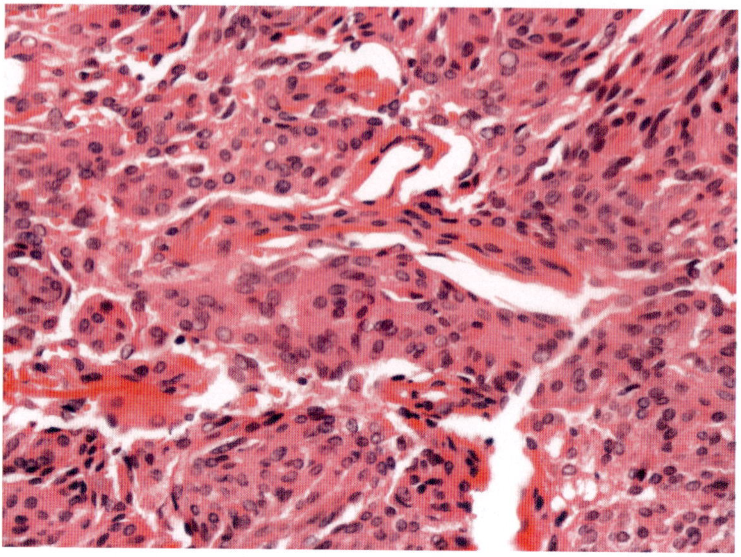

FIGURE 16.34 Most meningiomas of the middle ear are meningotheliomatous.

react with antibodies to EMA and vimentin.[143] Occasional cases have cells immunoreactive with antibodies to S100 protein. Rarely, immunoreactivity with antibodies to pankeratins is noted.

Rhabdomyosarcomas of the temporal bone represent up to 15% of all head and neck rhabdomyosarcomas.[144–147] They also sometimes involve the external ear. These tumors occur in young children with a mean age of 4 years. Patients typically present with hearing loss or pain. Hemorrhagic, friable tumor tissue may be noted extending into the external ear canal. Metastasis and involvement of the meninges are common at diagnosis. Almost all reported cases are embryonal and the histologic features are identical to those of the analogous tumors seen throughout the upper aerodigestive tract, discussed in detail in Chapter 9 (Fig. 16.35).

Eosinophilic granuloma or *Langerhans cell histiocytosis* is, perhaps, the most common hematolymphoid malignancy of the ear, occurring most often within the temporal bone and middle ear.[57,148] These tumors occur most often in infants, children and young adults. Lesions of the temporal bone can be either unifocal or represent one focus of systemic or multifocal forms of the disease. Unifocal disease usually presents in older children or young adults, and lesions are either discovered incidentally with imaging for some other process or due to symptoms secondary to local mass effect. Multifocal or systemic disease presents in infants or children with systemic symptoms such as fever, rash, hepatosplenomegaly, lymphadenopathy, and cytopenias.

Microscopic sections of Langerhans cell histiocytosis classically appear hypercellular with a mixed inflammatory infiltrate rich in histiocytes, neutrophils, lymphocytes, and eosinophils.[148] Langerhans cells

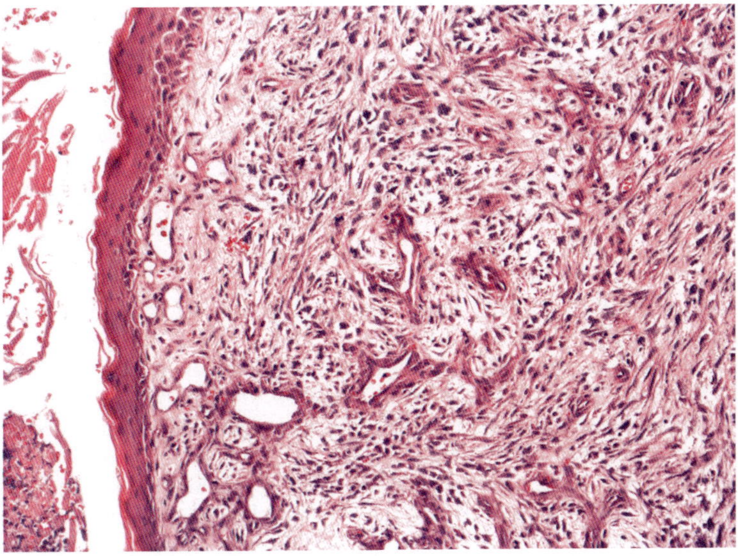

FIGURE 16.35 Embryonal rhabdomyosarcomas of the temporal bone are similar to their counterparts found elsewhere.

are critical for the diagnosis. These histiocytic-appearing cells are usually abundant. They have a moderate amount of granular or vacuolated eosinophilic cytoplasm with large, folded, and indented nuclei that often resemble beans. Occasional mitotic figures may be present, but abundant cytologic atypia, mitotic activity, or necrosis should lead one to consider another diagnosis. Neoplastic cells react strongly and diffusely with antibodies to langerin, S100 protein, and CD1a, and variably with antibodies to CD45, lysozyme, and CD68.

Many other neoplasms may rarely involve the middle ear or temporal bone.[61,116,129] Benign nevi and vascular neoplasms such as lobular capillary hemangiomas have been reported here as have many different malignancies including lymphomas, melanomas, and various sarcomas. Metastases occur here as well and careful history taking is key for their diagnoses often coupled with the use of immunohistochemical stains.[149,150] Criteria used for the diagnosis of these lesions at other, more common sites should be applied here as required.

REFERENCES

1. Brownstein MH, Wanger N, Helwig EB. Accessory tragi. *Arch Dermatol.* 1971;104:625-631.
2. Olsen KD, Maragos NE, Weiland LH. First branchial cleft anomalies. *Laryngoscope.* 1980;90:423-436.
3. Gyure KA, Thompson LD, Morrison AL. A clinicopathological study of 15 patients with neuroglial heterotopias and encephaloceles of the middle ear and mastoid region. *Laryngoscope.* 2000;110:1731-1735.

4. Levy RA, Platt N, Aftalion B. Encephalocele of the middle ear. *Laryngoscope.* 1971;81:126-130.
5. Manolidis S. Dural herniations, encephaloceles: an index of neglected chronic otitis media and further complications. *Am J Otolaryngol.* 2002;23:203-208.
6. Mischke RE, Brackmann DE, Gruskin P. Salivary gland choristoma of the middle ear. *Arch Otolaryngol.* 1977;103:432-434.
7. Saeger KL, Gruskin P, Carberry JN. Salivary gland choristoma of the middle ear. *Arch Pathol Lab Med.* 1982;106:39-40.
8. Slater DN, Timperley WR, Smith CM. Heterotopic middle ear gliomatosis. *Histopathology.* 1988;12:230-231.
9. Wine CJ, Metcalf JE. Salivary gland choristoma of the middle ear and mastoid. *Arch Otolaryngol.* 1977;103:435-436.
10. Bennett M, Warren F, Jackson GC, Kaylie D. Congenital cholesteatoma: theories, facts, and 53 patients. *Otolaryngol Clin North Am.* 2006;39:1081-1094.
11. Ferlito A. A review of the definition, terminology and pathology of aural cholesteatoma. *J Laryngol Otol.* 1993;107:483-488.
12. Potsic WP, Korman SB, Samadi DS, Wetmore RF. Congenital cholesteatoma: 20 years' experience at The Children's Hospital of Philadelphia. *Otolaryngol Head Neck Surg.* 2002;126:409-414.
13. Sculerati N, Bluestone CD. Pathogenesis of cholesteatoma. *Otolaryngol Clin North Am.* 1989;22:859-868.
14. Richter GT, Lee KH. Contemporary assessment and management of congenital cholesteatoma. *Curr Opin Otolaryngol Head Neck Surg.* 2009;17:339-345.
15. Beers SL, Abramo TJ. Otitis externa review. *Pediatr Emerg Care.* 2004;20:250-256.
16. Nager GT. *Pathology of the Ear and Temporal Bone.* Baltimore: Williams and Wilkins; 1993.
17. Neal GD, Gates GA. Invasive pseudomonas osteitis of the temporal bone. *Am J Otol.* 1983;4:332-337.
18. Zaky DA, Bentley DW, Lowy K, Betts RF, Douglas RG Jr. Malignant external otitis: a severe form of otitis in diabetic patients. *Am J Med.* 1976;61:298-302.
19. Sweeney CJ, Gilden DH. Ramsay Hunt syndrome. *J Neurol Neurosurg Psychiatry.* 2001;71:149-154.
20. Smith JA, Danner CJ. Complications of chronic otitis media and cholesteatoma. *Otolaryngol Clin North Am.* 2006;39:1237-1255.
21. Windle-Taylor PC, Bailey CM. Tuberculous otitis media: a series of 22 patients. *Laryngoscope.* 1980;90:1039-1044.
22. Hirsch BE. Infections of the external ear. *Am J Otolaryngol.* 1992;13:145-155.
23. Ho T, Vrabec JT, Yoo D, Coker NJ. Otomycosis: clinical features and treatment implications. *Otolaryngol Head Neck Surg.* 2006;135:787-791.
24. Paulose KO, Al Khalifa S, Shenoy P, Sharma RK. Mycotic infection of the ear (otomycosis): a prospective study. *J Laryngol Otol.* 1989;103:30-35.
25. Goette DK. Chondrodermatitis nodularis chronica helicis: a perforating necrobiotic granuloma. *J Am Acad Dermatol.* 1980;2:148-154.
26. Metzger SA, Goodman ML. Chondrodermatitis helicis: a clinical re-evaluation and pathological review. *Laryngoscope.* 1976;86:1402-1412.
27. Santa Cruz DJ. Chondrodermatitis nodularis helicis: a transepidermal perforating disorder. *J Cutan Pathol.* 1980;7:70-76.
28. Heffner DK, Hyams VJ. Cystic chondromalacia (endochondral pseudocyst) of the auricle. *Arch Pathol Lab Med.* 1986;110:740-743.
29. Lazar RH, Heffner DK, Hughes GB, Hyams VK. Pseudocyst of the auricle: a review of 21 cases. *Otolaryngol Head Neck Surg.* 1986;94:360-361.